Ellis's Clinical Anatomy

To my wife, Wendy, and to my late parents
H. E.

To my wife, Neila, and to my late parents
V. M.

Ellis's Clinical Anatomy

Applied Anatomy for Medical Students, Clinicians in Training, and Allied Health Professionals

HAROLD ELLIS
CBE, MA, DM, MCh, FRCS, FRCP, FRCOG, FRCR, FACS (Hon)
Formerly Clinical Anatomist, Guy's, King's and St Thomas' School of Biomedical Sciences;
Emeritus Professor of Surgery, Charing Cross and Westminster Medical School, London;
Formerly Examiner in Anatomy, Primary FRCS (Eng)

VISHY MAHADEVAN
MBBS, PhD, FRCSEd, FDSRCSEng (Hon), FRCS
Emeritus Professor of Surgical Anatomy
The Royal College of Surgeons of England
Lincoln's Inn Fields
London;
Formerly Barbers' Company Professor of Anatomy & Professor & Head of Anatomy
The Royal College of Surgeons of England, London
Member of the Court of Examiners, RCS England

FIFTEENTH EDITION

WILEY

This edition first published 2027

Edition History
Harold Ellis (1960, 1962, 1966, 1969, 1971, 1977, 1977, 1983, 1992, 1992, 2002, 2006); Harold Ellis and Vishy Mahadevan (2010); John Wiley & Sons Ltd (2013, 2019).

Registered Offices
John Wiley & Sons, Inc., 111 River Street, Hoboken, NJ 07030, USA
John Wiley & Sons Ltd, New Era House, 8 Oldlands Way, Bognor Regis, West Sussex, PO22 9NQ, UK

For details of our global editorial offices, customer services, and more information about Wiley products visit us at www.wiley.com.

The manufacturer's authorized representative according to the EU General Product Safety Regulation is Wiley-VCH GmbH, Boschstr. 12, 69469 Weinheim, Germany, e-mail: Product_Safety@wiley.com.

Wiley also publishes its books in a variety of electronic formats and by print-on-demand. Some content that appears in standard print versions of this book may not be available in other formats.

Library of Congress Cataloging-in-Publication Data

Names: Ellis, Harold, 1926– author | Mahadevan, Vishy author
Title: Ellis's clinical anatomy : applied anatomy for medical students, clinicians in training, and allied health professionals / Harold Ellis CBE, MA, DM, MCh, FRCS, FRCP, FRCOG, FRCR FACS (Hon), Vishy Mahadevan MBBS, PhD, FRCSEd, FDSRCSEng (Hon), FRCS.
Description: 15th edition. | Hoboken, NJ : Wiley, 2027. | Includes bibliographical references and index.
Identifiers: LCCN 2026006333 (print) | LCCN 2026006334 (ebook) | ISBN 9781394217458 paperback | ISBN 9781394217472 adobe pdf | ISBN 9781394217465 epub
Subjects: LCSH: Human anatomy
Classification: LCC QM23.2 .E43 2027 (print) | LCC QM23.2 (ebook)
LC record available at https://lccn.loc.gov/2026006333
LC ebook record available at https://lccn.loc.gov/2026006334

Cover Design: Wiley
Cover Images: Trust me bro/Shutterstock, sasirin pamai/Shutterstock, sciencepics/Shutterstock, benote/Shutterstock, PIC4U/stock.adobe.com, Matthieu/stock.adobe.com

Set in 9/12pt Palatino LTStd by Straive, Pondicherry, India

Printed in Singapore

M126376130726

In Memoriam

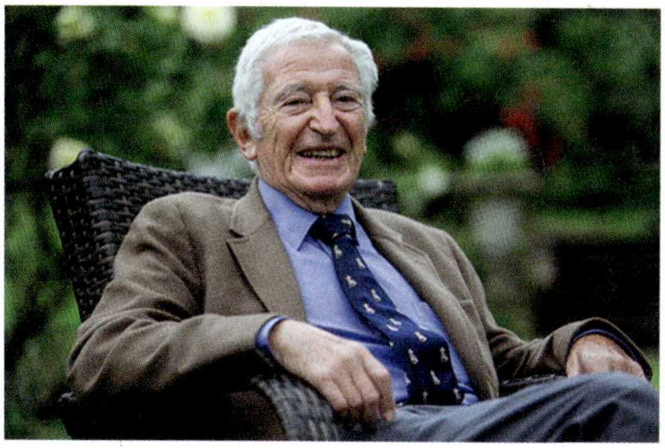

It is with great sadness and a profound sense of loss to announce the passing of Professor Harold Ellis CBE FRCS, the original and senior author of *Clinical Anatomy*. He had not long crossed his landmark 100th birthday.

Professor Ellis was a Surgeon, Academic, Anatomist and Educator of great distinction, eminence and international renown. He was undoubtedly one of the notable figures in the world of surgery during the latter half of the 20th century.

Professor Ellis was a gifted and charismatic teacher and orator. His contribution to surgical and anatomical literature was prodigious. He authored and/or edited over 25 books, in addition to publishing numerous articles in surgical journals.

The first of the many books he wrote was Clinical Anatomy. Professor Ellis conceived of the need for such a book while still a trainee surgical registrar in Oxford. The book was published in 1960. It was Professor Ellis's intention that the book should be a distillate of clinically relevant anatomical information that could readily be put to use on the wards and in the operating theatre. It was also his intention that the book should be slender enough to be carried about easily and written in an unpretentious and conversational style.

In recognition of his phenomenal contribution to the surgical profession, particularly in the field of education, both nationally and internationally, Professor Ellis was awarded numerous accolades including visiting Professorships, fellowships, eponymous medals and, in 1987, the CBE, from Her Majesty Queen Elizabeth II.

To quote the late William Arthur Ward, the celebrated American motivational writer – 'A Good teacher explains, a Superior teacher demonstrates and a Great teacher inspires'.

Professor Harold Ellis was all three rolled into one – he always explained, often demonstrated and, above all, he always inspired!

Professor Ellis was aware that this edition of the book was in preparation but sadly did not live to see it appear in print.

It is to Professor Harold Ellis CBE FRCS – my mentor, benefactor, inspirational colleague and my very dear and irreplaceable friend that I dedicate my efforts in bringing this edition to fruition.

Vishy Mahadevan

Contents

Part 3: The Upper Limb

Preface to the Fifteenth Edition

More than 15 years ago, when CLINICAL ANATOMY, then in its 11th edition, was approaching its 50th birthday, Professor Harold Ellis invited me to join him as co-editor and co-author of the proposed 12th edition of the legendary textbook, thereby simultaneously, conferring on me a great honour and paying me a huge compliment. The 12th edition was due to be launched in 2010 to mark the fiftieth anniversary of the book, first published in 1960. With the publication of the Golden Jubilee edition, history was made in 2010, for never before in the history of English-language medical publishing had one and the same author carried a book through 50 years of its existence! An extraordinary personal achievement and landmark for Professor Ellis. Fifteen years on and two further editions later, CLINICAL ANATOMY, now in its 65th year, is soon to appear as the 15th edition. Professor Ellis has entrusted the revision and rewriting of this new edition, entirely to me.

I feel honoured yet again and I can only hope that I will prove myself worthy of the trust placed in me by Professor Ellis.

Remaining faithful to the principles that have always guided this book, I have striven to maintain, describe and emphasize the clinical relevance and clinical application of Anatomy throughout the text. I have also undertaken an extensive and thorough revision of the entire text, culling all that is now deemed out of date and irrelevant to contemporary clinical practice. A substantial amount of new material has been introduced. While the anatomy of the human body is in itself relatively unchanging, the manner in which the anatomy is explored, studied, described and, where necessary, reconstructed is often influenced by technological advances. We hope these are reflected in this edition.

We hope also that this book will continue to remain popular and be of help to undergraduate students of medicine and allied health sciences throughout the English-speaking world and to postgraduate trainees, in particular those preparing for the MRCS examination.

Vishy Mahadevan
March 2026

Preface to the First Edition

Experience of teaching clinical students at three medical schools has convinced me that there is still an unfortunate hiatus between the anatomy which the student learns in his pre-clinical years and that which he later encounters in the wards and operating theatres.

This book attempts to bridge this gap. It does so by highlighting those features of anatomy which are of clinical importance, in medicine and midwifery as well as in surgery. It presents the facts which a student might reasonably be expected to carry with him during his years on the wards, through final examinations and into his post-graduate years; it is designed for the clinical student.

Anatomy is a vast subject and therefore, in order to achieve this goal, I have deliberately carried out a rigorous selection of material so as to cover only those of its thousands of facts which I consider form the necessary anatomical scaffolding for the clinician. Wherever possible practical applications are indicated throughout the text – they cannot, within the limitations of a book of this size, be exhaustive, but I hope that they will act as signposts to the student and indicate how many clinical phenomena can be understood and remembered on simple anatomical grounds.

Harold Ellis
Oxford, 1960

Acknowledgements to the Fifteenth Edition

We wish to thank our many professional colleagues (far too many to mention individually) drawn from the fields of Surgery and Anatomy for their careful perusal and scrutiny of the text in the previous edition of this book and for their many thoughtful, constructive and helpful comments. Their observations and suggestions have informed many of the revisions implemented in this edition.

We wish also to thank the many students, undergraduates and postgraduates, who have taken the trouble to send us several useful suggestions, many of which we have acted upon during the preparation of this new edition.

Our eternal thanks to Jane Fallows whose skilfully produced illustrations and depictions we continue to use in this edition.

CT and MRI scans were provided by Dr Sheila Rankin and Dr Jeremy Rabouhans of the Department of Radiology at Guy's Hospital and by Professor Adrian Dixon of Addenbrooke's Hospital, Cambridge. Our thanks to all three.

We are grateful to the following authors for permission to reproduce illustrations:

The late Lord Brock for Figs 20 and 21 (from *Lung Abscess*); and

The late Professor R. G. Harrison for Figs 12, 32 and 67 (from *A Textbook of Human Embryology*).

Our profuse gratitude to Alex Antony Sabu for his invaluable editorial advice and help and for his ever-reassuring manner. Also to Alex and his editorial team, in particular, Jamila Niroop, our heartfelt gratitude for their diligence in scrutinizing and editing the text in the latter stages of the production of this volume.

Finally, we wish to express our debt and gratitude to Amanda Sleeth, Catriona King, Calee Sears, Ella Elliott and the staff of Wiley Blackwell for their guidance, support and unfailing help.

Vishy Mahadevan
Harold Ellis
March 2026

Acknowledgements to the First Edition

I wish to thank Dr Max Cowan of the Department of Anatomy, Oxford, who has given freely of advice and criticism in the production of this book.

My colleagues – the registrars and house surgeons at the Radcliffe Infirmary – have kindly perused and commented on the text and have given valuable help in proof-reading.

The majority of the illustrations are by Miss Margaret McLarty and Miss Audrey Arnott; I must thank them sincerely for all their care.

I am grateful to the following authors for permission to reproduce illustrations:

Sir Russell Brock for Fig. 15 (from *Lung Abscess*); Professor R. G. Harrison for Figs 10, 23, 53, 67 and 155 (from *A Textbook of Human Embryology*); Professor David Sinclair for Figs 69, 92, 95, 97, 100–1, 105, 107, 114, 126, 132, 137, 139, 177 and 181 (from *An Introduction to Functional Anatomy*); and Professor Sheila Sherlock for Fig. 55 (from *Diseases of the Liver and Biliary System*).

The illustrations for an anatomical textbook are inevitably a costly item, yet I was anxious that this book should be within the budget of the students for whom it is primarily intended. It is therefore a pleasure to acknowledge here the generosity of Upjohn of England Ltd in contributing towards the cost of the blocks: their gesture will be widely appreciated.

To my sister, Mrs L. Witte, go my grateful thanks for invaluable secretarial assistance. Finally, I wish to express my debt to Mr Per Saugman and staff at Blackwell Scientific Publications for guiding the hesitant steps of the beginner.

Harold Ellis

Part 1
The Thorax

Introduction

The clinical anatomy of the thorax, together with the anatomy of radiological and other imaging techniques of the thorax, are in daily use in clinical practice. The routine clinical examination of the patient's chest is little more than an exercise in relating the deep structures of the thorax to the chest wall. Moreover, several commonly undertaken procedures – chest aspiration, insertion of a chest drain or of a subclavian line and placement of a cardiac pacemaker, for example – have their basis, and their safe performance, in sound anatomical knowledge.

Surface anatomy and surface markings

Much of the working life of an experienced clinician is spent in relating the patient's surface anatomy to underlying deep structures (Fig. 1; see also Figs 11, 22).

The following bony prominences can usually be palpated in the living subject (corresponding vertebral levels are given in brackets):

- superior angle of the scapula (T2);
- upper border of the manubrium sterni, the suprasternal notch (T2/3);
- spine of the scapula (T3);
- sternal angle (of Louis) – the transverse ridge at the manubriosternal junction (T4/5);
- inferior angle of the scapula (T8); it also overlies the 7th rib;
- xiphisternal joint (*T8*/9);
- lowest part of the costal margin – 10th rib (the subcostal plane/line passes through L3).

Note from Fig. 1 that the manubrium sterni corresponds to the 3rd and 4th thoracic vertebrae and overlies the aortic arch and that the body of the sternum corresponds to the 5th–8th thoracic vertebrae and overlies the heart.

Since the 1st and 12th ribs are difficult to feel, the ribs should be enumerated from the 2nd costal cartilage, which articulates with the sternum invariably and exactly at the level of the angle of Louis. Indeed, the only infallible way of counting the ribs accurately is to begin by identifying the unmistakable sternal angle. The second costal cartilage is readily identified at that level on either side, and thereafter the subsequent ribs may be enumerated, in sequence. It is advisable always to identify the ribs and intercostal spaces alongside the sternal edge initially before tracking them laterally.

Owing to the natural kyphosis (dorsal convexity) of the thoracic part of the vertebral column, the spinous processes of all the thoracic vertebrae can normally be palpated in the midline posteriorly.

The position of the *nipple* varies considerably in the female, but in the male, it usually overlies the 4th intercostal space approximately 10 cm (4 in) from the midline. The *apex beat*, which marks the lowest and outermost point at which the cardiac impulse can be felt, is normally in the 5th left intercostal space 9 cm (3.5 in) from the midline and within the midclavicular line. (This corresponds to a point just below and medial to the nipple in the male, but it is always preferable and advisable to use bony rather than soft-tissue landmarks as points of reference.)

The *trachea* is palpable in the suprasternal notch midway between the medial ends of the two clavicles.

The trachea (Figs 1, 2)

The trachea commences in the neck at the level of the lower border of the cricoid cartilage (C6) and runs vertically downwards to end below the level of the sternal angle of Louis (T4/5), just to the right of the midline, by dividing to form the right and left main bronchi. In the erect position and in full inspiration the level of bifurcation is at T6.

The pleura (Figs 2, 3)

The *cervical pleura* can be marked out on the surface by a curved line drawn from the sternoclavicular joint to the junction of the medial and middle thirds of the ipsilateral clavicle; the apex of the pleura is approximately 2.5 cm (1 in) above the medial third of the clavicle. This fact is easily explained by the natural slope of the first rib due to the head of the rib being at a higher level than the anterior end of the rib. The obliquity of the plane of the superior thoracic aperture is merely a consequence of this natural inclination of the first rib. It is important to be aware of this because the pleura can be punctured (with consequent pneumothorax) by a penetrating wound in the root of the neck – and this includes inadvertent injuries caused by the surgeon's knife and the

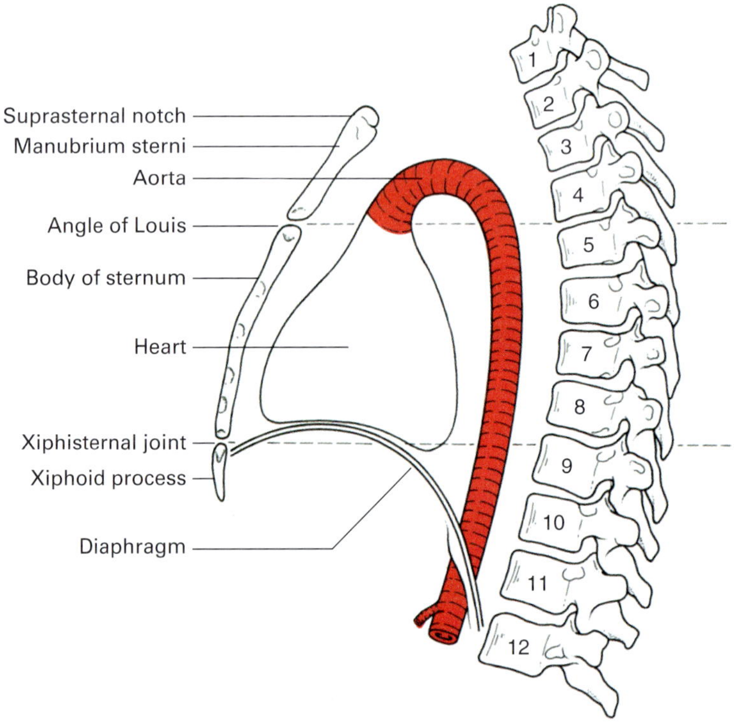

Fig. 1 Lateral view of the thorax – its surface markings and vertebral levels. (Note that a horizontal plane at the level of the angle of Louis (T4/5) demarcates the lower boundary of the superior mediastinum, the upper margin of the fibrous pericardium and the commencement and termination of the aortic arch.)

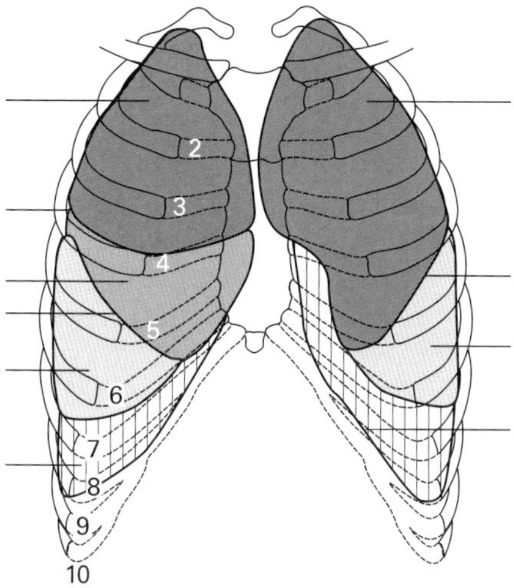

Fig. 2 The surface markings of the lungs and pleura – anterior view.

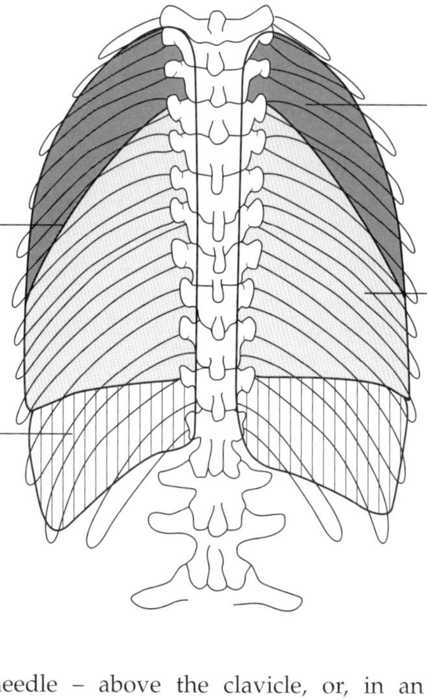

Fig. 3 The surface markings of the lungs and pleura – posterior view.

anaesthetist's needle – above the clavicle, or, in an attempted subclavian vein catheterization, below the clavicle. The lines of pleural reflexion pass from behind the sternoclavicular joint on each side to meet in the midline at the level of 2nd costal cartilage (the angle of Louis). The right pleural edge then passes vertically downwards to the level of the 6th costal cartilage and then crosses:

- the 8th rib in the midclavicular line;
- the 10th rib in the midaxillary line;
- the 12th rib at the lateral border of the erector spinae.

On the left side the pleural edge arches laterally at the 4th costal cartilage and descends lateral to the border of the sternum, owing, of course, to its lateral displacement by the heart; apart from this, its relationships are those of the right side.

The pleura descends just below the 12th rib margin at the medial extremity of the rib. Obviously, in this situation, the pleura may be inadvertently injured when making a loin incision to expose the kidney or for procedures such as adrenalectomy or drainage of a subphrenic abscess.

The lungs (Figs 2, 3)

The surface projection of the lung is somewhat less extensive than that of the parietal pleura as outlined previously, and in addition it varies quite considerably with the phase of respiration. The *apex* of the lung closely follows the line of the cervical pleura and the surface marking of the *anterior border of the right lung* corresponds to that of the right mediastinal pleura. On the left side, however, the *anterior border* has a distinct notch (the *cardiac notch*) that passes behind the 5th and 6th costal cartilages. The *lower border* of the lung has an excursion of as much as 5–8 cm (2–3 in) between the extremes of respiration, but in the neutral position (midway between inspiration and expiration) it lies along a line which crosses the 6th rib in the midclavicular line, the 8th rib in the midaxillary line and reaches the 10th rib adjacent to the vertebral column posteriorly.

The *oblique fissure*, which divides the lung into upper and lower lobes, is indicated on the surface by a line drawn obliquely downwards and outwards from 2.5 cm (1 in) lateral to the spine of the 3rd thoracic vertebra along the 5th intercostal space to the 6th costal cartilage approximately 4 cm (1.5 in) from the midline. This can be represented approximately by abducting the shoulder to its full extent; the line of the oblique fissure then corresponds to the position of the medial border of the scapula.

The surface marking of the *transverse fissure* (separating the middle and upper lobes of the right lung) is a line drawn horizontally along the 4th right costal cartilage to meet the oblique fissure where the latter crosses the 5th rib.

The heart (Fig. 4)

The outline of the heart can be represented on the surface by a trapezoid (i.e. an irregular quadrangle) bounded by the following four points (Fig. 4):

1 2nd *left* costal cartilage 1.25 cm (0.5 in) from the left edge of the sternum;
2 3rd *right* costal cartilage 1.25 cm (0.5 in) from the right sternal edge;
3 6th *right* costal cartilage 1.25 cm (0.5 in) from the sternum;
4 5th *left* intercostal space 9 cm (3.5 in) from the midline (corresponding to the apex beat).

The *left border* of the heart (indicated by a curved line joining points 1 and 4) is formed almost entirely by the left ventricle (the auricular appendage of the left atrium peeping around this border superiorly); the *lower border* (the horizontal line joining points 3 and 4) corresponds to the right ventricle and the apical part of the left ventricle; the *right border* (marked by the line joining points 2 and 3) is formed by the right atrium (see Fig. 24a). The superior border runs obliquely joining points 1 and 2 and corresponds to the roots of the two great vessels, namely the pulmonary trunk and the aorta.

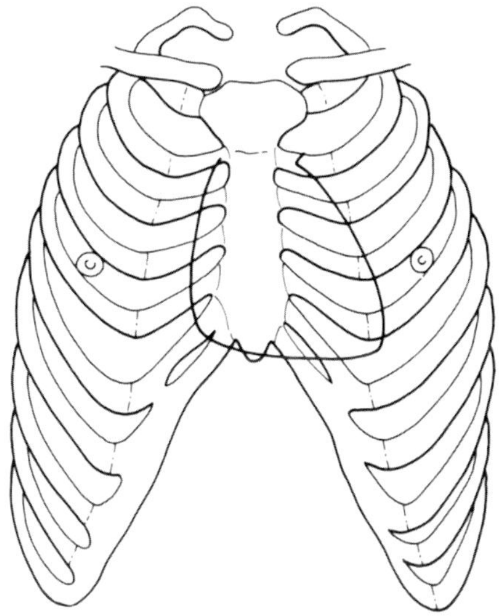

Fig. 4 The surface markings of the heart (see text).

An approximate representation of the size and position of your own heart is given by placing your clenched right fist palmar surface inwards immediately inferior to the manubriosternal junction. Note that the heart is approximately the size of the subject's fist, lies behind the body of the sternum (therefore anterior to thoracic vertebrae 5–8) and bulges over to the left side.

The surface markings of the vessels of the thoracic wall are of importance if these structures are to be avoided when performing aspiration of the chest. The *internal thoracic* (*internal mammary*) *vessels* run vertically downwards behind the costal cartilages 1.25 cm (0.5 in) from the lateral border of the sternum. The intercostal vessels lie immediately below their corresponding ribs (the vein above the artery) so that it is safe to pass a needle immediately *above* a rib, but hazardous to pass it immediately *below* (see Fig. 8).

The thoracic cage

The thoracic cage is formed, posteriorly, by the twelve thoracic vertebrae and intervening intervertebral discs that collectively make up the thoracic region of the vertebral column. On both sides are the twelve ribs and eleven intercostal spaces, while anteriorly is the sternum (with the lateral edge of the sternum receiving the costal cartilages on either side). Above, the thoracic cavity communicates through the superior aperture of the thoracic cage with the root of the neck; below, it is separated from the abdominal cavity by the diaphragm (Fig. 1). Amusingly, the superior aperture of the thoracic cage is termed the 'thoracic inlet' by anatomists, while clinicians (especially vascular surgeons, neurosurgeons and radiologists) refer to the same aperture as the 'thoracic outlet'. Thus, the clinical condition termed **'thoracic outlet syndrome'** implies an abnormality in the vicinity of the superior thoracic aperture and may be defined as a **sustained, symptomatic and pathological** compression of neurovascular structures in the root of the neck.

The thoracic vertebrae

See 'The vertebral column', page 347. See also page 350 and Fig. 227.

The ribs

The greater part of the thoracic cage is formed by the twelve pairs of ribs. Of these, the first seven are connected anteriorly by way of their costal cartilages to the sternum, the cartilages of the 8th, 9th and 10th articulate each with the cartilage of the rib above and the last two ribs are free anteriorly ('floating ribs').

Each typical rib (Fig. 5) has a *head* bearing two articular facets, for articulation with the upper demifacet on the side of the body of the numerically corresponding thoracic vertebra and the lower demifacet of the vertebra above (see Fig. 227). Thus, the head of the third rib articulates with the third vertebral body and with the vertebral body above (i.e. the second vertebral body). The head continues laterally as a stout *neck*, which gives attachment to the costotransverse ligaments. Lateral to the neck is a *tubercle* with a rough non-articular portion and a smooth facet, for articulation with the transverse process of the numerically corresponding vertebra. Still more laterally, the shaft of the rib takes an angled turn anteriorly. This point, known as the angle of the rib, demarcates the lateral limit of attachment of the erector spinae muscle. Beyond the angle the shaft of the rib is gently curved (convex outwards) and is flattened from side to side, presenting lateral and medial surfaces.

The 1st, 2nd, 10th, 11th and 12th ribs are spoken of as 'atypical' ribs. The following are the significant features of the 'atypical' ribs.

The *1st rib* (Fig. 6) is flattened from above downwards. It is not only the flattest but also the shortest and most highly curved of all the ribs. It has a prominent *tubercle* on the inner border of its upper surface for the insertion of scalenus anterior. In front of this tubercle, the subclavian vein crosses the rib; behind the tubercle is the *subclavian groove*, where the subclavian artery and lowest trunk of the brachial plexus lie in relation to the bone. This is one of the sites where the anaesthetist can infiltrate the plexus with local anaesthetic to achieve a brachial plexus block.

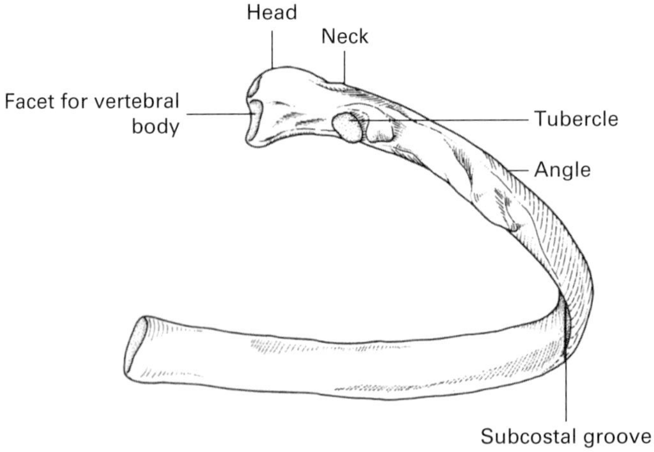

Fig. 5 A typical rib.

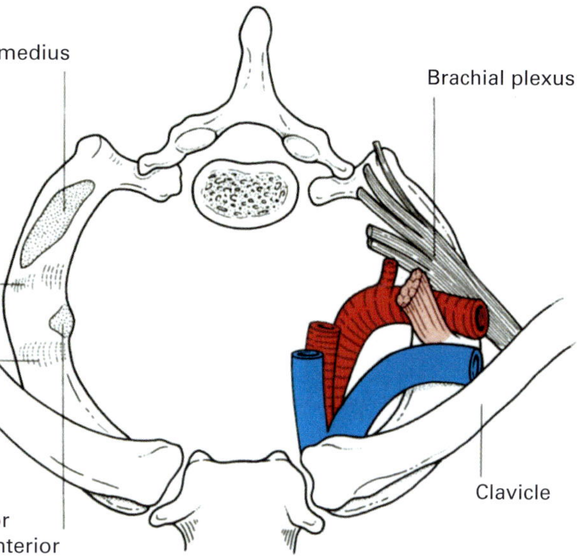

Fig. 6 Structures crossing the first rib.

Crossing the front of the neck of the first rib vertically and lying from medial to lateral are the sympathetic trunk, the superior intercostal artery (from the costocervical trunk) and the large branch of the first thoracic nerve to the brachial plexus.

The *2nd rib* is much less curved than the 1st and approximately twice as long.

The *10th rib* has only one articular facet on the head.

The *11th* and *12th ribs* (*the so-called 'floating ribs'*) are short, have no tubercles and only a single facet on the head. The 11th rib has a slight angle and a shallow subcostal groove; the 12th has neither of these features.

CLINICAL FEATURES

Rib fractures

The chest wall of the child is highly elastic, and therefore fractures of the ribs in children are rare. In adults, the ribs may be fractured by direct impact or indirectly by crushing injuries; in the latter, the rib tends to give way at its weakest part in the region of its angle. As might be expected, the upper two ribs, which are protected by the clavicle, and the lower two ribs, which have no bony attachments anteriorly and are cushioned by nearby muscles, are the ones that are least often injured.

In a severe crush injury to the chest two or more adjacent ribs may sustain fractures both in front and behind resulting in a segment of the thoracic cage becoming detached from the rest of the rib cage ('stove-in chest'). With each inspiration, this loose segment (termed a 'Flail segment') sucks in; with each expiration, it blows out, thereby displaying paradoxical respiratory movement. The associated swinging movements of the mediastinum may produce severe shock in the patient, and this injury calls for urgent treatment by insertion of a chest drain with underwater seal, followed by endotracheal intubation, or tracheostomy, combined with positive pressure ventilation.

Coarctation of the aorta (see Fig. 34b and page 44)

In coarctation of the aorta, the intercostal arteries derived from the aorta receive blood from the superior intercostals (from the costocervical trunk of the subclavian artery), from the anterior intercostal branches of the internal thoracic artery (arising from the subclavian artery) and from the arteries anastomosing around the scapula. Together with the communication between the internal thoracic and inferior epigastric arteries, they provide the principal collaterals between the aorta above and below the block. In consequence, the intercostal arteries undergo dilatation and tortuosity and erode the lower borders of the corresponding ribs to give the characteristic irregular *notching of the ribs*, which is very useful in the radiographic confirmation of this aortic lesion.

Cervical rib

A cervical rib (Fig. 7) occurs in 0.5% of subjects and is bilateral in half of these. It is attached to the transverse process of the 7th cervical vertebra and articulates with the 1st (thoracic) rib or, if short, has a free distal extremity which usually attaches by a fibrous strand to the (normal) first rib. Pressure of such a rib on the lowest trunk of the brachial plexus arching over it may produce paraesthesiae along the ulnar border of the forearm and wasting of the small muscles of the hand (T1). Less commonly, vascular changes, even gangrene, may be caused by pressure of the abnormal rib on the overlying subclavian artery. This results in post-stenotic dilatation of the vessel distal to the rib in which a thrombus may form, and from which emboli may be thrown off. A cervical rib is one of many causes of thoracic outlet syndrome.

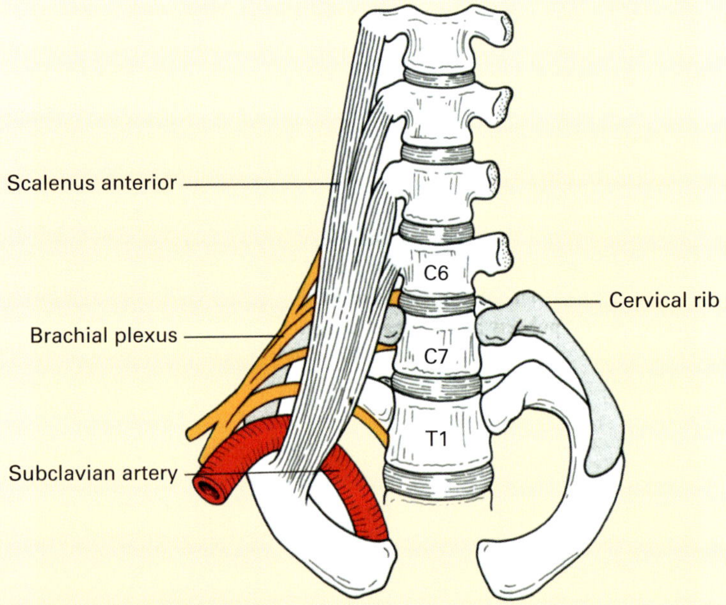

Fig. 7 Bilateral cervical ribs. On the right side the brachial plexus is seen arching over the rib, its lowest trunk being stretched by the rib. The subclavian artery may also be pressed upon by the underlying cervical rib.

The costal cartilages

These bars of hyaline cartilage serve to connect the upper seven ribs directly to the side of the sternum and the 8th, 9th and 10th ribs each to the cartilage of the rib immediately above. The cartilages of the 11th and 12th ribs merely end in the abdominal musculature of the vicinity.

CLINICAL FEATURES

1 The cartilage adds considerable resilience to the thoracic cage and protects the sternum and ribs by making them less susceptible to fractures.
2 In old age (and sometimes also in young adults) the costal cartilages undergo progressive ossification; they then become radio-opaque and may give rise to some confusion when examining a chest radiograph of an elderly patient.

The sternum

This dagger-shaped bone, which forms the anterior part of the thoracic cage, consists of three parts. The *manubrium* is quadrangular in outline and provides articulation for the clavicles and for the 1st and 2nd costal cartilages on either side. It is situated opposite the 3rd and 4th thoracic vertebrae. At the level of the disc between T4 and T5 it articulates with the body of the sternum by means of a secondary cartilaginous joint. When viewed in profile this articulation is seen to be an angled articulation, with the manubrium subtending an obtuse angle with the body of the sternum. It is for this reason that the manubriosternal articulation is known synonymously as the sternal angle and angle of Louis. It is because of this pronounced angle that the manubriosternal junction is always palpable as a prominent ridge spanning the width of the sternum at that level. Articulating with the sternum invariably and precisely at this level, on either side, is the corresponding 2nd costal cartilage.

The body of the sternum, also known as mesosternum, lies opposite T5–T8 vertebrae. It is composed of four pieces or 'sternebrae' arranged vertically, which fuse between puberty and 25 years of age. Its lateral border is notched for articulation with costal cartilages 2nd to 7th (inclusive). *The xiphoid process* is the smallest part of the sternum and usually remains cartilaginous well into adult life. The cartilaginous manubriosternal joint and the joint between the xiphoid and the body of the sternum may become ossified in later life.

CLINICAL FEATURES

1 The attachment of the resilient and somewhat elastic costal cartilages goes a long way towards protecting the sternum from injury. Nevertheless, a sufficiently powerful indirect force, transmitted from a fracture dislocation of the thoracic spine, may be associated with a sternal fracture. Road traffic accidents in which the driver of a car

sustains a forceful thrust to the anterior chest wall from the steering wheel, may result in displacement of the relatively mobile body of the sternum backwards from the relatively fixed manubrium, with the possibility of cardiac tamponade or cardiac contusion.

2 In a sternal puncture a wide-bore needle is pushed through the thin layer of cortical bone covering the sternum into the highly vascular spongy bone beneath, and a specimen of bone marrow aspirated with a syringe.

3 In operations on the thymus gland, and occasionally for a retrosternal goitre, it is necessary to split the manubrium in the midline in order to gain access to the superior mediastinum. A complete vertical split of the whole sternum (median sternotomy) is one of the standard approaches to the heart and great vessels used in cardiac surgery.

The intercostal spaces

There are slight variations between the different intercostal spaces, but typically each space is bridged by a three-ply arrangement of muscular sheets (comparable to the three-ply arrangement of muscles in the anterolateral part of the abdominal wall) and an associated neurovascular bundle (Fig. 8). The muscles of the intercostal space are:

1 the *external intercostal*, the fibres of which pass downwards and forwards from the rib above to the rib below and reach from the vertebrae behind to the costochondral junction in front, where muscle is replaced by the *anterior intercostal membrane*;

2 the *internal intercostal*, the fibres of which run downwards and backwards from the rib above to the rib below. The internal intercostal muscle extends laterally from the sternal edge to the angles of the ribs where muscle is replaced by the *posterior intercostal membrane*;

3 the *innermost intercostal layer* is made up of three discontinuous strands of muscle, all of which lie in the same plane.

Just as in the anterior abdominal wall, the nerves and vessels of the thoracic wall lie in the interval between the middle and innermost layers of muscles. This is the neurovascular plane of the chest wall. The neurovascular bundle consists, from above downwards, of vein, artery and nerve, the vein lying in a groove on the undersurface of the corresponding rib (remember: v, a, n).

The vessels comprise the posterior and anterior intercostal arteries and veins.

The *posterior intercostal arteries* of the lower nine spaces are direct branches of the descending thoracic aorta, while the first two posterior intercostal arteries are derived from the superior intercostal branch of the costocervical trunk, the only branch of the second part of the subclavian artery. Each runs forwards in the subcostal groove to anastomose with the anterior intercostal artery. Each has a number of branches to adjacent muscles, to the skin and to the spinal cord. The corresponding veins are mostly tributaries of the azygos and hemiazygos veins. The first posterior intercostal vein drains into the brachiocephalic or vertebral vein. On the left, the 2nd and 3rd veins often join to form a superior intercostal vein, which crosses the aortic arch to drain into the left brachiocephalic vein.

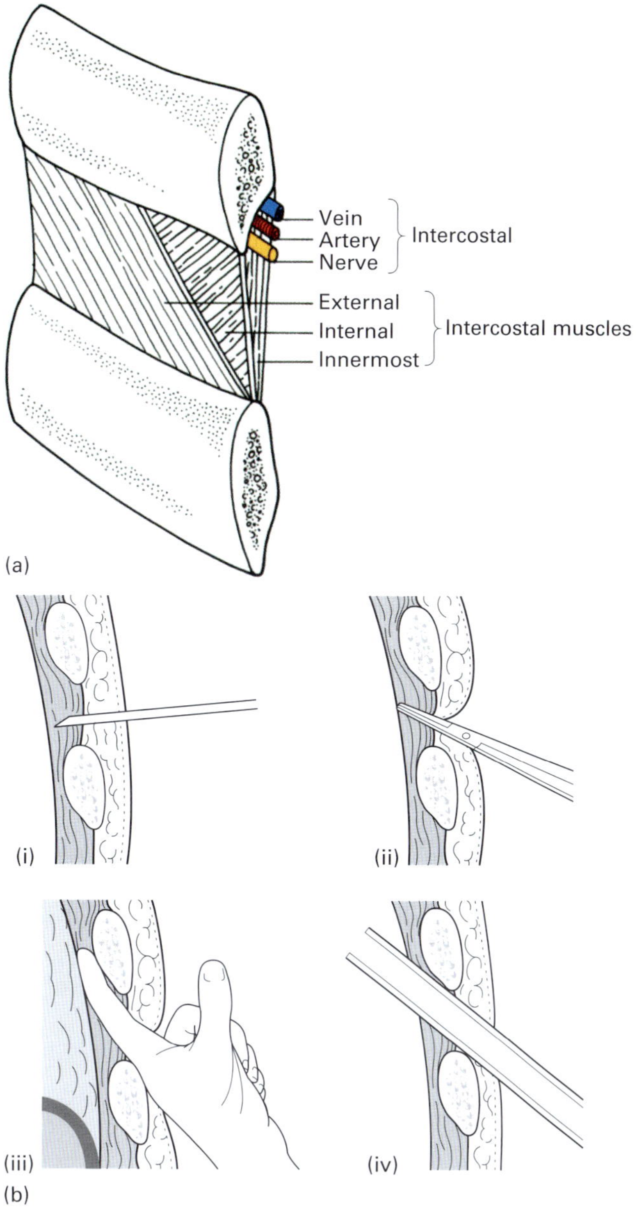

Fig. 8 (a) The anatomy of an intercostal space. (Note that a needle passed into the chest immediately *above* a rib will avoid the neurovascular bundle.) (b) Steps in the insertion of a chest drain. (i) Local anaesthetic is infiltrated into an intercostal space. (ii) Incision followed by blunt dissection allows access to the pleura. (iii) A finger is passed through the incision to clear the lung away. (iv) A chest tube is passed into the pleural cavity.

The *anterior intercostal arteries* are branches of the internal thoracic artery (1st–6th space) or of its musculophrenic branch (7th–9th spaces). The lowest two spaces have only posterior intercostal arteries. Perforating branches pierce the upper five or six intercostal spaces; those of the 2nd–4th spaces are large in the female and supply the breast.

The *intercostal nerves* are the anterior primary rami of the thoracic nerves, each of which gives off a collateral muscular branch and lateral and anterior cutaneous branches for the innervation of the thoracic and abdominal walls (Fig. 9).

CLINICAL FEATURES

1 Local irritation of the intercostal nerves by such conditions as Pott's disease of the thoracic vertebrae (tuberculosis) may give rise to pain that is referred to the front of the chest or abdomen in the region of the peripheral termination of the nerves.
2 Local anaesthesia of an intercostal space is easily produced by infiltration around the intercostal nerve trunk and its collateral branch – a procedure known as intercostal nerve block.
3 Insertion of an emergency chest drain, for example for a traumatic haemopneumothorax, is performed through the 5th intercostal space, somewhat anterior to the midaxillary line. Under local anaesthetic, an incision is made through the skin and subcutaneous tissue. The rest of the procedure is carried out by blunt dissection over the upper edge of the lower rib. In this way, injury to the intercostal bundle in the subcostal groove is avoided (Fig. 8a). A finger is passed into the pleural space to ensure that there are no lung adhesions in the vicinity and to confirm that the pleural cavity is entered. A chest tube is then placed into the pleural space, connected to an underwater drain and firmly sutured in place (Fig. 8b).
4 In a conventional posterolateral thoracotomy (e.g. for a pulmonary lobectomy) an incision is made along the line of the 5th or 6th rib; the periosteum over a segment of the rib is elevated, thus protecting the neurovascular bundle, and a sufficient length of the rib is excised. Access to the lung or mediastinum is then gained through the intercostal space, which can be opened out considerably owing to the elasticity of the thoracic cage.

The diaphragm

The diaphragm is the dome-shaped septum dividing the thoracic from the abdominal cavity. It is present only in mammals. It comprises two portions: a peripheral muscular part that arises from the inner aspect of the margins of the inferior aperture of the thoracic cage (termed by anatomists as the 'thoracic outlet') and a centrally placed aponeurosis (Fig. 10).

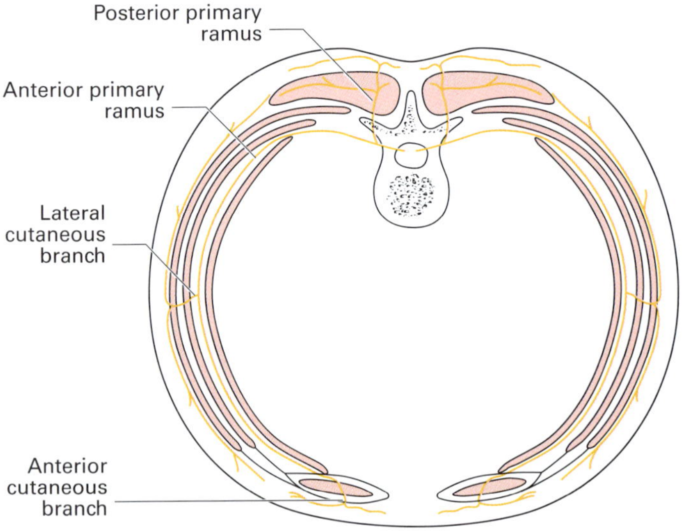

Fig. 9 Diagram of a typical spinal nerve and its relationship to the body wall.

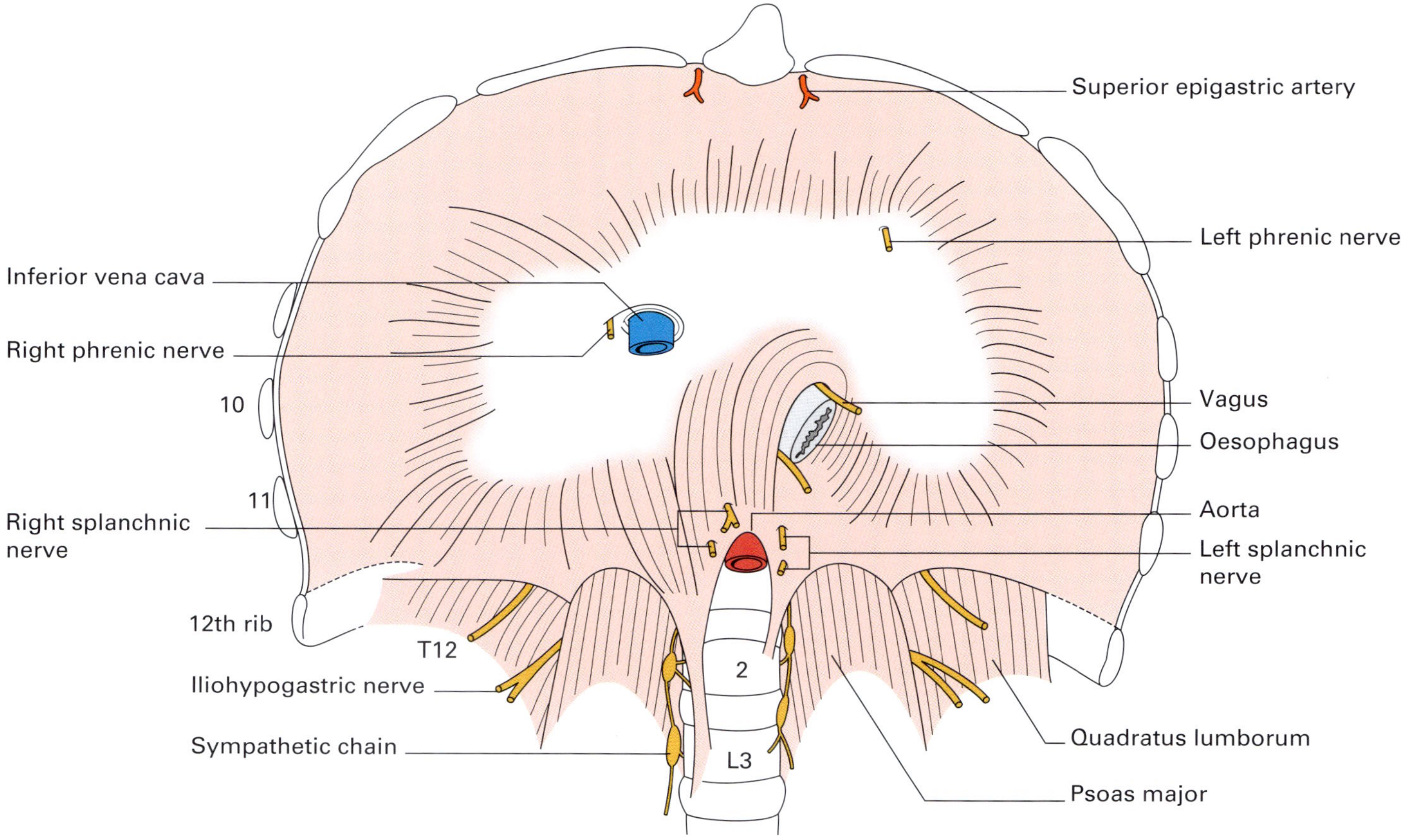

Fig. 10 The diaphragm – inferior aspect. The three major orifices, from above downwards, transmit the inferior vena cava, oesophagus and aorta.

The muscular fibres are arranged in three parts:

1 A *vertebral part* from the crura and from the arcuate ligaments. The *right crus* arises from the front of the bodies of the upper three lumbar vertebrae and intervertebral discs; the *left crus* is attached to only the first two lumbar vertebrae. The arcuate *ligaments* are a series of fibrous arches, the *medial* being a thickening in the fascia covering psoas major and the *lateral* being a thickening in the fascia overlying quadratus lumborum. The tendinous medial borders of the two crura join each other in front of the aorta to form the *median arcuate ligament*.
2 A *costal part* is attached to the inner aspect of the lower six ribs and their costal cartilages.
3 A *sternal portion* consists of two small slips from the deep surface of the xiphisternum.

The central tendon, into which the muscular fibres are inserted, is trefoil in shape and, superiorly, is partially fused with the undersurface of the fibrous pericardium.

The diaphragm receives its motor innervation entirely and exclusively from the right and left phrenic nerves (C3, C4, C5), whose long course from the neck follows the embryological migration of the muscle of the diaphragm from the cervical region (see 'The development of the diaphragm and the anatomy of diaphragmatic hernia'). Injury or operative transection of this nerve results in paralysis and permanent elevation of the ipsilateral half of the diaphragm.

Radiographically, paralysis of the diaphragm is recognized by its abnormal elevation and by its paradoxical movement: instead of descending on inspiration, it is forced upwards by pressure from the abdominal viscera.

The sensory nerve fibres from the central part of the diaphragm also run in the phrenic nerve; hence, irritation of the diaphragmatic pleura (in pleurisy) or of the peritoneum on the undersurface of the diaphragm by subphrenic collections of pus or blood produces referred pain in the corresponding cutaneous area, the shoulder tip.

The peripheral part of the diaphragm, including the crura, receives sensory (proprioceptive) fibres from the lower intercostal nerves.

Openings in the diaphragm

The three main openings in the diaphragm (Figs 10, 11) are:

1 The *aortic* (at the level of T12), which transmits the abdominal aorta, the thoracic duct and often the azygos vein. The aortic opening lies in the midline.
2 The *oesophageal* (T10), which is situated within the muscular fibres of the left and right crura of the diaphragm and transmits, in addition to the oesophagus, branches of the left gastric artery and vein and the two vagi. The oesophageal opening lies slightly to the left of the midline.
3 The *opening for the inferior vena cava* (IVC) (T8), which is situated in the central tendon and also transmits the right phrenic nerve. The vena caval opening lies slightly to the right of the midline.

In addition to these structures, the greater and lesser splanchnic nerves (see page 52) pierce the crura and the sympathetic chain passes behind the diaphragm deep to the medial arcuate ligament to reach the posterior abdominal wall.

The development of the diaphragm and the anatomy of diaphragmatic hernia

The diaphragm is formed (Fig. 12) by fusion in the embryo of the following elements:

1 the septum transversum (forming the central tendon);
2 the dorsal oesophageal mesentery;

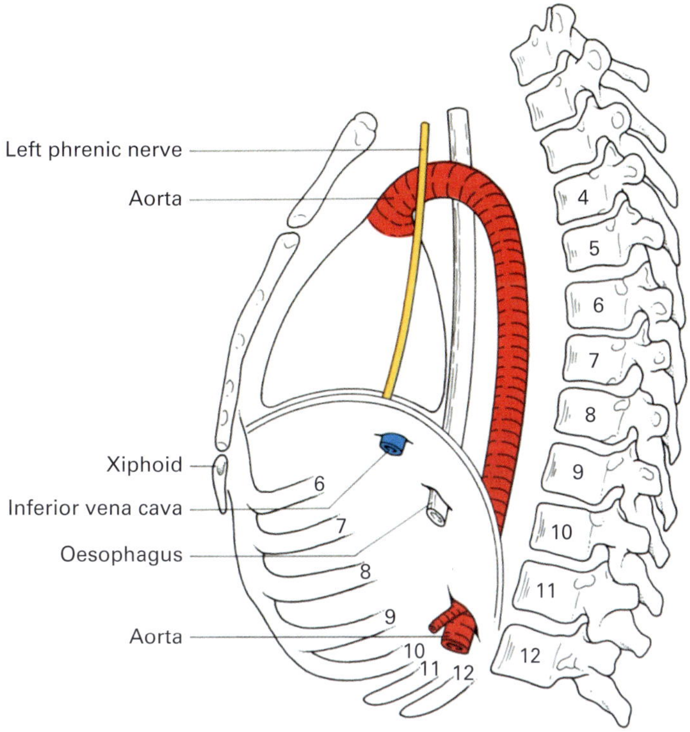

Fig. 11 Schematic lateral view of the diaphragm to show the levels at which it is pierced by major structures.

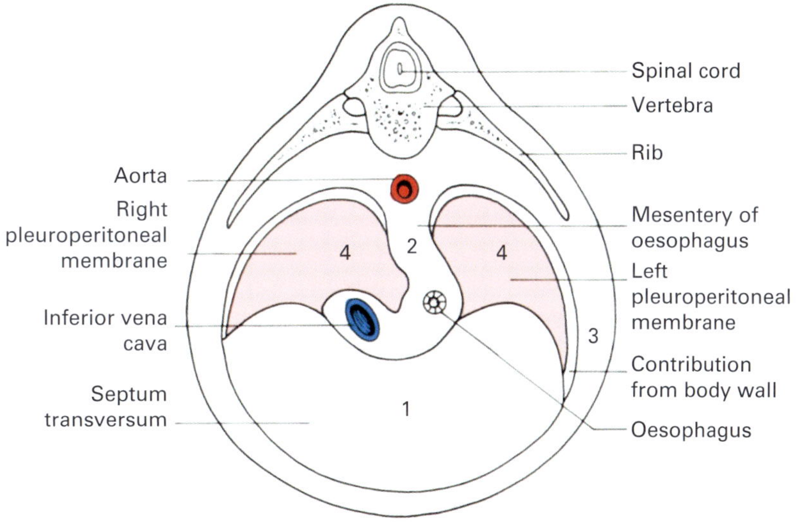

Fig. 12 The development of the diaphragm, showing the four elements contributing to the diaphragm – (1) the septum transversum, (2) the dorsal mesentery of the oesophagus, (3) the body wall and (4) the pleuroperitoneal membrane.

3 a peripheral rim derived from the body wall;

4 the pleuroperitoneal membranes, which close the fetal communication between the pleural and peritoneal cavities.

The septum transversum is the mesoderm which, in early development, lies in front of the head end of the embryo. With the folding off of the head, this mesodermal mass is carried ventrally and caudally, to lie in its definitive position at the anterior part of the diaphragm. During this migration, the cervical myotomes and nerves contribute

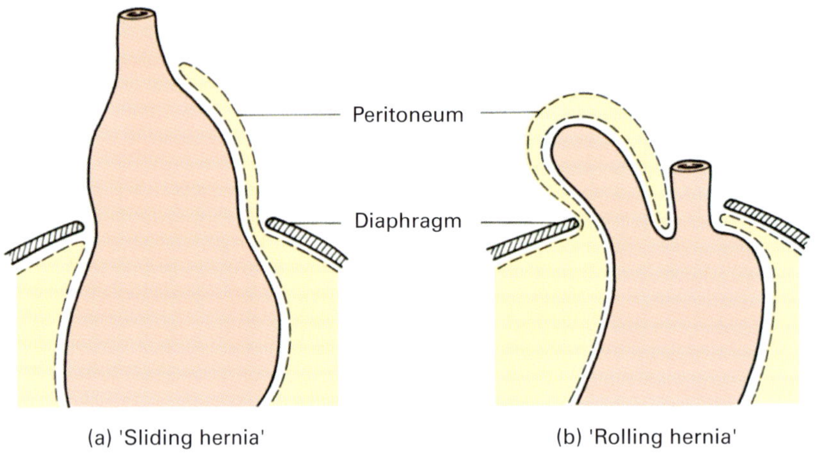

Fig. 13 (a) A sliding hiatus hernia. (b) A rolling hiatus hernia.

muscle and nerve supply, respectively, thus accounting for the long course of the phrenic nerve (C3, C4 and C5) from the neck to the diaphragm.

Given such a complex embryological journey undertaken by the diaphragm, it is somewhat surprising that congenital abnormalities of the diaphragm are relatively uncommon.

However, defects in the structure and integrity of the diaphragm can occur, giving rise to a variety of congenital hernias through the diaphragm. These may be:

1 through the foramen of Morgagni – anteriorly between the xiphoid and costal origins;
2 through the foramen of Bochdalek – the pleuroperitoneal canal – lying posterolaterally;
3 through a deficiency of the whole central tendon (occasionally such a hernia may be traumatic in origin);
4 through a congenitally large oesophageal hiatus.

Far more common than congenital hernias are the *acquired* hiatus hernias (classified into sliding and rolling hernia). These are found in patients usually of middle age in whom weakening and widening of the oesophageal hiatus of the diaphragm has occurred (Fig. 13).

In the *sliding hernia* the upper stomach and lower oesophagus slide upwards into the chest through the lax hiatus, when the patient lies down or bends over; the competence of the gastro-oesophageal junction is often disturbed with consequent reflux of gastric secretions into the oesophagus when lying down or bending over. This may be followed by oesophagitis with associated heartburn, bleeding and possible stricture formation.

In the *rolling hernia* (which is far less common) the gastro-oesophageal junction remains in its normal subdiaphragmatic position, but the fundus of the stomach rolls up through the hiatus to lie in front of the oesophagus; hence, the alternative term of para-oesophageal hernia. In such a case there may be epigastric discomfort, eructation and even dysphagia, but *no* reflux because the lower oesophageal sphincter mechanism is not compromised.

The movements of respiration

During inspiration the movements of the chest wall and diaphragm result in an increase in all diameters of the thorax. This, in turn, brings about an increase in the negative intrapleural pressure and an expansion of the lung tissue. Conversely, in expiration the relaxation of the respiratory muscles and the elastic recoil of the lung reduce the thoracic capacity and force air out of the lungs.

Quiet *inspiration* is brought about almost entirely by active contraction of the diaphragm with very little chest movement. Confirm this on yourself; your hands on your chest will show minimal movement as you breathe quietly. As respiratory movement grows deeper, the contraction of the intercostal muscles raises the ribs. The first rib remains relatively stationary, ribs 2–6 principally increase the anteroposterior diameter of the thorax (the pump handle movement), while the corresponding action of the lower ribs is to increase the transverse diameter of the thoracic cage (the bucket handle movement). Again, confirm this on your own chest during deep inspiration. In progressively deeper inspiration, more and more of the diaphragmatic musculature is called into play. On radiographic screening of the chest, the diaphragm will be seen to move approximately 2.5 cm (1 in) in quiet inspiration and up to 6–10 cm (2.5–4 in) on deep inspiration.

Normal quiet expiration is brought about by elastic recoil of the elevated ribs and passive relaxation of the contracted diaphragm. In deeper expiration, the abdominal muscles have an important part to play – they contract vigorously, compress the abdominal viscera, raise the intra-abdominal pressure and force the relaxed diaphragm upwards. Indeed, diaphragmatic movement accounts for approximately 65% of air exchange, whereas chest movement accounts for the remaining 35%.

In deep and forced inspiration, additional 'accessory muscles of respiration' are called into play. These are the muscles attached to the thorax that are normally used in movements of the arms and the head. The accessory muscles of respiration include pectoralis major, serratus anterior, latissimus dorsi, the scalene muscles and sternocleidomastoid.

The pleurae

The two pleural cavities are totally separate from each other (Fig. 2). Each *pleural sac* consists of two layers: a *visceral layer* intimately related to the surface of the lung, and a *parietal layer* lining the inner aspect of the chest wall, the upper surface of the diaphragm and the sides of the pericardium and mediastinum. The visceral layer is firmly attached to the underlying lung. In contrast, the parietal pleura is separated from its overlying structures by a loose, thin layer of connective tissue, the extrapleural fascia (endothoracic fascia), which enables the surgeon to strip the parietal pleura easily from the chest wall. The two layers are continuous with each other in front of and behind the root of the lung, but below the root, the pleura hangs down in a loose fold, the *pulmonary ligament*, which forms a 'dead space' for distension of the pulmonary veins. The surface markings of the pleura and lungs have already been described in the section on surface anatomy.

Each pleural sac is in effect a closed sac that is invaginated from its medial aspect by the corresponding lung. Notice that even in forced maximal inspiration, the lungs do not completely obliterate the space in the pleural cavity.

CLINICAL FEATURES

1 Normally the two pleural layers are in close apposition with the space between them containing just a thin layer of fluid which acts as a lubricant enabling the two pleural

layers to glide against each other. Abnormally however, the pleural space (pleural cavity) may fill with air (pneumothorax), blood (haemothorax) or pus (empyema).

2 Since the parietal pleura is segmentally innervated by the intercostal nerves, inflammation of the pleura results in pain referred to the cutaneous distribution of these nerves (i.e. to the thoracic wall or, in the case of the lower intercostal nerves, to the anterior abdominal wall, which may mimic an acute abdominal emergency).

The lower respiratory tract

The trachea (Figs 14, 15)

The trachea is approximately 11.5 cm (4.5 in) in length and nearly 2.5 cm (1 in) in diameter. It commences at the lower border of the cricoid cartilage (C6) and terminates by bifurcating somewhat below the level of the sternal angle of Louis (T4/5) to form the right and left main bronchi. (In the living subject, the level of bifurcation varies slightly with the phase of respiration; in deep inspiration it descends to T6 or even T7, and in expiration it rises to T4.)

Relations

Lying partly in the neck and partly in the thorax (superior mediastinum), its relations are as follows.

Cervical

- Anteriorly – the isthmus of the thyroid gland, inferior thyroid veins, sternohyoid and sternothyroid muscles.
- Laterally – the lobes of the thyroid gland and the common carotid artery (within its sheath) lying on either side.

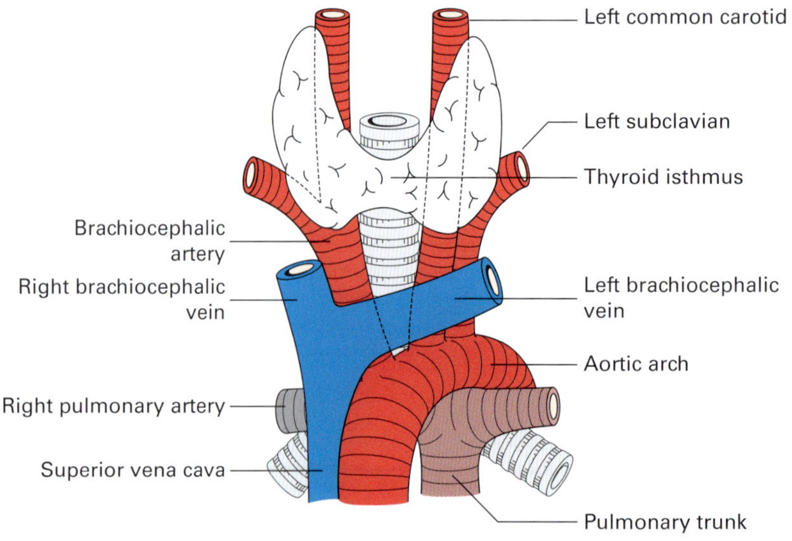

Fig. 14 The trachea and its anterior relationships.

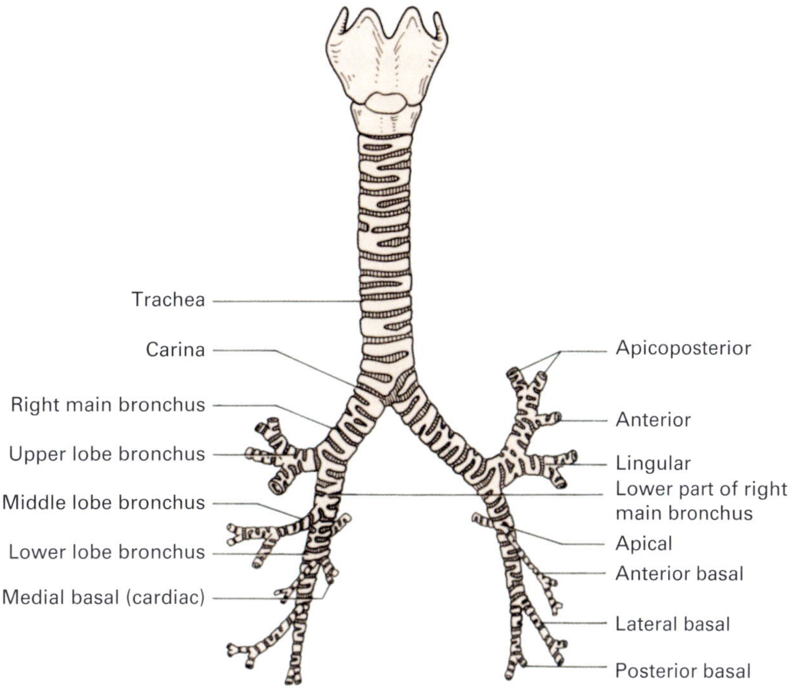

Fig. 15 The trachea and main bronchi viewed from the front.

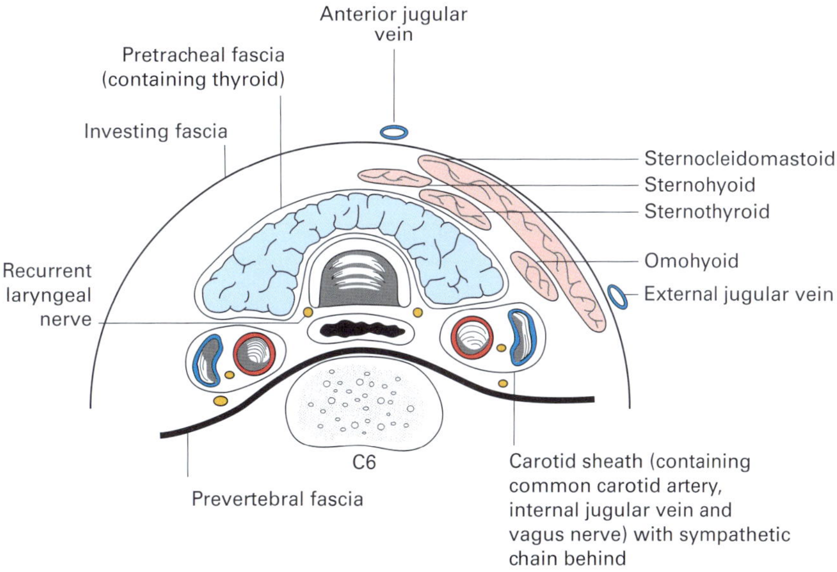

Fig. 16 The cervical part of the trachea and its environs in transverse section (through the 6th cervical vertebra) (viewed from below).

- Posteriorly – the oesophagus with the recurrent laryngeal nerve lying in the groove between the oesophagus and trachea (Fig. 16).

Thoracic

- Anteriorly – commencement of the brachiocephalic artery and left common carotid artery, both arising from the arch of the aorta, the left brachiocephalic vein and the thymus.

- Posteriorly – oesophagus and left recurrent laryngeal nerve.
- To the left – arch of the aorta, left common carotid and left subclavian arteries, left recurrent laryngeal nerve and pleura.
- To the right – vagus, azygos vein and pleura (Fig. 17).

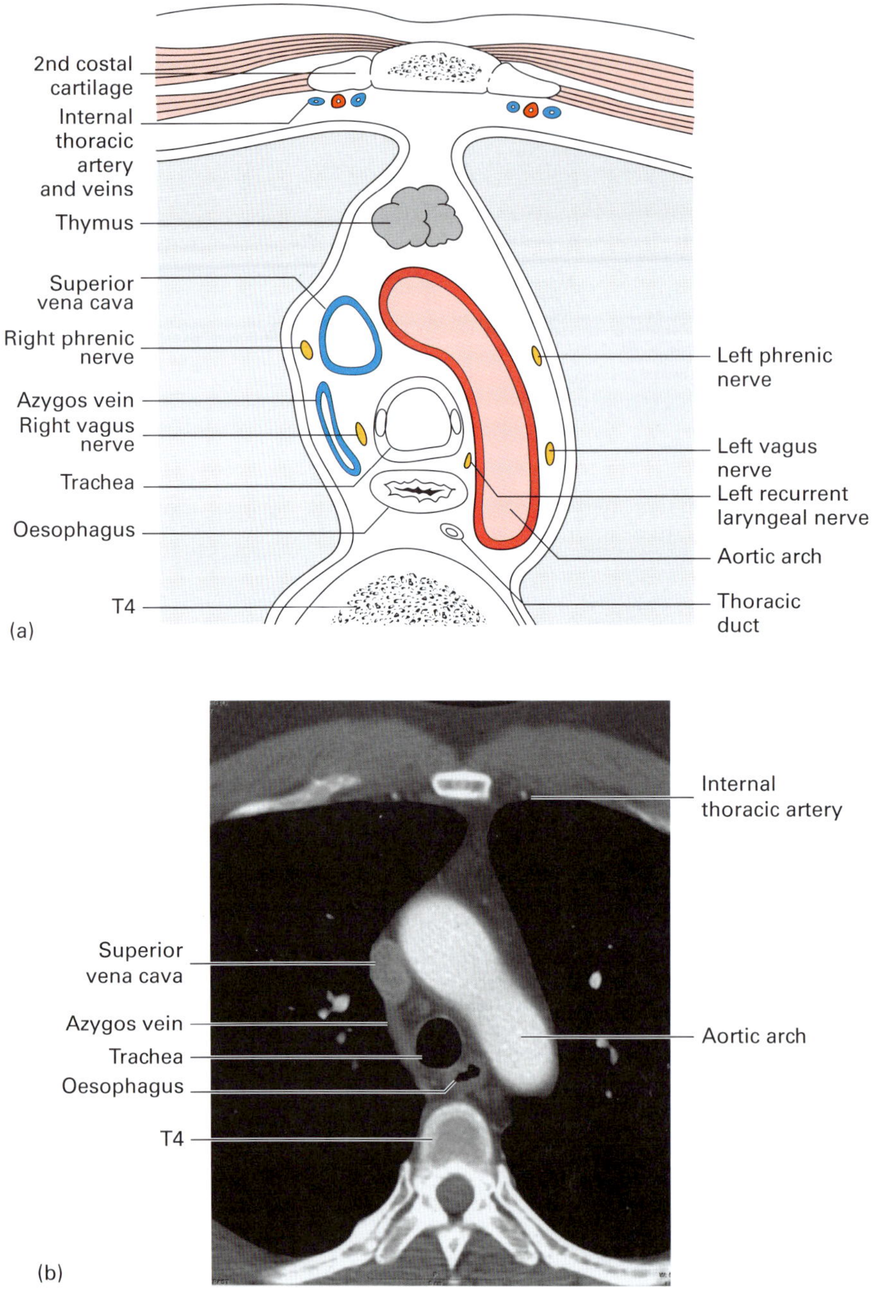

Fig. 17 (a) The thoracic part of the trachea and its environs in transverse section (through the 4th thoracic vertebra) (viewed from below). (b) CT scan (axial view) of the superior mediastinum at a level corresponding to that in (a) (Dr Sheila Rankin).

Structure

The patency of the trachea is maintained by a series of 15–20 U-shaped strips of hyaline cartilage (called tracheal 'rings'). Posteriorly, where the cartilage is deficient, the trachea is flattened and its wall completed by fibrous tissue and a sheet of smooth muscle (the trachealis). Within, it is lined by a ciliated columnar epithelium with many goblet cells.

CLINICAL FEATURES

Radiology

Since it contains air, the trachea is more radiolucent than the neighbouring structures and is seen in posteroanterior and lateral radiographs as a dark area passing downwards, backwards and slightly to the right. In the elderly, calcification of the tracheal rings is not uncommon.

Displacement

The trachea may be compressed or displaced by pathological enlargement of the neighbouring structures, particularly the thyroid gland and the arch of the aorta.

'Tracheal tug'

The intimate relationship between the arch of the aorta and the trachea and left bronchus is responsible for the physical sign known as 'tracheal tug', characteristic of aneurysms of the aortic arch.

Tracheostomy

Tracheostomy may be required for laryngeal obstruction (diphtheria, tumours, inhaled foreign bodies), for the evacuation of excessive secretions (severe postoperative chest infection in a patient who is too weak to cough effectively) and for long-term artificial ventilation for patients with spinal cord injuries or those with severe chest injuries. It is important to note that respiration is further assisted by considerable reduction of the dead-space air.

The neck is extended and the head held exactly in the midline by an assistant. A vertical incision is made downwards from the cricoid cartilage, passing between the anterior jugular veins. Alternatively, a more cosmetic transverse skin crease incision, placed halfway between the cricoid and suprasternal notch, is employed. A hook is thrust under the lower border of the cricoid to steady the trachea and pull it forwards. The pretracheal fascia is split longitudinally, the isthmus of the thyroid either pushed upwards or divided between clamps and the cartilage of the trachea clearly exposed. A circular opening is then made into the trachea to admit the tracheostomy tube.

In children the neck is relatively short and the left brachiocephalic vein may come up above the suprasternal notch so that dissection is rather more difficult and dangerous. This difficulty is made greater because the child's trachea is softer and more mobile than the adult's and is, therefore, not so readily identified and isolated. Its softness means that care must be taken, in incising the child's trachea, not to let the scalpel plunge through and damage the underlying oesophagus.

In contrast, the trachea may be ossified in the elderly and small bone shears may be required to open into it.

The golden rule of tracheostomy – based entirely on anatomical considerations – is *stick exactly to the midline*. If this dictum is not obeyed, major vessels may be in jeopardy.

Cricothyroid puncture is now frequently used in the emergency management of upper respiratory obstruction (see page 305 and Fig. 204).

The bronchi (Fig. 15)

The *right main bronchus* is wider, shorter and more vertical than the left. It is approximately 2.5 cm (1 in) long and passes directly to the root of the lung at the level of T5 vertebra. Before entering the lung, it gives off its *upper lobe branch* and then passes below the pulmonary artery to enter the hilum of the lung. It has two important relations: the azygos vein, which arches over it from behind to reach the superior vena cava, and the pulmonary artery, which lies first below and then anterior to it.

The *left main bronchus* is nearly 5 cm (2 in) long and passes downwards and outwards below the arch of the aorta, in front of the oesophagus and descending aorta. Unlike the right main bronchus, it gives off no branches until it enters the hilum of the lung, which it reaches opposite T6. The pulmonary artery spirals over the bronchus, lying first anteriorly and then above it.

CLINICAL FEATURES

1 The greater width and more vertical course of the right main bronchus accounts for the greater tendency for foreign bodies and aspirated material to pass into the right bronchus (and thence especially into the middle and lower lobes of the right lung) rather than into the left lung. Note that this also applies to an endotracheal tube which, if too long for the size of the patient's trachea, will be pushed down into the right main bronchus. This must be kept in mind particularly when intubating a neonate or an infant.

2 The inner aspect of the whole of the trachea, the main and lobar bronchi and the commencement of the segmental bronchi can be seen at bronchoscopy.

3 Widening and distortion of the angle between the right and left main bronchi (the carina) as seen at bronchoscopy may be a grave prognostic sign, as it may signify carcinomatous involvement of the tracheobronchial lymph nodes around the bifurcation of the trachea.

The lungs (Figs 18, 19)

Each lung is conical in shape, having a blunt apex that reaches above the sternal end of the 1st rib, a concave base overlying the diaphragm, an extensive costovertebral (outer) surface moulded to the form of the chest wall and a mediastinal (inner) surface that faces and is indented by the fibrous pericardium.

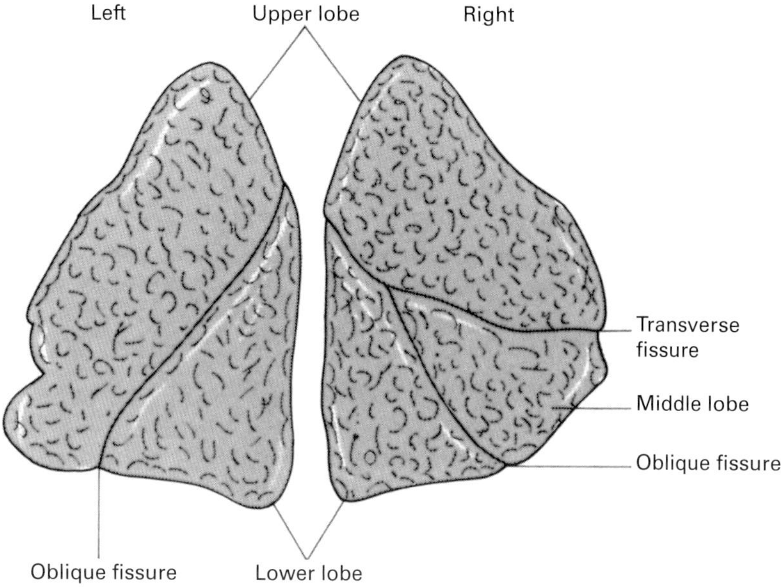

Fig. 18 The lungs, lateral aspects.

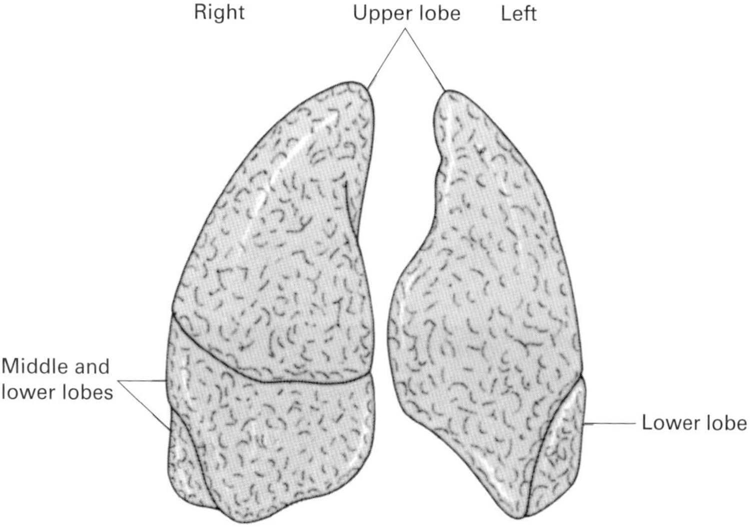

Fig. 19 The lungs, anterior aspects.

The right lung is somewhat shorter in height than the left; this is because it is pushed upwards by the higher right dome of the diaphragm, itself pushed up by the underlying liver. However, although shorter than the left, the right lung is actually the bulkier and heavier of the two because the size of the left lung is reduced by the considerable indentation on its medial aspect produced by the heart.

The right lung is divided into three lobes – the upper, middle and lower – by the oblique and horizontal fissures. The left lung has only an oblique fissure and hence only two lobes – an upper and a lower. There appears to be no physiological advantage in the fact that the lungs are lobed. However, the lobes are of considerable interest:

1 'lobar pneumonia', caused by *Pneumococcus*, affects an individual lobe;
2 a plug of mucus, tumour or an inhaled foreign body may block an individual lobar bronchus and produce a lobar collapse, as residual air in the occluded lobe is gradually and progressively absorbed.
3 as each lobe possesses its own bronchus and blood supply, the surgeon can perform a *lobectomy* in suitable cases.

Study Figs 2, 3 and also Figs 18, 19 and note an important error in current terminology: the so-called 'upper lobe' on each side is actually anterosuperior and the 'lower lobe' is more accurately described as being posteroinferior! When you examine the front of a patient's chest, you are listening, on the left side, almost exclusively to the *upper* lobe of the lung. On the right side, you are examining the upper lobe down to the level of the 4th intercostal space and, below that, the *middle* lobe. Only a relatively small part of the lower lobe can be assessed from the front. To examine the *lower* lobe of a patient – a common site for postoperative pulmonary collapse, for example – the posterior aspect of the chest must be examined, from the 3rd intercostal space downwards. Note also that a stab wound through the back of the chest, going through the 4th intercostal space, is likely to injure the lower, not upper, lobe!

Blood supply

Mixed venous blood is returned to the lungs by the pulmonary arteries; the air passages are themselves supplied by the bronchial arteries, which are small branches of the descending thoracic aorta. The *bronchial arteries*, although small, are of great clinical importance. They maintain the blood supply to the lung parenchyma after pulmonary embolism, so that, if the patient recovers, lung function returns to normal.

The *superior* and *inferior pulmonary veins* return oxygenated blood to the left atrium, while the *bronchial veins* drain into the azygos system.

Lymphatic drainage

The lymphatics of the lung drain centripetally from the pleura towards the hilum. From the *bronchopulmonary lymph nodes* in the hilum, efferent lymph channels pass to the *tracheobronchial nodes* at the bifurcation of the trachea, thence to the *paratracheal nodes* and the mediastinal lymph trunks to drain usually directly into the brachiocephalic veins or, rarely, indirectly via the thoracic duct or the right lymphatic duct.

Nerve supply

The innervation of the lung is via the pulmonary plexus at its hilum. This conveys sympathetic (T2–T5 or T6) and parasympathetic (vagal, X) fibres. The sympathetic fibres are bronchodilator to the bronchial muscles – hence the use of sympathomimetic drugs in asthma. The vagal fibres carry signals from stretch receptors in the lungs and provide secretomotor fibres to the mucous glands.

The bronchopulmonary segments of the lungs (Figs 20, 21)

A knowledge of the finer arrangement of the bronchial tree is an essential prerequisite to intelligent appreciation of lung radiology, to interpretation of bronchoscopic findings and to the surgical resection of lung segments. Each lobe of the lung is subdivided into a small number of bronchopulmonary segments, each of which is supplied by a segmental bronchus and a segmental branch of the pulmonary artery. Each bronchopulmonary segment is a functionally independent and anatomically discrete segment of the pulmonary lobe. The segments are wedge-shaped with their apices at the pulmonary hilum and bases at the lung surface; if excised accurately along their boundaries (which are marked by intersegmental veins), there is little

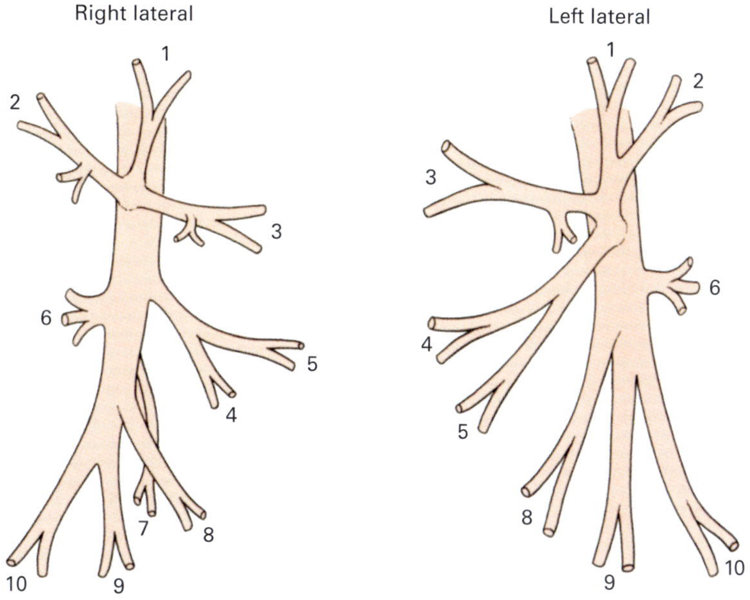

Right
Upper lobe
1 Apical bronchus
2 Posterior bronchus
3 Anterior bronchus

Middle lobe
4 Lateral bronchus
5 Medial bronchus

Lower lobe
6 Apical bronchus
7 Medial basal (cardiac) bronchus
8 Anterior basal bronchus
9 Lateral basal bronchus
10 Posterior basal bronchus

Left
Upper lobe
1, 2 } Apicoposterior bronchus
3 Anterior bronchus

Lingula
4 Superior bronchus
5 Inferior bronchus

Lower lobe
6 Apical bronchus
8 Anterior basal bronchus
9 Lateral basal bronchus
10 Posterior basal bronchus

Fig. 20 The named divisions of the main bronchi.

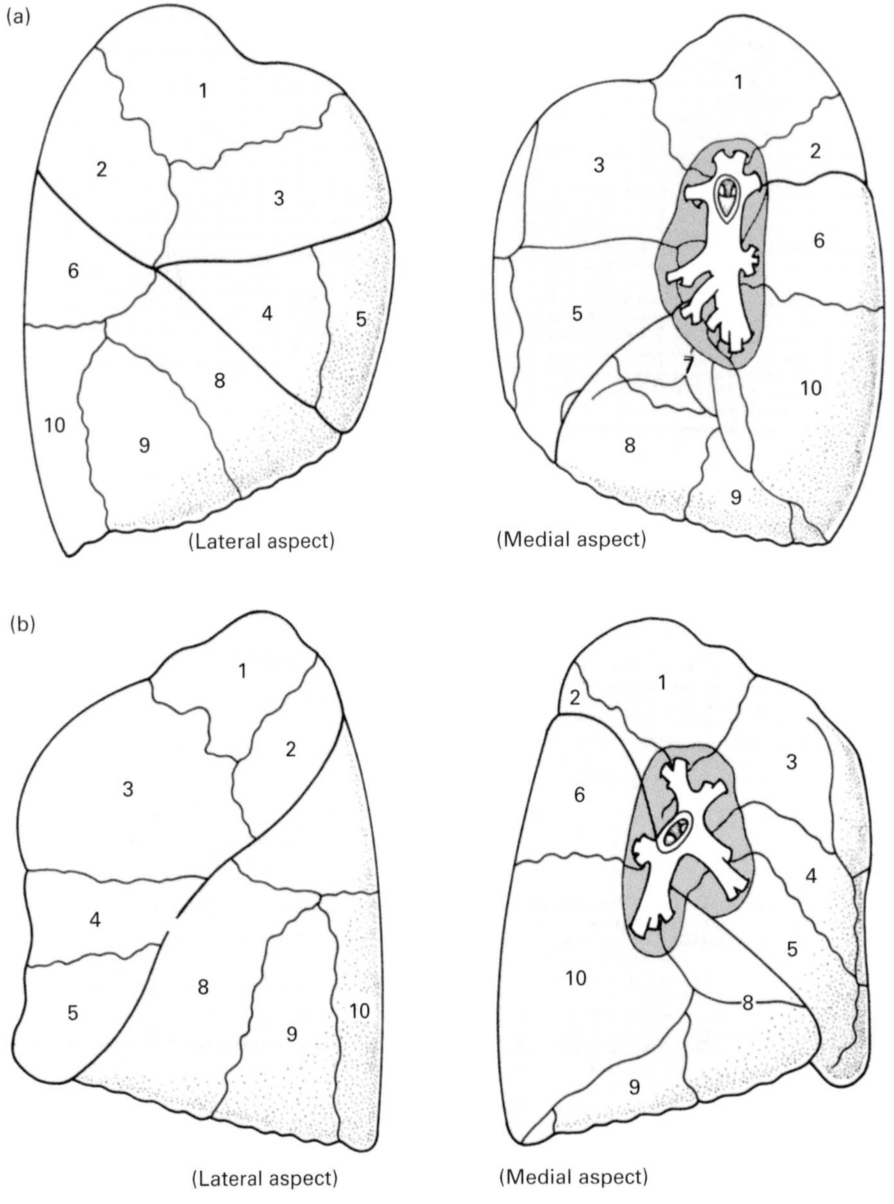

Fig. 21 (a) The segments of the right lung. (b) The segments of the left lung.

bleeding or alveolar air leakage from the raw lung surface. There are typically ten bronchopulmonary segments in each lung. However, owing to confluence of two or more segmental bronchi in the lung, *the left lung* may appear, on occasion, to possess just nine or eight segments.

The names and arrangements of the bronchi are given in Table 1; each bronchopulmonary segment takes its title from that of its supplying segmental bronchus (listed in the right-hand column of the table).

Table 1 The named divisions of the main bronchi

Right main bronchus	Upper lobe bronchus	Apical	
		Posterior	
		Anterior	
	Middle lobe bronchus	Lateral	
		Medial	
	Lower lobe bronchus	Apical	
		Basal →	Medial basal
			Anterior basal
			Lateral basal
			Posterior basal
Left main bronchus	Upper lobe bronchus	Apicoposterior	
		Anterior	
	↓ Lingular bronchus	Superior	
		Inferior	
	Lower lobe bronchus	Apical	
		Basal →	Anterior
			Lateral
			Posterior

The left upper lobe has a *lingular segment*, supplied by the *lingular bronchus* from the main upper lobe bronchus. This segment is equivalent to the *right middle lobe*, whose bronchus arises as a branch from the main bronchus. Apart from this, differences between the two sides are very slight; on the left, the upper lobe bronchus gives off a combined apicoposterior segmental bronchus and an anterior segmental bronchus, whereas, on the right side, the three segmental branches are separate.

On the right also there is a small medial (or cardiac) lower lobe bronchus that is absent on the left, the lower lobes being otherwise mirror images of each other.

The mediastinum

Together, the two pleural sacs (each enclosing an air-filled lung) occupy two-thirds to three-quarters of the volume of the thoracic cavity. The central part of the thoracic cavity between the two pleural sacs is termed the mediastinum (from the Latin for 'middle partition'). Thus, the mediastinum is bounded anteriorly, by the sternum; posteriorly, by the entire length of the thoracic part of the vertebral column; inferiorly, by the upper surface of the diaphragm; on either side, by the medial aspect of the corresponding pleural sac; and superiorly, by the oblique plane of the superior aperture of the thoracic cage or thoracic outlet.

For descriptive purposes the mediastinum is divided into two parts – the superior mediastinum and the inferior mediastinum, by an imaginary horizontal plane drawn at the level of the sternal angle. When projected to the vertebral column this plane, the *transverse thoracic plane* is seen to meet the vertebral column at the level of the disc between T4 and T5 vertebrae.

Located in its entirety within the inferior mediastinum is the fibrous pericardium. Based on the location of the fibrous pericardium, the inferior mediastinum is further

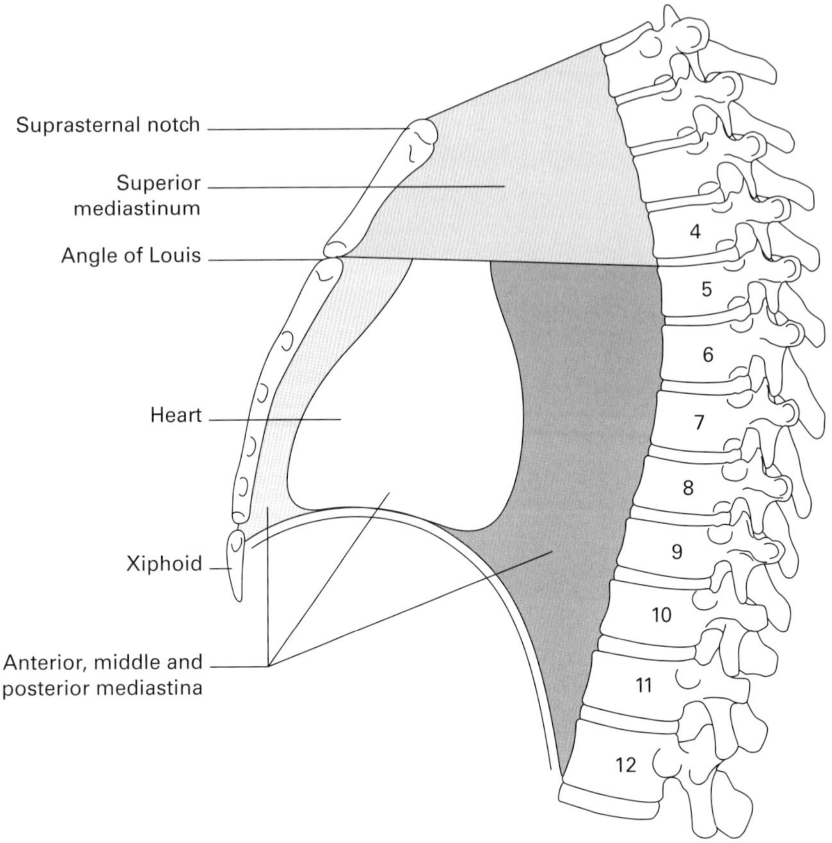

Fig. 22 The subdivisions of the mediastinum.

subdivided into three regions: **the anterior mediastinum** (in front of the fibrous pericardium), **the posterior mediastinum** behind the fibrous pericardium (between the fibrous pericardium and the lower eight thoracic vertebrae) and **the middle mediastinum** comprising the fibrous pericardium itself with its contents (Fig. 22).

The following are the principal contents of each of the subdivisions of the mediastinum:

The superior mediastinum contains the aortic arch and the origins of the three great vessels (brachiocephalic artery, left common carotid artery and left subclavian artery) that arise from the aortic arch. Behind the aortic arch is the trachea, behind which is the oesophagus. Behind the oesophagus is the thoracic vertebral column. In front of the aortic arch and its branches is the left brachiocephalic vein on its way to join the right brachiocephalic vein to form the superior vena cava within the right side of the superior mediastinum. Also coursing through the superior mediastinum are the right and left vagi and right and left phrenic nerves. Within the left side of the superior mediastinum are the thoracic duct and the left recurrent laryngeal nerve, hooking around the aortic arch before coursing superiorly into the neck in the tracheo-oesophageal groove.

Completing the list of structures in the superior mediastinum are the all-important mediastinal lymph nodes and thymic remnants.

The anterior mediastinum is bounded anteriorly by the posterior surface of the body of the sternum and bounded posteriorly by the fibrous pericardium. The anterior mediastinum contains the sternopericardial ligaments (superior and inferior). These are strands of fibrous tissue running from the sternum to blend with the fibrous pericardium.

The posterior mediastinum lies between the fibrous pericardium in front and the thoracic vertebral column behind (T5 to T12 vertebrae inclusive). Its upper boundary is the transverse thoracic plane and its inferior boundary is the upper surface of the diaphragm. The lateral boundary on either side is the medial surface of the corresponding pleural sac.

The contents of the posterior mediastinum include the descending thoracic aorta and its branches, the oesophagus with the vagal trunks running on its wall, the ganglionated right and left sympathetic trunks, the splanchnic nerves arising from the bilateral sympathetic trunks, the azygos, hemiazygos and accessory hemiazygos veins and their tributaries, the thoracic duct and the posterior mediastinal lymph nodes.

The middle mediastinum comprises the fibrous pericardium and its contents: the heart, ascending aorta and the pulmonary trunk. The four pulmonary veins and the terminations of the superior and inferior venae cavae are also contents of the middle mediastinum as are the right and left phrenic nerves which run on the surface of the fibrous pericardium.

The roots of the right and left lungs are also regarded as contents of the middle mediastinum.

The pericardium

The heart and the roots of the great vessels are contained within the conical *fibrous pericardium*, the apex of which is fused with the adventitia of the great vessels (the pulmonary trunk and the ascending aorta) and the base of which is fused with the central tendon of the diaphragm. Anteriorly the fibrous pericardium is related to the body of the sternum (to which it is attached by the sternopericardial ligaments), to the 3rd–6th costal cartilages and to the anterior borders of the lungs. Posteriorly, it is related to the oesophagus, descending thoracic aorta and vertebrae T5–T8, and on either side to the roots of the lungs, the mediastinal pleura and the phrenic nerves.

The pericardial cavity is the potential space between the visceral and parietal layers of the pericardium. Just like the pleural and peritoneal cavities, it is lubricated by a film of serous fluid. Following trauma it may fill with blood (haemopericardium).

The inner aspect of the fibrous pericardium is lined by the *parietal layer of serous pericardium*. This, in turn, is reflected around the roots of the great vessels to become continuous with the *visceral layer* or *epicardium*. The lines of pericardial reflexion are marked on the posterior surface of the heart (Fig. 23) by the *oblique sinus*, bounded by the IVC and the four pulmonary veins, which form a recess between the left atrium and the pericardium, and the *transverse sinus* between the superior vena cava and left atrium behind and the pulmonary trunk and aorta in front.

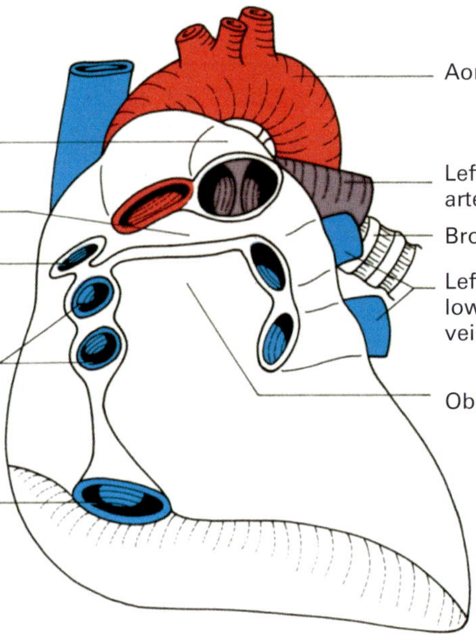

Fig. 23 The transverse and oblique sinuses of the pericardium. The heart has been removed from the pericardial sac, which is seen in anterior view.

The heart (Fig. 24)

Its great importance means no excuse need be offered for dealing with the heart in considerable detail.

The heart is irregularly conical in shape, and it is placed obliquely in the middle mediastinum. Viewed from the front, portions of all the heart chambers can be seen. The right border is formed entirely by the right atrium, the left border partly by the auricular appendage of the left atrium but mainly by the left ventricle and the inferior border chiefly not only by the right ventricle but also by the lower part of the right atrium and the apex of the left ventricle.

The bulk of the anterior surface is formed by the right ventricle, which is separated from the right atrium by the vertical atrioventricular groove and from the left ventricle by the anterior interventricular groove.

The inferior or *diaphragmatic surface* consists of the right and left ventricles separated by the posterior interventricular groove, and the portion of the right atrium that receives the IVC.

The base or *posterior surface* is quadrilateral in shape and is formed mainly by the left atrium with the openings of the pulmonary veins and, to a lesser extent, by the right atrium, and partly also by a strip of the posterior aspect of the left ventricle.

Chambers of the heart

Right atrium (Fig. 25a)

The right atrium receives the superior vena cava in its upper and posterior part, the IVC and coronary sinus in its lower part and the anterior cardiac veins (draining much of the front of the heart) anteriorly. Running more or less vertically downwards between

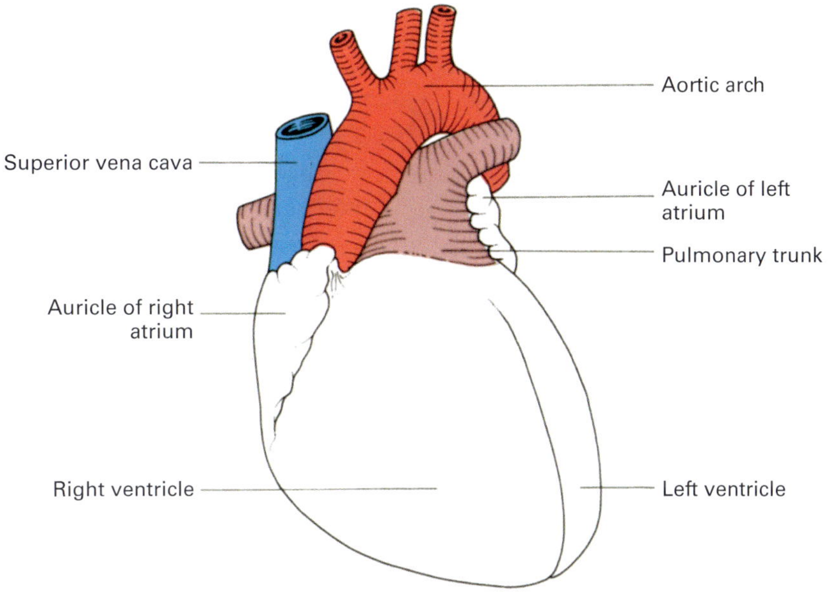

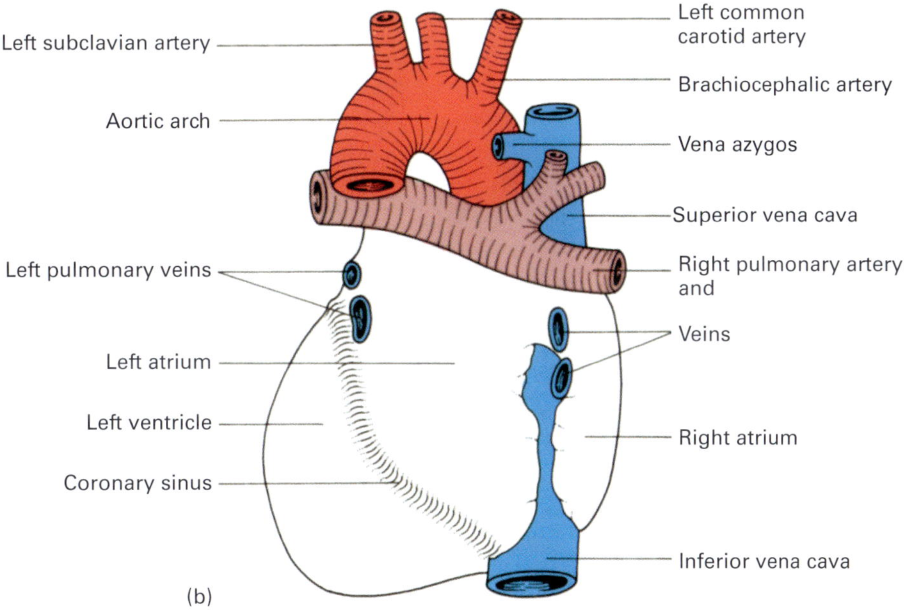

Fig. 24 The heart – (a) anterior and (b) posterior aspects.

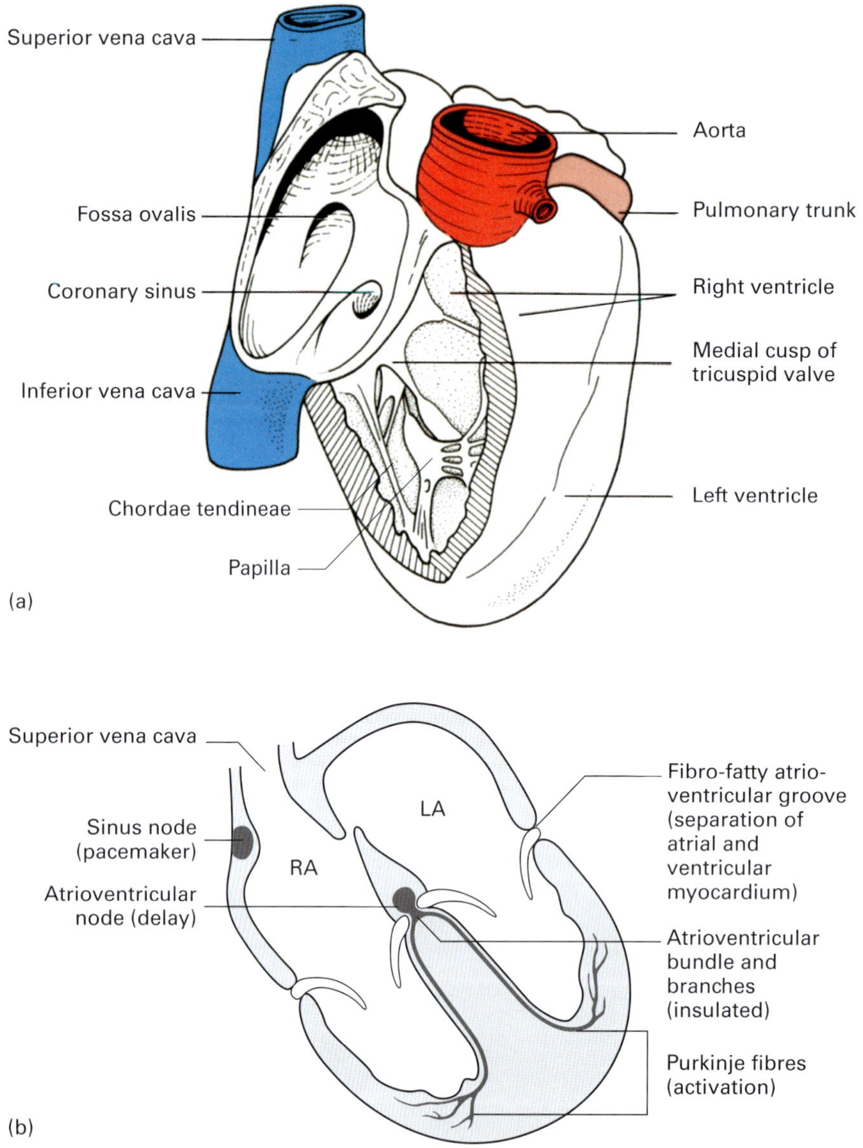

Fig. 25 (a) The interior of the right atrium and ventricle. (b) The conducting system of the heart. LA, left atrium; RA, right atrium.

the venae cavae is a distinct muscular ridge, the *crista terminalis* (indicated on the outer surface of the atrium by a shallow groove – the *sulcus terminalis*). This ridge separates the smooth-walled posterior part of the right atrium, derived from the sinus venosus, from the rough-walled anterior portion which is prolonged into the *auricular appendage* and which is derived from the true fetal atrium (see page 39).

The trabeculations in the rough-walled part of the atrium are produced by parallel columns of muscle termed *musculi pectinati* (*pectinate muscles*); 'pectinate' comes from the Latin for 'like a comb'. The same term applies to the columns of muscle seen in the auricular appendage of the left atrium.

The openings of the IVC and the coronary sinus are guarded by rudimentary valves; that of the IVC being continuous with the *annulus ovalis* around the shallow depression on the atrial septum, the *fossa ovalis*, which marks the site of the fetal *foramen ovale*.

Right ventricle (Fig. 25)

The right ventricle is joined to the right atrium by way of the vertically disposed *tricuspid valve*, and with the pulmonary trunk through the pulmonary valve. A muscular ridge, the *infundibulo ventricular crest*, between the atrioventricular and pulmonary orifices, separates the 'inflow' and 'outflow' tracts of the ventricle. The inner aspect of the inflow tract is marked by the presence of a number of irregular muscular elevations (*trabeculae carneae*), from some of which the *papillary muscles* project into the lumen of the ventricle and find attachment to the free borders of the cusps of the tricuspid valve by way of the *chordae tendineae*.

When the ventricle contracts in systole, the papillary muscles shorten, the chordae tendineae are pulled upon and the tricuspid valve is prevented from prolapsing into the right atrium. (The same mechanism, of course, takes place with the mitral valve of the left ventricle.) Rupture of a papillary muscle, following an adjacent myocardial infarction, will allow prolapse of the affected cusp to occur into the atrium at each systole, with consequent regurgitation of blood into the atrium and possible cardiac failure.

The *moderator band* is a muscular bundle crossing the right ventricular cavity from the interventricular septum to the anterior wall and is of some importance since it conveys the right branch of the atrioventricular bundle to the ventricular muscle.

The outflow tract of the ventricle or *infundibulum* is smooth-walled and is directed upwards and to the right towards the pulmonary trunk. The pulmonary orifice is guarded by the *pulmonary valve*, comprising three semilunar cusps.

Left atrium

The left atrium is rather smaller than the right but has somewhat thicker walls. On the upper part of its posterior wall it presents the openings of the four pulmonary veins, and on its septal surface there is a shallow depression corresponding to the fossa ovalis of the right atrium. As on the right side, the main part of the cavity is smooth-walled but the inner surface of the auricle is marked by a number of ridges due to the underlying pectinate muscles.

Left ventricle (Fig. 26)

The left ventricle communicates with the left atrium by way of the *mitral valve* (so-called because it vaguely resembles a bishop's mitre), which possesses a large anterior and a smaller posterior cusp attached to papillary muscles of the ventricular wall by chordae tendineae. With the exception of the fibrous *vestibule* immediately below the aortic orifice, the wall of the left ventricle is marked by thick trabeculae carneae.

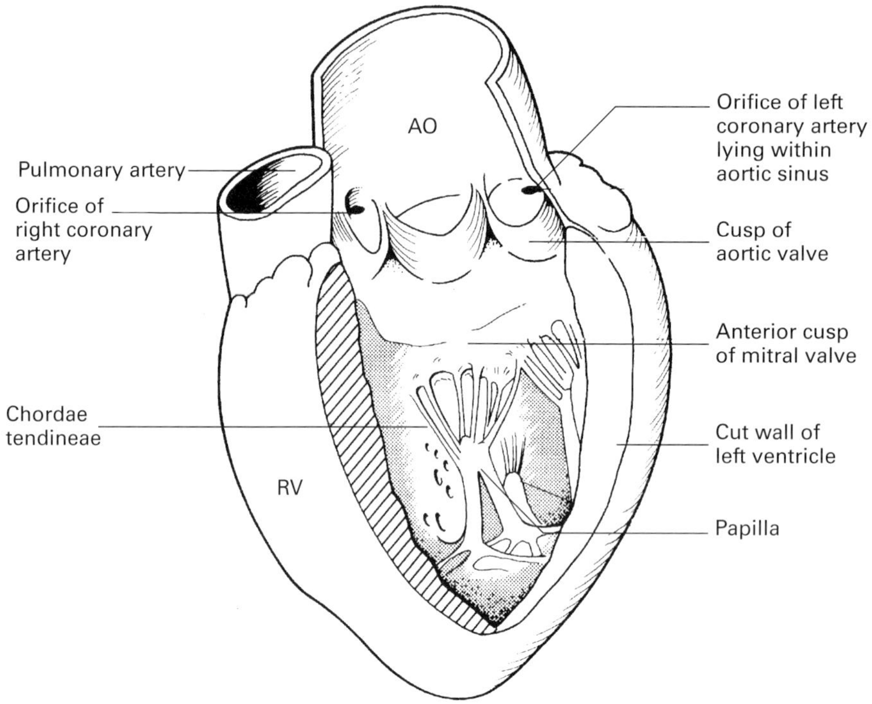

Fig. 26 The interior of the left ventricle. AO, aorta; RV, right ventricle.

The term 'cusps' applied to the tricuspid and mitral valves is somewhat misleading. It suggests that, as in the aortic and pulmonary valves, these are individual structures and separate from each other (Fig. 26). In fact, the tricuspid and mitral valves can be compared to circular curtains that hang down from each atrioventricular orifice, and that descend into the lumen of the ventricle with three drapes on the right side and two drapes on the left, held in place by chordae tendineae.

The aortic orifice is guarded by the three semilunar cusps of the *aortic valve*, immediately above which are the dilated *aortic sinuses*. The mouths of the right and left coronary arteries are seen in the anterior and left posterior sinuses, respectively. These two aortic sinuses are more commonly known as the right and left aortic sinuses, respectively: the former opening into the right coronary artery and the latter into the left coronary artery. The third aortic sinus is known, in the terminology of the cardiologist, as the *non-coronary sinus* implying that it does not give rise to a coronary artery. In diastole, blood refluxing into the aortic sinuses sets up turbulent flow, which helps to close the valve. The same mechanism applies to the pulmonary valve. In addition, on the left, blood refluxes in diastole into the two coronary artery ostia, placed within the sinuses, so that cardiac perfusion takes place in the ventricular diastolic phase of the cardiac cycle. This is an ingenious piece of engineering; since, in the absence of this arrangement, it would be almost impossible for ventricular cardiac muscle perfusion to take place when this muscle is firmly contracted in systole.

The conducting system of the heart (Fig. 25b)

This consists of specialized cardiac muscle found in the sinuatrial node and in the atrioventricular node and bundle. The heart beat is initiated in the *sinus* (or *sinuatrial*) *node* (the 'pacemaker of the heart'), situated in the upper part of the crista terminalis just to the right of the opening of the superior vena cava into the right atrium. From there the cardiac impulse spreads throughout the atrial musculature to reach the *atrioventricular node* lying in the atrial septum immediately above the opening of the coronary sinus. The impulse is then conducted to the ventricles by way of the specialized tissue of the *atrioventricular bundle* (*of His*). This bundle divides at the junction of the membranous and muscular parts of the interventricular septum into its right and left branches, which run immediately beneath the endocardium to activate all parts of the ventricular musculature. The bundle of His is made up of specialized large, pale, striated muscle fibres (the cells of Purkinje).

The blood supply to the heart (Fig. 27)

The heart's blood supply is derived from the right and left coronary arteries, whose main branches lie in each of the interventricular and atrioventricular grooves.

The *right coronary artery* arises from the right (anterior) aortic sinus and passes forwards between the pulmonary trunk and the right atrium to descend in the right atrioventricular groove. At the inferior border of the heart it continues along the atrioventricular groove to anastomose with the left coronary artery at the posterior interventricular groove. It gives off a *marginal branch* along the lower border of the heart and the *posterior interventricular branch* which runs forwards in the interventricular groove on the surface of the heart to anastomose near the apex of the heart with the corresponding branch of the left coronary artery.

The *left coronary artery*, which is larger than the right, arises from the left (left posterior) aortic sinus. Passing first behind and then to the left of the pulmonary trunk, it reaches

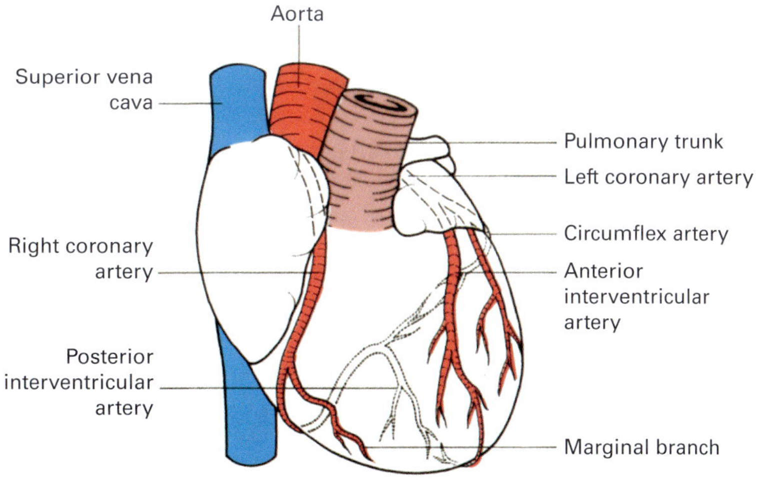

Fig. 27 The coronary arteries. (Dotted vessels lie posteriorly.)

the left atrioventricular groove, in which it runs laterally round the left border of the heart as the *circumflex artery* to reach the posterior interventricular groove. Its most important branch, given off less than 2.5 cm (1 in) from its origin, is the *anterior interventricular artery*, which supplies the anterior aspect of both ventricles and passes around the apex of the heart to anastomose with the posterior interventricular branch of the right coronary artery. Note that the sinuatrial node is usually supplied by the right coronary artery, although the left coronary artery takes over this role in approximately one-third of subjects.

Although anastomoses occur between the terminations of the right and left coronary arteries, these are usually inefficient, and the arteries are best regarded as end arteries. Thrombosis in one or other of these vessels leads to ischaemia or infarction of the area of heart muscle supplied (myocardial ischaemia/infarction).

The venous drainage of the heart (Fig. 28)

The bulk of the venous drainage of the heart is achieved by veins that accompany the coronary arteries and that open into the right atrium. The rest of the blood drains by means of small veins (*venae cordis minimae*) directly into the cardiac cavity.

The coronary sinus lies in the posterior atrioventricular groove and opens into the right atrium just to the left of the mouth of the IVC.

It receives:

1 the *great cardiac vein* which runs in the anterior interventricular groove;
2 the *middle cardiac vein* in the inferior interventricular groove;
3 the *small cardiac vein* – accompanying the marginal artery along the lower border of the heart;
4 the *oblique vein* – descends obliquely on the posterior aspect of the left atrium.

The *anterior cardiac veins* (up to three or four in number) cross the anterior atrioventricular groove, drain much of the anterior surface of the heart and open directly into the right atrium.

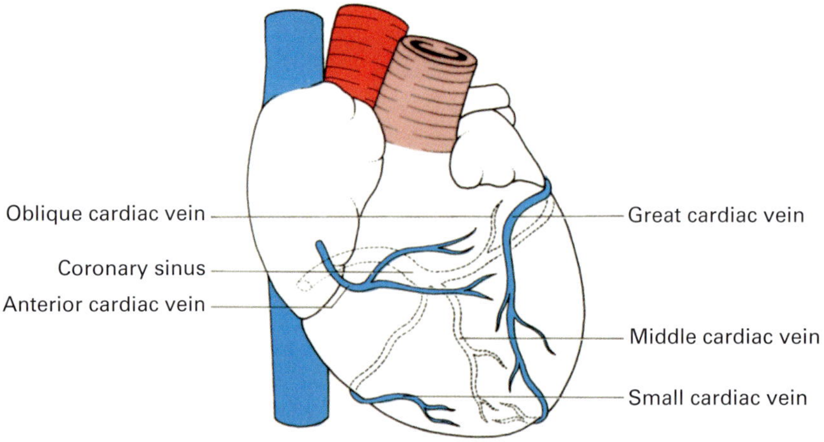

Fig. 28 The coronary veins. (Dotted vessels lie posteriorly.)

Nerve supply

The nerve supply of the heart is derived from the vagus (parasympathetic cardio-inhibitor) and the cervical and upper five thoracic sympathetic ganglia (cardio-accelerator) by way of superficial and deep cardiac plexuses. Cardiac pain (as in coronary thrombosis) may be experienced centrally in the chest but commonly may be referred to the neck ('angina'), left arm and epigastrium via T1 to T5 sympathetic afferent nerves. (See also page 423.)

The development of the heart

The primitive heart is a single tube which soon shows grooves demarcating the *sinus venosus, atrium, ventricle* and *bulbus cordis* from behind forwards. As this tube enlarges a kink occurs so that its caudal end, receiving venous blood, comes to lie behind its cephalic end with its emerging arteries (Fig. 29).

The sinus venosus later absorbs into the atrium and the bulbus becomes incorporated into the ventricle so that, in the fully developed heart, the atria and great veins come to lie posterior to the ventricles and the roots of the great arteries.

The boundary tissue between the primitive single atrial cavity and single ventricle grows out as a *dorsal* and a *ventral endocardial cushion* that meet in the midline, thus dividing the common atrioventricular orifice into a right (tricuspid) and left (mitral) orifice.

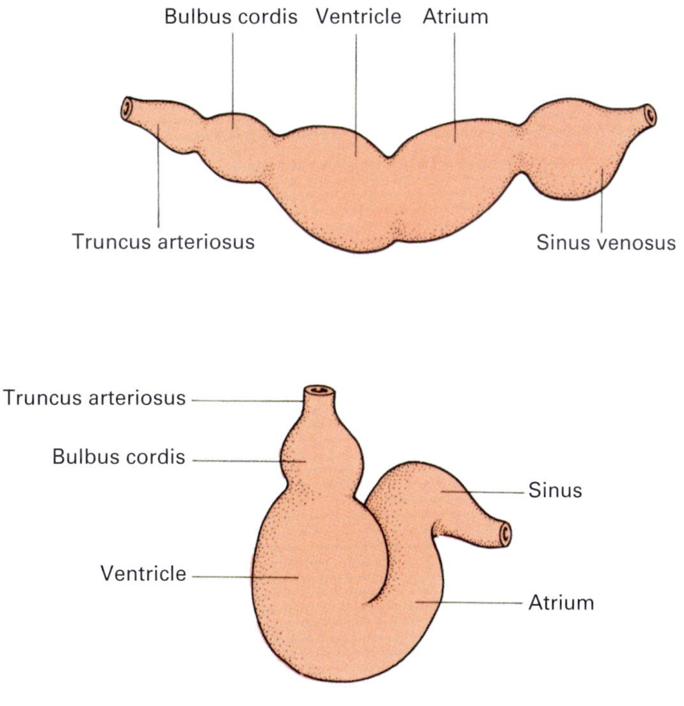

Fig. 29 The coiling of the primitive heart tube into its definitive form.

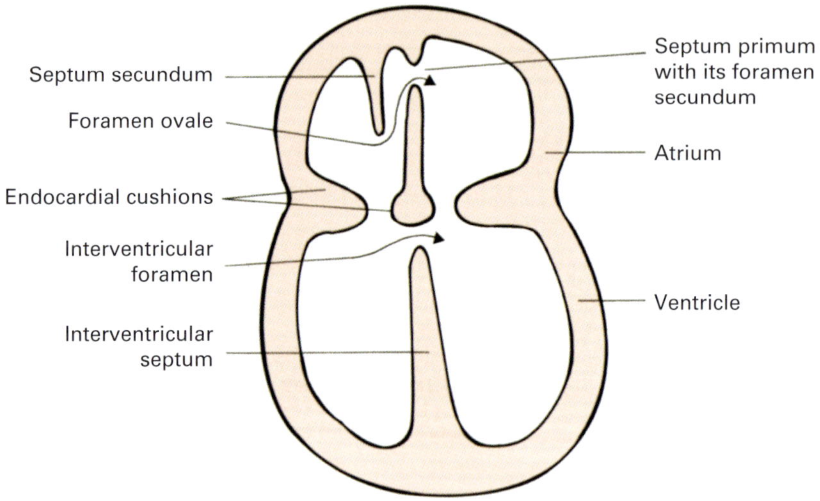

Fig. 30 The development of the chambers of the heart. (Note the septum primum and septum secundum that form the interatrial septum, leaving the foramen ovale as a valve-like opening passing between them.)

The division of the primitive atrium into two is a complicated process but an important one in the understanding of congenital septal defects (Fig. 30). A partition, the *septum primum*, grows downwards from the posterior and superior walls of the primitive common atrium to fuse with the endocardial cushions. Before fusion is complete, however, a hole appears in the upper part of this septum which is termed *the foramen secundum in the septum primum.*

A second membrane, the *septum secundum*, then develops to the right of the primum but this is never complete; it has a free lower edge that does, however, extend low enough for this new septum to overlap the foramen secundum in the septum primum and hence to close it.

The two overlapping defects in the septa form the valve-like *foramen ovale*, which shunts blood from the right to the left heart in the fetus (see 'The fetal circulation'). After birth, this foramen usually becomes completely fused, leaving only the fossa ovalis on the septal wall of the right atrium as its memorial. In approximately 10% of adult subjects, however, a probe can still be insinuated through an anatomically patent, although functionally sealed, foramen.

Division of the ventricle is commenced by the upgrowth of a fleshy septum from the apex of the heart towards the endocardial cushions. This stops short of dividing the ventricle completely, and thus it has an upper free border, forming a temporary interventricular foramen. At the same time, the single truncus arteriosus is divided into the aorta and pulmonary trunk by a *spiral septum* (hence the spiral relations of these two vessels), which grows downwards to the ventricle and fuses accurately with the upper free border of the ventricular septum. This contributes the small *pars membranacea septi*, which completes the separation of the ventricle in such a way that blood on the left of the septum flows into the aorta and on the right into the pulmonary trunk.

The primitive *sinus venosus* absorbs into the right atrium so that the venae cavae draining into the sinus come to open separately into this atrium. The smooth-walled part of the adult atrium represents the contribution of the sinus venosus; the pectinate part represents the portion derived from the primitive atrium and is termed the *auricle* or the *auricular appendage* of the right atrium (Fig. 24a).

Rather similarly, the adult left atrium has a double origin. The original single pulmonary venous trunk entering the left atrium becomes absorbed into it and donates the smooth-walled part of this chamber with the pulmonary veins entering as four separate openings; the trabeculated part of the definitive left atrium is the remains of the original atrial wall. This forms the *auricle* or the *auricular appendage* of the left atrium (Fig. 24a).

The development of the aortic arches and their derivatives (Fig. 31)

Emerging from the bulbus cordis is a common arterial trunk termed the *truncus arteriosus*, from which arise six pairs of aortic arches, equivalent to the arteries supplying the gill clefts of the fish. These arteries curve dorsally around the pharynx on either side and join to form two longitudinally placed dorsal aortae that fuse distally into the descending aorta.

The 1st and 2nd arches disappear; the 3rd arches become the carotids. The 4th arch on the right becomes the brachiocephalic and right subclavian artery; on the left, it differentiates into the definitive aortic arch, gives off the left subclavian artery and links up distally with the descending aorta.

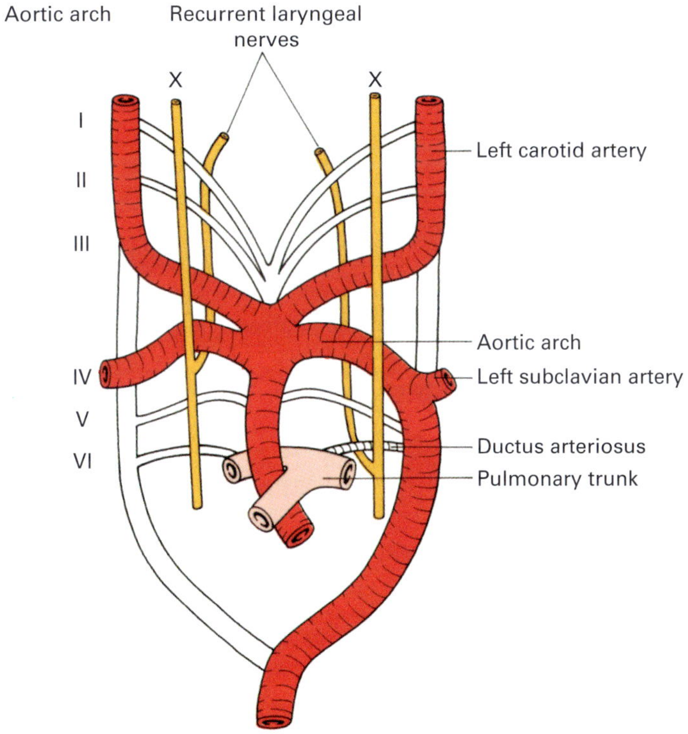

Fig. 31 The aortic arches and their derivatives. This diagram explains the relationship of the right recurrent laryngeal nerve to the right subclavian artery and the left nerve to the aortic arch and the ligamentum arteriosum (or to a persistent ductus arteriosus).

The 5th arch artery is rudimentary and disappears.

When the truncus arteriosus splits longitudinally to form the ascending aorta and pulmonary trunk, the 6th arch artery, unlike the others, remains linked with the latter and forms the right and left pulmonary arteries. On the left side this arch retains its connection with the dorsal aorta to form the *ductus arteriosus* (the ligamentum arteriosum of adult anatomy).

This asymmetrical development of the aortic arches accounts for the different course taken by the recurrent laryngeal nerve on each side. In the early fetus the vagus nerve lies lateral to the primitive pharynx, separated from it by the aortic arches. What are to become the recurrent laryngeal nerves pass medially, caudal to the aortic arches, to supply the developing larynx. With elongation of the neck and caudal migration of the heart, the recurrent nerves are caught up and dragged down by the descending aortic arches. On the right side, the 5th arch and distal part of the 6th arch become absorbed, leaving the nerve to hook round the 4th arch (i.e. the right subclavian artery). On the left side, the nerve remains looped around the persisting distal part of the 6th arch (the ligamentum arteriosum), which is overlapped and dwarfed by the arch of the aorta (Fig. 31).

The fetal circulation (Fig. 32)

The circulation of the blood in the embryo is a remarkable example of economy in nature and results in the shunting of well-oxygenated blood from the placenta to the brain and the heart, leaving relatively desaturated blood for less essential structures.

Blood is returned from the placenta by the umbilical vein to the IVC and thence the right atrium, most of it bypassing the liver in the *ductus venosus* (see page 98). Relatively little mixing of oxygenated and deoxygenated blood occurs in the right atrium since the valve overlying the orifice of the IVC serves to direct the flow of oxygenated blood from that vessel through the *foramen ovale* into the left atrium, while the deoxygenated stream from the superior vena cava is directed through the tricuspid valve into the right ventricle. From the left atrium the oxygenated blood (together with a small amount of deoxygenated blood from the lungs) passes into the left ventricle and hence into the ascending aorta for the supply of the brain and heart via the vertebral, carotid and coronary arteries.

As the lungs of the fetus are inactive, most of the deoxygenated blood from the right ventricle is short-circuited by way of the *ductus arteriosus* from the pulmonary trunk into the descending aorta. This blood supplies the abdominal viscera and the lower limbs and is shunted to the placenta, for oxygenation, along the *umbilical arteries* arising from the internal iliac arteries.

At birth, expansion of the lungs leads to an increased blood flow in the pulmonary arteries; the resulting pressure changes in the two atria bring the overlapping *septum primum* and *septum secundum* into apposition, which effectively closes off the foramen ovale. At the same time active contraction of the muscular wall of the ductus arteriosus results in a functional closure of this arterial shunt and, in the course of the next 2–3 months, its complete obliteration. Similarly, ligature of the umbilical cord is followed by thrombosis and obliteration of the umbilical vessels.

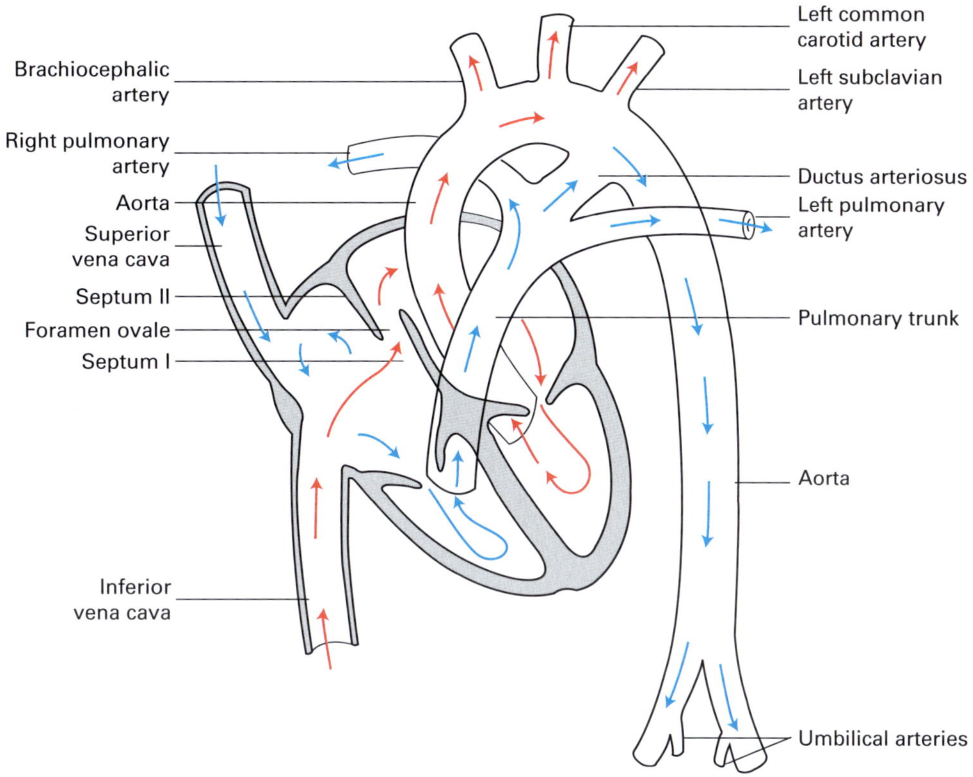

Fig. 32 The fetal circulation. The red arrows denote oxygenated blood.

The obliterated umbilical artery is represented by the *medial umbilical ligament*, leading from the superior vesical branch of the internal iliac artery on either side, across the deep aspect of the lower anterior abdominal wall to the umbilicus. The obliterated umbilical vein becomes the *ligamentum teres*, which runs in the free edge of the falciform ligament to the liver (see Fig. 69).

Congenital abnormalities of the heart and great vessels

The complex development of the heart and major arteries accounts for the multitude of congenital abnormalities that may affect these structures, either alone or in combination.

Dextrorotation of the heart means that this organ and its emerging vessels lie as a mirror image to the normal anatomy. It may be associated with reversal of all the intra-abdominal organs; one of the authors (H.E.) has seen a student correctly diagnose acute appendicitis as the cause of a patient's severe *left* iliac fossa pain because he found that the apex beat of the heart was on the right side!

Septal defects

At birth, the septum primum and septum secundum are forced together, closing the flap valve of the foramen ovale. Fusion usually takes place approximately 3 months after birth. In approximately 10% of subjects, this fusion may be incomplete. However, the two septa overlap and this patency of the foramen ovale is of no functional significance. If the septum secundum is too short to cover the foramen secundum in the septum primum, an *atrial septal defect* persists after the septum primum and septum secundum are pressed together at birth. This results in an *ostium secundum defect*, which allows shunting of blood from the left to the right atrium. This defect lies high up in the atrial wall and is relatively easy to close surgically. A more serious atrial septal defect results if the septum primum fails to fuse with the endocardial cushions. This *ostium primum defect* lies immediately above the atrioventricular boundary and may be associated with a defect of the pars membranacea septi of the ventricular septum. In such a case, the child is born with both an atrial and ventricular septal defect.

Occasionally, the ventricular septal defect is so huge that the ventricles form a single cavity, giving a *trilocular heart*.

Congenital pulmonary stenosis may affect the trunk of the pulmonary artery, its valve or the infundibulum of the right ventricle. If stenosis occurs in conjunction with a septal defect, the compensatory hypertrophy of the right ventricle (developed to force blood through the pulmonary obstruction) develops a sufficiently high pressure to shunt blood through the defect into the left heart; this mixing of the deoxygenated right heart blood with the oxygenated left-sided blood results in the child being *cyanosed at birth*.

The commonest combination of congenital abnormalities causing cyanosis is *Fallot's tetralogy* (Fig. 33). This results from unequal division of the truncus arteriosus by the spiral septum, resulting in a stenosed pulmonary trunk and a wide aorta that overrides the orifices of both the ventricles. The displaced septum is unable to close the interventricular septum, which results in a ventricular septal defect. Right ventricular hypertrophy develops as a consequence of the pulmonary stenosis. Cyanosis results from the shunting of large amounts of unsaturated blood from the right ventricle through the ventricular septal defect into the left ventricle and also directly into the aorta.

A *persistent ductus arteriosus* (Fig. 34a) is a relatively common congenital defect. If left uncorrected, it causes progressive work hypertrophy of the left heart and pulmonary hypertension.

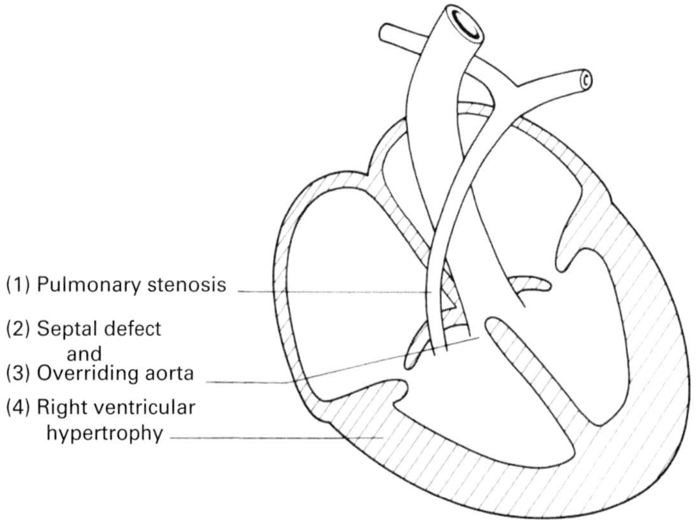

Fig. 33 The tetralogy of Fallot.

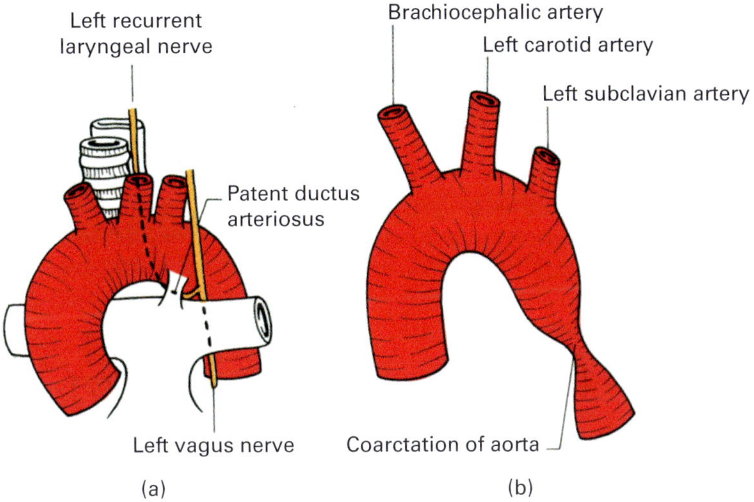

Fig. 34 (a) Persistent ductus arteriosus – showing its close relationship to the left recurrent laryngeal nerve. (b) Coarctation of the aorta.

Aortic coarctation (Fig. 34b) is thought to be due to an abnormality of the obliterative process that normally occludes the ductus arteriosus. There may be an extensive obstruction of the aorta from the left subclavian artery to the ductus, which is widely patent and maintains the circulation to the lower parts of the body; often, there are multiple other defects and frequently infants so afflicted die at an early age. More commonly, there is a short segment involved in the region of the ligamentum arteriosum or still patent ductus. In these cases, circulation to the lower limbs is maintained via collateral arteries around the scapula anastomosing with the intercostal arteries and via the link-up between the superior epigastric artery (a terminal branch of the internal thoracic artery) and the inferior epigastric – artery, a branch of the external iliac artery, which takes place in the posterior rectus sheath.

Clinically, this circulation may be manifest by enlarged vessels being palpable around the scapular margins; radiologically, dilatation of the engorged intercostal arteries results in notching of the inferior borders of the ribs.

Abnormal development of the primitive aortic arches may result in the aortic arch being on the right or actually being double. An abnormal right subclavian artery may arise from the dorsal aorta and pass behind the oesophagus – a rare cause of difficulty in swallowing (*dysphagia lusoria*).

Rarely, the division of the truncus into the aorta and pulmonary artery is incomplete, leaving an *aorta–pulmonary window*, the most unusual congenital fistula between the two sides of the heart.

The superior mediastinum

This is bounded in front by the manubrium sterni and behind by the upper four thoracic vertebrae (T1 to T4 inclusive) (Fig. 22). Above, it is in direct continuity with the root of the neck, and, below, it is continuous with the three subdivisions of the inferior mediastinum. Its principal contents are: the arch of aorta, the origins of the three great vessels arising from the aortic arch, the left and right brachiocephalic veins, the commencement of the superior vena cava, trachea, oesophagus, thymus, thoracic duct, right and left vagal nerves, left recurrent laryngeal nerve, the right and left phrenic nerves and lymph nodes (Fig. 17).

The *arch of the aorta* has an oblique trajectory and is directed anteroposteriorly from right to the left; its three great branches, the *brachiocephalic artery*, *left common carotid artery* and *left subclavian artery*, ascend to the thoracic outlet, the first two forming a 'V' around the trachea. The *brachiocephalic veins* lie in front of the arteries, the left running obliquely across the superior mediastinum and the right vertically downwards; the two unite behind the right half of the manubrium to form the *superior vena cava*. Posterior to the aortic arch lies the trachea, behind which is the oesophagus lying in front of the thoracic vertebral column.

The thymus (Fig. 17)

Of paramount importance as an immunological organ and crucial to the development, maturation and regulation of cell-mediated immunity is the thymus gland.

The thymus is a soft, bi-lobed organ that lies anteriorly in the superior mediastinum, closely related to the left brachiocephalic vein, and extends downwards into the anterior part of the inferior mediastinum.

The gland is large in the fetus and young child, and at that age may extend upwards into the neck even as far as the lower pole of the thyroid gland. From about the time of adolescence the thymus begins to shrink and by adulthood the gland appears as fibro-fatty nodules. Moreover, although it is pink and glandular in the fetus and child, it becomes increasingly infiltrated with fat in later years; in adults, it is distinguishable from surrounding fat only by its distinct capsule.

The oesophagus

The oesophagus, which is 25 cm (10 in) long, extends from the level of the lower border of the cricoid cartilage at the level of the 6th cervical vertebra to the cardiac orifice of the stomach (Fig. 35).

Course and relations

Cervical

In the neck it commences in the median plane and deviates slightly to the left as it approaches the thoracic inlet. The trachea and the thyroid gland are its immediate anterior relations, the 6th and 7th cervical vertebrae and the prevertebral muscles covered by prevertebral fascia are behind it, and on either side it is related to the common carotid arteries and the recurrent laryngeal nerves. On the left side it is also related to the subclavian artery and the terminal part of the thoracic duct (Fig. 16).

Thoracic

The thoracic part traverses first the superior and then the posterior mediastinum. From being somewhat over to the left, it returns to the midline at T5 then passes downwards, forwards and to the left to reach the oesophageal opening in the diaphragm (T10). For convenience, the relations of this part are given in sequence from above downwards.

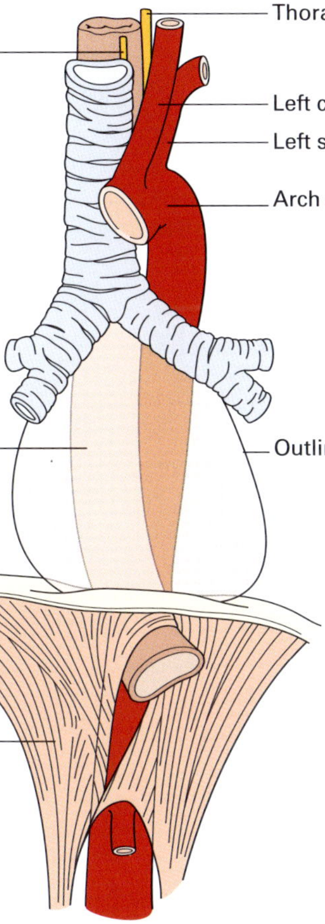

Fig. 35 The oesophagus and its relations.

Anteriorly (Fig. 35), it is crossed by the trachea, the left bronchus (which constricts it), the pericardium (separating it from the left atrium) and the diaphragm.

Posteriorly lie the thoracic vertebrae, the thoracic duct, the azygos vein and its tributaries and, near the diaphragm, the descending aorta.

On the left side (see Fig. 38) it is related to the left subclavian artery, the terminal part of the aortic arch, the left recurrent laryngeal nerve, the thoracic duct and the left pleura. In the posterior mediastinum it relates to the descending thoracic aorta before this passes posteriorly to the oesophagus above the diaphragm.

On the right side (see Fig. 39) there is the pleura and the azygos vein. Below the root of the lung the vagi form a plexus on the oesophagus, the left vagus lying anteriorly, the right posteriorly.

In the abdomen, passing forwards through the opening in the right crus of the diaphragm, the oesophagus comes to lie in the oesophageal groove on the posterior surface of the left lobe of the liver, covered by peritoneum on its anterior and left aspects. Behind it is the left crus of the diaphragm. It has a short course of approximately 3 cm (1.2 in) before it enters the stomach at the *cardiac orifice* (see Fig. 49).

Structure

The oesophagus is made of:

1 an outer connective tissue sheath of areolar tissue;
2 a muscular layer of outer longitudinal and inner circular fibres that are striated in the upper two-thirds and smooth in the lower one-third;
3 a submucous layer containing mucous glands;
4 a mucosa of stratified squamous epithelium passing abruptly into the columnar epithelium of the stomach.

Lower oesophageal sphincter mechanism

There is no anatomical sphincter of thickened circular muscle at the lower end of the human oesophagus, although such a sphincter can be demonstrated in a number of animal species. Nevertheless, a sphincter mechanism clearly exists at the lower end of the oesophagus, as evidenced by the fact that lying down or bending over does not result in gastric contents being refluxed back into the oesophagus. The 'sphincter' can, however, relax to allow vomiting and belching. The lower oesophageal sphincter mechanism is a complex affair, comprising:

1 a physiological high-pressure zone at the terminal few centimetres of the oesophagus, which can be demonstrated on oesophageal manometry;
2 a pinch-cock effect of the crural sling of the diaphragm (Fig. 10);
3 the positive intra-abdominal pressure acting on the short abdominal segment of the oesophagus;
4 the valve-like effect of the obliquity of the oesophago-gastric angle (see Fig. 49);
5 the plug-like action of a rosette of mucosal folds (seen on oesophago-gastroscopy) at the cardiac orifice.

Failure of this sphincter mechanism may result in *reflux oesophagitis*. The patient complains of 'heartburn', the feeling of an unpleasant burning pain behind the sternum, on bending over or lying down, often accompanied by reflux of gastric contents into the mouth. This is often associated with the presence of a sliding hiatus hernia (see page 18), but may occur even if no such hernia can be demonstrated.

Blood supply, lymphatic drainage and radiology of the oesophagus

Blood supply is from the inferior thyroid artery, branches of the descending thoracic aorta and the left gastric artery. The veins from the cervical part drain into the inferior thyroid veins, from the thoracic portion into the azygos vein and from the abdominal portion partly into the azygos and partly into the left gastric veins. This is by far the most important of the portocaval anastomoses (see page 92).

The *lymphatic drainage* is from a peri-oesophageal lymph plexus into the posterior mediastinal nodes, which drain both into the supraclavicular nodes and into nodes around the left gastric vessels. It is not uncommon to be able to palpate hard, fixed supraclavicular nodes in patients with advanced oesophageal cancer.

Radiographically, the oesophagus may be studied on films taken after a barium swallow. These show the oesophagus lying in the retrocardiac space just in front of the vertebral column. Anteriorly, the normal oesophagus is indented from above downwards by the three most important structures that cross it – the arch of the aorta, the left bronchus and the left atrium.

CLINICAL FEATURES

1 For oesophagoscopy, measurements are made from the upper incisor teeth; the three important levels 17 cm (7 in), 28 cm (11 in) and 43 cm (17 in) corresponding to the commencement of the oesophagus, the point at which it is crossed by the left bronchus and the point where it goes through the oesophageal hiatus of the diaphragm, respectively.

2 The first and last of these three points also indicate the two narrowest parts of the oesophagus: the sites at which, as might be expected, swallowed foreign bodies are most likely to become obstructed and strictures are most likely to occur after swallowing corrosive fluids.

3 The anastomosis between the azygos (systemic) and left gastric (portal) venous tributaries in the oesophageal veins is of great importance. In portal hypertension these veins distend into large collateral channels, *oesophageal varices*, which may then rupture with severe haemorrhage (probably as a result of peptic ulceration of the overlying mucosa).

4 In days prior to the advent of modern imaging techniques (CT and MRI scans) use was made of the close relationship between the oesophagus and the left atrium in determining the degree of left atrial enlargement in mitral stenosis; a barium swallow would show marked backward displacement of the oesophagus caused by the dilated atrium.

5 The oesophagus in the posterior mediastinum is best approached surgically from the right side, as the only major structure crossing the field is the vena azygos. The very lower end of the intrathoracic oesophagus, however, is approached from the left side (as, for example, in surgery for achalasia cardia).

Development of the oesophagus

The oesophagus develops from the distal part of the primitive foregut. From the floor of the foregut also differentiate the larynx and trachea, first as a groove (the laryngotracheal groove) which then converts into a tube, a bud on each side of which develops and ramifies into the lung.

This close relationship between the origins of the oesophagus and trachea accounts for the relatively common malformation in which the upper part of the oesophagus ends blindly while the lower part opens into the lower trachea at the level of T4 (*oesophageal atresia with tracheo-oesophageal fistula*). Less commonly, the upper part of the oesophagus opens into the trachea, or oesophageal atresia occurs without concomitant fistula into the trachea. Rarely, there is a tracheo-oesophageal fistula without atresia (Fig. 36).

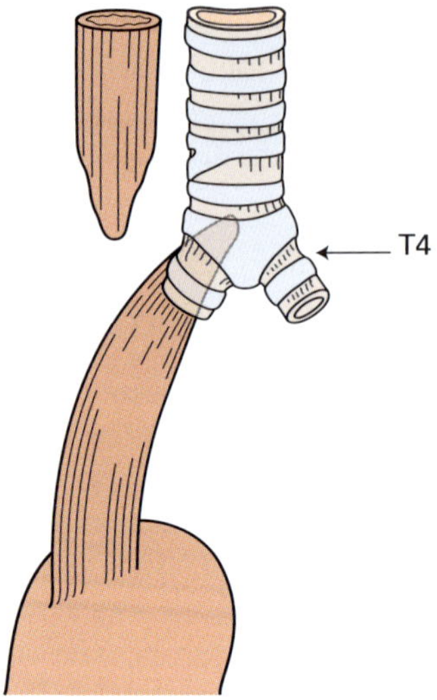

Fig. 36 The usual form of oesophageal stenosis. The upper oesophagus ends blindly; the lower oesophagus communicates with the trachea at the level of the 4th thoracic vertebra.

The thoracic duct (Figs 37, 212)

The *cisterna chyli* lies between the abdominal aorta and right crus of the diaphragm. It drains lymphatics from the abdomen and the lower limbs, then passes upwards through the aortic opening to become the *thoracic duct*. This ascends behind the oesophagus, inclines to the left of the oesophagus at the level of T5, then runs upwards behind the carotid sheath, descends over the subclavian artery and drains into the commencement of the left brachiocephalic vein (see Fig. 212).

The left *jugular*, *subclavian* and *mediastinal lymph trunks*, draining the left side of the head and neck, upper limb and thorax, respectively, usually join the thoracic duct, although they may open directly into the adjacent large veins at the root of the neck.

The thoracic duct thus usually drains the whole lymphatic field below the diaphragm and the left half of the lymphatics above it.

On the right side, the right subclavian, jugular and mediastinal trunks may open independently into the great veins. Usually the subclavian and jugular trunks first join into a *right lymphatic duct*; this may be joined by the mediastinal trunk so that all three then have a common opening into the origin of the right brachiocephalic vein.

CLINICAL FEATURES

1 The lymphatics may become blocked by infection and fibrosis due to *Microfilaria bancrofti*. This usually results in lymphoedema of the legs and scrotum, but occasional involvement of the main channels of the trunk and thorax is followed by chylous ascites, chyluria and chylous pleural effusion.
2 The thoracic duct may be damaged during block dissection of the neck. If noticed at operation, the injured duct should be ligated; lymph then finds its way into the venous system by anastomosing channels. If the accident is missed, there follows an unpleasant chylous fistula in the neck.

3 Tears of the thoracic duct have also been reported as a complication of fractures of the thoracic vertebrae to which, in its lower part, the duct is closely related. It may also be damaged in mobilizing the oesophagus at oesophagectomy. Such injuries are followed by a chylothorax.

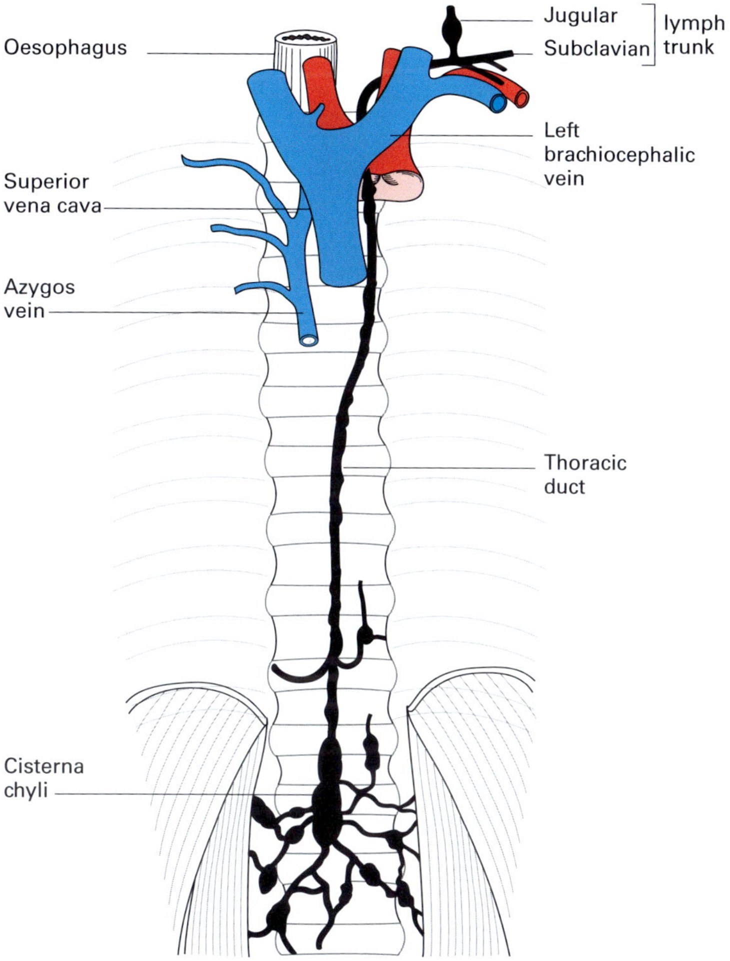

Fig. 37 The course of the thoracic duct.

The thoracic sympathetic trunk (Fig. 38a,b)

The ganglionated thoracic sympathetic chain lies lateral to the vertebral bodies, extrapleurally, in much the same way as does the descending thoracic aorta. It may therefore be regarded as a content of the posterior mediastinum.

As the downward continuation of the cervical sympathetic chain, the ganglionated thoracic sympathetic chain crosses:

- the neck of the first rib;
- the heads of the 2nd–10th ribs;
- the bodies of the 11th and 12th thoracic vertebrae.

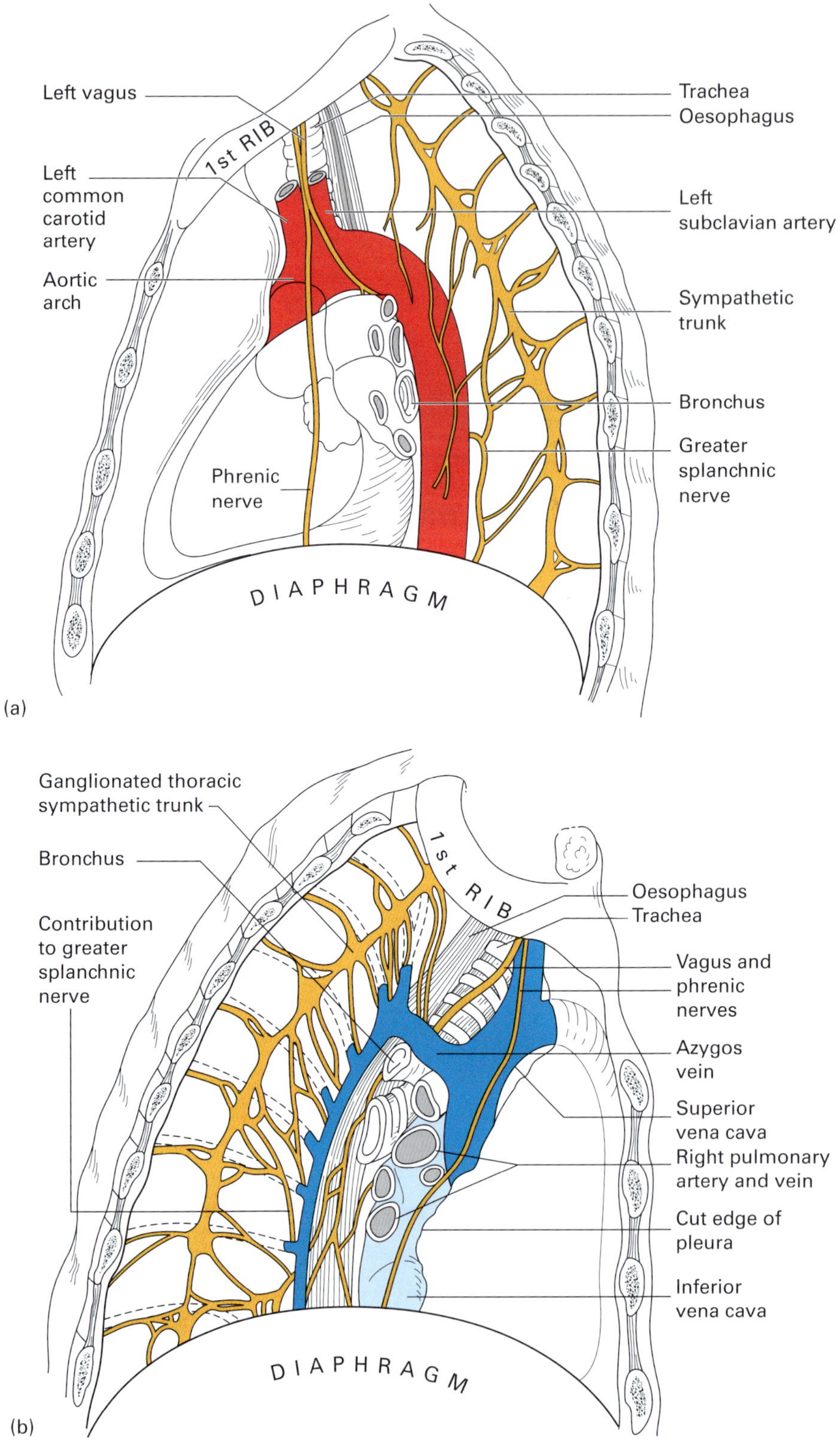

Fig. 38 (a) The left thoracic sympathetic trunk with a display of the left mediastinum. (b) The right thoracic sympathetic trunk with a display of the right mediastinum.

It then passes behind the medial arcuate ligament of the diaphragm to continue as the lumbar sympathetic trunk.

The thoracic chain bears a ganglion for each spinal nerve; the first frequently joins the inferior cervical ganglion to form the *stellate ganglion*. Each ganglion receives a white ramus communicans containing preganglionic fibres from its corresponding spinal nerve and donates back a grey ramus, bearing postganglionic fibres.

Branches

1 Sympathetic fibres are distributed to the skin with each of the thoracic spinal nerves.
2 Postganglionic fibres from T1–T5 are distributed to the thoracic viscera – the heart and great vessels, the lungs and the oesophagus.
3 Mainly preganglionic fibres from T5–T12 form the *splanchnic nerves*, which pierce the crura of the diaphragm and pass to the coeliac, superior mesenteric, inferior mesenteric and renal ganglia, from which they are relayed as postganglionic fibres to the abdominal viscera. These splanchnic nerves are classically divided into:
   - *greater splanchnic* (T5–T10);
   - *lesser splanchnic* (T10–T11);
   - *least splanchnic* (T12).

However, although these fibres do indeed arise from the T5–T12 ganglia, their exact arrangement is very variable.

The splanchnic nerves lie medial to the sympathetic trunk on the bodies of the thoracic vertebrae and are quite easily visible through the parietal pleura. (For their important distribution, see page 422.)

CLINICAL FEATURES

A high spinal anaesthetic will produce temporary hypotension by paralysing the sympathetic (vasoconstrictor) preganglionic outflow from spinal segment T5 downwards, passing to the abdominal viscera.

On the examination of a chest radiograph

The following features should be examined in every radiograph of the chest.

'Centering' and density of film

The sternal ends of the two clavicles should be equidistant from the shadow of the vertebral spines. The assessment of the density of the film can be learned only by experience, but in a 'normal' film the bony cage should be clearly outlined and the larger vessels in the lung fields clearly visible.

General shape

Any abnormalities in the general form of the thorax (scoliosis, kyphosis and the barrel chest of emphysema, for example) should always be noted before other abnormalities are described.

Bony cage

The thoracic vertebrae should be examined first, then each of the ribs in turn (counting conveniently from their posterior ends and comparing each one with its fellow of the opposite side) and finally clavicles and scapulae. Unless this procedure is carried out systematically, important diagnostic clues (e.g. the presence of a cervical rib, or notching of the ribs by enlarged anastomotic vessels) are liable to be missed.

The domes of the diaphragm

These should be examined for height and symmetry and the nature of the cardiophrenic and costophrenic angles observed.

The mediastinum

The outline of the mediastinum should be traced systematically. Special note should be made of the size of the heart, of mediastinal shift and of the vessels and nodes at the hilum of the lung.

Lung fields

Again, systematic examination of the lung fields visible in each intercostal space is necessary if slight differences between the two sides are not to be overlooked.

Abnormalities

When this scheme has been carefully followed, any abnormalities in the bony cage, the mediastinum or lung fields should now be apparent. They should then be defined anatomically as accurately as possible and checked, where necessary, by reference to a film taken from a different angle.

Radiographic appearance of the heart

For the appearance of the heart as seen at fluoroscopy, reference should be made to a standard work in radiology or cardiology. In the present account, only the more important features of the heart and great vessels that can be seen in standard posteroanterior views of the chest and CT and MR images will be described.

The heart and great vessels in anteroposterior radiographs (Fig. 39)

The greater part of the 'mediastinal shadow' in an anteroposterior film of the chest is formed by the heart and great vessels. These should be examined as follows.

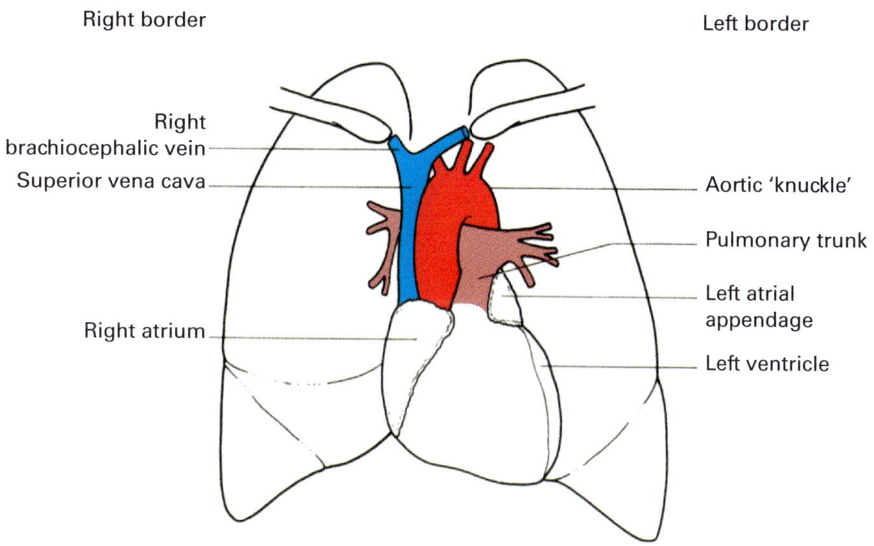

Fig. 39 A tracing of a chest radiograph to show the composition of the right and left borders of the mediastinal shadow.

Size and shape of the heart

Normally the transverse diameter should not exceed half the total width of the chest, but since it varies widely with bodily build and the position of the heart, these factors must also be assessed. The *shape* of the cardiac shadow also varies a good deal with the position of the heart, being long and narrow in a vertically disposed heart and broad and rounded in the so-called horizontal heart.

The cardiac outline

Each 'border' of the cardiac shadow should be examined in turn. The *right border* of the mediastinal shadow is formed from above downwards by the right brachiocephalic vein, the superior vena cava and the right atrium. Immediately above the heart, the *left border* of the mediastinal shadow presents a well-marked projection, the *aortic knuckle*, which represents the arch of the aorta seen 'end-on'. Beneath this there are, successively, the shadows due to the pulmonary trunk (or the infundibulum of the right ventricle), the auricle of the left atrium (left atrial appendage) and the left ventricle. The shadow of the inferior border of the heart blends centrally with that of the diaphragm, but on either side the two shadows are separated by the well-defined cardiophrenic angles.

Part 2
The Abdomen and Pelvis

Surface anatomy and surface markings

Clinical examination of the patient's abdomen requires not only skill and gentleness but also detailed knowledge of its anatomy.

Look at your own abdomen in the mirror, with your muscles tensed, or examine the abdomen of a moderately well-toned patient. The midline *linea alba* is evident, and, even more obvious, is the linea semilunaris on either side (see Fig. 41). The tendinous intersections of the rectus abdominis at the level of the umbilicus and halfway between the umbilicus and xiphoid are responsible for the six-pack appearance of the tensed rectus muscles in a well-toned subject.

Identify these landmarks on yourself or on a patient (Fig. 40).

The *xiphoid* and the *costal margin. The latter* extends from the 7th costal cartilage at the xiphoid to the tip of the 12th rib (although the latter is often difficult to feel); this margin bears a distinct step, which is the tip of the 9th costal cartilage.

The *iliac crest* ends in front at the *anterior superior iliac spine* from which the *inguinal ligament* (*Poupart's ligament*) passes downwards and medially to the *pubic tubercle*. Identify this tubercle by direct palpation and also by running the fingers along the adductor longus tendon (tensed by flexing, abducting and externally rotating the thigh) to its origin just inferior to the pubic tubercle.

In the male feel the firm *vas deferens* between the finger and thumb as it lies within the spermatic cord at the scrotal neck. Trace the vas upwards and note that it passes medial to the pubic tubercle and thence through the *external inguinal ring*, which can be felt by invaginating the scrotal skin with the fingertip.

Vertebral levels (Fig. 40a)

- T9 – *the xiphoid*.
- L1 – *the transpyloric plane of Addison*, as originally described, is a horizontal or transverse plane that lies halfway between the suprasternal notch and the upper edge of the pubic symphysis. As an approximate alternative, the transpyloric plane may also be defined as a horizontal plane that lies a hand's breadth below the xiphoid. This plane passes through the pylorus, the pancreatic neck, the duodenojejunal flexure, the fundus of the gall bladder, the tip of the 9th costal cartilage (felt as a distinct 'step' on the costal margin) and the hila of the kidneys. It also corresponds (in the adult) to the level of termination of the spinal cord.
- L3 – the *subcostal plane* is a horizontal plane at the level of the lowest part of the costal margin, which is the inferior margin of the 10th rib. The origin of the inferior mesenteric artery lies at this level.
- L4 – the *supracristal plane (supracristal line)* is a horizontal plane at the level of the summits of the iliac crests. This corresponds to the level of the bifurcation of the abdominal aorta. It is also a useful landmark in determining the level at which to introduce a needle for a lumbar puncture, since it is well below the level of the termination of the spinal cord, which is approximately at L1 (see page 381 and Fig. 245).
- The *umbilicus* is an inconstant landmark. In an adult of moderate build, the umbilicus lies at the junction of the L3 and L4 vertebrae. It is lower in the infant and, in an individual in whom the anterior abdominal wall is pendulous. It is higher in late pregnancy.

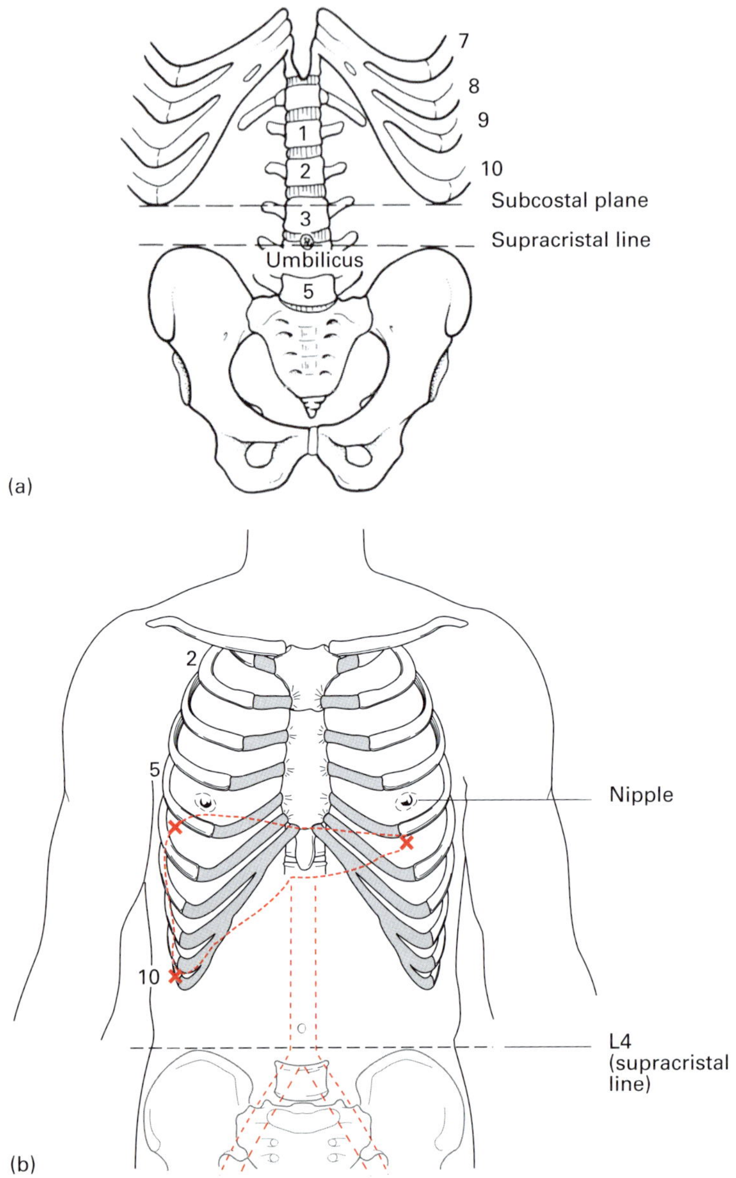

Xs mark the outline of the liver, which reaches from the right 5th intercostal space in the midaxillary line to the left 5th intercostal space in the midclavicular line, and from the latter to the lower margin of the right 10th rib

The aorta bifurcates at L4, which is in line with the summits of the iliac crests

Fig. 40 (a) Boundaries, bony landmarks and vertebral levels of the abdomen. (b) The surface markings of the liver and aorta.

Surface markings of individual viscera (Fig. 40b)

The abdominal viscera are inconstant in their position, but the surface markings of the following structures are of clinical value.

Liver

Mark the position of the right 10th rib in the midaxillary line (the costal border); mark the 5th right intercostal space in the midaxillary line; mark the left 5th intercostal space in the midclavicular line. Join these three points and you have outlined the position of the normal liver.

This is not palpable in the normal subject – what is often mistaken for the liver edge, especially in a muscular subject, is the rolled up anterior abdominal muscles gathered up by the examining fingers. Confirm this by percussion – the 'liver' will be resonant to percussion!

Spleen

This lies under cover of the left 9th, 10th and 11th ribs posteriorly, commencing 5 cm (2 in) from the posterior midline. It is approximately the size of the subject's cupped hand. The spleen must be enlarged to at least three times its normal size to be clinically palpable – and so, a spleen that is 'only just palpable' below the left costal margin is in fact a considerably enlarged one!

Gall bladder

The fundus of the gall bladder corresponds to the point where the lateral border of the right rectus abdominis cuts the costal margin; this is at the tip of the 9th right costal cartilage, felt as a distinct 'step' when the fingers are run along the costal margin.

Pancreas

The transpyloric plane defines the level of the neck of the pancreas, which overlies the vertebral column. From this landmark, the head can be imagined passing slightly downwards and to the right and the body and tail passing slightly upwards and to the left.

Aorta

In an individual of thin build who is not overly muscular, the pulsations of the abdominal aorta can be felt by firm downward palpation of the abdomen in the midline. Because of the lumbar lordosis, the lower part of the aorta is pushed forwards and is therefore more readily felt than its upper part. These pulsations terminate at the level of the aortic bifurcation at L4, which is demarcated by a line joining the summits of the right and left iliac crests – *the supracristal line* (Fig. 40). A pulsatile swelling detected below this level may be an iliac, but cannot be an aortic, aneurysm. (Consider also the possibility of transmitted pulsations through a pelvic mass.)

Kidneys

The lower pole of the normal right kidney may sometimes be felt in the thin subject on deep inspiration. Anteriorly, the hilum of the kidney lies in the transpyloric plane four or so finger-breadths from the midline. Posteriorly, the upper pole of the kidney lies deep to the 12th rib. The right kidney normally extends approximately 2.5 cm (1 in) lower than the left. Using these landmarks, the outlines of the kidneys can be projected onto either the anterior or posterior aspects of the abdomen.

The anterior abdominal wall

The outline of the anterior abdominal wall is approximately hexagonal. It is bounded superiorly by the arched costal margin, with the xiphoid at the summit of the arch. The lateral boundary on either side is arbitrarily the midaxillary line between the costal margin and the summit of the iliac crest. Inferiorly, on each side, the anterior abdominal wall is bounded in continuity by the anterior half of the iliac crest, inguinal ligament, pubic crest and pubic symphysis.

The anterior abdominal wall is a many-layered structure (Figs 41 and 42). From the surface inwards, the successive layers are skin, superficial fascia, a musculo-aponeurotic plane (comprising the rectus abdominis, anteriorly, and the obliques and transversus, anterolaterally), transversalis fascia, extraperitoneal adipose layer and parietal peritoneum.

Fasciae of the anterior abdominal wall

There is no deep fascia in the anterior abdominal wall, only the superficial fascia. (If there were, we would presumably be unable to take a deep breath or enjoy a large meal!) The superficial fascia of the anterior abdominal wall comprises two distinct layers: (1) An outer adipose layer immediately subjacent to the dermis and similar to superficial fascia elsewhere in the body. This layer is also sometimes referred to as *Camper's fascia*. (2) An inner (deeper) fibroelastic layer termed *Scarpa's fascia*. Scarpa's fascia is also known as the membranous layer of superficial fascia. Scarpa's fascia is more prominent and better defined in the lower half of the anterior abdominal wall. Also, it is more prominent in children (particularly infants) than in adults.

Above the level of the umbilicus, Scarpa's fascia is thinner and less prominent than in the lower abdomen. Nevertheless, it is a distinct layer that crosses superficial to the costal margin to become continuous with the retromammary fascia of the anterior chest wall. Traced laterally, Scarpa's fascia fades out beyond the midaxillary line. Inferiorly, Scarpa's fascia crosses superficial to the inguinal ligament and blends with the deep fascia of the upper thigh along the flexion crease, about 1–2 cm distal to the inguinal ligament. Below the level of the pubic symphysis, in the male, Scarpa's fascia is prolonged quite distinctly into the scrotum and around the penile shaft. This prolongation of Scarpa's fascia into the perineum is known as the *superficial perineal fascia* or *Colles' fascia*. The superficial perineal fascia is attached, posteriorly, to the perineal body and posterior margin of the perineal membrane and, laterally, to the everted ischiopubic

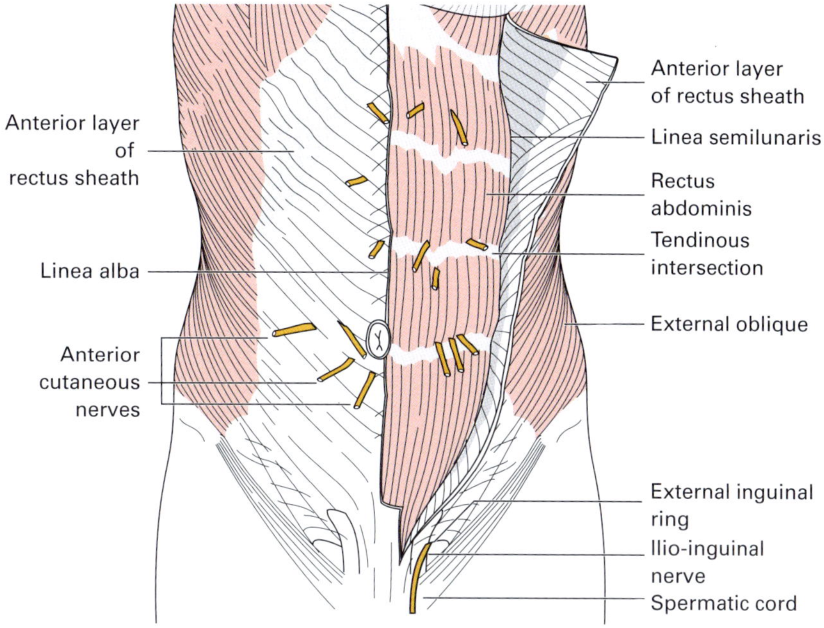

Fig. 41 Anterior abdominal wall. The anterior rectus sheath on the left side has been reflected laterally.

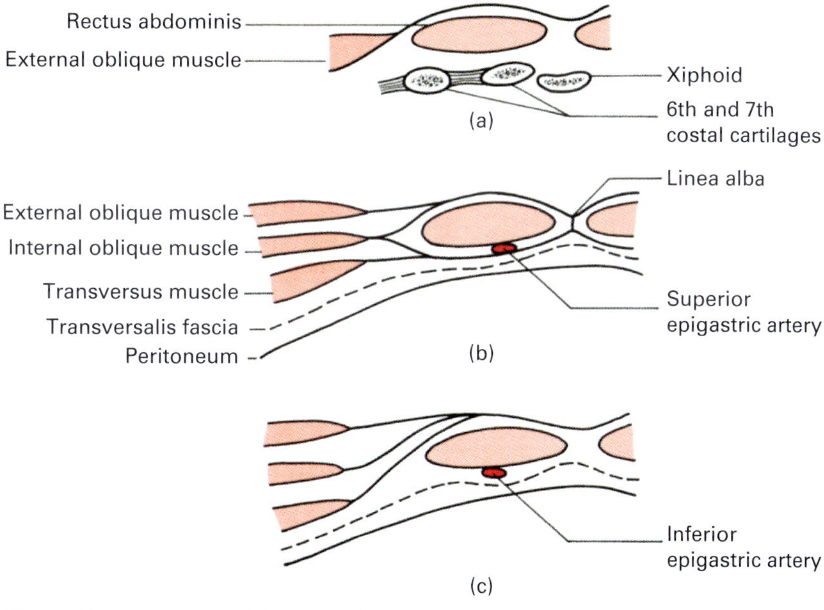

Fig. 42 The composition of the rectus sheath shown in transverse section (a) above the costal margin, (b) above the arcuate line and (c) below the arcuate line.

ramus on either side. It is because of these attachments that a rupture of the urethral bulb may be followed by extravasation of blood and urine into the scrotum, perineum and around the penile shaft and then into the lower abdomen *deep* to Scarpa's fascia. However, the extravasation will not extend into the thigh, owing to the attachment of Scarpa's fascia to the deep fascia of the upper thigh.

A similar but less distinct and less readily demonstrable extension of Scarpa's fascia into the perineum occurs in the female. As in the male, this extension is known as superficial perineal fascia.

The fatty layer (of Camper) is continuous with the superficial fat of the rest of the body.

Nerve supply

The segmental nerve supply of the anterior abdominal wall muscles and the overlying skin is derived from the spinal nerves T7–L1 (inclusive). This distribution can be mapped out approximately if it is remembered that the umbilicus is supplied by T10 and the groin and scrotum by L1 (via the ilio-inguinal and iliohypogastric nerves – see Fig. 137).

Before considering the musculo-aponeurotic plane of the anterior abdominal wall in detail, it may be helpful to describe briefly the fascial layers that lie deep to the muscles.

The *transversalis fascia* (fascia transversalis) is the name given to the anterior part of the general endoabdominal fibrous fascial layer that envelops the peritoneum. It is thicker and less expansile in the lower part of the anterior abdominal wall. The transversalis fascia is closely applied to the deep surface of the transversus abdominis muscle but is easily separable from the latter.

Extraperitoneal adipose layer also known as properitoneal fat is immediately deep to transversalis fascia and is interposed between the transversalis fascia and parietal peritoneum. The amount of fat in this layer varies between individuals. The extraperitoneal adipose layer offers little resistance to the spread of infection and, consequently, cellulitis secondary to surgical wound infections may spread rapidly within it.

The muscles of the anterior abdominal wall

These are of considerable practical importance because their anatomical arrangement has a considerable bearing on the manner in which all abdominal incisions and abdominal stomas are fashioned and sited.

The *rectus abdominis* (Fig. 41) arises along a 7.5 cm (3 in) slightly oblique line from the 5th, 6th and 7th costal cartilages and is inserted for a length of 2.5 cm (1 in) into the crest of the pubis. The rectus abdominis muscle features three transverse tendinous intersections; one at the level of the tip of the xiphoid, one at the level of the umbilicus and one halfway between the two.

These intersections occupy only the anterior half or so of the thickness of the rectus muscle and therefore are not evident on the posterior aspect of the muscle. Furthermore these intersections are firmly fused with the anterior wall of the rectus sheath. Posteriorly, the rectus muscle is completely free of the posterior layer of the rectus sheath. At each intersection, vessels from the superior epigastric artery and vein pierce the rectus.

The sheath which encloses the rectus muscle, is formed, to a large extent, by the aponeurotic expansions of the lateral abdominal muscles (Fig. 42):

(a) Above the costal margin, the anterior wall of the rectus sheath is made up of the external oblique aponeurosis alone; posteriorly the rectus muscle lies directly on the costal cartilages.

(b) From the costal margin to a point halfway between the umbilicus and pubic symphysis, the external oblique and the anterior lamina of the internal oblique aponeurosis form the anterior wall of the rectus sheath. The posterior wall of the sheath is formed by the blending of the posterior lamina of the split internal oblique aponeurosis and the aponeurosis of transversus abdominis.

(c) Below a point halfway between the umbilicus and pubic symphysis all three aponeuroses pass in front of the rectus so that the anterior sheath, below this level, is made up of the aponeuroses of the external oblique, internal oblique and transversus abdominis muscles (in that order from outside in) blended together. The posterior wall of the rectus sheath below this level is made up of the transversalis fascia alone (which in this situation is considerably thicker than elsewhere in the abdomen). Deep to the fascia transversalis is the extraperitoneal fat and the parietal peritoneum.

The posterior junction between (b) and (c) is marked by the *arcuate line (semicircular fold of Douglas)*, which is the lower border of the posterior aponeurotic part of the rectus sheath. At this point the inferior epigastric artery and vein (from the external iliac vessels) enter the sheath, pass upwards and within the substance of the rectus muscle, anastomose with the superior epigastric vessels, which are terminal branches of the internal thoracic artery and vein. The right and left rectus sheaths fuse in the midline to form the *linea alba* stretching from the xiphoid to the pubic symphysis.

The lateral muscles of the abdominal wall comprise the external and internal oblique and the transverse muscles. These correspond to the three layers of muscle of the intercostal spaces – external, internal and innermost intercostals. As in the anterior chest wall, the neurovascular plane of the anterior abdominal wall lies between the middle layer and inner layer (i.e. between the internal oblique and transversus abdominis muscle layers).

The attachments of the lateral abdominal wall muscles can be recalled easily if one bears in mind that these muscles fill the space between the costal margin above, the iliac crest below and the lumbar muscles, covered by lumbar fascia, behind. Anteriorly and medially, as already noted, they constitute the rectus sheath and thence blend into the linea alba from xiphoid to pubic symphysis.

The *obliquus externus abdominis* (external oblique) arises from the outer surfaces of the lower eight ribs and fans out into the xiphoid, anterior layer of rectus sheath and linea alba, the pubic crest, pubic tubercle and the anterior half of the iliac crest.

From the pubic tubercle to the anterior superior iliac spine its lower border rolls in on itself to form the *inguinal ligament (of Poupart)*.

The *obliquus internus abdominis* (internal oblique) arises from the lumbar fascia, the anterior two-thirds of the iliac crest and the lateral two-thirds of the inguinal ligament. It is inserted into the lowest six costal cartilages, linea alba and the pubic crest.

The *transversus abdominis* arises from the inner surfaces of the lowest six costal cartilages (interdigitating with the diaphragm), the lumbar fascia, the anterior two-thirds of the iliac crest and the lateral one-third of the inguinal ligament; it is inserted into the linea alba and the pubic crest.

Note that the external oblique passes downwards and forwards, the internal oblique upwards and forwards and the transversus, transversely. Note also that the external oblique has its posterior border free, but the deeper two muscles both arise posteriorly from the lumbar fascia.

The anatomy of abdominal incisions

The choice of incision for 'open' abdominal surgery is dictated by three main considerations: the need for adequate exposure of the peritoneal cavity for the required procedure, the need to preserve the innervation of the rectus abdominis muscle as also that of the anterolateral abdominal muscles and the need to employ an incision that is likely to heal in a timely and satisfactory manner without leaving an unsightly scar.

Midline incision

The midline incision is made through the linea alba. Superiorly, this is a relatively wide fibrous structure, but below the umbilicus it becomes extremely narrow and the surgeon may experience difficulty in finding the exact line of separation between the recti at this level. Being made of fibrous tissue only, it provides an almost bloodless line along which the abdomen can be opened rapidly and, if necessary, from one end to the other.

Paramedian incision

The paramedian incision is a vertical incision placed 2.5 cm (1 in) to 4 cm (1.5 in) lateral, and parallel, to the midline; the anterior rectus sheath is opened, the rectus displaced laterally and the posterior sheath, together with peritoneum, then incised. This incision has the advantage that, on suturing the peritoneum, the rectus slips back into place to cover and protect the peritoneal scar.

The adherence of the anterior sheath to the rectus muscle at its tendinous intersections means that the sheath must be dissected off the muscle at each of these sites, and at each of these a segmental vessel requires division. Having done this, the rectus is easily slid laterally from the posterior sheath from which it is quite free. The posterior sheath and the peritoneum form a tough membrane down to halfway between the pubis and umbilicus, but it is much thinner and more fatty below this level where, as we have seen, it loses its aponeurotic component and is made up of only transversalis fascia and peritoneum. The inferior epigastric vessels are seen passing anterior to the arcuate line of Douglas in the posterior sheath and may require division in a low paramedian incision.

The transrectus incision

Occasionally, the rectus muscle is split in the line of the paramedian incision. The rectus receives its nerve supply laterally and the muscle medial to the incision must, in consequence, be deprived of its innervation and undergo atrophy; it is an incision therefore best avoided.

Subcostal incision

The subcostal (Kocher) incision is used on the right side in biliary surgery, and on the left in exposure of the spleen. The skin incision commences at the midline and extends parallel to, and 2.5 cm (1 in) below, the costal margin.

The anterior rectus sheath is opened, the rectus muscle is divided and the posterior sheath with underlying adherent peritoneum incised. The relatively small 8th intercostal nerve branch to the rectus is sacrificed but the larger and more important 9th nerve, in the lateral part of the wound, is preserved. The divided rectus muscle is held by the intersections above and below and retracts very little. It subsequently heals by fibrous tissue. This incision is valuable in the patient with the wide subcostal angle. Where this angle is narrow, the paramedian incision is usually preferred.

A bilateral subcostal incision, with the two limbs of the incision meeting in the midline, is called a *rooftop incision,* and for many surgeons it is the incision of choice for the D-2 gastrectomy procedure.

The muscle split or gridiron approach to the appendix

The oblique skin incision centred at *McBurney's point* (two-thirds of the way laterally along the line from the umbilicus to the *right* anterior superior iliac spine) is now less popular than an almost transverse incision in the line of the skin crease forwards from, and 2.5 cm (1 in) above, the anterior superior iliac spine.

The aponeurosis of the external oblique is incised in the line of its fibres (obliquely downwards and medially); the internal oblique and transversus muscles are then split in the line of their fibres and retracted without the need to cut across either of the muscles. When closing the incision, these muscles are easily coapted, without compromising the function of the abdominal wall in the long term.

Transverse and oblique incisions

Incisions cutting through the lateral abdominal muscles do not cause significant damage to their rich motor innervation, and these incisions heal without causing weakness to the abdominal wall. They are useful, for example, in exposing the sigmoid colon or the caecum or, by displacing the peritoneum medially, extraperitoneal structures such as the ureter, sympathetic chain and the external iliac vessels.

Pfannenstiel incision

This is a useful incision in gynaecological surgery, caesarian section and open extraperitoneal exposure of the prostate and urinary bladder in the retropubic space. A curving transverse incision is made approximately 5 cm (2 in) above the pubic symphysis. The anterior rectus sheath is incised on either side in the line of the skin incision and the underlying rectus abdominis muscle, with the small triangular pyramidalis muscle, is dissected off the sheath on either side, retracted laterally and the peritoneum opened in the midline. Care is taken not to damage the bladder; first, by emptying it by catheterization before surgery and, second, by commencing the incision of the peritoneum at the upper end of the exposed peritoneum. The healed incision, lying in a skin crease and just within the line of the pubic hair, is inconspicuous.

Thoraco-abdominal incisions

An upper paramedian or upper oblique abdominal incision can be extended through the 8th or 9th intercostal space, the diaphragm incised and an extensive exposure achieved of both the upper abdomen and thorax. This is used, for example, on the left in removing growths of the upper stomach or lower oesophagus and on the right in resection of the right lobe of the liver.

Paracentesis abdominis

Intraperitoneal fluid collections can be evacuated via a cannula inserted through the abdominal wall. The bladder having been first emptied with a catheter, the cannula is introduced on a trocar either through the midline (where the linea alba is relatively bloodless) or lateral to McBurney's point (where there is no danger of wounding the inferior epigastric vessels). The coils of gut are not in danger in this procedure because they are mobile and are pushed away by the tip of the trocar. These two landmarks are also used for insertion of *ports* for laparoscopic surgery.

The inguinal canal (Fig. 43)

The inguinal canal represents the oblique passage taken through the lower abdominal wall by the testis and cord (the round ligament of the uterus in the female).

The inguinal canal is approximately 5 cm (2 in) long. It passes downwards and medially from the internal inguinal ring (deep inguinal ring) to the external inguinal ring (superficial inguinal ring) and lies parallel to, and immediately above, the medial half

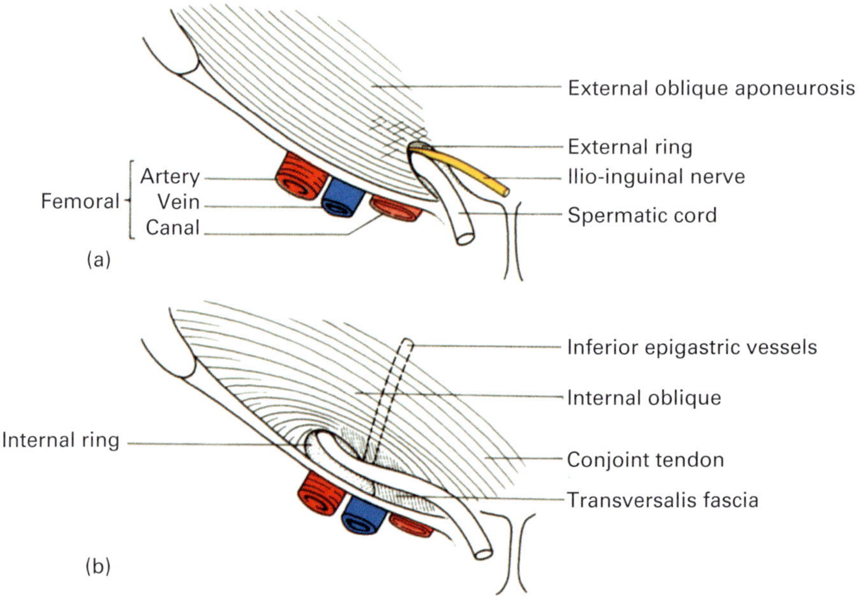

Fig. 43 The right inguinal canal (a) with the external oblique aponeurosis intact and (b) with the external oblique aponeurosis removed.

of the inguinal ligament. The internal inguinal ring is a discrete area of deficiency in the fascia transversalis, while the superficial inguinal ring is a well-defined V-shaped defect in the external oblique aponeurosis.

Boundaries of the inguinal canal

- *Anteriorly* – external oblique aponeurosis with the overlying Scarpa's fascia, subcutaneous fat and skin cover the full length of the canal; the internal oblique, lying deep to the external oblique aponeurosis reinforces the lateral one-third of the anterior wall.
- *Posteriorly* – the *conjoint tendon* forms the posterior wall of the canal medially, the transversalis fascia laterally. (The conjoint tendon represents the fused common insertion of the internal oblique and transversus onto the pubic crest and pectineal line. The transversalis fascia is the name given to the extraperitoneal fascia which, in the lower abdomen, is much thickened.)
- *Above* – arch the lowest fibres of the internal oblique and transversus abdominis.
- *Below* – lies the upper surface of the inrolled inguinal ligament.

The *internal (or deep) inguinal ring* represents the point at which the spermatic cord pushes through the transversalis fascia, dragging from it a covering which forms the *internal spermatic fascia*. This ring is demarcated medially by the inferior epigastric vessels passing upwards and medially from the external iliac artery and vein.

The *external (or superficial) ring* is a V-shaped defect in the external oblique aponeurosis and lies immediately above and medial to the pubic tubercle. As the cord traverses this opening, it carries the *external spermatic fascia* from the ring's margins.

In the male, the inguinal canal transmits the spermatic cord and the ilio-inguinal nerve. In the female, the canal is a much narrower channel and transmits only the round ligament of the uterus (which represents the gubernaculum testis of the male embryo, see page 126) together with the ilio-inguinal nerve. Nevertheless the round ligament of the uterus carries the same three fascial coverings that the spermatic cord does.

The *spermatic cord* comprises (Fig. 44):

- *three layers of fascia* – the *external spermatic fascia*, from the external oblique aponeurosis; the *cremasteric fascia*, from the internal oblique muscle (containing muscle fibres termed the *cremaster muscle*); the *internal spermatic fascia*, from the transversalis fascia;
- *three arteries* – the testicular artery (from the aorta); the cremasteric artery (from the inferior epigastric artery); the artery of the vas (from the inferior vesical artery);
- *three veins* – the pampiniform plexus of veins (draining the right testis into the inferior vena cava (IVC) and the left into the left renal vein), and the cremasteric vein and vein of the vas, which accompany their corresponding arteries;
- *three nerves* – the nerve to the cremaster muscle (from the genitofemoral nerve); sympathetic fibres from the T10 and T11 spinal segments; the ilio-inguinal nerve (strictly, *on* and not *in* the cord);
- *three other structures* – the vas deferens; lymphatics of the testis, which pass to the para-aortic lymph nodes; and the obliterated remains of the processus vaginalis.

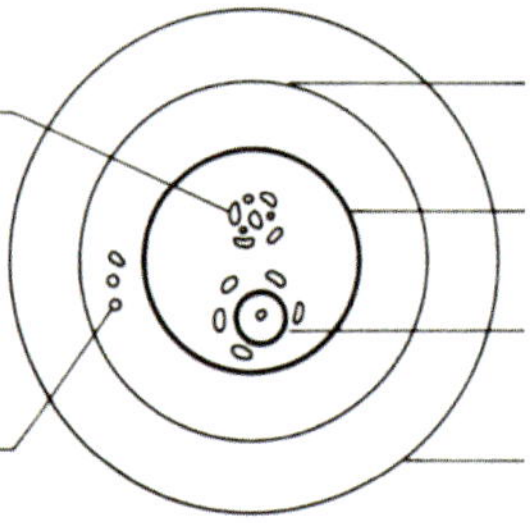

Fig. 44 Scheme of the spermatic cord and its contents, in transverse section.

CLINICAL FEATURES

An *indirect inguinal hernia* passes through the internal ring, along the canal and then, if large enough, emerges through the external ring and, in the male, descends into the scrotum. If reducible, such a hernia can be completely controlled by pressure with the fingertip over the internal ring, which lies 1.2 cm (0.5 in) above the mid-point of the inguinal ligament (a point halfway between the anterior superior iliac spine and the pubic tubercle).

If the hernia protrudes through the external ring, it can be felt to lie above and medial to the pubic tubercle and is thus differentiated from a femoral hernia emerging from the femoral canal, which lies below and lateral to this landmark (see Fig. 174).

A *direct inguinal hernia* pushes its way directly forwards through the posterior wall of the inguinal canal. Since it lies medial to the internal ring, it is not controlled by digital pressure applied immediately above the femoral pulse. Occasionally, a direct hernia becomes large enough to push its way through the external ring and then into the neck of the scrotum. This is so unusual that one can usually assume that a scrotal hernia is an indirect hernia.

The only certain way of determining the issue is at operation; the inferior epigastric vessels lie along the medial edge of the internal ring; therefore an indirect hernia sac will pass lateral and a direct hernia medial to these vessels. Quite often both a direct and an indirect hernia coexist; they bulge through on each side of the inferior epigastric vessels like the legs of a pair of pantaloons; hence the term *pantaloon hernia*!

Peritoneal cavity

The abdomen is the largest part of the trunk. It comprises the abdomen proper, superiorly, and the pelvis, inferiorly. The abdomen and pelvis contain a single cavity, the *abdomino-pelvic cavity* whose walls are lined on the inside with the parietal layer of peritoneum. The upper limit of the abdomino-pelvic cavity is the inferior surface of the dome-shaped diaphragm, while the inferior limit is the pelvic floor, a smaller and thinner muscular sheet than the diaphragm. The abdominal cavity is continuous with the pelvic cavity through the *pelvic brim*. On account of the pronounced forward tilt of the articulated bony pelvis, the plane of the pelvic brim lies obliquely downwards and forwards.

The epithelial lining of the primitive coelomic cavity of the embryo becomes the thoracic pleura and the abdominal peritoneum. Each is invaginated by ingrowing viscera that thus come to be covered by a serous membrane and to be packed snugly into a serous-lined cavity. The serous membrane applied to the surface of the viscus is the visceral layer, while the serous membrane lining the inner surface of the body wall is the parietal layer. The two are, of course, continuous with each other.

In the male, the peritoneal cavity is completely closed, but in the female, it is perforated by the lateral ends of the uterine tubes, which constitute a possible pathway of infection from the exterior into the peritoneal cavity.

To revise the complicated attachments of the peritoneum, it is best to start at one point and trace this membrane in an imaginary round-trip of the abdominal cavity, aided by Figs 45 and 46. A convenient point of departure is the parietal peritoneum of the anterior abdominal wall below the umbilicus. At this level the membrane is smooth apart from the shallow ridges formed by the median umbilical fold (the obliterated fetal urachus passing from the apex of the urinary bladder to the umbilicus), the bilateral, medial umbilical folds (the obliterated umbilical arteries passing to the umbilicus from the internal iliac arteries) and the bilateral, lateral umbilical folds (the peritoneum covering the inferior epigastric vessels).

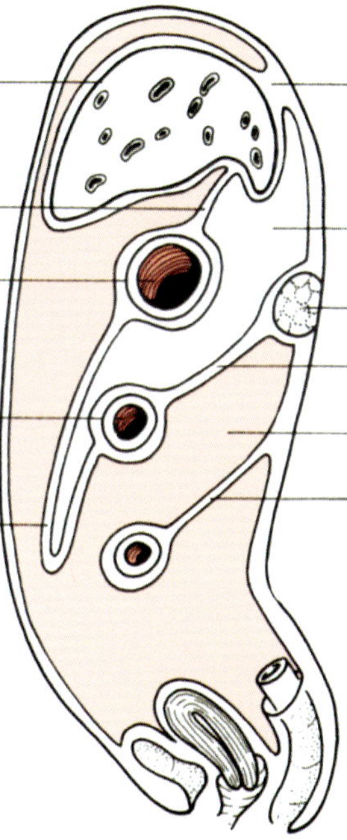

Fig. 45 The peritoneal cavity in longitudinal (sagittal) section (female).

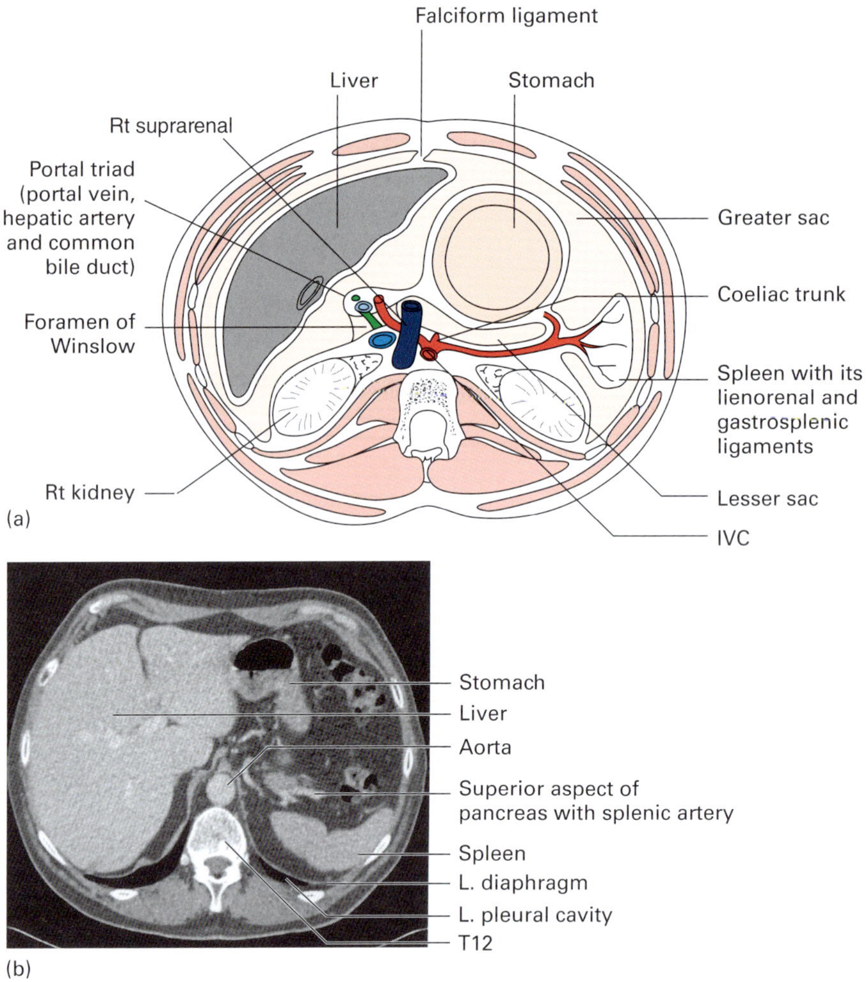

Fig. 46 (a) The peritoneal cavity in transverse section (through the foramen of Winslow), seen from below. (b) The corresponding CT scan through T12 (Dr Sheila Rankin).

A cicatrix can usually be felt and seen at the posterior aspect of the umbilicus, and from this the *falciform ligament* sweeps upwards and slightly to the right of the midline to the liver. In the free border of this ligament lies the *ligamentum teres* (the obliterated fetal left umbilical vein), which passes into the groove between the quadrate lobe and left lobe of the liver (see Fig. 69).

Elsewhere, the peritoneum sweeps over the inferior aspect of the diaphragm, to be reflected onto the liver (leaving a bare area demarcated by the *upper* and *lower coronary ligaments* of the liver) and onto the right margin of the abdominal oesophagus. After enclosing the liver (for further details, see page 99), the peritoneum descends from the porta hepatis as a double-layered sheet, the *lesser omentum*, to the lesser curve of the stomach. Here, the two layers (leaves) of the lesser omentum split to enclose the stomach, before meeting at the greater curve of the stomach to form the *greater omentum*. This loops downwards and then up again to attach to the length of the transverse colon, from which it hangs down like a long and wide apron.

The transverse colon, in turn, is enclosed within this peritoneum, which then passes upwards and backwards as the transverse mesocolon to the posterior abdominal wall, where it is attached along the anterior aspect of the head and body of the pancreas.

At the base of the transverse mesocolon, this double peritoneal sheet divides once again; the upper leaf passes upwards over the posterior abdominal wall to reflect onto the liver (at the bare area), the lower leaf passes over the lower part of the posterior abdominal wall to cover the pelvic viscera and to link up once again with the peritoneum of the anterior wall. This posterior layer is, however, interrupted by its being reflected along an oblique line running from the duodenojejunal flexure, above and to the left, to the ileocaecal junction, below and to the right, to form the *mesentery of the small intestine*.

The mesentery of the small intestine, the lesser and greater omenta and mesocolon all carry the vascular supply and lymphatic drainage of their contained viscera.

The *lesser sac* (Fig. 46) is the extensive pouch lying behind the lesser omentum and the stomach and projecting downwards (although usually this space is obliterated) between the layers of the greater omentum. Its left wall is formed by the peritoneum covering the medial surface of the spleen and completed by the two peritoneal folds extending from the hilar region of the spleen: the *gastrosplenic* and *splenorenal* (*lienorenal*) *ligaments*. The right extremity of the lesser sac opens into the general peritoneal cavity (the greater sac) via the *epiploic foramen* or *foramen of Winslow* (Fig. 47), which is a peritoneal window whose boundaries are as follows:

- *anteriorly* – the free edge of the lesser omentum, containing the common bile duct to the right, the hepatic artery to the left and the portal vein posteriorly;
- *posteriorly* – peritoneum overlying the IVC;
- *inferiorly* – peritoneum covering the first part of the duodenum, over which runs the hepatic artery before this ascends into the anterior wall of the foramen;
- *superiorly* – peritoneum covering the caudate process of the liver.

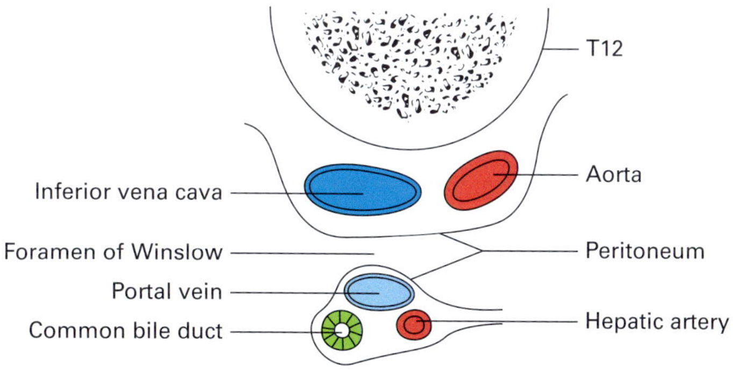

Fig. 47 The foramen of Winslow in transverse section (viewed from above).

CLINICAL FEATURES

1 Occasionally a loop of intestine passes through the foramen of Winslow into the lesser sac and becomes strangulated by the edges of the foramen. Notice that none of these important boundaries can be incised to release the strangulation; the bowel must be decompressed by a needle to allow its reduction.
2 It is important to the surgeon that the hepatic artery can be compressed with a vascular clamp applied across the free edge of the lesser omentum (which forms the anterior wall of the foramen of Winslow). If the cystic artery is torn during cholecystectomy, haemorrhage can be controlled by this manoeuvre (named after James Pringle), which then enables the damaged vessel to be identified and secured.

Intraperitoneal fossae

A number of fossae occur within the peritoneal cavity in which loops of bowel may become trapped and strangulated. Those of importance are:
1 the *lesser sac* – via the foramen of Winslow, described previously;
2 *paraduodenal fossa* – between the duodenojejunal flexure and the inferior mesenteric vessels;
3 *retrocaecal fossa* – in which the appendix frequently lies;
4 *intersigmoid fossa* – formed by the inverted 'V' attachment of the mesosigmoid.

The subphrenic spaces (Fig. 48)

Below the diaphragm are a number of potential spaces formed in relation to the attachments of the liver. One or more of these spaces may become filled with pus (a subphrenic abscess) walled off inferiorly by adhesions. There are five subdivisions of clinical importance.

The *right* and *left subphrenic spaces* lie between the diaphragm and the upper surface of the liver, separated from each other by the falciform ligament.

The *right* and *left subhepatic spaces* lie below the liver. The right subhepatic space is known also as the hepatorenal pouch or the *pouch of Morison*. It is bounded, posteriorly, by the *peritoneum overlying the fascial coverings of the right kidney; anterosuperiorly by the visceral surface of the right lobe of the liver and superiorly by the peritoneal reflexion between the liver and diaphragm*. It communicates anteriorly with the right subphrenic space around the anterior margin of the right lobe of the liver. Inferiorly, both the right subhepatic space and the right subphrenic space open into the general peritoneal cavity. Infected fluid, for example, from a perforated appendix or a perforated peptic ulcer can track upwards into either of the above-mentioned two spaces. The left subhepatic space is none other than the lesser sac. Also known as the omental bursa, the lesser sac communicates with the right subhepatic space through the foramen of Winslow (epiploic foramen). It may fill with fluid as a result of a perforation in the posterior wall of the stomach or from an inflamed or injured pancreas to form a pseudocyst of the pancreas.

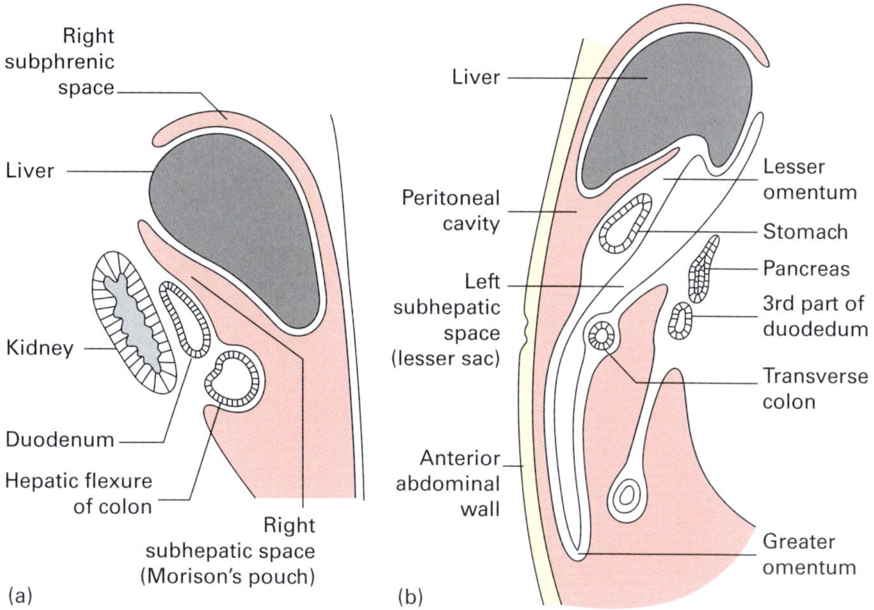

Fig. 48 The anatomy of (a) the right and (b) the left subphrenic spaces in sagittal section (each viewed from the lateral aspect).

The *right extraperitoneal space* lies between the bare area of the liver and the diaphragm. It may become involved in retroperitoneal infections or directly from a liver abscess.

Posterior subphrenic abscesses are drained by an incision below, or through the bed of, the 12th rib. A finger is then passed upwards and forwards between the liver and diaphragm to open into the abscess cavity. An anteriorly placed collection of pus below the diaphragm can alternatively be drained via an incision placed below and parallel to the costal margin. Nowadays, intra-abdominal fluid collections are, as a routine, drained percutaneously under ultrasound or CT-guided control.

The gastrointestinal tract

The stomach

The stomach is roughly J-shaped, although its size and shape vary considerably. It tends to be high and transverse in the obese short subject and to be elongated in the asthenic individual; even in the same person, its shape depends on whether it is full or empty, on the position of the body and on the phase of respiration. The stomach has two surfaces – the anterior and posterior; two curvatures – the greater and lesser; and two orifices – the cardia and pylorus (Fig. 49).

The stomach projects to the left, above the level of the cardiac orifice (or *cardia*), to form the dome-like gastric *fundus*. Along the lesser curve is a distinct notch, the *incisura*

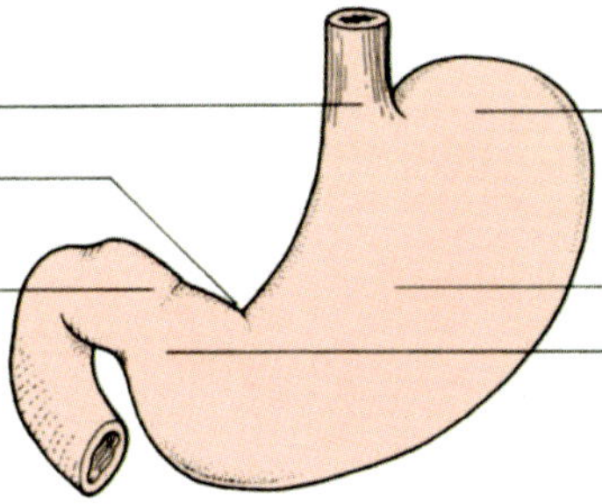

Fig. 49 The stomach and its subdivisions.

angularis. Between the cardiac orifice and the incisura is the body of the stomach, while the area between the incisura and the pylorus is the pyloric antrum. The junction of the pylorus with the duodenum is marked by a constriction externally and also by a constant vein that crosses it, the *prepyloric vein of Mayo*.

It is the body of the stomach that bears the HCl-secreting parietal cells. The antrum secretes the enzyme gastrin and its secretion is alkaline.

The thickened *pyloric sphincter* is easily felt and surrounds the lumen of the *pyloric canal*. The pyloric sphincter is an anatomical structure as well as a physiological mechanism. The cardia, on the other hand, although competent (gastric contents do not flow out of your mouth if you stand on your head), is not demarcated by a distinct anatomical sphincter. The exact nature of the cardiac sphincter action is still not fully understood, but the following mechanisms have been suggested, each supported by some experimental and clinical evidence.

1 Mucosal folds at the oesophagogastric junction act as a valve.
2 The acute angle of entry of the oesophagus into the stomach produces a valve-like effect.
3 The circular muscle of the lower oesophagus is a physiological, as distinct from an anatomical, sphincter.
4 The arrangement of the muscle fibres of the stomach around the cardia either acts as a sphincter or else maintains the acute angle of entry of the oesophagus into the stomach.
5 The right crus of the diaphragm acts as a 'pinch-cock' to the lower oesophagus as it pierces this muscle.
6 The positive intra-abdominal pressure compresses the walls of the short segment of the intra-abdominal oesophagus.

Relations (Fig. 50)

- *Anteriorly* – the abdominal wall, the left costal margin, the diaphragm and the left lobe of the liver;
- *Posteriorly* – the lesser sac, which separates the stomach from the pancreas, transverse mesocolon, left kidney, left suprarenal, the spleen and the splenic artery;
- *Superiorly* – the left dome of the diaphragm.

The lesser omentum is attached along the lesser curvature of the stomach; the greater omentum along the greater curvature. These omenta contain the vascular and lymphatic supply of the stomach.

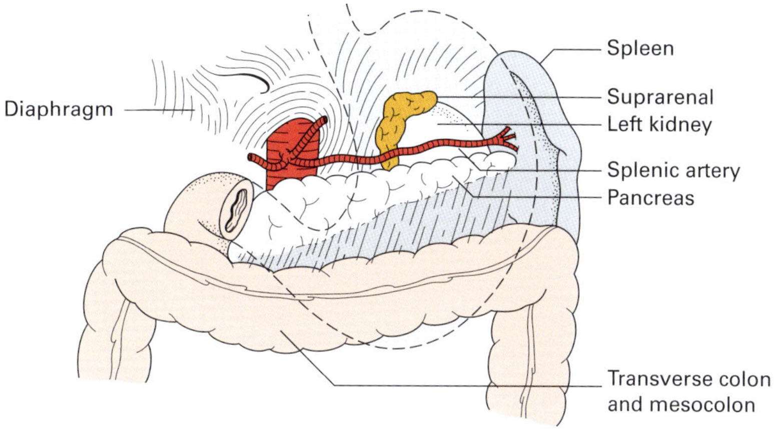

Fig. 50 The posterior relations of the stomach; the stomach (indicated by the dashed line) is superimposed upon its bed.

The *arterial supply* (Fig. 51) to the stomach is extremely rich and comprises:

- *the left gastric artery* – from the coeliac axis;
- *the right gastric artery* – from the hepatic artery;
- *the right gastro-epiploic artery* – from the gastroduodenal branch of the common hepatic artery;
- *the left gastro-epiploic artery* – from the splenic artery;
- *the short gastric arteries* – from the splenic artery.

The corresponding veins drain into the portal system.

The *lymphatic drainage* of the stomach accompanies its blood vessels. The stomach can be divided into three drainage zones (Fig. 52).

- *Area I* – the superior two-thirds of the stomach drains along the left and right gastric vessels to the aortic nodes.

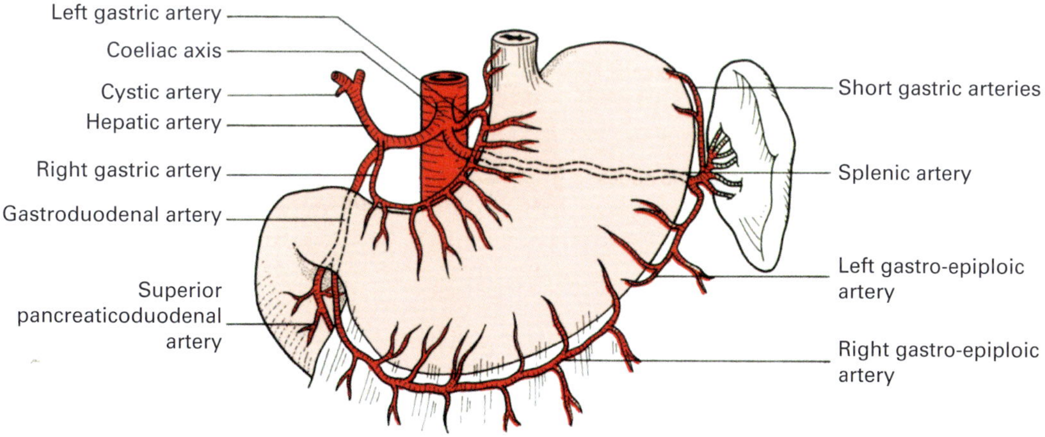

Fig. 51 The arterial supply of the stomach.

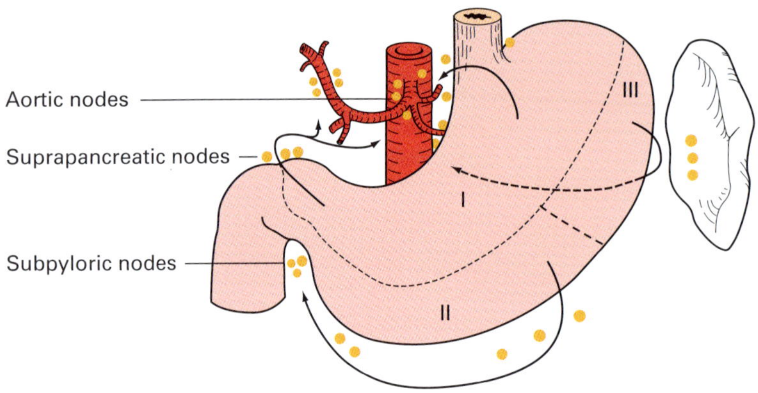

Fig. 52 The lymphatic drainage of the stomach.

- *Area II* – the right two-thirds of the inferior one-third of the stomach drain along the right gastro-epiploic vessels to the subpyloric nodes and thence to the aortic nodes.
- Area I drains along the right and left gastric vessels to the aortic nodes.
- Area II drains to the subpyloric and thence aortic nodes via lymphatics along the right gastro-epiploic vessels.
- Area III drains via lymphatics along the splenic vessels to the suprapancreatic nodes and thence to the aortic nodes.
- *Area III* – the left one-third of the greater curvature of the stomach drains along the short gastric and splenic vessels lying in the gastrosplenic and splenorenal ligaments, then, via the suprapancreatic nodes, to the aortic group.

This extensive lymphatic drainage and the technical impossibility of its complete removal is one of the serious problems in dealing with stomach cancer. Involvement of the nodes along the splenic vessels can be dealt with by removing the spleen, the gastrosplenic and splenorenal ligaments and the body and tail of the pancreas. Lymph nodes among the gastro-epiploic vessels are removed by excising the greater omentum. However, involvement of the nodes around the aorta and the head of the pancreas may render the growth incurable.

The vagal supply to the stomach (Fig. 53)

The anterior and posterior vagi enter the abdomen through the oesophageal hiatus. The anterior nerve lies close to the stomach wall but the posterior, and larger, nerve is at a little distance from it. The anterior vagus supplies branches to the cardia and lesser curve of the stomach and also a large hepatic branch. The posterior vagus gives branches to both the anterior and posterior aspects of the body of the stomach, but the bulk of the nerve forms the coeliac branch. This runs along the left gastric artery to the coeliac ganglion for distribution to the intestine, as far as the mid-transverse colon, and the pancreas.

The exact means by which the vagal fibres reach the stomach is of considerable practical importance to the surgeon. The gastric divisions of both the anterior and posterior vagi reach the stomach at the cardia and descend along the lesser curvature between

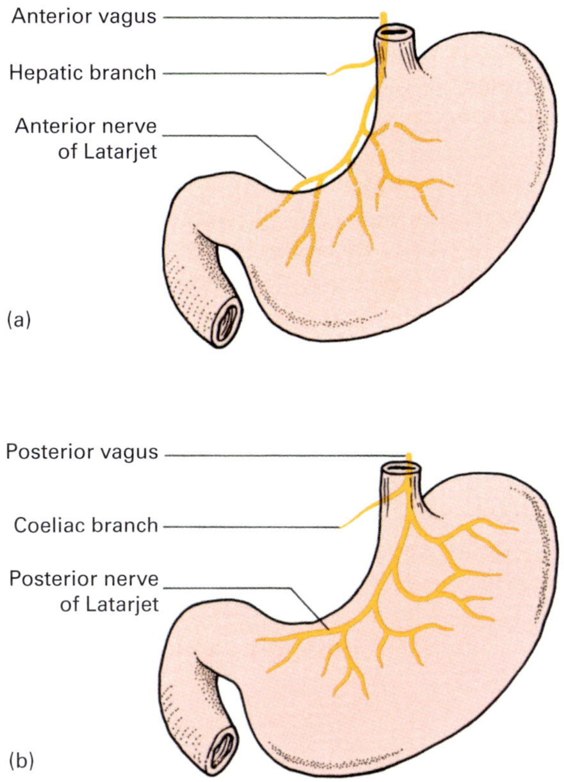

Fig. 53 The vagal supply to the stomach: (a) anterior vagus; (b) posterior vagus.

the anterior and posterior layers of the lesser omentum (the anterior and posterior nerves of Latarjet). The stomach is innervated by terminal branches from the anterior and posterior gastric nerves, and it is, therefore, possible to divide those branches that supply the acid-secreting body of the stomach and yet preserve the pyloric innervation (highly selective vagotomy).

The vagus constitutes the motor and secretory nerve supply for the stomach. When divided, in the operation of *vagotomy*, the neurogenic (reflex) gastric acid secretion is abolished but the stomach is, at the same time, rendered atonic so that it empties only with difficulty; because of this, total vagotomy must always be accompanied by some sort of drainage procedure, either a pyloroplasty (to enlarge the pyloric exit and render the pyloric sphincter incompetent) or a gastrojejunostomy (to drain the stomach into the proximal small intestine). Drainage can be avoided if the nerve of Latarjet is preserved, thus maintaining the innervation and function of the pyloric antrum (highly selective vagotomy). From the early 1990s onwards, the advent of powerful and effective pharmacological agents that inhibit gastric acid secretion, such as H-2 receptor antagonists and proton-pump inhibitors and the now-universal realization that acid-peptic disease (peptic ulcer disease) is often due to an infection by the bacterium *helicobacter pylori*, that can be eradicated by a course of antibiotics, has practically consigned to the history books, such surgical procedures as truncal vagotomy, and selective and highly selective vagotomies that were undertaken in the surgical management of peptic ulcer disease.

CLINICAL FEATURES

1 A posterior gastric ulcer or cancer may erode the pancreas, giving pain referred to the back. Ulceration into the splenic artery – a direct posterior relation – may cause torrential haemorrhage.

2 There may be adhesions across the lesser sac that bring the transverse mesocolon into intimate relationship with the stomach or greater omentum. In these circumstances, the middle colic vessels are in danger of damage during mobilization of the stomach for gastrectomy.

3 *Radiology of the stomach* (Fig. 54). A plain erect film of the abdomen reveals a bubble of air below the left diaphragm; this is gas in the stomach fundus. After the subject has swallowed radio-opaque contrast fluid, for example barium sulphate, the stomach can be seen and its position, movements and outline studied. The wide variations in the position and shape of the stomach that we have already mentioned have come to light principally as a result of such investigations.

By tipping the subject head-down, the opaque meal can be made to impinge against the cardia; incompetence of this sphincter mechanism will be demonstrated by seeing barium regurgitate into the oesophagus.

4 Upper GI endoscopy/gastroscopy: The mucosa of the air-inflated stomach can be inspected in the living subject through the gastroscope. With the modern fibreoptic instrument the whole of the gastric mucosa can be viewed, the duodenum examined and the common bile duct and the pancreatic duct cannulated for retrograde contrast-enhanced radiological study.

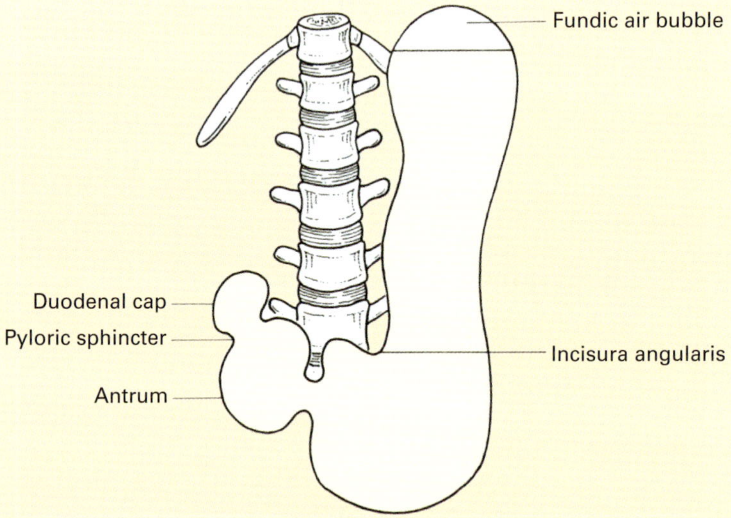

Fig. 54 Tracing of a barium meal radiograph of the stomach.

The duodenum

The duodenum curves in a C around the head of the pancreas and is 25 cm (10 in) long. At its origin from the pylorus it is completely covered with peritoneum for approximately 2.5 cm (1 in), but then becomes a retroperitoneal organ, only partially covered by serous membrane.

Relations (Figs 55, 56)

For descriptive purposes, the duodenum is divided into four sections.

The first part (5 cm (2 in)) ascends from the gastroduodenal junction, overlapped by the liver and gall bladder. Immediately posterior to it lie the portal vein, common bile duct and gastroduodenal artery, which separate it from the IVC.

The second part (7.5 cm (3 in)) descends in a curve around the head of the pancreas. It is crossed by the transverse colon and lies on the right kidney and ureter. Halfway along, its posteromedial aspect enters the common opening of the bile duct and the *main pancreatic duct* (*of Wirsung*) onto an eminence called the *duodenal papilla*. This common opening is guarded by the *sphincter of Oddi*. The *accessory pancreatic duct*

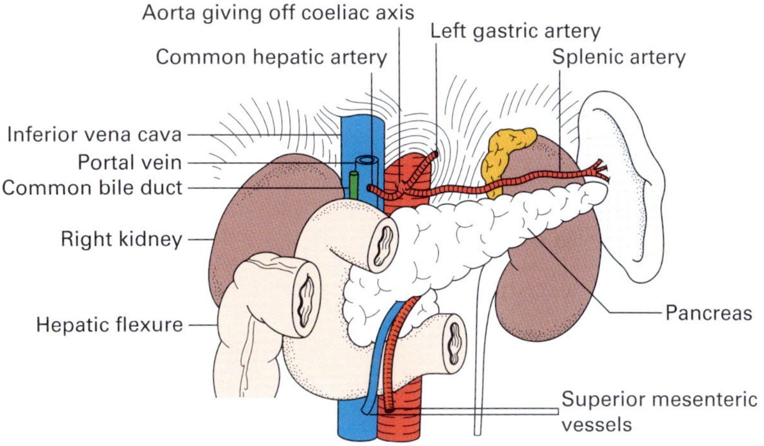

Fig. 55 The relations of the duodenum.

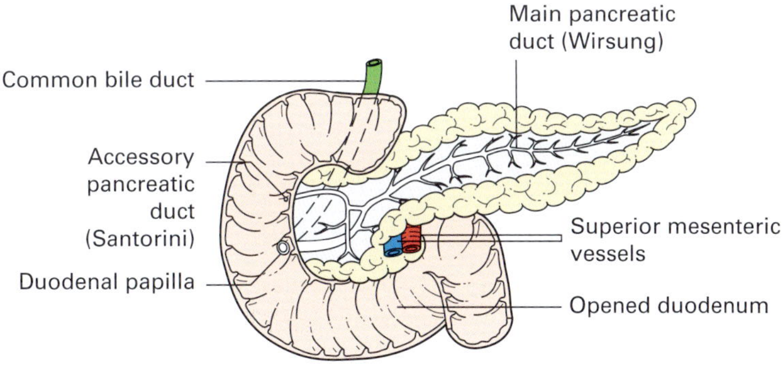

Fig. 56 The duodenum and pancreas dissected to show the pancreatic ducts and their orifices.

(*of Santorini*) opens into the duodenum a couple of cms proximal to the opening of the main duct.

The third part (10 cm (4 in)) runs transversely to the left, crossing the IVC, the aorta and the third lumbar vertebra. It is itself crossed anteriorly by the root of the mesentery and the superior mesenteric vessels. Its upper border hugs the pancreatic head.

The fourth part (2.5 cm (1 in)) ascends upwards and to the left to end at the duodenojejunal junction. The identity of the duodenal termination is confirmed by the presence of the *suspensory ligament of Treitz*, which is a well-marked peritoneal fold descending from the right crus of the diaphragm to the duodenojejunal junction, and by visualizing the inferior mesenteric vein, which ascends immediately to the left of the duodenojejunal junction to join the splenic vein behind the pancreas.

Blood supply

The superior pancreaticoduodenal artery arises from the gastroduodenal artery; the inferior pancreaticoduodenal artery originates as the first branch of the superior mesenteric artery. These vessels both lie in the curve between the duodenum and the head of the pancreas, supplying both structures. Interestingly, their anastomosis represents the site of the junction of the foregut (supplied by the coeliac artery) and the midgut (supplied by the superior mesenteric artery), at the level of the duodenal papilla (see page 80 and Fig. 56).

CLINICAL FEATURES

1 The first part of the duodenum is overlapped by the liver and gall bladder, either of which may adhere to, or even be eroded by, a duodenal ulcer. Moreover, a gallstone may be extruded from the fundus of a chronically inflamed gall bladder into the duodenum. The gallstone may then impact in the lower ileum as it traverses the gut to produce intestinal obstruction (*gallstone ileus*).
2 The pancreas, as the duodenum's most intimate relation, is readily invaded by a posterior duodenal ulcer. This should be suspected if the patient's pain radiates into the dorsolumbar region. Erosion of the gastroduodenal artery by such an ulcer results in severe haemorrhage.
3 Extensive dissection of a duodenum, scarred by severe ulceration, may damage the common bile duct, which passes behind the first part of the duodenum approximately 2.5 cm (1 in) from the pylorus.
4 The hepatic flexure of the colon crosses the second part of the duodenum and the latter may be damaged during a right hemicolectomy. Similarly, the right kidney lies directly behind this part of the duodenum, which may be injured in performing a right nephrectomy.
5 *Radiology of the duodenum*. Within a few minutes of swallowing a barium meal, the first part of the duodenum becomes visible as a triangular shadow termed the *duodenal cap*.

Every few seconds the duodenum contracts, emptying this cap, which promptly proceeds to fill again. It is in this region that the great majority of duodenal ulcers occur; an actual ulcer crater may be visualized, filled with barium, or deformity of the cap, produced by scar tissue, may be evident. The rest of the duodenum can also be seen, the shadow being floccular owing to the rugose arrangement of the mucosa.

6 *Mobilization of the duodenum*, together with the head of the pancreas and termination of the common bile duct, is performed by incising the peritoneum lateral to the second part of the duodenum and developing the avascular plane between these structures and the posterior abdominal wall – Kocher's manoeuvre (see also page 96).

Small intestine

The *length* of the small intestine varies from 3 to 10 m (10–33 feet) in different subjects; the average is some 6.5 m (24 feet). Resection of up to one-third or even half of the small intestine is compatible with a more-or-less normal life, and long-term survival has been reported with only 45 cm (18 in) of small intestine preserved.

The *mesentery* of the small intestine has a 15 cm (6 in) origin from the posterior abdominal wall, which commences at the duodenojejunal junction to the left of the 2nd lumbar vertebra, and passes obliquely downwards to the right sacro-iliac joint; it contains the superior mesenteric vessels, the lymph nodes draining the small gut and autonomic nerve fibres.

The upper half of the small intestine is termed the *jejunum*; the remainder is the *ileum*. There is no sharp demarcation between the two and the transition from one to the other is a gradual one. The bowel does, however, change its character from above downwards, the following points enabling the surgeon to determine the level of a loop of small intestine at operation.

1 The jejunum has a thicker wall as the circular folds of mucosa (*valvulae conniventes*) are larger and thicker more proximally.
2 The proximal small intestine is of greater diameter than the distal.
3 The jejunum tends to lie at the umbilical region; the ileum in the suprapubic region and pelvis.
4 The mesentery becomes thicker and more fat-laden from above downwards.
5 The mesenteric vessels form only one or two arcades to the jejunum, with long and relatively infrequent terminal branches passing to the gut wall. The ileum is supplied by shorter and more numerous terminal vessels arising from complete series of three, four or even five arcades (Fig. 57).

Large intestine

The large intestine is subdivided, for descriptive purposes, into:

- caecum with the appendix vermiformis;
- ascending colon (12–20 cm (5–8 in));
- hepatic flexure (right colic flexure);
- transverse colon (45 cm (18 in));

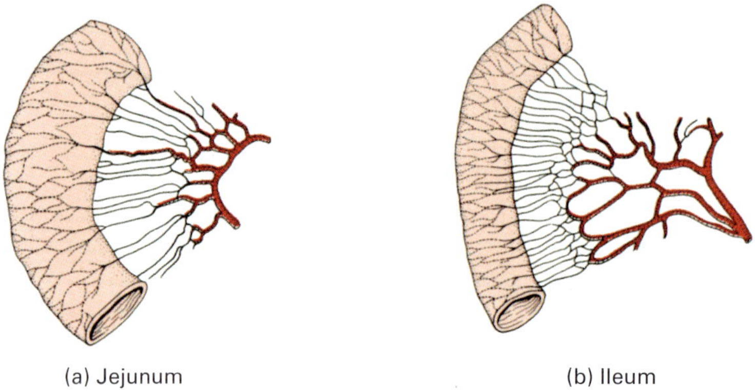

Fig. 57 The simple arterial arcades of the jejunum (a) compared with the complex arcades of the ileum (b).

- splenic flexure (left colic flexure);
- descending colon (22–30 cm (9–12 in));
- sigmoid colon (12–76 cm (5–30 in), average 38 cm (15 in));
- rectum (12 cm (5 in));
- anal canal (4 cm (1.5 in)).

The large bowel may vary considerably in length in different subjects; the average is approximately 1.5 m (5 feet).

The colon (but not the appendix, caecum or rectum) bears characteristic fat-filled peritoneal tags called *appendices epiploicae* scattered over its surface. These are especially numerous over the sigmoid colon and the distal part of the descending colon. Their function, if any, is obscure, but they may, in rare instances, undergo torsion, which is an unusual cause of acute abdominal pain.

The colon and caecum (but not the appendix or rectum) are marked by the presence of *taeniae coli*. These are three flattened bands commencing at the base of the appendix and running the length of the large intestine to end at the rectosigmoid junction. They represent band-shaped condensations of the longitudinal muscle in the wall of the large bowel; because the taeniae are approximately 30 cm (12 in) shorter than the gut to which they are attached, the colon becomes drawn into its typical sacculated shape. These sacculations (also known as haustrations) may be seen in a plain radiograph of the abdomen when the large bowel is distended. They appear as incomplete septa projecting into the gas shadow. The radiograph of distended small intestine, in contrast, characteristically has complete transverse lines across the bowel shadow owing to the transverse mucosal folds of the valvulae conniventes.

Peritoneal attachments

The transverse colon and sigmoid are each completely ensleeved in peritoneum and each is suspended from the posterior abdominal wall by its mesentery (transverse mesocolon and sigmoid mesocolon, respectively). The considerable mobility of the transverse and sigmoid colons within the abdominal cavity is due entirely to the presence of these generous suspensory mesenteries. The greater omentum descends from the greater curvature of the stomach and overlaps the entire length of the anterior aspect of the transverse colon. It is attached along the free border of the transverse colon. The strip of greater omentum extending between the greater curvature of the stomach and the free border of the transverse colon is referred to as the *gastrocolic omentum*.

Neither the ascending colon nor the descending colon possesses a mesentery. The posterior walls of both adhere directly to the posterior abdominal wall (although in rare instances, either may possess a mesocolon). The caecum is usually completely enveloped in visceral peritoneum and often possesses a very short post-caecal fold. However the caecum, like the ascending colon, may be devoid of peritoneum on its posterior surface. The appendix, although usually free within its own mesentery, occasionally lies extraperitoneally behind the caecum and ascending colon or adheres to the posterior wall of these structures.

The rectum is extraperitoneal on its posterior aspect in its upper third, posteriorly and laterally in its middle third and completely extraperitoneal in its lower third as it sinks below the pelvic peritoneum.

The appendix

The appendix arises from the posteromedial aspect of the caecum approximately 2.5 cm (1 in) below the ileocaecal valve; its length ranges from 1.25 cm (0.5 in) to 22 cm (9 in). In the fetus it is a direct outpouching of the caecum, but differential overgrowth of the lateral caecal wall results in its medial displacement.

The position of the appendix is extremely variable – more so than that of any other organ (Fig. 58). Most frequently (75% of cases) the appendix lies behind the caecum. The appendix is usually quite free in this position, although occasionally it lies beneath the peritoneal covering of the caecum. If the appendix is very long, it may actually extend behind the ascending colon and abut against the right kidney or the duodenum; in these cases, its distal portion lies extraperitoneally.

In approximately 20% of cases, the appendix lies just below the caecum or else hangs down into the pelvis. Less commonly, it passes in front of or behind the terminal ileum, or lies in front of the caecum or in the right paracolic gutter.

A long appendix has been known to ulcerate into the duodenum or perforate into the *left* paracolic gutter. It may well be said that 'the appendix is the only organ in the body that has no anatomy'.

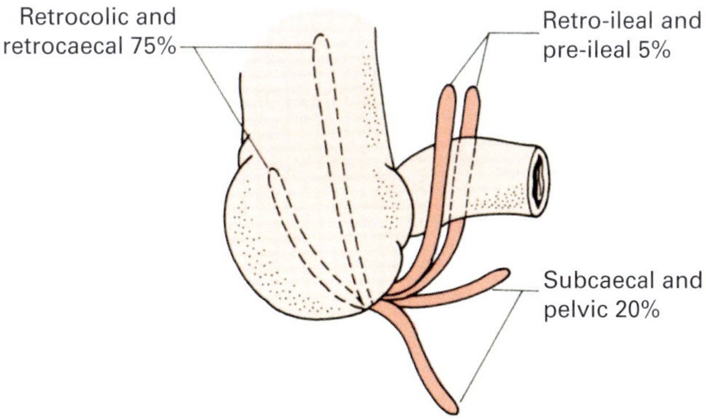

Fig. 58 The positions in which the appendix may lie, together with their approximate incidence.

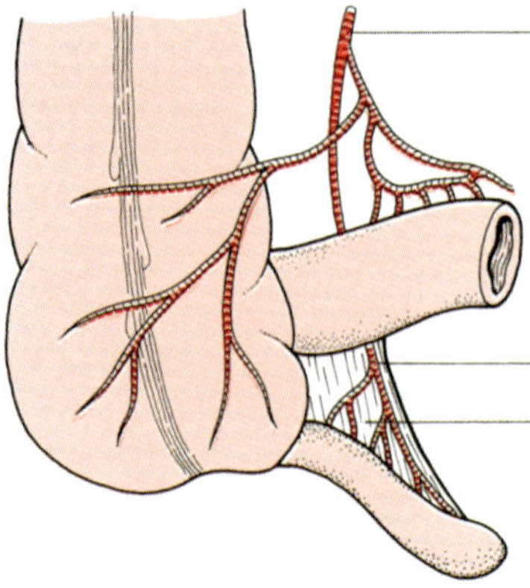

Fig. 59 The blood supply of the appendix.

The mesentery of the appendix, containing the appendicular branch of the ileocolic artery, descends behind the ileum as a triangular fold (Fig. 59). Another peritoneal sheet, the *ileocaecal fold*, passes to the appendix or to the base of the caecum from the front of the ileum. The ileocaecal fold is termed the *bloodless fold of Treves* although, in fact, it often contains a vessel and, if cut, proves far from bloodless.

CLINICAL FEATURES

1 The lumen of the appendix is relatively wide in the infant and is frequently completely obliterated in the elderly. Since obstruction of the lumen is the usual precipitating cause of acute appendicitis it is not unnatural, therefore, that appendicitis should be uncommon at the two extremes of life.

2 The appendicular artery represents the entire vascular supply of the appendix. It runs first in the edge of the appendicular mesentery and then, distally, along the wall of the appendix. Acute infection of the appendix may result in thrombosis of this artery with rapid development of gangrene and subsequent perforation. This is in contrast to acute cholecystitis, where the rich collateral vascular supply from the liver bed ensures the rarity of gangrene of the gall bladder even if the cystic artery becomes thrombosed.

3 *Appendicectomy* is usually performed through a muscle-splitting incision in the right iliac fossa (see 'The anatomy of abdominal incisions', page 65). The caecum is delivered into the wound and, if the appendix is not immediately visible, it is located by tracing the taeniae coli along the caecum – they fuse at the base of the appendix. When the caecum is extraperitoneal it may be difficult to bring the appendix up into the incision; this is facilitated by first mobilizing the caecum by incising the almost avascular peritoneum along its lateral and inferior borders.

The appendix mesentery, containing the appendicular vessels, is firmly tied and divided, the appendix base tied, the appendix removed and its stump invaginated into the caecum.

The rectum

The rectum is the direct continuation of the sigmoid colon and commences in front of the third segment of the sacrum and ends at the level of the apex of the prostate or, in the female, at the level of the lower end of the intrapelvic vagina, where the rectum traverses the pelvic floor to become continuous with the anal canal. The rectum is 10–12 cm (5 in) in length.

The rectum is straight in lower primates (hence its name) but is curved in man to conform to the ventral concavity of the sacrum. Thus the rectum runs downwards and backwards initially and then downwards and forwards to reach the levator hiatus (the gap in the pelvic floor between the two levator ani muscles through which the pelvic viscera pass inferiorly into the perineum).

Additionally, the rectum presents, externally, a succession of three smooth, laterally facing curves. The upper and lower curves are directed to the right and the middle curve to the left. Each of the three curves presents, on the inside, a transverse sickle-shaped muscular fold. These folds are known as rectal shelves or the valves of Houston. The inferior third of the rectum is somewhat dilated and is referred to as the ampulla.

The haustrations, appendices epiploicae and taeniae coli that characterize the sigmoid colon and other segments of the colon, are absent on the rectal wall.

Relations (Figs 60, 61)

The topographical relations of the rectum are important and must be kept in mind when carrying out a digital rectal examination (DRE). They provide the key to the local spread of rectal growths and are important considerations in procedures involving surgical resection of the rectum.

Posteriorly lie the sacrum and coccyx and the middle sacral artery, which are separated from it by extraperitoneal connective tissue containing the rectal vessels and lymphatics.

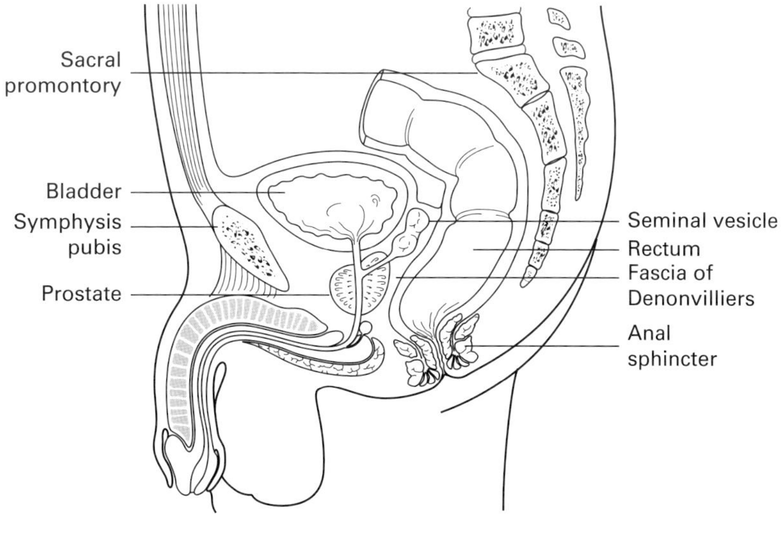

Fig. 60 Sagittal section of the rectum and its related viscera in the male.

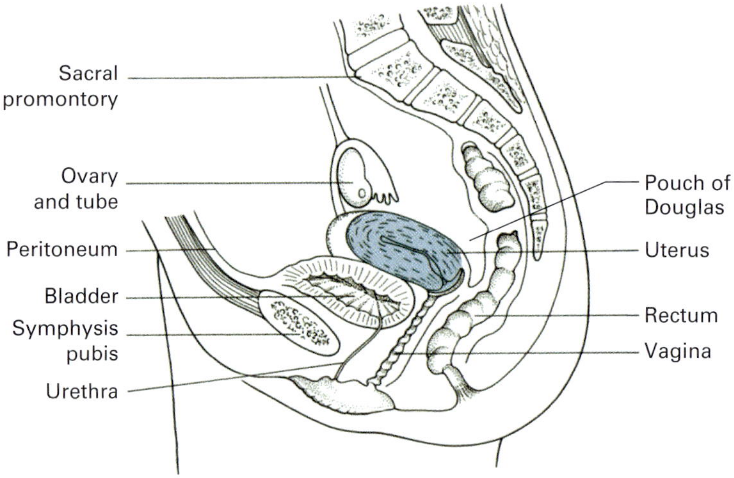

Fig. 61 Sagittal section of the rectum and its related viscera in the female.

The lower sacral nerves, emerging from the anterior sacral foramina, may be involved by growth spreading posteriorly from the rectum, resulting in severe sciatic pain.

Anteriorly, the upper two-thirds of the rectum are covered by peritoneum and relate to coils of small intestine which, in the female, lie in the cul-de-sac of the pouch of Douglas between the rectum and the uterus. In front of the lower one-third of the rectum lie the prostate, bladder base and seminal vesicles in the male, and the vagina in the female. A layer of fascia (*Denonvilliers*) separates the rectum from the anterior structures and forms the plane of dissection which must be sought when performing excision of the rectum.

Laterally, the rectum is related to and supported by the levator ani.

The anal canal (Fig. 62)

The anal canal is 4 cm (1.5 in) long and is directed downwards and backwards from the rectum to end at the anal orifice. The mid-anal canal represents the junction between the endoderm of the embryonic hindgut and the ectoderm of the embryonic

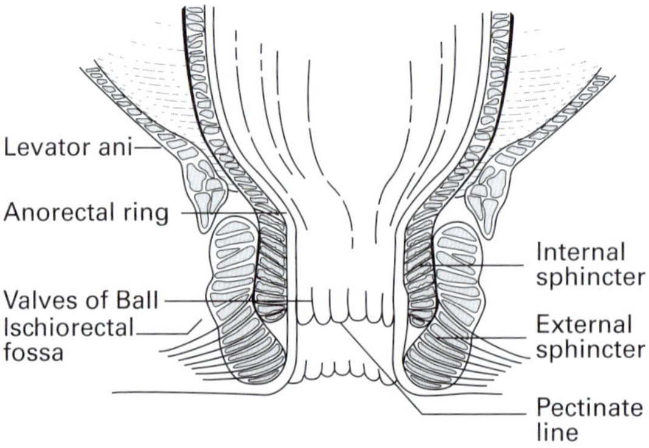

Fig. 62 The sphincters of the anus.

cutaneous invagination termed the proctodaeum. Failure of breakdown of the separating membrane results in *imperforate anus*. In the adult this embryonic junction is denoted by

1 The distal half of the anal canal is lined by stratified squamous epithelium and the proximal half by columnar epithelium; the latter presents vertical columns of mucosa (*the columns of Morgagni*) connected at their distal extremities by valve-like folds (*the valves of Ball*). A carcinoma originating in the upper anal canal is thus likely to be an adenocarcinoma, whereas that arising from the lower part is likely to be a squamous carcinoma.
2 The blood supply of the upper half of the anal canal may derive its blood supply in part from the superior rectal artery, derived from the inferior mesenteric artery (see Fig. 64), and its corresponding superior rectal vein, which drains into the inferior mesenteric vein, which, in turn, enters the splenic vein and thus drains into the portal vein (see Fig. 65). In contrast, the blood supply of the lower anal canal and the surrounding perianal skin is from the inferior rectal vessels, derived from the internal pudendal and, ultimately, the internal iliac artery and vein. The two venous systems communicate and therefore form one of the many anastomoses between the portal and systemic venous systems.
3 The lymphatics above this mucocutaneous junction drain along the superior rectal vessels to the lumbar nodes, whereas, below this line, drainage is to the inguinal nodes. A carcinoma of the rectum that invades the lower anal canal may thus metastasize to the groin nodes.
4 The nerve supply to the upper anal canal is via the autonomic plexuses; the lower part is supplied by the somatic inferior rectal nerve, a terminal branch of the pudendal nerve (see Fig. 97b). (The lower canal is therefore sensitive to the prick of a hypodermic needle, whereas injection of an internal haemorrhoid with sclerosant fluid, by passing a needle through the mucosa of the upper part of the canal, is painless.)

The anal sphincter

Forming the walls of the anal canal is a rather complicated muscle arrangement which constitutes a powerful sphincter mechanism (Fig. 62). This comprises:

- *the internal anal sphincter*, of involuntary muscle, which continues above with the circular muscle coat of the rectum;
- *the external anal sphincter*, of voluntary muscle, which surrounds the internal sphincter and which extends further downwards and curves medially to occupy a position below and slightly lateral to the lower rounded edge of the internal sphincter, close to the skin of the anal orifice. The lowermost, or subcutaneous, portion of the external sphincter is traversed by a fan-shaped expansion of the longitudinal muscle fibres of the anal canal that continue above with the longitudinal muscle of the rectal wall. At its upper end the external sphincter fuses with the fibres of levator ani.

In carrying out a DRE, the ring of muscle on which the flexed finger rests just over 2.5 cm (1 in) from the anal margin is the *anorectal ring*. This represents the deep part of the external sphincter where this blends with the internal sphincter and levator ani and demarcates the junction between the anal canal and the rectum.

The anal canal is related posteriorly to the fibrous tissue between it and the coccyx (the anococcygeal body), laterally to the *ischioanal fossa* on either side, containing fat, and anteriorly to the perineal body, which separates it from the bulb of the urethra in the male and the lower vagina in the female. Note that the ischiorectal fossa is now often referred to, more accurately, as the ischioanal fossa – it relates to the anal canal rather than the rectum.

Rectal examination

The following structures can be palpated by the finger passed *per rectum* in the normal patient:

1 *both sexes* – the anorectal ring (see previous section), coccyx and sacrum, ischioanal fossae and ischial spines;
2 *male* – prostate, rarely the healthy seminal vesicles;
3 *female* – perineal body, cervix and, occasionally, the ovaries.

Abnormalities which can be detected include:

1 *within the lumen* – faecal impaction and foreign bodies;
2 *in the wall* – rectal growths, strictures, granulomata, etc., but *not* haemorrhoids unless these are thrombosed;
3 *outside the rectal wall* – pelvic bony tumours, abnormalities of the prostate or seminal vesicle, distended bladder, uterine or ovarian enlargement, collections of fluid or neoplastic masses in the pouch of Douglas.

Do not be deceived by foreign objects placed in the vagina. The commonest are a tampon or a pessary.

During parturition, dilatation of the cervical os can be assessed by rectal examination since it can be felt quite easily through the rectal wall.

CLINICAL FEATURES

Haemorrhoids

Haemorrhoids (piles) are sustained, pathological engorgements of the submucosal arteriovenous cushions that are normally present in the upper half of the anal canal. Initially contained within the anal canal (1st degree), they gradually enlarge until they prolapse on defecation (2nd degree) and finally remain prolapsed through the anal orifice (3rd degree). Anatomically, each pile comprises: a venous plexus draining into one of the superior rectal veins; terminal branches of the corresponding superior rectal artery; and a covering of anal canal mucosa and submucosa. There are arteriovenous anastomoses between the vessels, since bleeding from piles is characteristically bright red. The so-called 'thrombosed external pile' is a small tense haematoma at the anal margin caused by rupture of a subcutaneous vein and is much better termed a *perianal haematoma*.

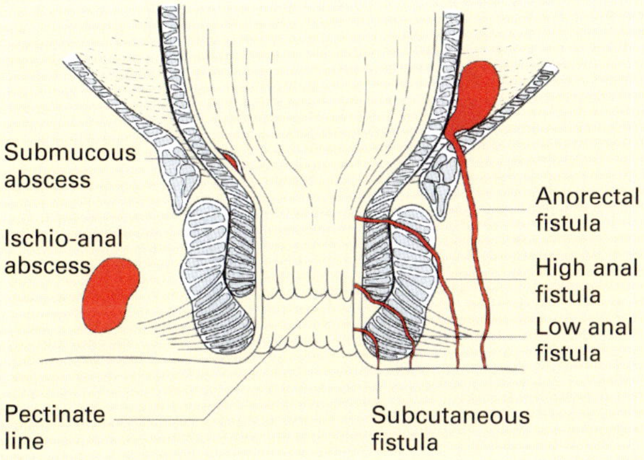

Fig. 63 The anatomy of perianal fistulae and abscesses.

Perianal abscesses (Fig. 63)

These may be localized beneath the anal mucosa (submucous), be beneath perianal skin (subcutaneous) or occupy the ischioanal fossa. Occasionally, abscesses lie in the pelvirectal space above levator ani, alongside the rectum, in an extraperitoneal location.

Fistulae (Fig. 63)

Anal fistulae usually result from rupture of perianal abscesses. They are classified anatomically and may be:

- *submucous* – confined to the tissues immediately below the anal mucosa;
- *subcutaneous* – confined to the perianal skin;
- *low level* – passing through the lower part of the superficial sphincter (most common);
- *high level* – passing through the deeper part of the superficial sphincter;
- *anorectal* – which has its track passing above the anorectal ring and which may or may not open into the rectum.

In laying open *fistulae in ano*, it is essential to preserve the anorectal ring if faecal incontinence is to be avoided. The lower part of the sphincter, on the other hand, can be divided quite safely without this risk.

Fissure *in ano*

This is a tear in the anal mucosa; over 90% occur posteriorly in the midline. The anatomical basis for this probably lies in the insertion of the superficial component of the external anal sphincter posteriorly into the coccyx; between the two limbs of the 'V' thus formed, the mucosa is relatively unsupported and may therefore be torn by a hard faecal mass at this site.

Arterial supply of the intestine

The alimentary tract develops from the foregut, midgut and hindgut; each with its principal artery. The foregut comprises the stomach and duodenum as far as the entry of the bile duct and is supplied by branches of the *coeliac axis*, which arises from the aorta at the T12 vertebral level (Fig. 51). The midgut extends from mid-duodenum to the distal transverse colon and is supplied by the *superior mesenteric artery* (Fig. 64) arising from the aorta at the level of L1. Its branches are:

1 the inferior pancreaticoduodenal artery;
2 jejunal and ileal branches – supplying the bulk of the small intestine;
3 the ileocolic artery – supplying the terminal ileum, caecum, the proximal part of the ascending colon and the appendix;
4 the right colic artery – supplying the distal ascending colon;
5 the middle colic artery – supplying the transverse colon.

The hindgut receives its supply from the *inferior mesenteric artery* (Fig. 64), arising from the aorta at L3 and giving the following branches:

1 the left colic artery – supplying the descending colon;
2 the sigmoid branches – supplying the sigmoid;
3 the superior rectal artery – supplying the rectum.

Lying within the inner margin of the colon, close to the bowel wall, is an extremely effective anastomotic arterial arcade known as the *marginal artery (of Drummond)* (Fig 64). This arcade links the colic branches of the superior and inferior mesenteric arteries. It is entirely due to the presence of an effective marginal artery that the inferior mesenteric artery is sacrificed in patients undergoing repair of an abdominal aortic aneurysm without jeopardizing the blood supply to the distal colon. Conversely, in some very elderly patients with advanced atheromatous disease, the marginal artery may be severely compromised, and this may lead to anastomotic ischaemia/dehiscence following bowel resection.

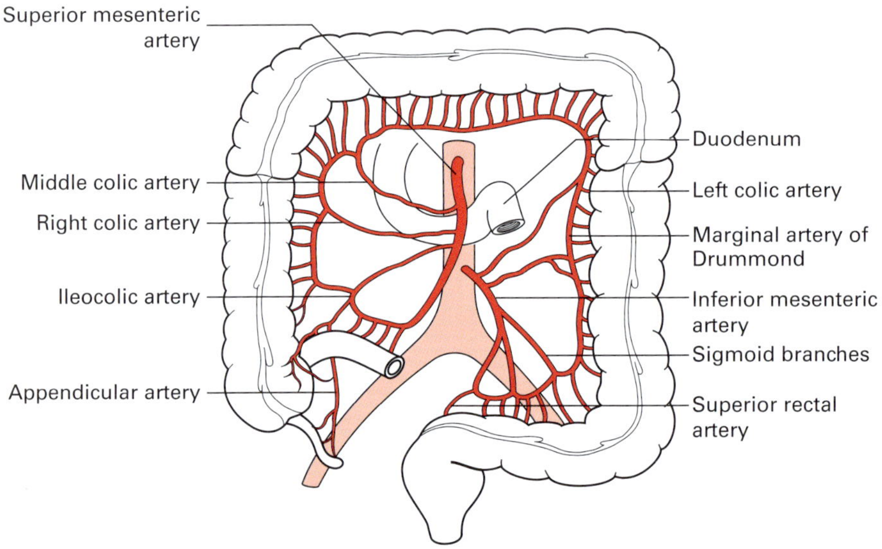

Fig. 64 The superior and inferior mesenteric arteries and their branches.

The portal system of veins

The portal venous system drains blood to the liver from the abdominal part of the alimentary canal (excluding the anal canal), the spleen, the pancreas and the gall bladder and its ducts.

The distal tributaries of this system correspond to, and accompany, the branches of the coeliac and the superior and inferior mesenteric arteries enumerated previously; only proximally (Fig. 65) does the arrangement differ.

The *inferior mesenteric vein* ascends above the point of origin of its artery to enter the splenic vein behind the pancreas.

The *superior mesenteric vein* joins the splenic vein behind the neck of the pancreas in the transpyloric plane to form the *portal vein*, which ascends behind the first part of the duodenum into the anterior wall of the foramen of Winslow and thence to the porta hepatis. Here the portal vein divides into right and left branches and breaks up into capillaries running between the lobules of the liver. These capillaries drain into the radicles of the hepatic vein through which they empty into the IVC.

Connections between the portal and systemic venous systems

Normally, portal venous blood traverses the liver as described previously and empties into the systemic venous circulation via the hepatic vein and IVC. This pathway may be blocked by a variety of causes, which are classified into:

- prehepatic, e.g. thrombosis or congenital obliteration of the portal vein;
- hepatic, e.g. cirrhosis of the liver;
- posthepatic, e.g. congenital stenosis of the hepatic veins.

If obstruction from any of these causes occurs, the portal venous pressure rises (*portal hypertension*) and collateral pathways open up between the portal and systemic venous systems.

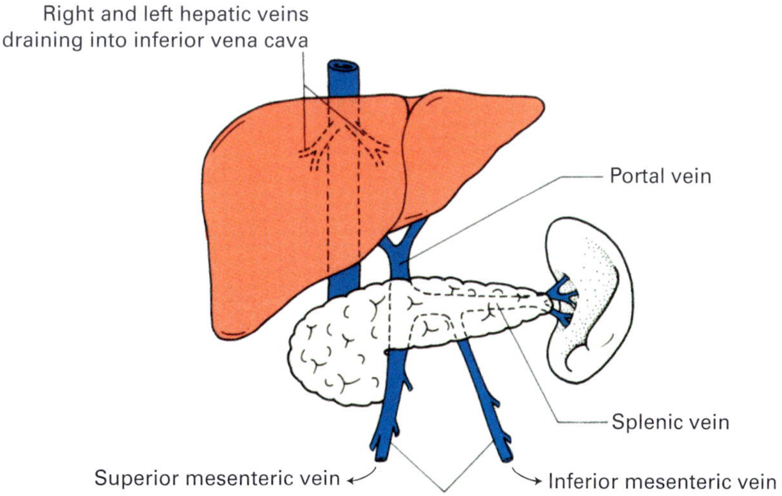

Fig. 65 The composition of the portal system.

These natural venous communications (known as portasystemic venous anastomoses) are:

1 between the oesophageal branch of the left gastric vein and the oesophageal veins of the azygos system (these *oesophageal varices* are the cause of the severe haematemesis that may occur in portal hypertension);
2 between the superior rectal branch of the inferior mesenteric vein and the inferior rectal veins draining into the internal iliac vein via its internal pudendal tributary;
3 between the portal tributaries in the mesentery and mesocolon and the retroperitoneal veins communicating with the renal, lumbar and phrenic veins;
4 between the portal branches in the liver and the veins of the abdominal wall via veins passing along the falciform ligament from the umbilicus (which may result in the formation of a cluster of dilated veins which radiate from the navel and which are called the *caput medusae*);
5 between the portal branches in the liver and the veins of the diaphragm across the bare area of the liver.

A striking feature of operations upon patients with portal hypertension is the extraordinary dilatation of every available channel between the two systems that renders such procedures extremely challenging and bloody.

Lymphatic drainage of the intestine (Fig. 66)

The arrangement of lymph nodes is relatively uniform throughout the small and large intestine. Numerous small nodes lying near, or even on, the bowel wall drain to intermediately placed and rather larger nodes along the vessels in the mesentery or mesocolon and thence to clumps of nodes situated near the origins of the superior and inferior mesenteric arteries. From these, efferent vessels link up to drain into the cisterna chyli.

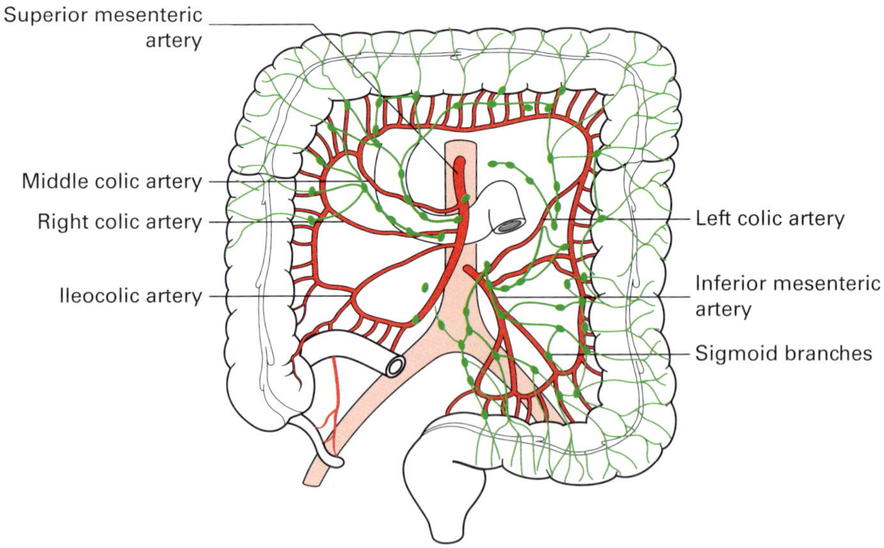

Fig. 66 Lymphatics and lymph nodes of the large intestine (coloured green).

The lymphatic drainage field of each segment of bowel corresponds fairly accurately to its blood supply. High ligation of the vessels to the involved segment of bowel with removal of a wide surrounding segment of mesocolon will, therefore, remove the lymph nodes draining the area. Division of the middle colic vessels and a resection of a generous wedge of transverse mesocolon, for example, would be performed for a malignant neoplasm of transverse colon.

The structure of the alimentary canal

The alimentary canal is made up of mucosa demarcated by the *muscularis mucosae* from the *submucosa*, the *muscle coat* and the *serosa* – the last being absent where the gut is extraperitoneal.

The oesophageal mucosa and that of the lower anal canal is lined with stratified squamous epithelium; elsewhere, it is columnar epithelium. At the cardio-oesophageal junction this transition is quite sharp, although occasionally columnar epithelium may line the lower oesophagus.

The gastric mucosa bears simple crypt-like glands projecting down to the muscularis mucosae. The pyloric antrum secretes an alkaline juice containing mucus and the hormone gastrin. The body of the stomach secretes pepsin and also HCl, the latter from the *oxyntic cells* lying sandwiched deeply between the surface cells. The stomach mucosa also produces intrinsic factor.

The mucosa of the duodenum and small intestine, as well as bearing crypt-like glands, projects into the bowel lumen in villous processes which greatly increase its surface area. The duodenum is distinguished by its crypts extending deep through the muscularis mucosae and opening into an extensive system of acini in the submucosa termed *Brunner's glands*.

The mucosa of the large intestine is lined by a profusion of mucus-secreting goblet cells; there are no villi.

The muscle layer (*muscularis propria*) of the alimentary tract is made up of an inner circular layer and an outer longitudinal layer of muscle. In the upper two-thirds of the oesophagus and at the anal margin this muscle is striated and voluntary; elsewhere it is smooth and involuntary. The stomach wall is reinforced by an innermost oblique coat of muscle, and the colon is characterized by the condensation of its outer longitudinal layer into three discrete bands termed taeniae coli that run along the entire length of the colon.

The autonomic nerve plexuses of Meissner and Auerbach lie, respectively, in the submucosal layer and in the muscle layer (between the inner circular and outer longitudinal muscle coats).

The development of the intestine and its congenital abnormalities (Fig. 67)

The primitive endodermal tube of the gut is divided into:

1 the foregut (supplied by the coeliac axis) extending as far as the entry of the bile duct into the duodenum;

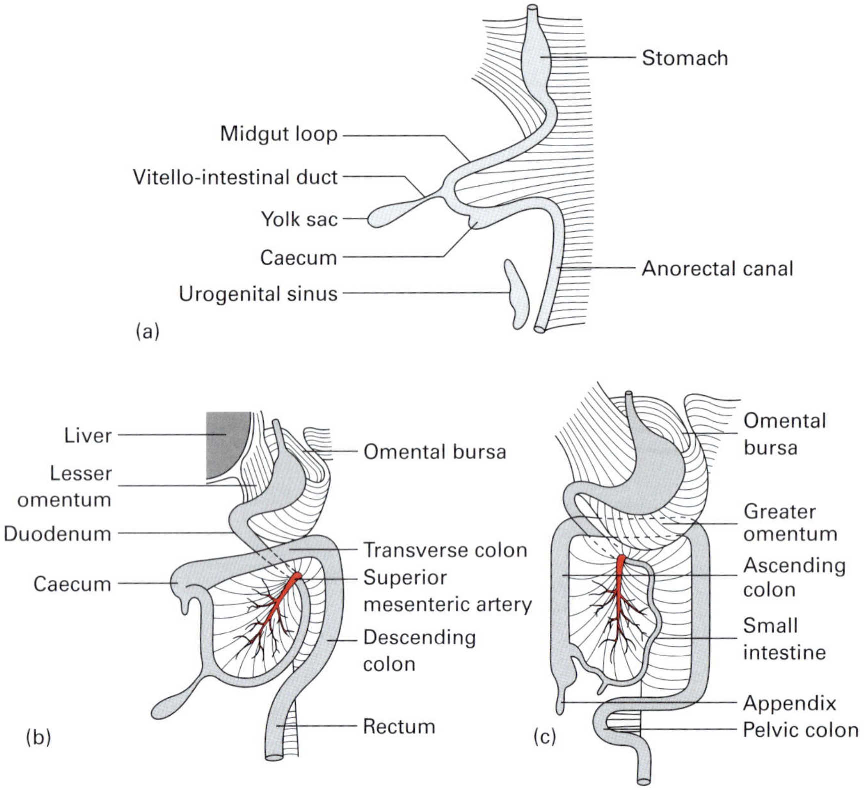

Fig. 67 Stages in rotation of the bowel. (a) The prolapsed midgut loop, seen in lateral view. (b) The midgut returns to the abdomen. (c) The caecum descends to its definitive position. Note the completion of stomach rotation with the formation of the lesser sac (omental bursa).

2 the midgut (supplied by the superior mesenteric artery) continuing as far as the distal transverse colon;

3 the hindgut (supplied by the inferior mesenteric artery) extending thence to the ectodermal part of the anal canal.

At an early stage rapid proliferation of the gut wall obliterates its lumen and this is followed by subsequent recanalization.

The foregut becomes rotated with the development of the lesser sac so that the original right wall of the stomach comes to form its posterior surface and the left wall its anterior surface. The vagi rotate with the stomach and therefore lie anteriorly and posteriorly to it at the oesophageal hiatus.

This rotation swings the duodenum to the right and the mesentery of this organ then blends with the peritoneum of the posterior abdominal wall – this blending process is termed *zygosis*.

The midgut enlarges rapidly in the 5 week fetus, becomes too large to be contained within the abdomen and herniates into the umbilical cord. The apex of this herniated bowel is continuous with the vitello-intestinal duct and the yolk sac, but this connection, even at this early stage of fetal life, is already reduced to a fibrous strand.

The axis of this herniated loop of gut is formed by the superior mesenteric artery, which demarcates a cephalic and a caudal limb. The cephalic element develops into the proximal small intestine; the caudal segment differentiates into the terminal 62 cm (2 feet) of ileum, the caecum and the colon as far as the junction of the middle and left thirds of the transverse colon.

A bud that develops on the caudal segment indicates the site of subsequent formation of the caecum; it may well be that this bud delays the return of the caudal limb in favour of the cephalic gut during the subsequent reduction of the herniated bowel.

At 10 weeks this return of the bowel into the abdominal cavity commences. The midgut loop first rotates anticlockwise through 90°.

The cephalic limb returns first, passing upwards and to the left into the space left available by the bulky liver. In doing so, this midgut passes *behind* the superior mesenteric artery (which thus comes to cross the third part of the duodenum) and also pushes the hindgut – the definitive distal colon – over to the left.

When the caudal limb returns, it lies in the only space remaining to it, superficial to, and above, the small intestine with the caecum lying immediately below the liver.

The caecum then descends into its definitive position in the right iliac fossa, dragging the colon with it. The transverse colon thus comes to lie in front of the superior mesenteric vessels and the small intestine.

Finally, the mesenteries of the ascending and descending parts of the colon blend with the posterior abdominal wall peritoneum by a process termed *zygosis*. This embryological fusion of peritoneal surfaces is of major surgical importance. Thus, in mobilizing the right or left colon, an incision is made along this avascular line of zygosis lateral to the bowel, allowing it to be mobilized with its mesocolon and blood supply. In a similar fashion, the duodenum, head of pancreas and termination of the common bile duct can be mobilized bloodlessly by incising the peritoneum along the right border of the duodenum – Kocher's manoeuvre (see page 82). Further mobilization of the third part of the duodenum, together with its second part and the pancreas, allows exposure of the abdominal aorta as far proximally as the level of its crossing by the left renal vein (see Fig. 108).

Numerous anomalies may occur in the highly complex developmental process.

1 *Atresia* or *stenosis of the bowel* may result from failure of recanalization of the lumen. Another cause of this may be damage to the blood supply to the bowel within the fetal umbilical hernia with consequent ischaemic changes. *Imperforate anus* – see page 87.

2 *Meckel's diverticulum* represents the remains of the embryonic vitello-intestinal duct (communication between the primitive midgut and yolk sac) and is, therefore, always on the anti-mesenteric border of the bowel. As an approximation to the truth it can be said to occur in 2% of subjects, twice as often in males as in females, to be situated at 62 cm (2 feet) from the ileocaecal junction and to be 5 cm (2 in) long. In fact, it may occur anywhere from 15 cm (6 in) to 3.5 m (12 feet) from the terminal ileum and may vary from a tiny stump to a 15 cm (6 in) long sac. Occasionally, the diverticulum ends in a whip-like solid strand.

As well as a diverticulum – the commonest form – this duct may persist as a fistula or band connecting the intestine to the umbilicus, as a cyst hanging from the anti-mesenteric border of the ileum or as a 'raspberry tumour' at the umbilicus, formed by the red mucosa of a persistent umbilical extremity of the diverticulum pouting at the navel (Fig. 68).

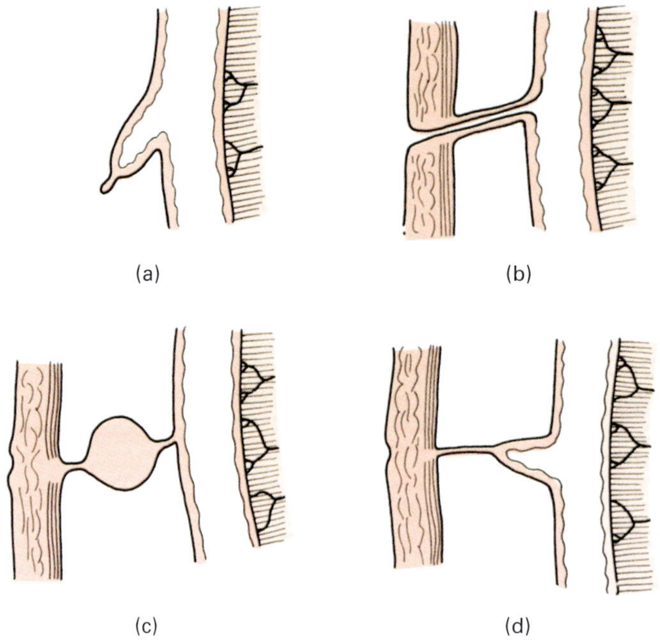

Fig. 68 Abnormalities associated with persistence of the vitello-intestinal tract. (a) Meckel's diverticulum. (b) Patent vitello-intestinal duct. (c) Cyst within a fibrous cord passing from the anti-mesenteric border of the intestine to the umbilicus. (d) Meckel's diverticulum with a terminal filament passing to the umbilicus.

The mucosa lining the diverticulum may contain islands of peptic epithelium with oxyntic (acid secreting) cells. Peptic ulceration of adjacent intestinal epithelium may then occur with haemorrhage or perforation.

3 The caecum may fail to descend; the peritoneal fold which normally seals it in the right iliac fossa passes, instead, across the duodenum and causes a neonatal intestinal obstruction. The mesentery of the small intestine in such a case is left as a narrow pedicle, which allows volvulus of the whole small intestine to occur (*volvulus neonatorum*).

4 Occasionally, reversed rotation occurs, in which the transverse colon comes to lie *behind* the superior mesenteric vessels with the duodenum in front of them; this may again be accompanied by extrinsic duodenal obstruction due to a peritoneal fold.

5 *Exomphalos* is persistence of the midgut herniation at the umbilicus after birth.

The gastrointestinal adnexae: liver, gall bladder and its ducts, pancreas and spleen

The liver (Fig. 69)

This is the largest solid organ in the body. It is related by its domed upper surface to the diaphragm, which separates it from the pleura, lungs, pericardium and heart. Its postero-inferior (or visceral) surface overlaps the abdominal oesophagus, the stomach

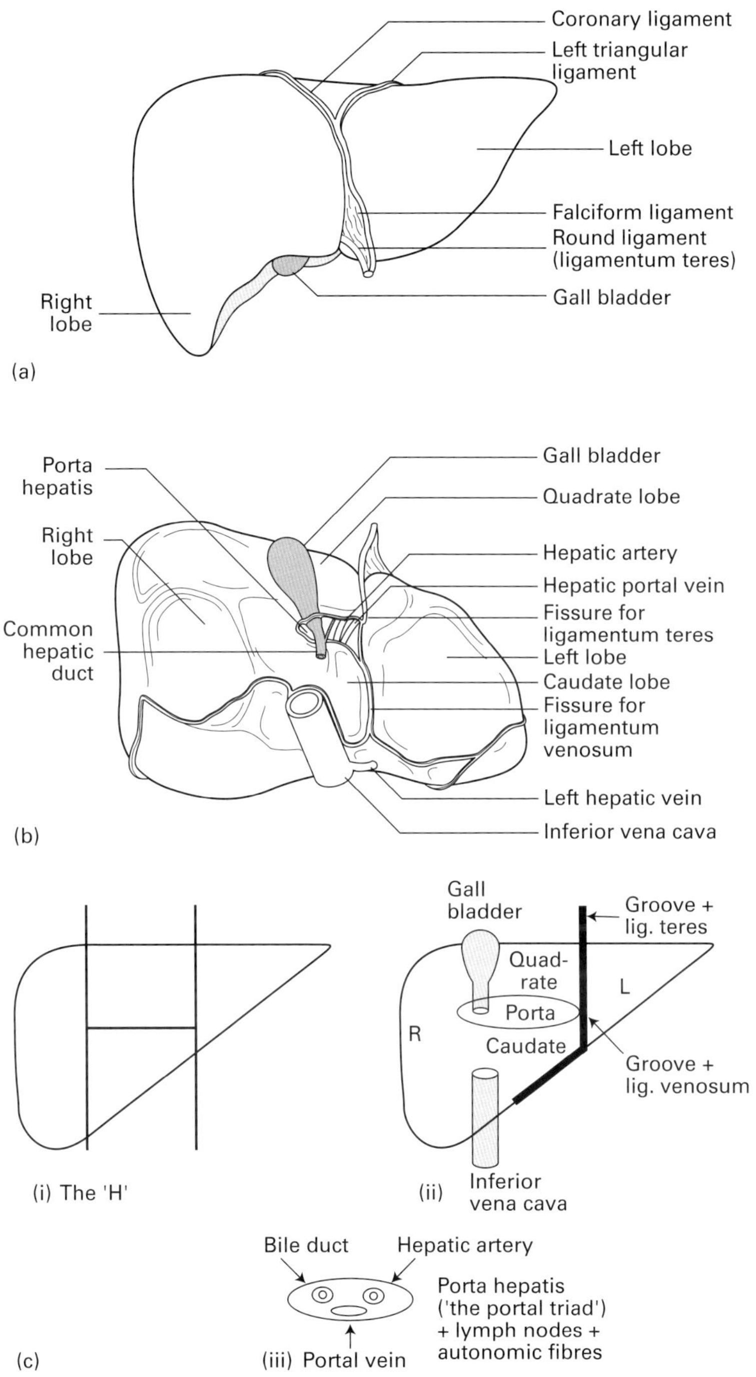

Fig. 69 The liver and its subdivisions. (a) Anterior aspect. (b) Inferior aspect. (c) The 'H'.

and the duodenum, the hepatic flexure of the colon and the right kidney and suprarenal, besides carrying the gall bladder.

The liver is divided into a larger right and small left lobe, separated superiorly by the falciform ligament and postero-inferiorly by an 'H'-shaped arrangement of fossae (Fig. 69b,c):

- *anteriorly and to the right* – the fossa for the gall bladder;
- *posteriorly and to the right* – the groove in which the IVC lies embedded;
- *anteriorly and to the left* – the fissure containing the ligamentum teres;
- *posteriorly and to the left* – the fissure for the ligamentum venosum.

The cross-bar of the 'H' is the *porta hepatis*. Two subsidiary lobes are marked out on the visceral aspect of the liver between the limbs of this 'H' – the *quadrate lobe* in front and the *caudate lobe* behind.

The *ligamentum teres* is the obliterated remains of the left umbilical vein which, *in utero*, carries oxygenated blood from the placenta to the fetus. The *ligamentum venosum* is the fibrous remnant of the fetal *ductus venosus* which shunts oxygenated blood from this left umbilical vein to the IVC, bypassing the liver. It is easy enough to realize, then, that the grooves for the ligamentum teres, ligamentum venosum and IVC, representing as they do the pathway of a fetal venous trunk, are continuous in the adult. See also 'The fetal circulation', page 42.

Lying in the porta hepatis (which is 5 cm (2 in) wide) are:

1 *the common hepatic duct* – anteriorly and to the right;
2 *the hepatic artery* – anteriorly and to the left;
3 *the portal vein* – posteriorly.

As well as these, autonomic nerve fibres (sympathetic from the coeliac axis and parasympathetic from the vagus), lymphatic vessels and lymph nodes are found there.

Peritoneal attachments

The liver is enclosed in peritoneum except for a small posterior bare area, demarcated by the peritoneum from the diaphragm reflected onto it as the upper and lower layers of the *coronary ligament*. To the right, these fuse to form the *right triangular ligament*.

The *falciform ligament* ascends to the liver from the umbilicus, somewhat to the right of the midline, and bears the ligamentum teres in its free border. The ligamentum teres passes into its fissure in the inferior surface of the liver, while the falciform ligament passes over the dome of the liver and then divaricates. Its right limb joins the upper layer of the coronary ligament and its left limb stretches out as the long narrow *left triangular ligament* which, when traced posteriorly and to the right, joins the lesser omentum in the upper end of the fissure for the ligamentum venosum.

The *lesser omentum* arises from the fissures of the porta hepatis and the ligamentum venosum and passes as a double-layered sheet to be attached along the anterior and posterior surfaces of the lesser curvature of the stomach.

Structure

The liver is made up of lobules, each with a solitary central vein that is a tributary of the hepatic vein, which, in turn, drains into the IVC. In the spaces between the lobules, termed *portal canals*, lie branches of the hepatic artery (bringing systemic blood) and the portal vein, both of which drain into the central vein by means of sinusoids traversing the lobule.

Branches of the *hepatic duct* also lie in the portal canals and receive fine bile capillaries from the liver lobules.

Segmental anatomy

The gross anatomical division of the liver into a right and left lobe, demarcated by a line passing from the attachment of the falciform ligament on its anterior surface to the fissures for the ligamentum teres and ligamentum venosum on its posterior surface, is simply a gross anatomical descriptive term with little functional significance. Studies of the distribution of the hepatic blood vessels and ducts have indicated that the true physiological division of the liver is into right and left functional 'hemi-livers' demarcated by a plane that passes through the fossa of the gall bladder and the fossa of the IVC. Although these two functional parts are not demarcated by any visible external line or feature on the dome of the liver, each has its own arterial and portal venous blood supply and separate biliary drainage. In this 'functional division' the quadrate lobe comes to be part of the left functional part of the liver along with the anatomical left lobe, while the caudate lobe lies partly in the left and partly in the right hemi-liver (Fig. 70).

The right and left physiological lobes of the liver can be further subdivided into a number of segments, four for each lobe (Fig. 70c). The student need not learn the details of these, but of course to the hepatic surgeon, carrying out a partial resection of the liver, knowledge of these segments, with their individual blood supply and biliary drainage, is of paramount importance.

At the hilum of the liver, the hepatic artery, portal vein and bile duct each divide into right and left branches, and there is little or no anastomosis between the divisions on the two sides (Fig. 71). From the region of the porta hepatis, the branches pass laterally and spread upwards and downwards throughout the liver substance, defining the morphological left and right lobes.

The hepatic veins (Figs 70c, 72)

These veins are large vessels and their distribution does not mirror that of the portal venous, hepatic arterial and bile duct systems already described. There are three major hepatic veins; a right vein, a central vein and a left vein. These pass upwards and backwards to drain into the IVC at the superior margin of the liver. Their terminations are somewhat variable, but usually the central hepatic vein enters the left hepatic vein near its termination. In other specimens it may drain directly into the cava. In addition, small hepatic venous tributaries run directly backwards from the substance of the liver to enter the vena cava more at points inferior to the levels at which the main hepatic veins join the IVC. Although these are not of great functional importance they do pose a challenge to the surgeon during the course of a right hepatic lobectomy.

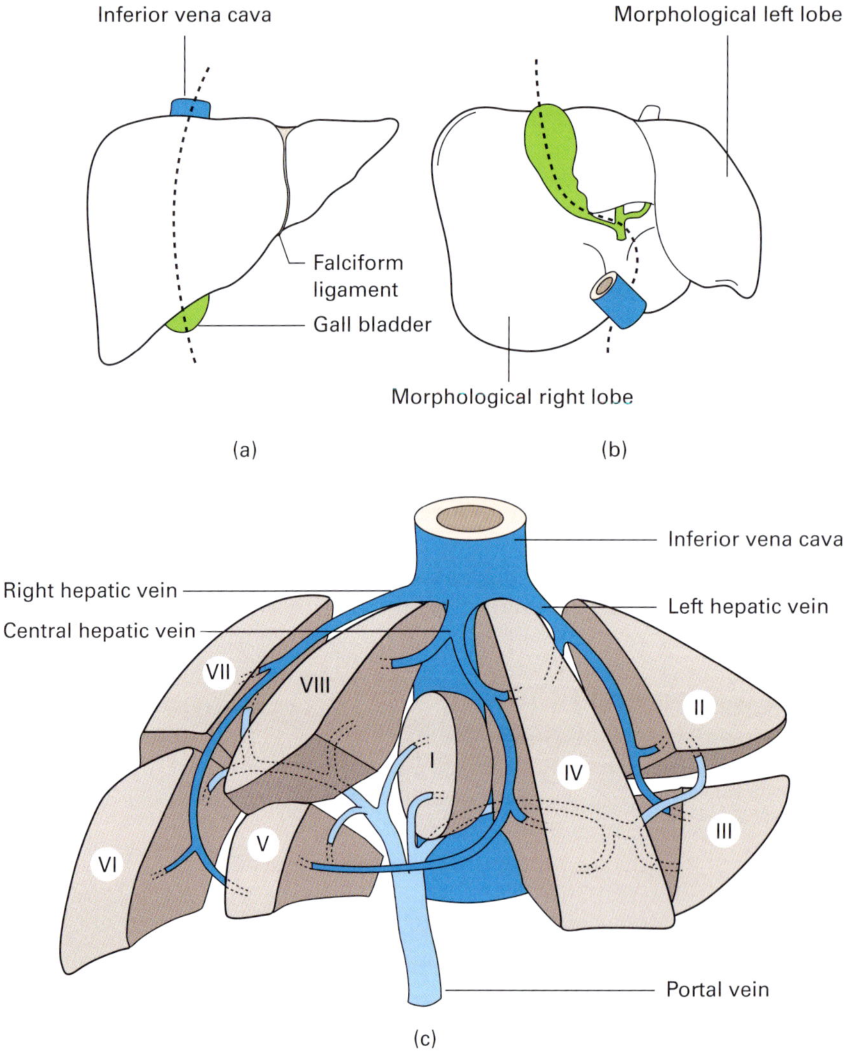

Fig. 70 The 'physiological' right and left lobes of the liver shown separated by the dotted line: (a) anterior and (b) inferior aspect. Note that the quadrate lobe is functionally a part of the left hemi-liver while the caudate lobe belongs to both the right and left parts of the liver. (c) The further segmental divisions of the liver.

The three principal hepatic veins have three zones of drainage corresponding roughly to the right, the middle and the left thirds of the liver. The plane defined by the falciform ligament corresponds to the boundary of the zones drained by the left and middle hepatic veins. Unfortunately for the surgeon, the middle hepatic vein lies just at the line of the principal plane of the liver between its right and left physiological lobes, and it is this fact which complicates the operation of right or left hepatic resection (Fig. 72).

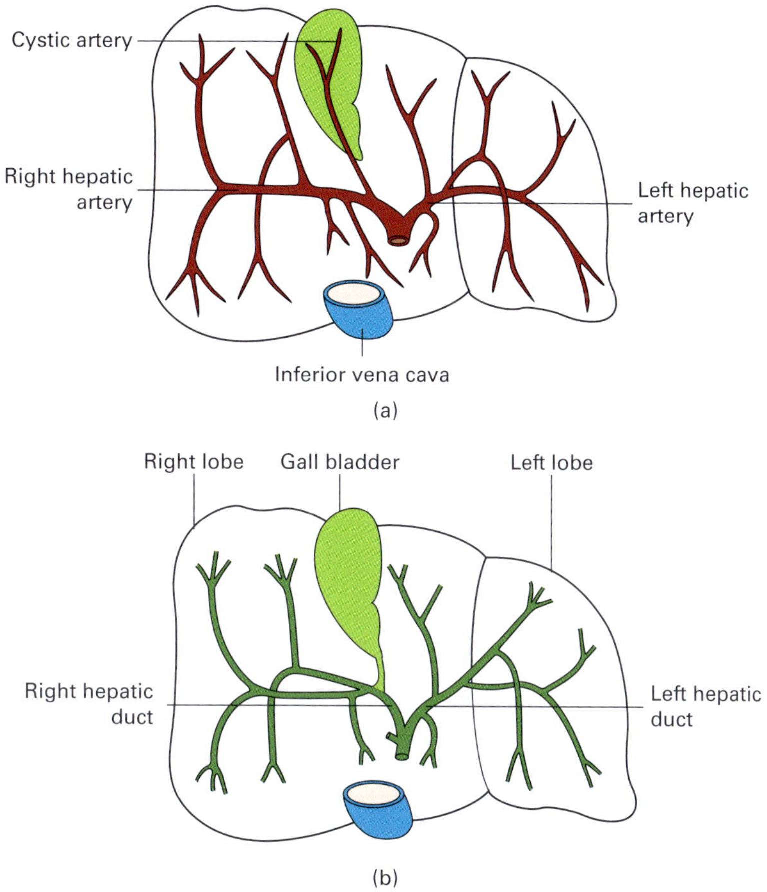

Fig. 71 (a) Distribution of hepatic arteries. (b) Distribution of hepatic biliary ducts. Note that the quadrate lobe is supplied exclusively by the left hepatic artery and drained by the left hepatic duct. The caudate lobe is supplied by each.

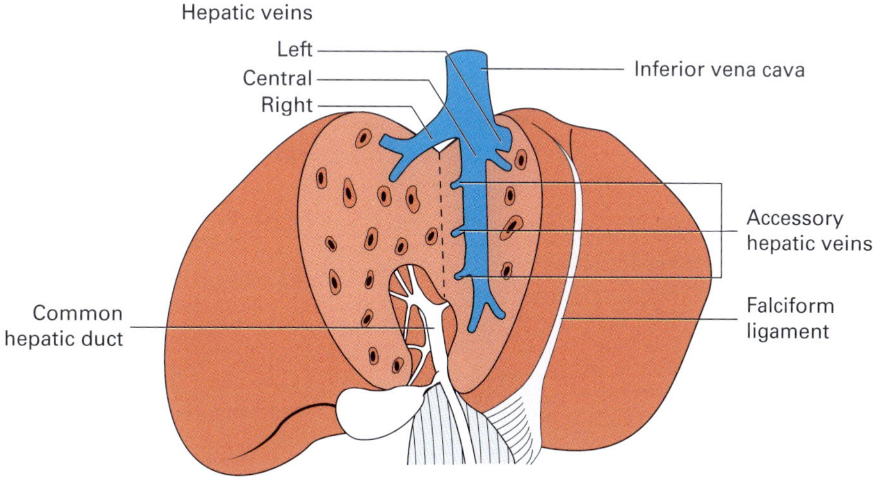

Fig. 72 Liver split open to demonstrate the tributaries of the hepatic vein.

The biliary system (Fig. 73)

The *right* and *left hepatic ducts* fuse in the porta hepatis to form the *common hepatic duct* (4 cm (1.5 in)). This joins with the *cystic duct* (4 cm (1.5 in)), draining the gall bladder, to form the *common bile duct* (10 cm (4 in)). The common bile duct commences approximately 2.5 cm (1 in) above the duodenum, then passes behind it to open at a papilla on the medial aspect of the second part of the duodenum. In this course the common duct either lies in a groove in the posterior aspect of the head of the pancreas or is actually buried in its substance.

As a rule, the termination of the common bile duct and that of the main pancreatic duct (of Wirsung) opens into a common vestibule, the *ampulla of Vater*, whose opening into the postero-medial wall of the second part of the duodenum is guarded by the *sphincter of Oddi*. Occasionally, the bile and pancreatic ducts open separately into the duodenum.

The common hepatic duct and the supraduodenal part of the common bile duct lie in the free edge of the lesser omentum, where they are related as follows (Fig. 47):

- *bile duct* – anterior to the right;
- *hepatic artery* – anterior to the left;
- *portal vein* – posterior;
- *IVC* – still more posterior, separated from the portal vein by the foramen of Winslow.

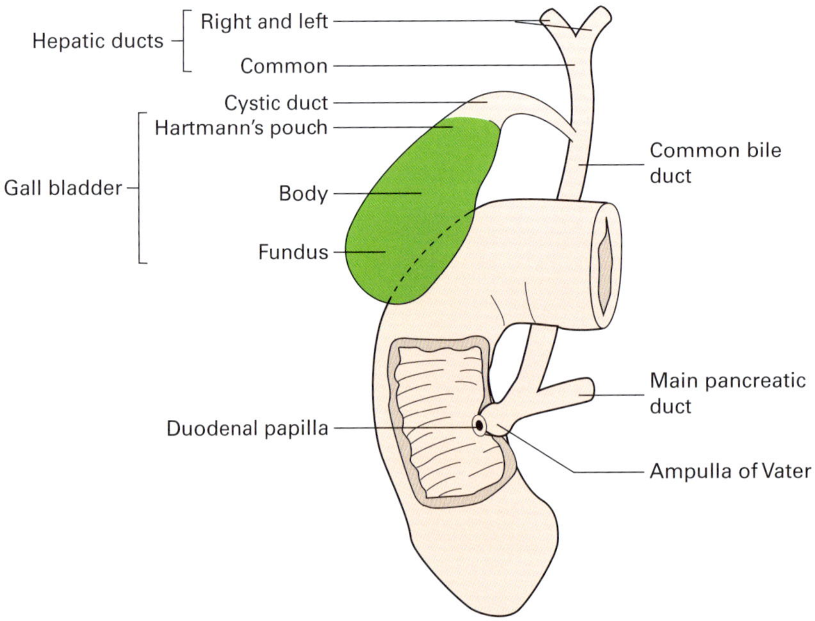

Fig. 73 The gall bladder and its duct system. (The anterior wall of the second part of the duodenum has been removed.)

The gall bladder (Fig. 73)

The gall bladder normally holds approximately 50 ml of bile and acts as a bile concentrator and reservoir. It also secretes mucus from the goblet cells in its wall. It lies in a fossa separating the right and quadrate lobes of the liver and is related inferiorly to the duodenum and transverse colon. (An inflamed gall bladder may occasionally ulcerate into either of these structures.)

For descriptive purposes, the organ is divided into the fundus, body and neck, the last opening into the cystic duct. In dilated and pathological gall bladders there is frequently a pouch present on the ventral aspect just proximal to the neck termed *Hartmann's pouch* in which gallstones may become lodged.

Blood supply (Fig. 74)

The gall bladder is supplied by the cystic artery (a branch usually of the right hepatic artery), which lies in the triangle made by the liver, the cystic duct and the common hepatic duct (Calot's triangle). Other vessels derived from the hepatic artery pass to the gall bladder from its bed in the liver. Interestingly, only rarely is there an accompanying vein to the cystic artery. Small veins pass from the gall bladder through its bed directly into tributaries of the right portal vein within the liver.

Nerve supply

The gall bladder and its ducts are supplied by afferent sympathetic (sensory) fibres from T7 via the splanchnic nerves. Biliary pain is experienced in the right upper abdomen and typically is referred to the lower pole of the right scapula (see also page 423). Motor fibres are conveyed in the hepatic branch of the anterior vagal trunk (Xth cranial nerve). Stimulation of the vagus by the sight, smell and taste of food results in contraction of the gall bladder.

Structure

The gall bladder wall and the sphincter of Oddi contain muscle, but there are only scattered muscle fibres throughout the remaining biliary duct system. The mucosa is lined throughout by columnar cells and bears mucus-secreting glands.

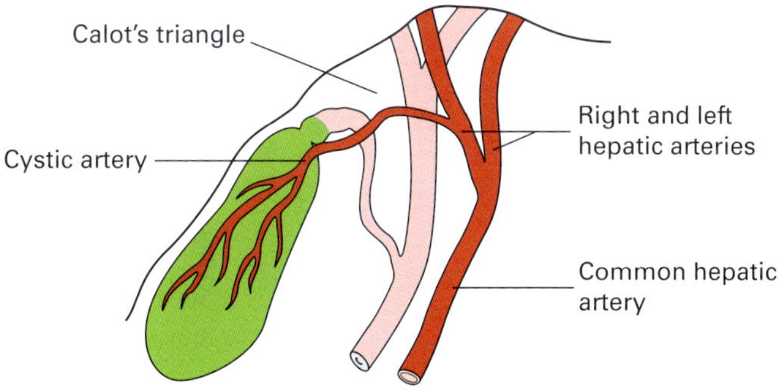

Fig. 74 The arterial supply of the gall bladder and Calot's triangle.

Development

The gall bladder and ducts are subject to numerous anatomical variations which are best understood by considering their embryological development. A diverticulum grows out from the ventral wall of the duodenum which differentiates into the hepatic ducts and the liver (see Fig. 76). Another diverticulum from the side of the hepatic duct bud forms the gall bladder and cystic duct.

Some variations are shown in Fig. 75.

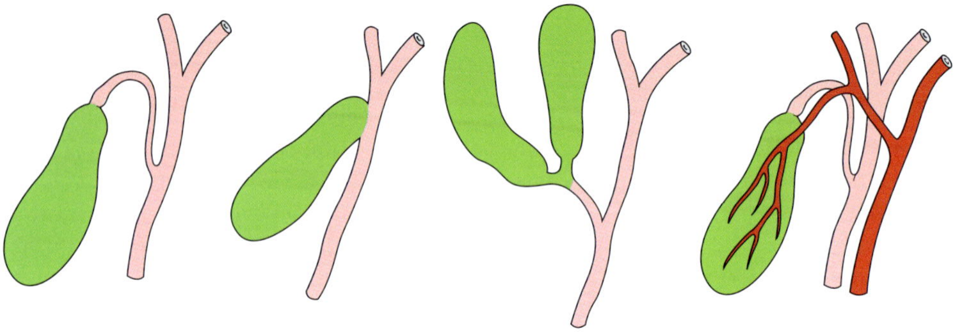

(a) (b) (c) (d)

Fig. 75 Some variations in biliary anatomy. (a) A long cystic duct joining the hepatic duct low down behind the duodenum. (b) Absence of the cystic duct – the gall bladder opens directly into the common hepatic duct. (c) A double gall bladder, the result of a rare bifid embryonic diverticulum from the hepatic duct. (d) The right hepatic artery crosses *in front* of the common hepatic duct; this occurs in 25% of cases.

CLINICAL FEATURES

1 Errors in gall bladder surgery are frequently the result of failure to appreciate the variations in the anatomy of the biliary system; it is important, therefore, before dividing any structures and removing the gall bladder, to have all three biliary ducts clearly identified, together with the cystic and hepatic arteries. The cystic artery is constantly found in Calot's triangle (Fig. 74), formed by the cystic duct, the common hepatic duct and the inferior aspect of the liver.

2 Haemorrhage during cholecystectomy may be controlled by compressing the hepatic artery (which gives off the cystic branch) between the finger and thumb where it lies in the anterior wall of the foramen of Winslow (Pringle's manoeuvre) (Fig. 47).

3 Gangrene of the gall bladder is rare because even if the cystic artery becomes thrombosed in acute cholecystitis there is a rich secondary blood supply coming in from the liver bed. Gangrene may occur in the unusual event of a gall bladder on an abnormally long mesentery undergoing torsion, which will destroy both its sources of blood supply.

4 Stones in the common duct can usually be removed endoscopically using a Dormia basket introduced after dividing the sphincter of Oddi. At other times, the common bile duct is explored via an incision in its supraduodenal portion. Sometimes a stone impacted at the ampulla of Vater must be approached via an incision in the second part of the duodenum. This last approach is also used when it is necessary to divide the sphincter of Oddi or to remove a tumour arising at the termination of the common bile duct.

The pancreas (Figs 55, 56)

The pancreas lies retroperitoneally in approximately the transpyloric plane. For descriptive purposes the pancreas is divided into the head, neck, body and tail.

Relations

The head lies in the C-curve of the duodenum and has an inferior projection, the *uncinate process*, which hooks behind the superior mesenteric vessels as these travel from behind the body of the pancreas into the root of the small intestinal mesentery.

Posterior to the pancreas from right to left lie the IVC, the commencement of the portal vein, the aorta (with the superior mesenteric artery arising therefrom), the crura of the diaphragm, the coeliac plexus, the left kidney and suprarenal gland. The tortuous splenic artery runs along the upper border of the pancreas. The splenic vein runs immediately behind the gland, receives the inferior mesenteric vein and joins the superior mesenteric to form the portal vein behind the pancreatic neck (Fig. 65).

To complete this list of important posterior relationships, the common bile duct either lies in a groove in the right extremity of the gland or is embedded in its substance, as it passes to open into the second part of the duodenum.

Anterior to the pancreas lies the lesser sac which separates the pancreas from the stomach. To the left, the pancreatic tail lies against the hilum of the spleen.

Blood supply

Blood is supplied from the splenic and the pancreaticoduodenal arteries; the corresponding veins drain into the portal system.

The lymphatics

The lymphatics drain into nodes which lie along its upper border, in the groove between its head and the duodenum, and along the root of the superior mesenteric vessels.

Structure

The pancreas macroscopically is lobulated and is contained within a fine capsule; these lobules are made up of alveoli of serous secretory cells draining via their ductules into the principal ducts. Between these alveoli lie the insulin-secreting *islets of Langerhans*.

The main duct of the pancreas (Wirsung) (Fig. 56) runs the length of the gland and usually opens at the ampulla of Vater along with the common bile duct; very occasionally, it drains separately into the duodenum.

The *accessory duct* (*of Santorini*) passes from the lower part of the head in front of the main duct, communicates with it and then opens into the duodenum above it. Occasionally it is absent.

Development (Fig. 76)

The pancreas develops from a larger dorsal diverticulum from the duodenum and a smaller ventral outpouching from the side of the common bile duct. The ventral pouch swings round posteriorly to fuse with the lower aspect of the dorsal diverticulum, trapping the superior mesenteric vessels between the two parts.

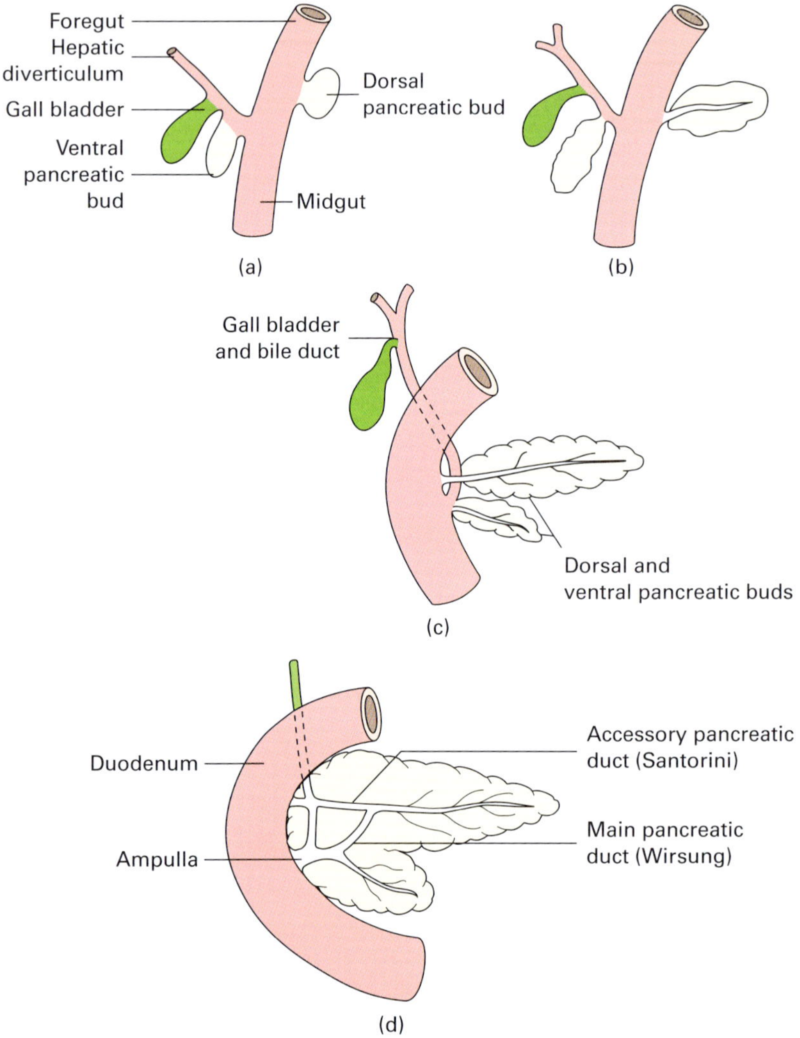

Fig. 76 Development of the intestinal adnexae.

The ducts of the two formative segments of the pancreas then communicate; that of the smaller takes over the main pancreatic flow to form the main duct, leaving the original duct of the larger portion of the gland as the accessory duct.

CLINICAL FEATURES

1 Rarely, the two developing segments of the pancreas completely surround the second part of the duodenum ('annular pancreas') and may produce duodenal obstruction.
2 Note from the posterior relations of the pancreas that a neoplasm of the head of the pancreas will produce obstructive jaundice by compressing the common bile duct. An extensive growth in the body of the gland may cause portal or IVC obstruction.
3 Anterior to the pancreas lies the stomach, separated from it by the lesser sac. This sac may become closed off and distended with fluid either from perforation of a posterior gastric ulcer or from the outpouring of fluid in acute pancreatitis, forming a *pseudocyst of the pancreas*. Such a collection may almost fill the abdominal cavity.

The spleen

The spleen is approximately the size of the cupped hand. It forms the left lateral extremity of the lesser sac. The spleen presents a concave medial surface and a reciprocally convex and rounded lateral surface. The medial surface of the spleen features a hilum through which vessels enter or leave the spleen. Passing from the hilar region of the spleen are two double-layered folds of peritoneum: the *gastrosplenic ligament* passes to the greater curvature of stomach (carrying the short gastric and left gastro-epiploic vessels) and the *splenorenal ligament* extends towards the ventral aspect of the left kidney. The splenorenal ligament conveys the splenic vessels and the tail of the pancreas.

Relations of the spleen (Fig. 77)

- *Posteriorly* – the left hemi-diaphragm, separating it from the pleura, left lung and the 9th, 10th and 11th ribs;
- *Anteriorly* – the stomach;
- *Inferiorly* – the splenic flexure of the colon;
- *Medially* – the lesser sac and the left kidney.

Blood supply

The splenic artery is one of the three main branches of the coeliac axis. While the splenic artery appears perfectly straight in lower animals and even the human infant, in human adults it is tortuous: the only artery to display this feature within the abdominal cavity. The splenic artery is thus easily identified on an aortogram or enhanced CT, as it is the only tortuous artery to be seen in the abdomen. The cause

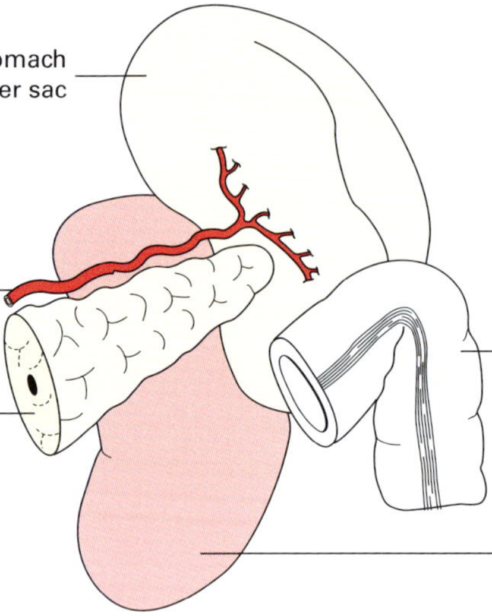

Fig. 77 The spleen and its immediate relations.

or significance of this is unknown. The splenic vein is joined by the superior mesenteric to form the portal vein.

Structure

The spleen represents the largest accumulation of reticulo-endothelial tissue in the body. It has a thin fibrous capsule, to which the peritoneum adheres intimately. The fibrous tissue of the capsule extends into the spleen to form a series of trabeculae between which lies the splenic pulp.

CLINICAL FEATURES

1 In performing a splenectomy the close relationship of the pancreatic tail to the splenic hilum and splenic pedicle must be remembered, lest it be inadvertently injured.
2 Note the close proximity of the lower ribs, the lowest part of the left lung and pleural cavity, the left diaphragm, the left kidney and the splenic flexure of the colon to the spleen; injuries to the left upper abdomen may damage any combination of these structures. Similarly, a stab wound of the posterior left chest may penetrate the diaphragm and tear the spleen. The spleen, with its thin tense capsule, is among the more commonly injured intra-abdominal viscera in blunt trauma to the abdomen.
3 Accessory spleens (one or more) may occur most commonly not only near the hilum but also in the tail of the pancreas, the mesentery of the spleen, the omentum, the small bowel mesentery, the ovary and even the testis. They occur in approximately one in ten subjects and, if left behind, may result in persistence of symptoms following splenectomy for congenital acholuric jaundice or thrombocytopenic purpura.

The urinary tract

The kidneys

The kidneys lie retroperitoneally on the posterior abdominal wall; the right kidney is 1.2 cm (0.5 in) lower than the left, presumably because of its downward displacement by the bulk of the liver. Each measures approximately 11 cm (4.5 in) long, 6 cm (2.5 in) wide and 4 cm (1.5 in) thick.

Relations (Figs 78, 79)

- *Posteriorly* – the diaphragm (separating pleura), quadratus lumborum, psoas, transversus abdominis, the 12th rib and three nerves – the subcostal (T12), iliohypogastric and ilio-inguinal (L1).
- *Anteriorly* – the right kidney is related to the liver, the second part of the duodenum (which may be opened accidentally in performing a right nephrectomy) and the ascending colon. In front of the left kidney lie the stomach, the pancreas and its vessels, the spleen and the descending colon. The suprarenals sit on each side as a cap on the kidney's upper pole.

The medial aspect of the kidney presents a deep vertical slit, the *hilum*, which transmits, from before backwards, the renal vein, the renal artery, the renal pelvis and, usually, a subsidiary branch of the renal artery. Lymphatics and nerves also enter the hilum, the latter being sympathetic, mainly vasomotor, fibres.

The *renal pelvis* is subject to considerable anatomical variations (Fig. 80); it may lie completely outside the substance of the kidney (even to the extent of having part of the major calyces extrarenal) or may be almost buried in the renal hilum. All gradations exist between these extremes. If a calculus is lodged in the renal pelvis, its removal is comparatively simple when this is extrarenal, and it is correspondingly difficult when the pelvis is hidden within the substance of the kidney.

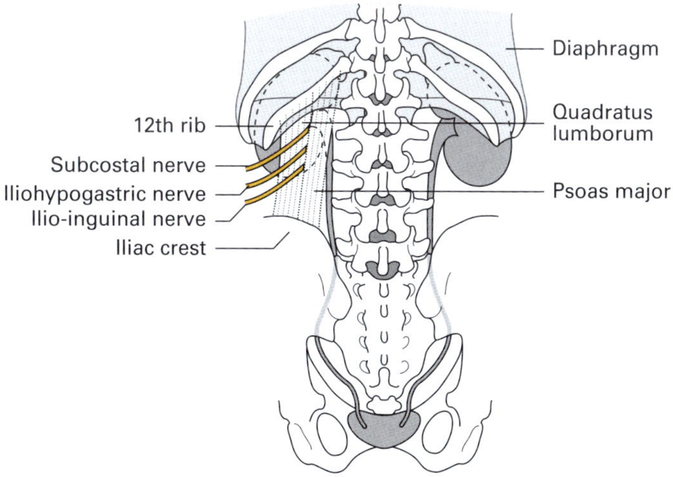

Fig. 78 The posterior relations of the kidney (viewed from behind).

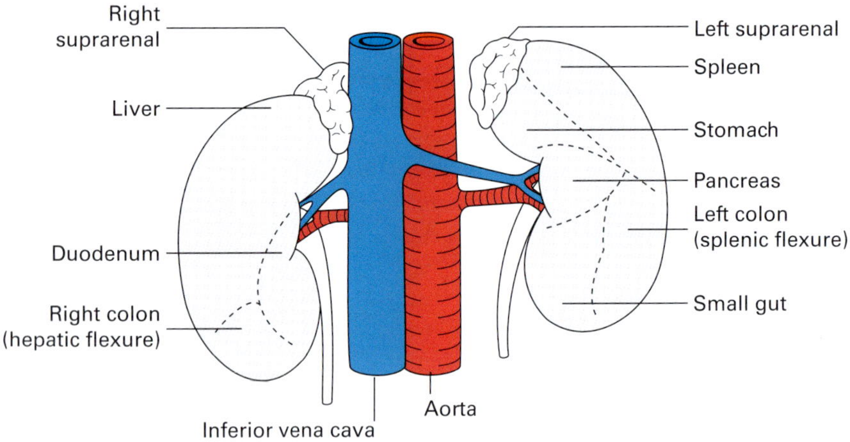

Fig. 79 The anterior relations of the kidneys.

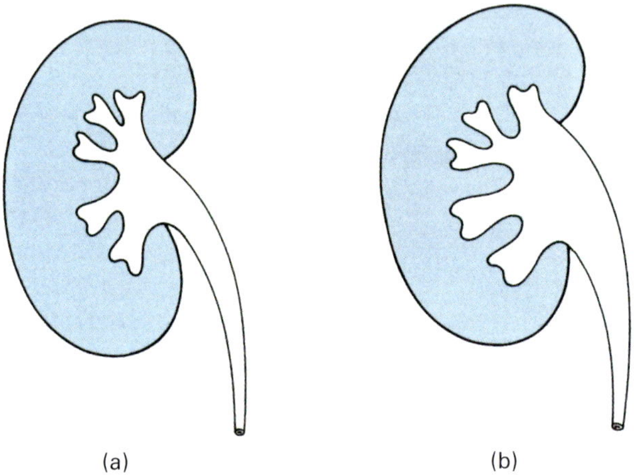

Fig. 80 Variations in the renal pelvis. (a) The pelvis is buried within the renal parenchyma – pyelolithotomy difficult. (b) The pelvis protrudes generously – pyelolithotomy easy.

Within the kidney, the renal pelvis receives two or three *major calyces*, each of which receives a number of *minor calyces*. Each of these, in turn, is indented by a papilla of renal tissue, and it is here that the collecting tubules of the kidney discharge urine into the conducting part of the urinary tract.

Each kidney lies within a fatty cushion (*perinephric fat*) that is contained in the *renal fascia* (Fig. 81). Superiorly, the renal fascia blends with the fascia on the undersurface of the diaphragm. However, just above the upper pole of the kidney, the renal fascia encloses the suprarenal gland within a separate compartment. This allows a nephrectomy to be performed without disturbing the suprarenal gland. Medially, the renal fascia blends with the retroperitoneal fascial layers that extend in front of, and posterior to the aorta and IVC. Laterally, the renal fascia blends with the endoabdominal fascia. Only inferiorly does it remain relatively open – tracking around the ureter into the pelvis.

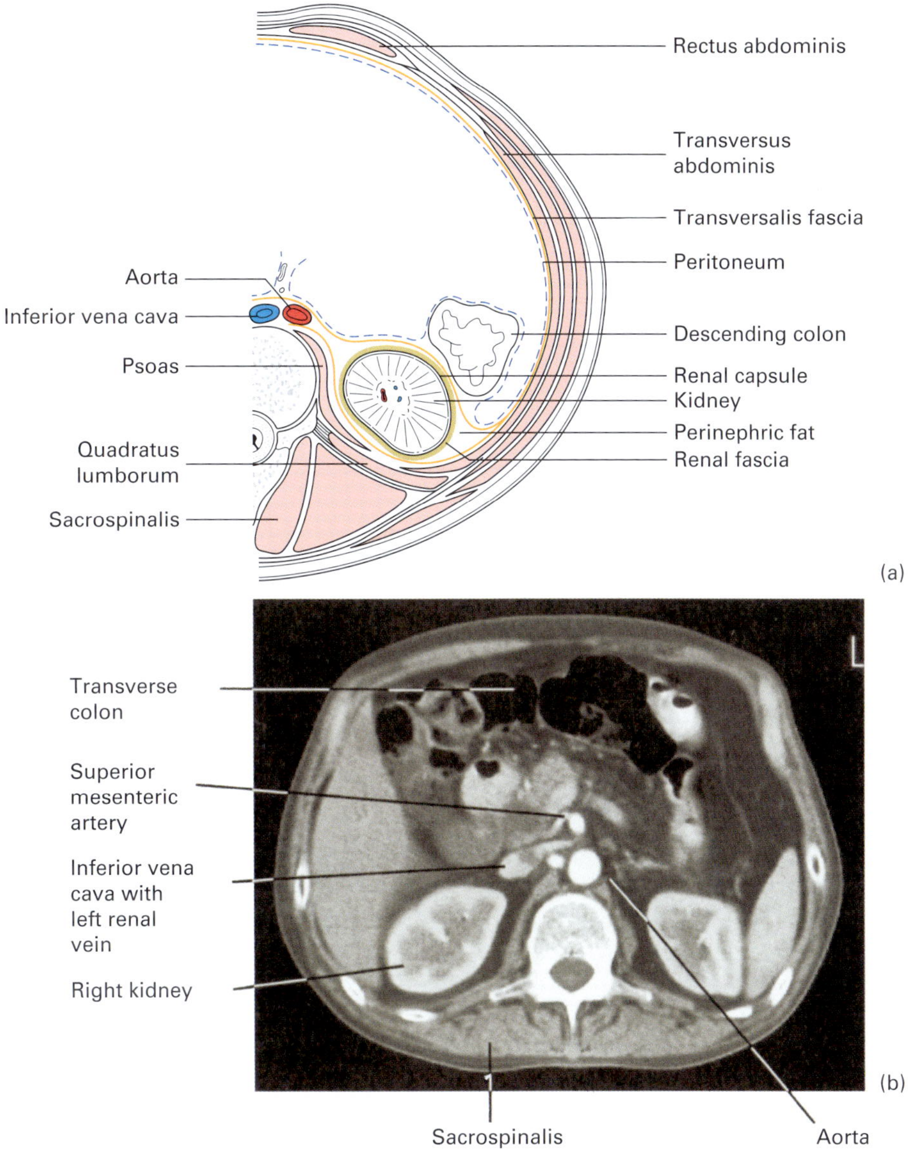

Fig. 81 (a) Transverse section (seen from below) demonstrating the fascial compartments of the kidney. (b) CT scan of the same region. Note that CT scans, by convention, are viewed from below, so that the aorta, for example, is seen on the right side. The blood vessels have been enhanced by an intravenous injection of contrast (Dr Sheila Rankin).

Thus the kidney has three concentric coverings:

1 the outermost covering being the renal fascia;
2 the intermediate covering being the perinephric fat;
3 the innermost covering being the fibrous renal capsule. This capsular layer can be stripped off readily from the surface of a normal kidney but adheres firmly to an organ that is the seat of chronic inflammation.

Blood supply

The *renal arteries (right and left)* arise directly from the abdominal aorta. The *renal veins* (both right and left) drain directly into the IVC. The *left renal vein* passes in front of the aorta immediately below the origin of the superior mesenteric artery to reach the IVC. The *right renal artery* passes behind the IVC to reach the right kidney.

Lymphatic drainage

Lymphatics drain directly to the para-aortic lymph nodes.

CLINICAL FEATURES

1 The highly vascular kidney is not infrequently ruptured by closed trauma, e.g. a kick in the loin. The capsule is torn and blood extravasates into the perinephric fat space. This is usually *'tamponaded'* by the renal fascia, and the bleeding controlled. Only if this fascial layer is ruptured, does haemorrhage continue and surgery may become necessary. The midline attachment of the renal fascia prevents extravasation to the opposite side.

2 In hypermobility of the kidney ('floating kidney'), this organ can be moved up and down in its fascial compartment but not from side to side. To a lesser degree, it is in this plane that the normal kidney moves during respiration.

3 *Exposure of the kidney via the loin.* An oblique incision is usually favoured midway between the 12th rib and the iliac crest, extending laterally from the lateral border of erector spinae. Latissimus dorsi and serratus posterior inferior are divided and the free posterior border of external oblique is identified, enabling this muscle to be split along its fibres. Internal oblique and transversus abdominis are then divided, revealing peritoneum anteriorly, which is pushed forwards. The renal fascial capsule is then brought clearly into view and is opened. The subcostal nerve and vessels are usually encountered in the upper part of the incision and are preserved. If more room is required, the lateral edge of quadratus lumborum may be divided and also the 12th rib excised, care being taken to push up, but not to open, the pleura, which crosses the medial half of the rib.

The ureter

The ureter is 25 cm (10 in) long and comprises its abdominal, pelvic and intravesical portions.

The *abdominal ureter* lies on the medial edge of psoas major (which separates it from the tips of the transverse processes of L2–L5) and then crosses into the pelvis at the bifurcation of the common iliac artery in front of the sacro-iliac joint. Anteriorly, the right ureter is covered at its origin by the second part of the duodenum and then lies lateral to the IVC and behind the posterior peritoneum. It is crossed by the testicular (or ovarian), right colic and ileocolic vessels. The left ureter is crossed by the testicular (or ovarian) and left colic vessels and then passes above the pelvic brim, behind the mesosigmoid and sigmoid colon to cross the common iliac artery immediately above its bifurcation.

The *pelvic ureter* runs on the lateral wall of the pelvis in front of the internal iliac artery to just in front of the ischial spine; it then turns forwards and medially to enter the bladder. In the male, it lies above the seminal vesicle near its termination and is crossed superficially by the vas deferens (see Fig. 85). In the female, the ureter passes above the lateral fornix of the vagina 1.25 cm (0.5 in) lateral to the supravaginal portion of the cervix and lies below the broad ligament and uterine vessels (see Fig. 102).

The *intravesical ureter* passes obliquely through the wall of the bladder for 2 cm (0.75 in); the vesical muscle and obliquity of this course produce, respectively, a sphincteric and valve-like arrangement at the termination of this duct.

Blood supply

The ureter receives a rich segmental blood supply from all available arteries along its course: the aorta, and the renal, testicular (or ovarian), internal iliac and inferior vesical arteries.

CLINICAL FEATURES

1 The ureter is readily identified in life by its thick muscular wall which is seen to undergo worm-like (vermicular) writhing movements, particularly if gently stroked or squeezed.

2 Throughout its abdominal and the upper part of its pelvic course, it adheres to the overlying peritoneum (through which it can be seen in the thin subject), and this fact is used in exposing the ureter – as the parietal peritoneum is dissected upwards, the ureter comes into view sticking to its posterior aspect.

3 The ureter is relatively narrowed at three sites:
- at the junction of the renal pelvis and ureter (pelvi-ureteric junction);
- at the pelvic brim;
- at the ureteric orifice (narrowest of all).

4 A ureteric calculus is likely to lodge at one of these three levels.

5 In searching for a ureteric stone on a plain radiograph of the abdomen, one must imagine the course of the ureter in relation to the bony skeleton (Fig. 82). It lies along the tips of the transverse processes, crosses in front of the sacro-iliac joint, swings out to the ischial spine and then passes medially to the bladder. An opaque shadow along this line is suspicious of calculus. This course of the ureter is readily studied by examining a radiograph showing a radio-opaque ureteric catheter *in situ*.

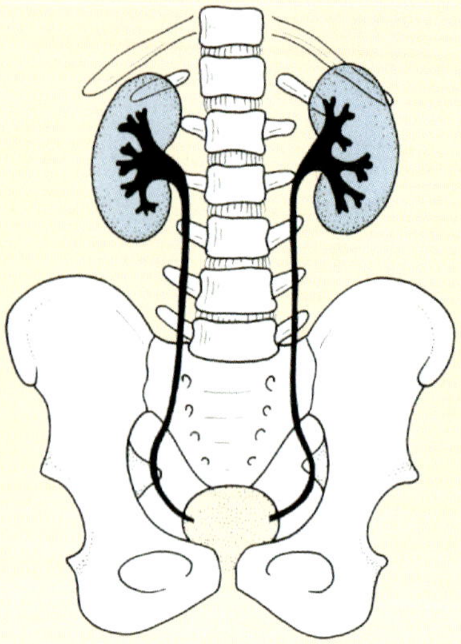

Fig. 82 Drawing from an intravenous pyelogram to show the relationship of the ureters to the bony landmarks.

The embryology and congenital abnormalities of the kidney and ureter (Fig. 83)

The kidney and ureter are mesodermal in origin and develop in an unusual manner of considerable interest to the comparative anatomist.

The *pronephros*, of importance in the lower vertebrates, is transient in humans, but the distal part of its duct receives the tubules of the next renal organ to develop, the *mesonephros*, and now becomes the *mesonephric* or *Wolffian duct*. The mesonephros itself then disappears except for some of its ducts, which form the efferent tubules of the testis. For further details of the fates of the mesonephros and mesonephric duct, see page 154.

A diverticulum then appears at the lower end of the mesonephric duct which develops into the *metanephric duct*; on top of the latter a cap of tissue differentiates to form the definitive kidney or *metanephros*. The metanephric duct develops into the ureter, pelvis, calyces and collecting tubules; the metanephros into the glomeruli and the proximal part of the renal duct system.

The mesonephric duct now loses its renal connection, atrophies in the female (remaining only as the epoophoron) but persists in the male, to become the epididymis and vas deferens.

The kidney first develops in the pelvis and then migrates upwards. Its blood supply is first obtained from the common iliac artery but, during migration, a series of vessels form to supply it, only to involute again when the renal artery takes over this duty.

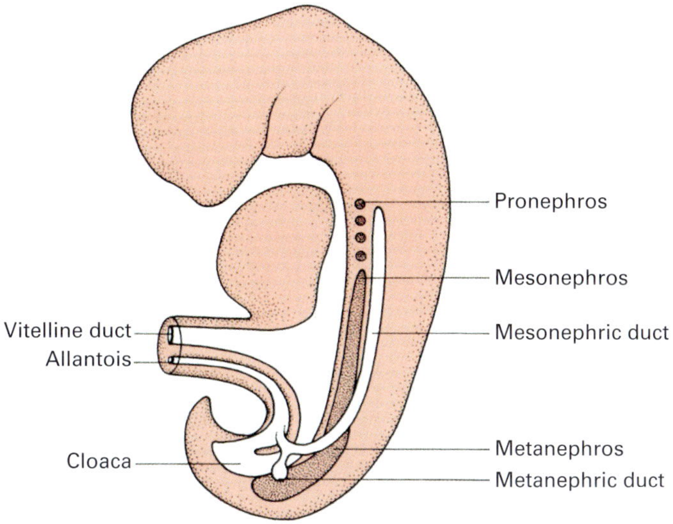

Fig. 83 Development of the pro-, meso- and metanephric systems (after Langman).

Developmental abnormalities (Fig. 84)

1 It is common for one or more distally placed arteries to persist (*aberrant renal arteries*) and one may even run to the kidney from the common iliac artery.
2 Occasionally the kidney will fail to migrate cranially, resulting in a persistent *pelvic kidney*.
3 The two metanephric masses may fuse in development, forming a *horseshoe kidney* linked across the midline.
4 In one in 2400 births there is complete failure of development of one kidney (*congenital absence of the kidney*).
5 *Congenital polycystic kidneys* (which are nearly always bilateral) are believed to result from failure of metanephric tissue to link up with some of the metanephric duct collecting tubules; blind ducts therefore form which subsequently become distended with fluid. This theory of origin does not explain their occasional association with multiple cysts of the liver, pancreas, lung and ovary.
6 The mesonephric duct may give off a double metanephric bud so that two ureters may develop on one or both sides. These ureters may fuse into a single duct anywhere along their course or open separately into the bladder (where the *upper* ureter enters *below* the *lower* ureter).

Rarely, the extra ureter may open ectopically into the vagina or urethra resulting in urinary incontinence.

The urinary bladder (Figs 60, 61, 85)

The capacity of the urinary bladder in the normal adult is variable, the average being approximately 300 ml. In cases of retention of urine, the adult bladder distends from the pelvic cavity into the abdomen, stripping the peritoneum upwards from the

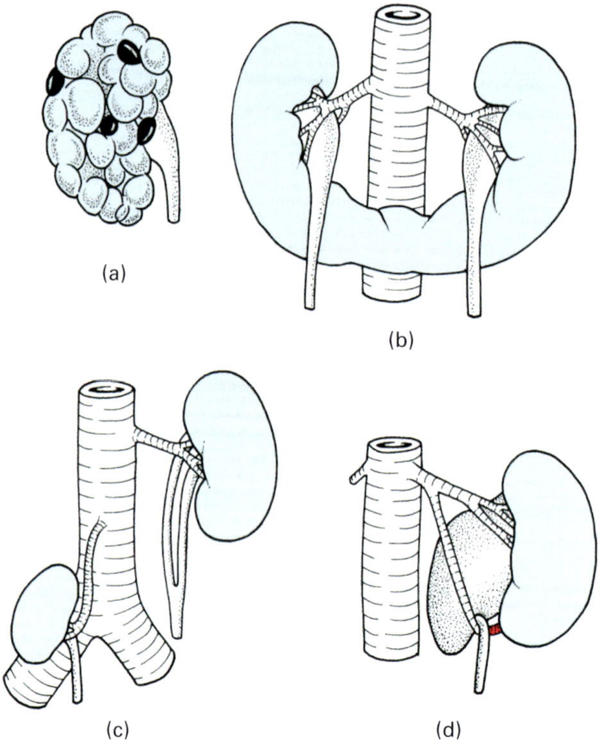

Fig. 84 Renal abnormalities. (a) Polycystic kidney. (b) Horseshoe kidney. (c) Pelvic kidney (right) and double ureter (left). (d) Aberrant renal artery and associated hydronephrosis.

anterior abdominal wall. The surgeon utilizes this fact in carrying out an extraperitoneal incision or suprapubic puncture into the bladder. In children up to the age of approximately 3 years, the pelvis is relatively small and the bladder is, in fact, intra-abdominal although still extraperitoneal.

Relations

- *Anteriorly* – the pubic symphysis.
- *Superiorly* – the bladder is covered by peritoneum with coils of small intestine and sigmoid colon lying against it. In the female, the body of the uterus flops against its posterosuperior aspect.
- *Posteriorly* – in the male the rectum, the termination of the vasa deferentia and the seminal vesicles; in the female, the vagina and the supravaginal part of the cervix.
- *Laterally* – the levator ani and obturator internus.

The neck of the bladder fuses with the prostate in the male; in the female it lies directly on the pelvic fascia surrounding the short urethra.

The muscle coat of the bladder is formed by a criss-cross arrangement of bundles; when these undergo hypertrophy in chronic obstruction (due to an enlarged prostate, for example) they account for the typical trabeculated 'open weave' appearance of the bladder wall, readily seen through a cystoscope.

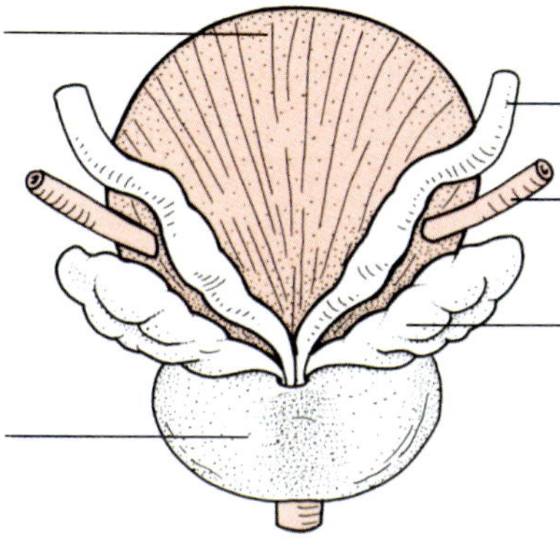

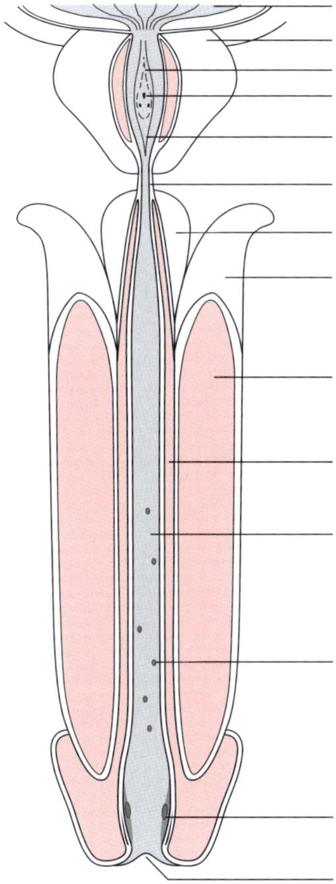

Fig. 85 (a) The prostate, seminal vesicles and vasa shown in a posterior view of the bladder. (b) The prostate and urethra in vertical section.

The circular component of the muscle coat condenses as an (involuntary) *internal urethral sphincter* around the internal urethral meatus.

Cystoscopy

The interior of the bladder and its three orifices (the internal urethral meatus and the two ureteric orifices) are easily inspected by means of a cystoscope. The ureteric orifices lie 2.5 cm (1 in) apart in the empty bladder, but, when this is distended for cystoscopic examination, the distance between the ureteric orifices may increase to 5 cm (2 in). The submucosa and mucosa of most of the bladder are only loosely adherent to the underlying muscle and are thrown into folds when the bladder is empty, smoothing out during distension of the organ. Over the *trigone*, the triangular area bounded by the ureteric orifices and the internal urethral meatus, the mucosa is adherent and remains smooth even in the empty bladder.

Between the ureters, a raised fold of mucosa can be seen that is called the *interureteric ridge*, which is produced by an underlying bar of muscle.

Blood supply

Blood is supplied from the superior and inferior vesical branches of the internal iliac artery. The vesical veins form a perivesical venous plexus which drains into the internal iliac veins, bilaterally.

Lymphatic drainage

Lymphatics drain alongside the vesical blood vessels to the iliac and then para-aortic nodes.

Nerve supply

Efferent parasympathetic fibres from S2 to S4 accompany the vesical arteries to the bladder. They convey motor fibres to the muscles of the bladder wall (the detrusor muscle) and inhibitory fibres to the internal urethral sphincter in the bladder neck. Sympathetic efferent fibres are said to be inhibitory to the bladder muscles and motor to its sphincter, although they may be mainly vasomotor in function, so that normal filling and emptying of the bladder are probably regulated largely by its parasympathetic innervation. The external urethral sphincter is made up of striated muscle. It is also concerned in the control of micturition and is supplied by the pudendal nerve (S2, S3, S4). Sensory fibres from the bladder, which are stimulated by distension, are conveyed in both the sympathetic and parasympathetic nerves, the latter pathway being the more important.

The urethra

The male urethra (Fig. 85b)

The male urethra in the adult is approximately 20 cm (8 in) long and is divided into the following successive segments, in proximo-distal sequence.

Pre-prostatic, prostatic, membranous and spongiose

The *pre-prostatic urethra* commences at the internal urethral orifice in the bladder neck and is about 1 cm in length. It is surrounded by the bladder neck sphincter also known as the internal urethral sphincter. This sphincter is composed of smooth muscle and is innervated by the sympathetic nerves.

The *prostatic urethra* is approximately 3 cm (1.25 in) in length, and as its name implies, traverses the prostate. Its posterior wall bears a longitudinal elevation termed the *urethral crest*, on each side of which is a shallow depression, the *prostatic sinus*, into which the 15–20 prostatic ducts empty. At approximately the middle of the crest is a prominence termed the *colliculus seminalis* (*verumontanum*) into which opens the *prostatic utricle*. This is a blind tract, approximately 0.5 cm (0.25 in) long, running downwards from the substance of the median lobe of the prostate. It is believed to represent the male equivalent of the uterus, a remnant of the paramesonephric duct (see page 154). On either side of the orifice of the prostatic utricle open the right and left *ejaculatory ducts*, each formed by the union of the ipsilateral duct of the seminal vesicle and the terminal part of the vas deferens.

The *membranous urethra* is 2 cm (0.75 in) long and is situated in the deep perineal pouch. It traverses the external urethral sphincter (the voluntary sphincter of the urethra) and the perineal membrane which covers the superficial aspect of the sphincter.

The *spongiose urethra* is 15 cm (6 in) long and is situated in the superficial perineal pouch. It traverses the corpus spongiosum of the penis. It first passes upwards and forwards to lie below the pubic symphysis and then, in the flaccid penis, bends downwards and forwards. The spongiose urethra is subdivided into the following parts. The initial part of the spongiose urethra, immediately distal to the membranous urethra, is known as the *bulbar urethra*. This is succeeded by the *pendulous* or *penile urethra*, which in turn is succeeded by the terminal segment of the urethra, the *glanular urethra*.

The prostatic urethra is the widest and most readily dilatable segment of the male urethra. The least dilatable segment is the membranous urethra. Usually, the narrowest part of the urethra is within the glanular urethra, a few millimetres proximal to the external urethral orifice, where a small mucosal fold hanging from the dorsal wall of the urethra compromises the urethral lumen.

CLINICAL FEATURES

1 Where the urethra passes beneath the pubis is a common site for it to be ruptured by a fall astride a sharp object, which crushes it against the edge of the symphysis.
2 The external orifice is the narrowest part of the urethra and a calculus may lodge there. Immediately within the meatus, the urethra dilates into a terminal fossa whose roof bears a mucosal fold (the *lacuna magna*), which may catch the tip of a catheter. Instruments should always be introduced into the urethra beak downwards for this reason.

The female urethra

The female urethra is 4 cm (1.5 in) long; it traverses the sphincter urethrae and lies immediately in front of, indeed embedded in the anterior wall of, the vagina. Its external meatus opens 2.5 cm (1 in) behind the clitoris. The sphincter urethrae in the female is a tenuous structure and vesical control appears to depend mainly on the intrinsic sphincter of condensed circular muscle fibres of the urinary bladder.

The mucosa of the urinary tract

The renal pelvis and calyceal system, ureter, bladder and urethra are lined by transitional epithelium as far as the entry of the ejaculatory ducts in the prostatic urethra. Transitional epithelium is exclusive to the conducting part of the urinary tract and is not found anywhere else in the body. It is also known as *uroepithelium* or *urothelium* since it has a uniform appearance. Furthermore the entire field lined with urothelium is susceptible to the effects of carcinogenic influences and pathological processes, e.g. the development of papillomata. The remainder of the urethra has a columnar lining except at its termination, where the epithelium becomes stratified squamous.

Radiology of the urinary tract

The renal contours can often be identified on a soft-tissue radiograph of the abdomen (plain X-ray). Intravenous injection of iodine-containing compounds excreted by the kidney will produce an outline of the calyces and the ureter (intravenous urogram). When the injection medium enters the bladder, a cystogram is obtained (Fig. 82).

Further information can be obtained by passing a catheter up the ureter through a cystoscope and injecting radio-opaque fluid to fill the pelvis and calyceal system (retrograde pyelogram). Similarly, injection of such fluid into the urethra or bladder may be used for the radiographic study of these viscera.

The kidneys are beautifully delineated in transverse section on computed tomography (CT) scans (Fig. 81b, and see Figs 110 and 111).

The male genital organs

The prostate (Fig. 85)

This is a pyramidal, fibromuscular and glandular organ, 3 cm (1.25 in) long, which surrounds the prostatic urethra. It resembles the size and shape of a chestnut.

Relations (Fig. 60)

- *Superiorly* – the prostate is continuous with the neck of the bladder. The urethra enters the upper aspect of the prostate near its anterior border.

- *Inferiorly* – the apex of the prostate rests on the external sphincter of the urethra, which lies within the deep perineal pouch.
- *Anteriorly* – lies the pubic symphysis separated from the prostate by the extraperitoneal fat of the *cave of Retzius* or *retropubic space*. Close against the prostate in this space lies the periprostatic plexus of veins. Near the apex of the prostate, the *puboprostatic ligament* (a condensation of fibrous tissue) passes forwards from the prostate to the pubis.
- *Posteriorly* – lies the rectum separated from the prostate by the rectovesical septum or *fascia of Denonvilliers*.
- *Laterally* – on either side lies the corresponding levator ani.

The ejaculatory ducts enter the upper posterior part of the gland to open into the urethra at the *colliculus seminalis* or verumontanum, one on either side of the prostatic utricle, demarcating a *median prostatic lobe* lying between these three ducts. In benign prostatic hyperplasia (but not in the normal prostate), a shallow posterior *median groove* (which can be felt on DRE) further divides the prostate into left and right *lobes*. Anterior to the urethra, the prostate consists of a narrow isthmus only.

The prostatic capsules (Fig. 86)

These are normally two, pathologically three, in number.

1 *The true capsule* – a thin fibrous sheath which surrounds the gland.
2 *The false capsule* – condensed extraperitoneal fascia which continues into the fascia surrounding the bladder and blends with the rectovesical fascia of Denonvilliers posteriorly. Between layers 1 and 2 lies the periprostatic venous plexus.
3 *The pathological capsule* – when benign 'adenomatous' hypertrophy of the prostate takes place, the normal peripheral part of the gland becomes compressed into a capsule around the enlarging hypertrophied mass (Fig. 86). In performing an enucleation of the prostate, the plane between the adenomatous mass and this compressed peripheral tissue is entered, the 'tumour' enucleated and a condensed rim of healthy prostate tissue, lying deep to the true capsule, left behind. The prostatic venous plexus, lying external to the true capsule, is thus undisturbed.

Blood supply

The arterial supply of the prostate is derived from the right and left inferior vesical arteries (each being a branch of the corresponding internal iliac artery). The inferior vesical artery gives off a prostatic artery which enters the prostate at its lateral aspect.

The veins form a periprostatic plexus, which receives the dorsal vein of the penis and drains into the internal iliac vein on each side. Some of the venous drainage passes to the plexus of veins lying in front of the vertebral bodies and within the vertebral canal. These veins are valveless and constitute the *valveless vertebral veins of Batson*. This communication may explain the readiness with which carcinoma of the prostate spreads to the pelvic bones and vertebrae.

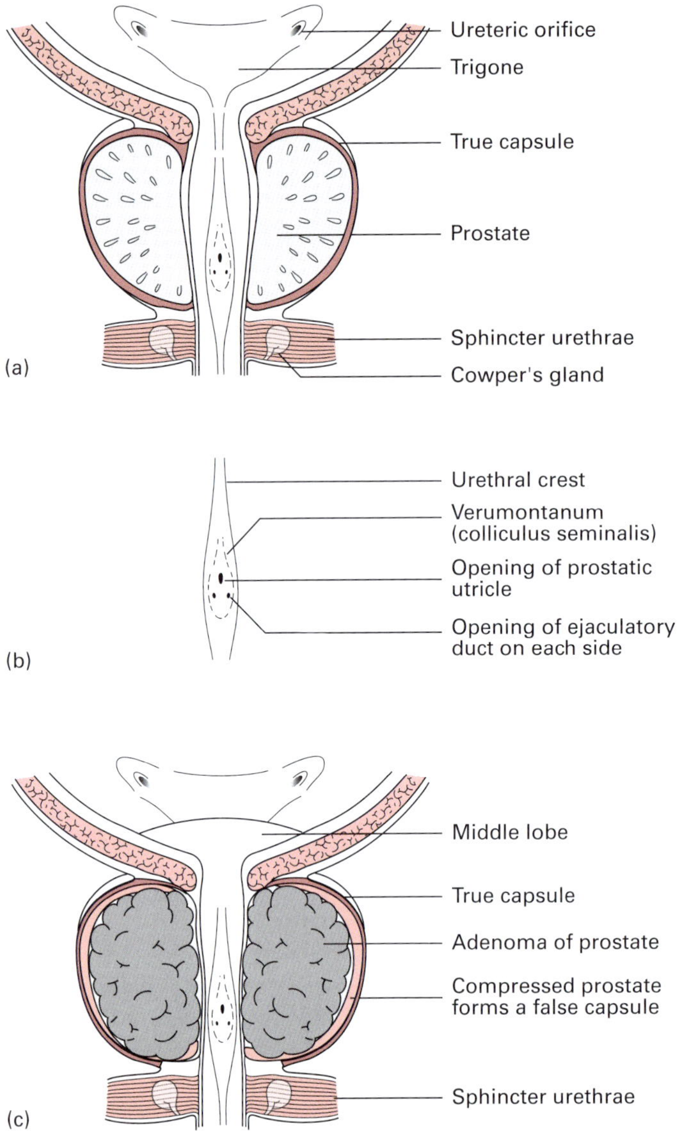

Fig. 86 The surgical anatomy of prostatectomy. (a) The normal prostate in vertical section. (b) Detail of the prostatic urethra. (c) A prostatic adenoma (benign hypertrophy) compresses the normal prostatic tissue into a false capsule.

CLINICAL FEATURES

1 Prostatectomy for benign prostatic hyperplasia involves removal of the hyperplastic mass of glandular tissue from the surrounding normal prostate, which is compressed as a thin rim around it – a false capsule (Fig. 86). This is usually performed

transurethrally by means of an operating cystoscope armed with a cutting diathermy loop. During this procedure, the verumontanum (colliculus seminalis) is an important landmark. The surgeon keeps the resection proximal to this structure in order not to damage the urethral sphincter. 'Open prostatectomy' is hardly ever undertaken these days but may be indicated in the extremely rare event of an excessively enlarged prostate causing bladder outflow obstruction. For open prostatectomy the gland may be approached retropubically, transvesically or transperineally.

2 After the age of 45 years or so, some degree of prostatic hyperplasia is practically inevitable; it is as much a feature of ageing as is greying of the hair. Usually the lateral lobes are affected, and such enlargement is readily detected on DRE. The median lobe may also be involved in this process or may be enlarged without the lateral lobes being affected. In such instances, symptoms of bladder outflow obstruction may occur (because of the valve-like effect of this hypertrophied lobe lying over the internal urethral orifice) without prostatic enlargement being detectable on DRE.

Anterior to the urethra the prostate consists of a narrow fibromuscular isthmus containing little, if any, glandular tissue. Benign glandular hypertrophy of the prostate, therefore, never affects this part of the organ.

3 The fascia of Denonvilliers is important surgically; in excising the rectum, it is the plane to be sought after in order to mobilise the rectum away from the prostate and urethra without damaging these structures. A carcinoma of the prostate often invades this fascial layer, but invasion of the rectal wall is unusual.

The scrotum

The scrotum is the pouch in which lie the testes and their coverings. Also in the scrotum are the epididymides, each epididymis with its associated vas, and the blood vessels and lymphatics that supply these structures. In cryptorchidism, as might be expected, this pouch is not well developed.

The skin of the scrotum is thin, pigmented, rugose and marked by a longitudinal median raphe. It is richly endowed with sebaceous glands, and consequently a common site for sebaceous cysts, which are often multiple. The subcutaneous tissue contains no fat but does contain the involuntary *dartos muscle*.

CLINICAL FEATURES

The scrotal subcutaneous tissue (superficial fascia) is continuous with the fasciae of the anterior abdominal wall and perineum and therefore extravasations of urine or blood deep to this plane will gravitate into the scrotum. The scrotum is divided by a septum into right and left compartments, but this septum is incomplete superiorly so extravasations of fluid into this sac tend to be bilateral.

The lax tissues of the scrotum and its dependent position cause it to fill readily with oedema fluid in cardiac or renal failure. Such a condition must be carefully differentiated from extravasation or from a scrotal swelling due to a hernia or hydrocele.

Testis and epididymis (Figs 87, 88)

The left testis lies at a lower level than the right within the scrotum; rarely, this arrangement is reversed. Each testis is contained by a white fibrous capsule, the *tunica albuginea*, and each is invaginated anteriorly into a double serous covering, the *tunica vaginalis*, just as the intestine is invaginated anteriorly into the peritoneum.

Along the posterior border of the testis, rather to its lateral side, lies the *epididymis*, which is divided into an expanded head, a body and a pointed tail inferiorly. Medially, there is a distinct groove, the *sinus epididymis*, between it and the testis. The epididymis is covered by the tunica vaginalis except at its posterior margin, which is free or, so to say, 'extraperitoneal'.

The testis and epididymis each bear at their upper extremities a small stalked body, termed, respectively, the *appendix testis* and *appendix epididymis* (*hydatid of Morgagni*). The appendix testis is a remnant of the upper end of the paramesonephric (Müllerian) duct; the appendix epididymis is a remnant of the mesonephros.

These structures, being stalked, are liable to undergo torsion.

Blood supply

The testicular artery arises from the aorta at the level of the renal vessels. It anastomoses with the artery to the vas, supplying the vas deferens and epididymis, which arises from the inferior vesical branch of the internal iliac artery. This cross-connection means that ligation of the testicular artery is not necessarily followed by testicular atrophy.

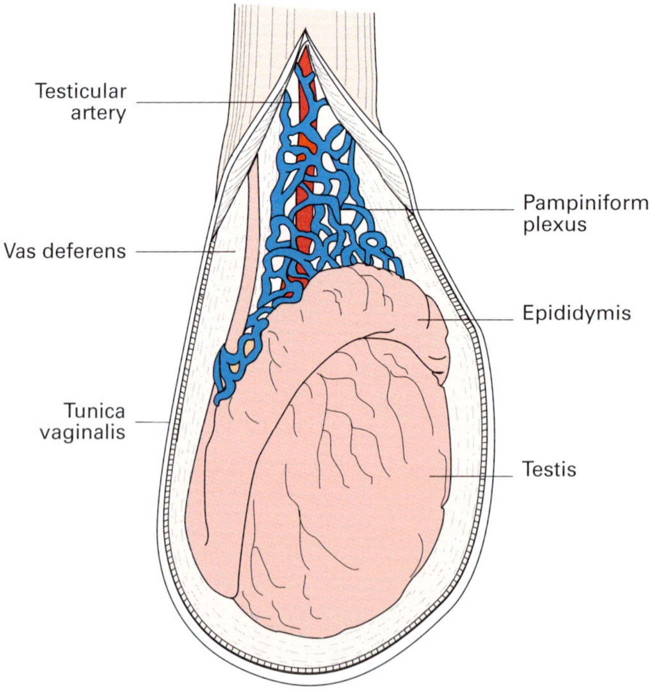

Fig. 87 Testis and epididymis.

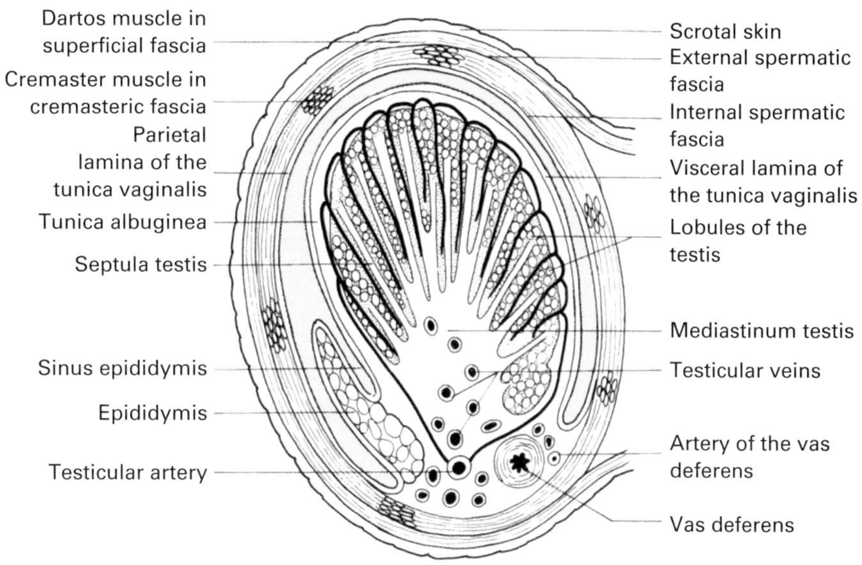

Fig. 88 Transverse section of the testis.

The pampiniform plexus of veins becomes a single vessel, the testicular vein, in the region of the internal ring. On the right, this drains into the IVC; on the left, into the renal vein.

Lymphatic drainage

The lymphatic drainage of the testis obeys the usual rule: it accompanies the venous drainage and thus passes to the para-aortic lymph nodes at the level of the renal vessels. Free communication occurs between the lymphatics on either side; there is also a plentiful anastomosis with the para-aortic intrathoracic nodes and, in turn, with the cervical nodes, so that spread of malignant disease from the testis to the nodes at the root of the neck is not rare.

Nerve supply

T10 and T11 sympathetic fibres via the renal and aortic plexus. These convey afferent (pain) fibres – hence referred pain from the testis to the loin and groin.

Structure

The testis is divided into 200–300 lobules, each containing one to three *seminiferous tubules*. Each tubule is some 62 cm (2 feet) in length when teased out and is thus obviously highly coiled and convoluted in order to be accommodated within the testis. The tubules anastomose posteriorly into a plexus termed the *rete testis* from which approximately a dozen fine *efferent ducts* arise, pierce the tunica albuginea at the upper part of the testis and pass into the head of the epididymis, which is actually formed by these efferent ducts coiled within it. The efferent ducts fuse to form a considerably convoluted single tube that constitutes the body and tail of the epididymis.

Development of the testis

This is important and is the key to several features which are of clinical interest.

The testis arises from a germinal ridge of mesoderm in the posterior wall of the abdomen just medial to the mesonephros (Fig. 83) and links up with the epididymis and vas, which differentiate from the mesonephric duct. As the testis enlarges, it also undergoes a caudal migration according to the following timetable:

3rd month (of fetal life)	reaches the iliac fossa;
7th month	traverses the inguinal canal;
8th month	reaches the external ring;
9th month	descends into the scrotum.

A mesenchymal strand, the *gubernaculum testis*, extends from the caudal end of the developing testis along the course of its descent to blend into the scrotal fascia. The exact role of this structure in the descent of the testis is not known; theories are that it acts as a guide (*gubernaculum* = rudder) or that its swelling dilates the inguinal canal and scrotum.

In the third fetal month, a prolongation of the peritoneal cavity invades the gubernacular mesenchyme and projects into the scrotum as the *processus vaginalis*. The testis slides into the scrotum posterior to this, projects into it and is therefore clothed front and sides with peritoneum. About the time of birth this processus obliterates, leaving the testis covered by the tunica vaginalis. Very rarely, fragments of adjacent developing organs – spleen or suprarenal – are caught up and carried into the scrotum along with the testis.

CLINICAL FEATURES

1 The testis arises in the vicinity of the mesonephros at the level of the L2/3 vertebrae and during embryological development drags its vascular, lymphatic and nerve supply from this region. Pain from the kidney is often referred to the scrotum and, conversely, testicular pain may radiate to the loin.

2 When searching for secondary lymphatic spread from a neoplasm of the testis, the upper abdomen must be palpated carefully for enlarged para-aortic nodes; because of cross-communications, these may be present on either side. Mediastinal and cervical nodes may also become involved. Inguinal lymph nodes are only involved if the tumour invades the scrotal skin and thereby invades the scrotal lymphatics which drain to the inguinal nodes.

3 Rarely, a rapidly developing *varicocele* (dilatation of the pampiniform plexus of veins) is said to be a presenting sign of a tumour of the left kidney which, by invading the renal vein, blocks the drainage of the left testicular vein. Most examples of varicocele are, however, idiopathic; why the vast majority are on the left side is unknown, but theories are that the left testicular vein is compressed by a loaded sigmoid colon, obstructed by angulation at its entry into the renal vein or even that it is put into spasm by adrenaline (epinephrine)-rich blood entering the renal vein from the suprarenal vein!

4 The testis may fail to descend and may rest anywhere along its course – intra-abdominally, within the inguinal canal, at the external ring or high in the scrotum. Failure to descend must be carefully distinguished from retraction of the testis; it is common in children for contraction of the cremaster muscle to draw the testis up into the superficial inguinal pouch – a potential space deep to the superficial fascia over the external ring. Gentle pressure from above, or the relaxing effect of a hot bath, coaxes the testis back into the scrotum in such cases. Occasionally the testis descends, but into an unusual (*ectopic*) position; most commonly, the testis passes laterally after leaving the external ring to lie superficial to the inguinal ligament, but it may be found in front of the pubis, in the perineum or in the upper thigh. In these cases (unlike the undescended testis), the cord is long and replacement into the scrotum without tension presents no surgical difficulty.

5 Abnormalities of the obliteration of the processus vaginalis lead to a number of extremely common surgical conditions, of which the *indirect inguinal hernia* is the most important.

This variety of hernia may be present at birth or develop in later life; in the latter circumstance, it is probable that the processus vaginalis has persisted as a narrow empty sac and that development of the hernia results from excessive strain due to a persistent cough or straining at micturition or at stool, which forces abdominal contents into this peritoneal recess.

In infants, the sac frequently has the testis lying in its wall (congenital inguinal hernia), but this is unusual in older patients.

The closed-off tunica vaginalis may become distended with fluid to form a *hydrocele*, which may be idiopathic (primary) or secondary to disease in the underlying testis. The anatomical classification of hydroceles is into the following groups (Fig. 89):

- *vaginal* – confined to the scrotum and so-called because it distends the tunica vaginalis;
- *congenital* – communicating with the peritoneal cavity;
- *infantile* – extending upwards to the internal ring;
- *hydrocele of the cord* – confined to the cord.

Notice that, from the anatomical point of view, a hydrocele (apart from one of the cord) must surround the front and sides of the testis since the tunica vaginalis bears this relationship to the testis. A cyst of the epididymis, in contrast, arises from the efferent ducts of the epididymis and must therefore lie above and behind the testis. This point enables a clinical distinction to be made between these two common types of scrotal cysts.

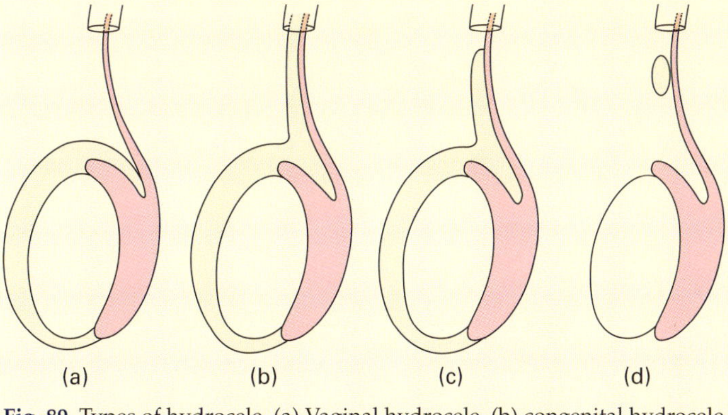

Fig. 89 Types of hydrocele. (a) Vaginal hydrocele, (b) congenital hydrocele, (c) infantile hydrocele, (d) hydrocele of the cord. (The tube at the upper end of each diagram represents the internal inguinal ring. Yellow, hydrocele; brown, vas and epididymis.)

Vas deferens (ductus deferens) (Fig. 85)

This tube is 45 cm (18 in) long (a length that is thought also to be the approximate length in adults, of the thoracic duct, the spinal cord and the femur, and the distance from the incisor teeth to the oesophagogastric junction).

The vas is the continuation of the epididymis. It ascends from the tail of the epididymis to the neck of the scrotum and traverses the inguinal canal before coming to lie upon the lateral wall of the pelvis. Here, lying immediately outside the peritoneum of the lateral wall, it extends almost to the ischial tuberosity before turning medially to approach the base of the urinary bladder. Here, it joins the more laterally placed seminal vesicle to form the *(common) ejaculatory duct*, which traverses the prostate to open into the prostatic urethra at the verumontanum just to the side of the utricle.

CLINICAL FEATURES

Infection may track from the bladder and urethra along the vas to the epididymis (acute epididymitis).

The operation of bilateral vasectomy is a commonly undertaken procedure for male sterilization. The vas is identified by its very firm consistency, which has been likened to whipcord and may also be likened to fine plastic tubing.

The seminal vesicles

These are coiled sacculated tubes 5 cm (2 in) long which can be unravelled to three times that length. They lie, one on each side, extraperitoneally at the bladder base, lateral to the termination of the vasa, and just above the base (upper surface) of the prostate. Each has common drainage with its neighbouring vas via the ejaculatory duct (Fig. 85). In spite of their name, they do not act as receptacles for semen, although their secretions do contribute considerably to the volume of seminal fluid.

CLINICAL FEATURES

The vesicles can be felt on rectal examination if enlarged and/or inflamed as may occur in association with acute epididymitis, and as may also occur in seminal vesiculitis associated with tuberculous infection of the male genital tract.

The penis

The penis, the scrotum and scrotal contents collectively make up the male external genitalia and these are located in the urogenital triangle (urogenital region) of the perineum, or more precisely, in the superficial perineal pouch of the urogenital triangle of the perineum. Besides being the male organ of copulation, the penis also contains the longest segment of the urethra, namely the spongiose urethra (Fig. 85b).

The penis is made up of three elongated, cylindrical columns of spongy, erectile tissue; a central column termed the corpus spongiosum which contains the urethra, immediately dorsal to the corpus spongiosum, and lying side by side are the two corpora cavernosa (singular, corpus cavernosum). The corpus spongiosum extends distally beyond the two corpora cavernosa becoming expanded at its distal extremity into the acorn-shaped glans penis. The latter has the external urethral orifice at its tip. Proximally, the two corpora cavernosa taper off into the crura, while the proximal end of the corpus spongiosum expands into the bulb (Fig. 96). Each crus is firmly attached to the inner surface of the ischiopubic ramus of its side and is covered by the corresponding ischiocavernosus muscle, while the bulb of the penis is firmly attached to the superficial surface of the perineal membrane and is covered by the right and left bulbospongiosus muscles. The two crura and the midline bulb collectively form the *root of the penis*. Followed distally, the root continues as the shaft of the penis which in turn expands at its distal extremity as the glans penis. The glans penis contains a high concentration of nerve endings and is a very sensitive area and thus an important source of sexual arousal. The ridged proximal edge of the glans is called the corona. The circumferential groove immediately proximal to the corona is the coronal sulcus. The relatively loose skin of the penis that is folded forwards over the glans is called the prepuce or foreskin, and it is this fold of skin that is excised in the procedure called circumcision.

The two corpora cavernosa and the corpus spongiosum have their individual arteries of supply. These are derived from the right and left internal pudendal arteries, in turn derived from the corresponding internal iliac artery. Venous drainage is largely via the dorsal vein of the penis which runs posteriorly beneath the subpubic arch to drain into the prevesical venous plexus.

The bony and ligamentous pelvis

The pelvis is made up of the innominate bones, the sacrum and the coccyx, bound to each other by dense ligaments.

The os innominatum (Fig. 90)

Examine the bone and revise the following structures.

The *ilium* with its *iliac crest* running between the *anterior* and *posterior superior iliac spines;* below each of these are the corresponding *inferior spines*. Well-defined ridges on its lateral surface are the strong muscle markings of the glutei. Its inner aspect bears the large *auricular surface*, which articulates with the sacrum. The *iliopectineal line* runs forwards from the apex of the auricular surface and demarcates the *true* from the *false pelvis*.

The pubis comprises the body and the superior and inferior pubic rami.

The *ischium* has a vertically disposed *body*, bearing the *ischial spine* on its posterior border that demarcates an upper (greater) and lower (lesser) sciatic notch. The inferior pole of the body bears the *ischial tuberosity*, then projects forwards almost at right angles into the *ischial ramus* to meet the inferior pubic ramus.

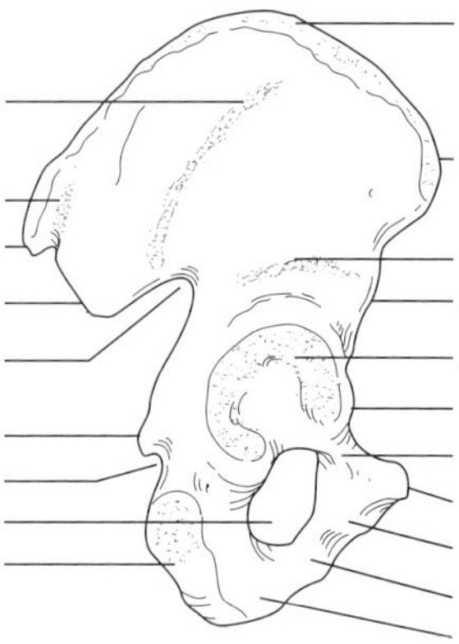

Fig. 90 Lateral view of the os innominatum.

The *obturator foramen* lies bounded by the body and rami of the pubis and the body and ramus of the ischium.

All three bones meet and fuse at the *acetabulum*, which forms the socket for the femoral head, for which it bears a wide crescentic articular surface.

The pelvis is tilted in the erect position so that the plane of its inlet is at an angle 60° to the horizontal. (To place a pelvis into this position, hold it against a wall so that the anterior superior spine and the top of the pubic symphysis both touch it.)

The sacrum (Fig. 91)

The sacrum is made up of five fused vertebrae and is roughly triangular. The anterior border of its upper part is termed the *sacral promontory* and is readily felt at laparotomy.

Its anterior aspect presents a *central mass*, a row of four *anterior sacral foramina* on each side (transmitting the upper four sacral anterior primary rami), and, lateral to these, the *lateral masses* of the sacrum. The superior aspect of the lateral mass on each side forms a fan-shaped surface termed the *ala*.

Note that the central mass is roughly rectangular – the triangular shape of the sacrum is due to the rapid shrinkage in size of the lateral masses of the sacrum from above down.

Posteriorly lies the *sacral canal*, continuing the vertebral canal, bounded by short pedicles, strong laminae and diminutive spinous processes. Perforating through from the sacral canal is a row of four *posterior sacral foramina* on each side. Inferiorly, the canal terminates in the *sacral hiatus*, which transmits the 5th sacral nerve. On either side of the lower extremity of the hiatus lie the *sacral cornua*. These can easily be palpated by the finger immediately above the natal cleft.

On its lateral aspect, the sacrum presents an *auricular facet* for articulation with the corresponding surface of the ilium.

The 5th lumbar vertebra may occasionally fuse with the sacrum in whole or in part (sacralization of L5); alternatively, the 1st sacral segment may be partially or completely separated from the rest of the sacrum (lumbarization of S1). The posterior arch of the sacrum is occasionally bifid.

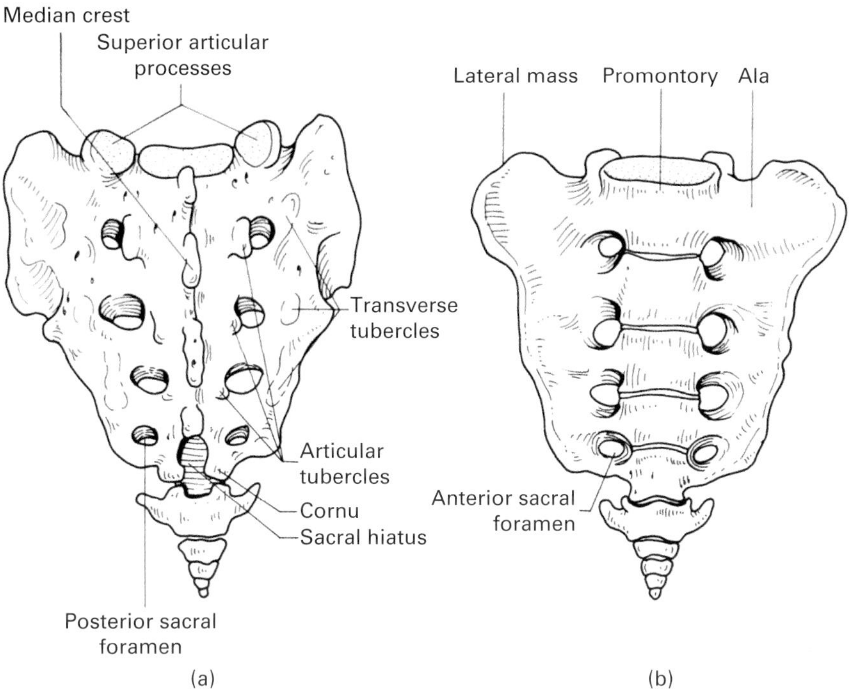

Fig. 91 The sacrum in: (a) posterior and (b) anterior views.

Note that the dural sheath terminates distally at the second piece of the sacrum. Beyond this the sacral canal is filled with the fatty tissue of the extradural space, the cauda equina and the filum terminale. (For sacral block, see page 137.)

The coccyx

This is made up of three to five fused vertebrae articulating with the sacrum; occasionally, the first segment remains separate. It represents, of course, the tail of more primitive animals.

The functions of the pelvis

1 It protects the pelvic viscera.
2 It supports the weight of the body, which is transmitted through the vertebrae, thence through the sacrum, across the sacro-iliac joints to the innominate bones and then to the femora in the standing position or to the ischial tuberosities when sitting. (The sacro-iliac joint is reinforced for this task as will be described in the next section.)
3 During walking the pelvis swings from side to side by a rotatory movement at the lumbosacral articulation, which occurs together with similar movements of the lumbar intervertebral joints. Even if the hip joints are fixed, this swing of the pelvis enables the patient to walk reasonably well.

4 As with all but a few small bones in the hand and foot, the pelvis provides attachments for muscles.
5 In the female it provides bony support for the birth canal.

Joints and ligamentous connections of the pelvis

The *symphysis pubis* is the name given to the cartilaginous joint between the pubic bones. Each pubic bone is covered by a layer of hyaline cartilage and is connected across the midline by a dense layer of fibrocartilage. The centre of the latter may break down to form a cleft-like joint space which, however, is not seen before the first decade and which is not lined by a synovial membrane.

The joint is surrounded and strengthened by fibrous ligaments, especially above and below.

The *sacro-iliac joints* are the articulations between the auricular surfaces of the sacrum and ilium on each side and are true synovium-lined and cartilage-covered joints.

The sacrum 'hangs' from these joints supported by the extremely dense *posterior sacro-iliac ligaments* lying posteriorly to the auricular joint surfaces. These support the whole weight of the body, tending to drag the sacrum forwards into the pelvis and, not surprisingly, are the strongest ligaments in the body.

Their action is assisted by an interlocking of the grooves between the auricular surfaces of the sacrum and ilium.

The *sacrotuberous ligament* passes from the ischial tuberosity to the side of the sacrum and coccyx.

The *sacrospinous ligament* passes from the ischial spine to the side of the sacrum and coccyx.

These two ligaments help to define two important exits from the pelvis:

1 *the greater sciatic foramen* – formed by the sacrospinous ligament and the greater sciatic notch;
2 *the lesser sciatic foramen* – formed by the sacrotuberous ligament and the lesser sciatic notch.

Note. There is a useful surface landmark in this region – the dimple constantly seen on each side immediately above the buttock – which defines:

1 the posterior superior iliac spine;
2 the centre of the sacro-iliac joint;
3 the level of the second sacral segment;
4 the level at which the dural sheath of the spinal meninges terminates.

Differences between the male and female pelvis (Fig. 92)

The pelvis demonstrates a large number of sex differences associated principally with two features: first, the heavier build and stronger muscles in the male, accounting for the stronger bone structure and better defined muscle markings in this sex; second,

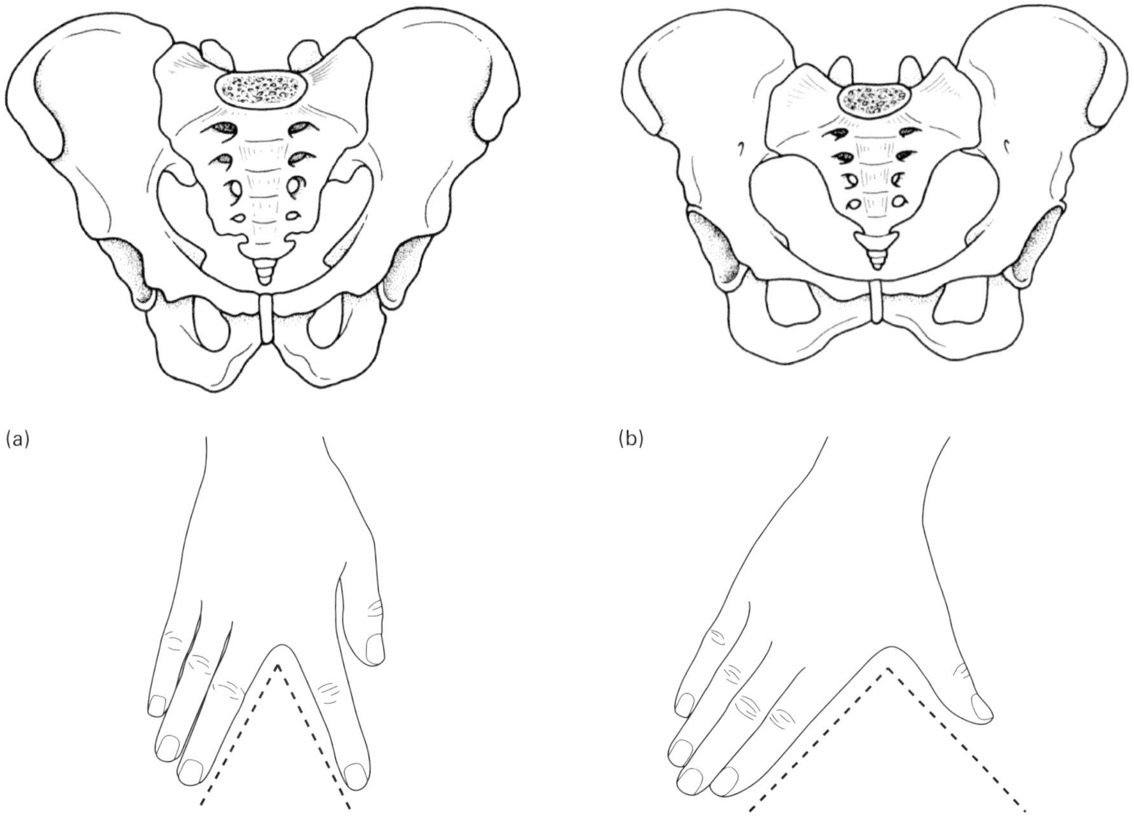

Fig. 92 (a) Male and (b) female pelvis compared.

the comparatively wider and shallower pelvic cavity in the female, correlated with its role as the bony part of the birth canal.

The sex differences are summarized in Table 2.

When looking at a radiograph of the pelvis, the sex is best determined by three features:

1 the pelvic inlet, which is heart-shaped in the male, oval in the female;
2 the angle between the inferior pubic rami, which is narrow in the male, wide in the female. In the former, it corresponds almost exactly to the angle between the index and middle fingers when these are held apart; in the latter, the angle equals that between the fully extended thumb and the index finger. This is a particularly reliable feature;
3 the soft-tissue shadow of the penis and scrotum can usually be seen or, if not, the dense shadow of the lead screen used to shield the testes from harmful radiation.

Table 2 Comparison of male and female pelvis

	Male	Female
General structure	Heavy and thick	Light and thin
Joint surfaces	Large	Small
Muscle attachments	Well marked	Rather indistinct
False pelvis	Deep	Shallow
Pelvic inlet	Heart-shaped	Oval
Pelvic canal	'Long segment of a short cone', i.e. long and tapered	'Short segment of a long cone', i.e. short with almost parallel sides
Pelvic outlet	Comparatively small	Comparatively large
1st piece of sacrum	The superior surface of the body occupies nearly half the width of the sacrum	Oval superior surface of the body occupies approximately one-third of the width of the sacrum
Sacrum	Long and narrow, with smooth concavity	Short, wide, flat and curving forwards in the lower part
Sacro-iliac articular facet (auricular surface)	Extends well down the 3rd piece of the sacrum	Extends down only to the upper border of the 3rd piece
Subpubic angle (between inferior pubic rami)	'The angle between the middle and index fingers'	'The angle between the thumb and the index finger'
Inferior pubic ramus	Presents a strong everted surface for attachment of the crus of the penis	This marking is not present
Acetabulum	Large	Small
Ischial tuberosities	Inturned	Everted
Obturator foramen	Round	Oval

Obstetrical pelvic measurements (Fig. 93)

The figures for the measurements of the inlet, mid-cavity and outlet of the true pelvis are readily committed to memory in the form shown in Table 3.

The *transverse diameter of the outlet* is assessed clinically by measuring the distance between the ischial tuberosities along a plane passing across the anus; the *anteroposterior outlet diameter* is measured from the pubis to the sacrococcygeal joint. The most useful measurement clinically is, however, the *diagonal conjugate* – from the lower border of the pubic symphysis to the promontory of the sacrum. This normally measures 12.5 cm (5 in); from the practical point of view, it is not possible in the normal pelvis to reach the sacral promontory on vaginal examination either readily or without discomfort to the patient.

Another useful clinical guide is the *subpubic arch*: the examiner's four knuckles (i.e. his clenched fist) should rest comfortably between the ischial tuberosities below the pubic symphysis.

Note that these measurements are all of the bony pelvis; the 'dynamic pelvis' of the birth canal, in fact, is narrowed by the pelvic musculature, the rectum and the thickness of the uterine wall. Today accurate imaging techniques enable exact measurements to be made of the bony pelvis.

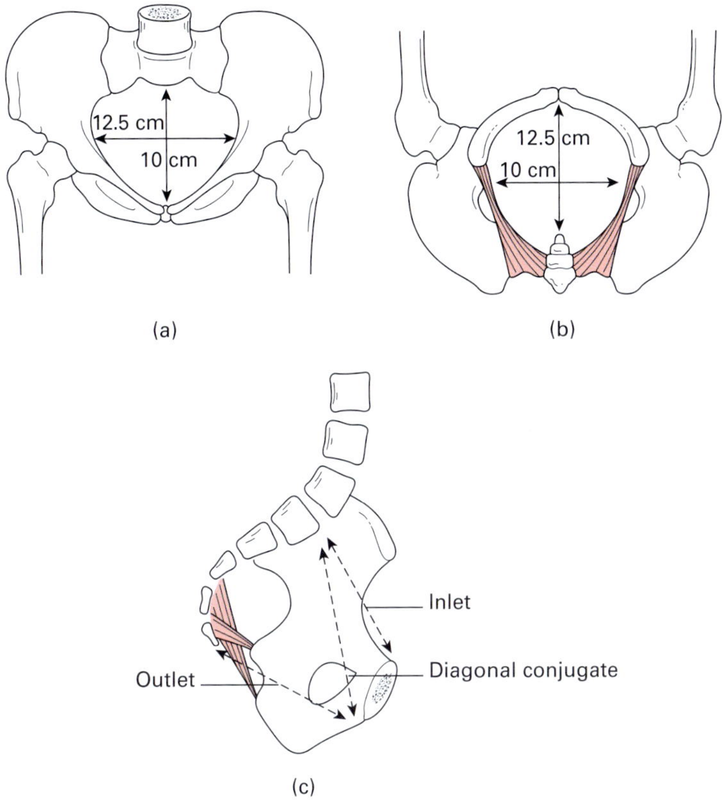

Fig. 93 The measurements of the female pelvis. (a) The inlet; (b) the outlet. (c) Lateral view to show the diagonal conjugate.

Table 3 Obstetrical pelvic measurements

	Transverse	Oblique	Anteroposterior
Inlet	12.5cm (5 in)	11.5cm (4.5 in)	10cm (4 in)
Mid-pelvis	11.5cm (4.5 in)	11.5cm (4.5 in)	11.5cm (4.5 in)
Outlet	10cm (4 in)	11.5cm (4.5 in)	12.5cm (5 in)

Variations of the pelvic shape (Fig. 94)

The shapes of the female pelvis may be classified (after Caldwell and Moloy) as follows.

1 The normal pelvis and its variants

- *Gynaecoid* – normal (most common variety in Caucasian women).
- *Android* – the masculine type of pelvis.
- *Platypelloid* – shortened in the anteroposterior diameter, increased in the transverse diameter (the 'non-rachitic flat pelvis').
- *Anthropoid* – resembling that of an anthropoid ape with a much lengthened anteroposterior diameter and a shortened transverse diameter.

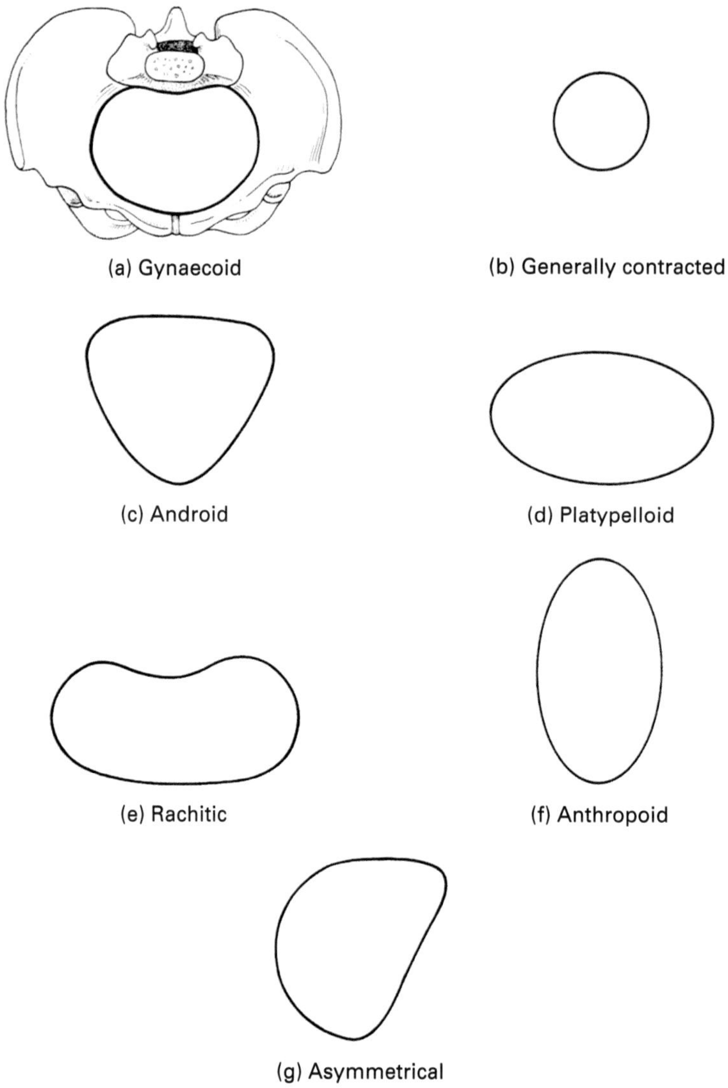

Fig. 94 Pelvic variations and abnormalities – shown as diagrammatic outlines of the pelvic inlet.

2 Symmetrically contracted pelvis

That of a small woman but with a symmetrical shape.

3 The rachitic flat pelvis

The sacrum is rotated so that the sacral promontory projects forwards and the coccyx tips backwards. The anteroposterior diameter of the inlet is therefore narrowed, but that of the outlet is increased. This deformity is typical of rickets, the result of vitamin D deficiency.

4 The asymmetrical

Asymmetry can be due to a variety of causes such as scoliosis, longstanding hip disease (e.g. congenital dislocation), poliomyelitis, pelvic fracture, congenital abnormality due to thalidomide and the *Naegele pelvis*, which is due to the congenital absence of one wing of the sacrum or its destruction by disease.

CLINICAL FEATURES

Fractures of the pelvis

These may be isolated lesions due to a localized blow or may be displacements of part of the pelvic ring due to compression injuries. Lateral compression usually results in fractures through both pubic rami on each side, or both rami on one side with dislocation at the symphysis; anteroposterior compression may be followed by dislocation at the symphysis or fractures through the pubic rami accompanied by dislocation at the sacro-iliac joint.

Displacement of part of the pelvic ring must, of course, mean that the ring has been broken in two places.

Falls upon the leg may force the head of the femur through the acetabulum, the so-called central dislocation of the hip. Isolated fractures may be produced by local trauma, especially to the iliac wing, sacrum and pubis.

Associated with pelvic fractures one must always consider soft-tissue injuries to the bladder, urethra and rectum, which may be penetrated by spicules of bone or torn by wide displacements of the pelvic fragments.

Occasionally in these pelvic displacements the iliolumbar branch of the internal iliac artery is ruptured as it crosses above the sacro-iliac joint; this may be followed by a severe or even fatal extraperitoneal haemorrhage.

Sacral (caudal) anaesthesia

The sacral hiatus, between the last piece of sacrum and coccyx, can be entered by a needle which pierces the skin, fascia and the tough posterior sacrococcygeal ligament to enter the sacral canal. The hiatus can be defined by palpating the sacral cornua on either side (Fig. 91) immediately above the natal cleft.

Anaesthetic solutions injected here will spread readily in the semi-liquid extradural fat to bathe the spinal roots emerging from the dural sheath, which terminates at the level of the 2nd sacral segment. The perineal anaesthesia can be used for low forceps delivery, episiotomy and repair of a perineal tear.

The muscles of the pelvic floor and perineum

The canal of the bony pelvis is closed inferiorly by a diaphragm of muscles and fasciae termed the *pelvic floor* or *pelvic diaphragm*, which the rectum, urethra and, in the female, the vagina must traverse to reach the perineum. The muscles are divided into (1) the

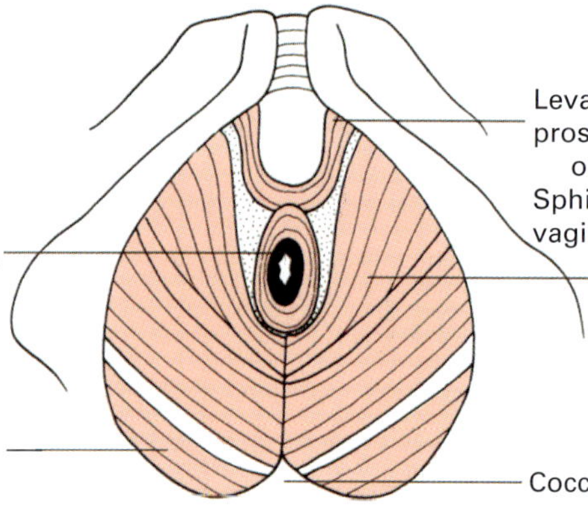

Fig. 95 Levator ani – inferior aspect. It forms the 'diaphragm of the pelvis'.

pelvic diaphragm, formed by the levator ani and the coccygeus, and (2) the *muscles* of (a) the anterior (urogenital) perineum and (b) the posterior (anal) perineum.

Levator ani (Fig. 95) is the largest and most important muscle of the pelvic floor. It arises from the posterior aspect of the body of the pubic bone, the fascia of the side wall of the pelvis (covering obturator internus) and the spine of the ischium. From this wide origin it sweeps down in a series of loops:

1 to form a sling around the prostate (*levator prostatae*) or vagina (*sphincter vaginae*), inserting into the perineal body;
2 to form a sling around the rectum and also insert into, and reinforce the deep part of, the anal sphincter at the anorectal ring (*puborectalis*);
3 the posterior fibres are attached to the sides of the coccyx and to a median fibrous raphe, which stretches between the apex of the coccyx and the anorectal junction.

(Note that the *coccygeus* is in the same tissue plane as levator ani. It corresponds almost exactly with the sacrospinous ligament, which it overlies, and the latter is commonly regarded as a degenerate part of the muscle. The muscle is well developed and the ligament is often missing in those mammals with a mobile tail.)

The muscle acts as the principal support of the pelvic floor, has a sphincter action on the rectum and vagina and assists in increasing intra-abdominal pressure during defecation, micturition and parturition.

Its deep aspect is related to the pelvic viscera and its perineal aspect forms the inner wall of the ischioanal fossa (see 'The posterior (anal) perineum').

The perineum (Figs 93b, 95, 96 & 97a)

The perineum is the very lowest part of the trunk. It is situated immediately below the pelvic floor (levator ani). The lateral boundary of the perineum on each side is the inner aspect of the very proximal end of the corresponding thigh. The inferior parts of the buttocks also contribute to the lateral boundary of the perineum. When the thighs and buttocks of the patient are parted as in the lithotomy position, the perineum may be pictured as lying within the osseo-ligamentous framework of the inferior pelvic aperture. This framework has a diamond-shaped outline (Fig. 93b). The four angles of the diamond are as follows: the anterior angle is the inferior edge of the pubic symphysis (the subpubic angle), the posterior angle is the tip of the coccyx and the lateral angle on either side is the corresponding ischial tuberosity. Incidentally all four angles of the 'diamond' are readily palpable on clinical examination. The four sides of the diamond are as follows: anterolaterally are the right and left ischiopubic rami, and posterolaterally are the inferior edges of the right and left sacrotuberous ligaments.

A transverse line drawn between the anterior ends of the right and left ischial tuberosities is seen to divide the perineum into two triangular regions. The anterior triangular area is the smaller of the two and is known as the urogenital triangle (urogenital region) of the perineum, while the larger posterior triangular area is known as the anal triangle (anal region) of the perineum.

The anal triangle of the perineum is similar in design in the two sexes and contains the centrally located anal canal flanked by the right and left ischioanal (ischiorectal) fossae.

The urogenital triangle, in both sexes, contains the external genitalia and the distal urethra.

The urogenital triangle of perineum (Figs 96, 97)

Stretching across the width of the urogenital triangle of the perineum from the inner surface of one ischiopubic ramus to the other is a distinct, tough fascial sheet termed the perineal membrane. The perineal membrane is quadrangular in outline and is confined to the urogenital triangle of the perineum. It serves to demarcate the two principal subdivisions of the urogenital triangle: the deep perineal pouch and the

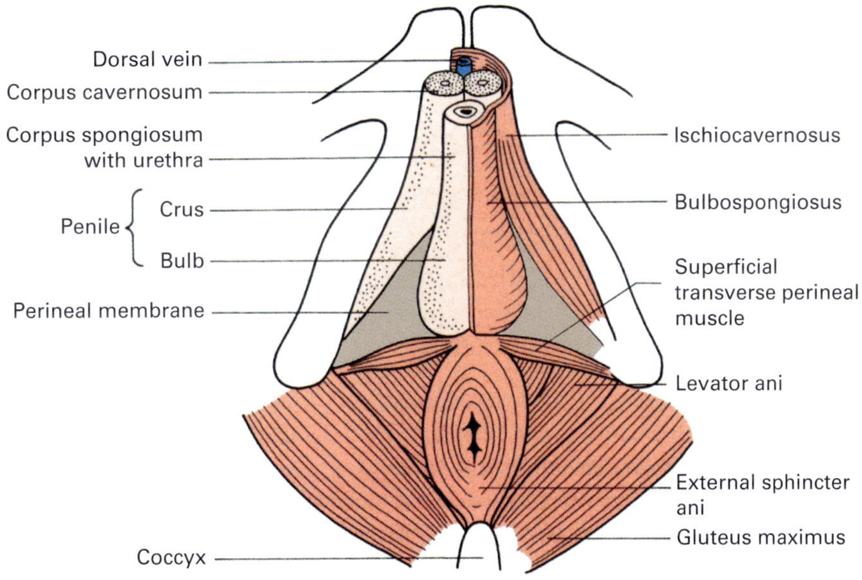

Fig. 96 The male perineum – on the right side the muscles of the urogenital region of the perineum have been dissected away.

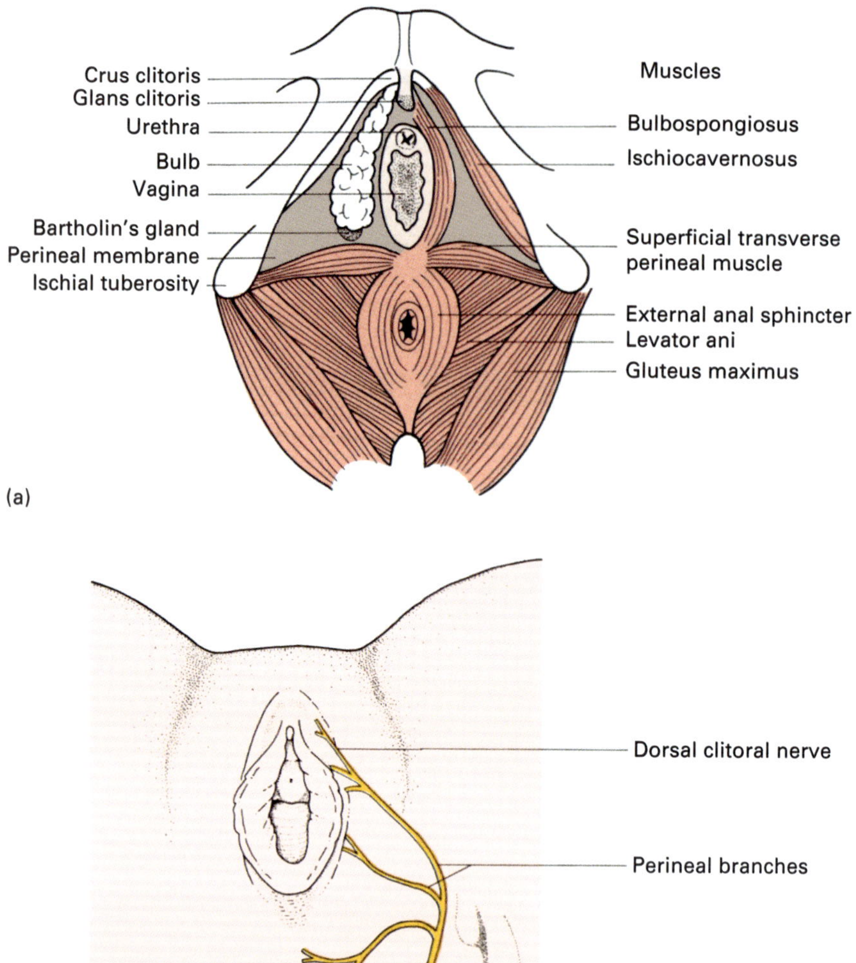

Fig. 97 (a) The female perineum – on the right side the muscles of the anterior perineum have been dissected away. (b) Distribution of the pudendal nerve to the female perineum.

superficial perineal pouch. The former lies deep to (i.e. above) the perineal membrane and is limited above, by the inferior surface of the pelvic floor (levator ani). The deep perineal pouch contains the membranous urethra, external urethral sphincter and the deep transverse perineal muscles. Additionally in the male, the bulbo-urethral glands (Cowper's glands) are situated in the deep perineal pouch, posterolateral to the membranous urethra.

The superficial perineal pouch lies superficial to (i.e. below) the perineal membrane.

This demarcation into superficial and deep pouches is more apparent in the male than in the female (owing to the perineal membrane being a more readily demonstrable entity in the male). The external genitalia both in the male and in the female are situated entirely in the superficial perineal pouch. The male external genital organs comprise the penis and spongiose urethra, muscles associated with the root of the penis, scrotum and scrotal contents. The female external genital organs (known collectively as the vulva) comprise the mons pubis, labia majora and minora, clitoris, vaginal vestibule and associated structures.

The perineal body (central perineal tendon)

This fibromuscular node-like structure lies in the midline at the junction of the anterior (urogenital region) and posterior (anal region) perineum. It is the point where several perineal muscles meet and interdigitate: the external anal sphincter, the bulbospongiosus, the transverse perineal muscles (deep and superficial) and fibres of levator ani.

The anal triangle of the perineum (Figs 97, 98)

This is the triangle lying between the right and left ischial tuberosities and between the inferior edges of the sacrotuberous ligaments on each side and the coccyx, posteriorly. It contains the anal canal with its external sphincter and, on either side, the corresponding ischioanal fossa. The anal canal has been described earlier.

The *ischioanal fossa* (Fig. 98) is of considerable surgical importance as it is frequently the site of abscess formation. The boundaries of the ischioanal fossa are:

- *laterally* – the fascia over the inner aspect of obturator internus (i.e. the side wall of the pelvis); contained in this wall within a fascial tunnel termed the *pudendal* or *Alcock's canal* are the pudendal vessels and nerve which give off, respectively, the inferior rectal vessels and nerve, which supply the external sphincter and perianal skin, then pass forwards to supply the structures in the urogenital region of the perineum;

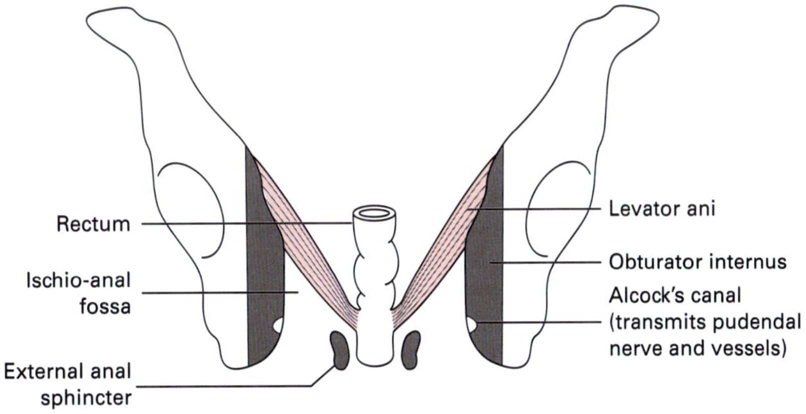

Fig. 98 The ischiorectal fossa (more accurately called the ischioanal fossa).

- *superiorly and medially* – the fascia on the inferior surface of levator ani and the external anal sphincter, respectively;
- *posteriorly* – the sacrotuberous ligament covered posteriorly by gluteus maximus;
- *anteriorly* – the urogenital perineum;
- *floor* – skin and subcutaneous fat.

CLINICAL FEATURES

1 The fossa contains coarsely lobulated fat. It is important to note that the ischioanal fossae communicate with each other behind the anal canal – infection in one may therefore pass to the other.

Infection of this space may occur from boils or abrasions of the perianal skin, or from lesions within the rectum and anal canal, especially infection of the branched anal glands, approximately six in number, which lie immediately above the valves of Ball (see page 87 and Fig. 62). Occasionally, it may follow from pelvic infection bursting through levator ani or, rarely, via the bloodstream. The fossa contains no important structures and can, therefore, be incised without fear when infected.

2 The pudendal nerves can be blocked in Alcock's canal on either side to give useful regional anaesthesia in obstetrical forceps delivery (Fig. 97 and see page 266).

The female genital organs

The vulva

The *vulva* (or *pudendum*) is the collective term applied to denote the female external genitalia.

The *labia majora* are the prominent hair-bearing folds extending back from the *mons pubis* to meet posteriorly in the midline of the perineum. They are the equivalent of the male scrotum.

The *labia minora* lie deep to the labia majora as lips of soft skin which meet posteriorly in a sharp fold, the *fourchette*. Anteriorly, they split to enclose the *clitoris*, forming an anterior *prepuce* and posterior *frenulum*.

The *vestibule* is the area enclosed by the labia minora and contains the *urethral orifice* (which lies immediately behind the clitoris) and the *vaginal orifice*.

The vaginal orifice is guarded in the virgin by a thin mucosal fold, the *hymen*, which is perforated to allow the egress of the menses, and may have an annular, semilunar, septate or cribriform appearance. Rarely, it is imperforate and menstrual blood distends the vagina (haematocolpos). At first coitus the hymen tears, usually posteriorly or posterolaterally, and after childbirth nothing is left of it but a few remnant tags termed *carunculae myrtiformes*.

Bartholin's glands (the greater vestibular glands) are a pair of lobulated, pea-sized, mucus-secreting glands lying deep to the posterior parts of the labia majora. They are impalpable when healthy but become obvious when inflamed or distended. Each drains by a duct 2.5 cm (1 in) long which opens into the groove between the hymen and the posterior part of the labium minus.

Anteriorly, each gland is overlapped by the *bulb of the vestibule* – a mass of cavernous erectile tissue equivalent to the bulbus spongiosum of the male. This tissue passes forwards, under cover of bulbospongiosus, around the sides of the vagina to the roots of the clitoris.

CLINICAL FEATURES

At childbirth the introitus may be enlarged by making an incision in the perineum (*episiotomy*). This starts at the fourchette and extends posterolaterally on the right side for 3 cm (1.5 in). The skin, vaginal epithelium, subcutaneous fat, perineal body and superficial transverse perineal muscle are incised. After delivery the episiotomy is carefully repaired in layers.

The vagina (Fig. 99)

The vagina surrounds the cervix of the uterus, then passes downwards and forwards through the pelvic floor to open into the vestibule.

The cervix projects into the anterior part of the vault of the vagina so that the continuous gutter surrounding the cervix is shallow anteriorly (where the vaginal wall is 7.5 cm (3 in) in length) and is deep posteriorly (where the vaginal wall is 10 cm (4 in) long). This continuous circumferential gutter is, for convenience of description, divided into the anterior, posterior and lateral *fornices*.

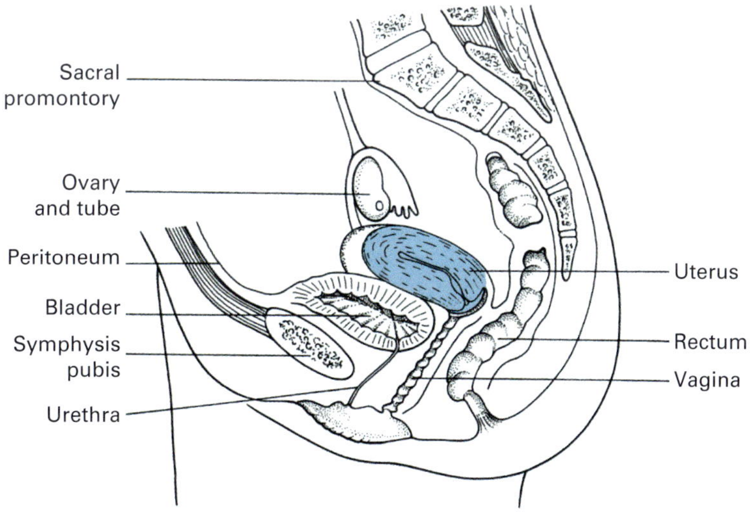

Fig. 99 Sagittal section of the uterus and its relations.

Relations

- *Anteriorly* – the base of the bladder and the urethra (which is embedded in the anterior vaginal wall).
- *Posteriorly* – from below upwards, the anal canal (separated by the perineal body), the rectum and then the peritoneum of the pouch of Douglas, which covers the *upper quarter of the posterior vaginal wall.*
- *Laterally* – levator ani, pelvic fascia and the *ureters*, which lie *immediately above the lateral fornices.*

Blood supply

Arterial supply is from the internal iliac artery via its vaginal, uterine, internal pudendal and middle rectal branches.

A venous plexus drains via the vaginal veins into the internal iliac vein.

Lymphatic drainage (see Fig. 103)

- Upper third to the external and internal iliac nodes.
- Middle third to the internal iliac nodes.
- Lower third to the superficial inguinal nodes.

Structure

A stratified squamous epithelium lines the vagina and the vaginal cervix; it contains no glands and is lubricated partly by cervical mucus and partly by desquamated vaginal epithelial cells. In nulliparous women the vaginal wall is rugose, but it becomes smoother after childbirth. The rugae of the anterior wall are situated transversely; this allows for filling of the bladder and for intercourse. In contrast, the rugae on the posterior wall run longitudinally. This allows for sideways stretching to accommodate a rectum distended with stool and for the passage of the fetal head.

Beneath the epithelial coat is a thin connective tissue layer separating it from the muscular wall, which is made up of a criss-cross arrangement of involuntary muscle fibres. This muscle layer is ensheathed in a fascial capsule that blends with adjacent pelvic connective tissues, so that the vagina is firmly supported in place.

In old age the vagina shrinks in length and diameter. The cervix projects far less into it so that the fornices all but disappear.

The uterus (Figs 99, 100)

The uterus is a pear-shaped organ, 7.5 cm (3 in) in length, made up of the *fundus*, *body* and *cervix*. The *Fallopian* (*uterine*) *tubes* enter into each supero-lateral angle of the body (the *cornu*), above which lies the fundus.

The body of the uterus narrows to a waist termed the *isthmus*, continuing into the *cervix* which is embraced about its middle by the vagina; this attachment delimits a supravaginal and vaginal part of the cervix.

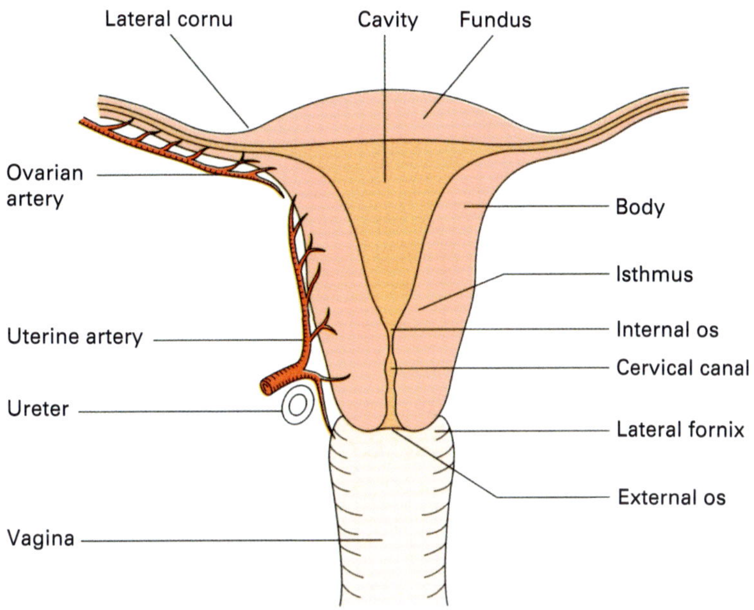

Fig. 100 Coronal section of the uterus and vagina. Note the important relationships of the ureter and uterine artery.

The isthmus is 1.5 mm wide. The anatomical *internal os* marks its junction with the uterine body, but its mucosa is histologically similar to the endometrium. The isthmus is that part of the uterus which becomes the lower segment in pregnancy.

The cavity of the uterine body is triangular in coronal section, but in the sagittal plane it is no more than a slit. This cavity communicates via the internal os with the *cervical canal*, which, in turn, opens into the vagina by the *external os*.

The nulliparous external os is circular, but after childbirth it becomes a transverse slit with an anterior and a posterior lip.

The non-pregnant cervix has a much firmer consistency than the pregnant cervix.

In fetal life the cervix is considerably larger than the body; in childhood (the *infantile uterus*) the cervix is still twice the size of the body but, during puberty, the uterus enlarges to its adult size and proportions by relative overgrowth of the body. The adult uterus is bent forwards on itself at about the level of the internal os to form an angle of 170°; this is termed *anteflexion of the uterus*. Moreover, the axis of the cervix forms an angle of 90° with the axis of the vagina – *anteversion of the uterus*. The uterus thus lies in an almost horizontal plane.

In *retroversion of the uterus*, the axis of the cervix is directed upwards and backwards. Normally, on vaginal examination the lowermost part of the cervix to be felt is its anterior lip; in retroversion, either the os or the posterior lip becomes the presenting part.

In *retroflexion* the axis of the body of the uterus passes upwards and backwards in relation to the axis of the cervix.

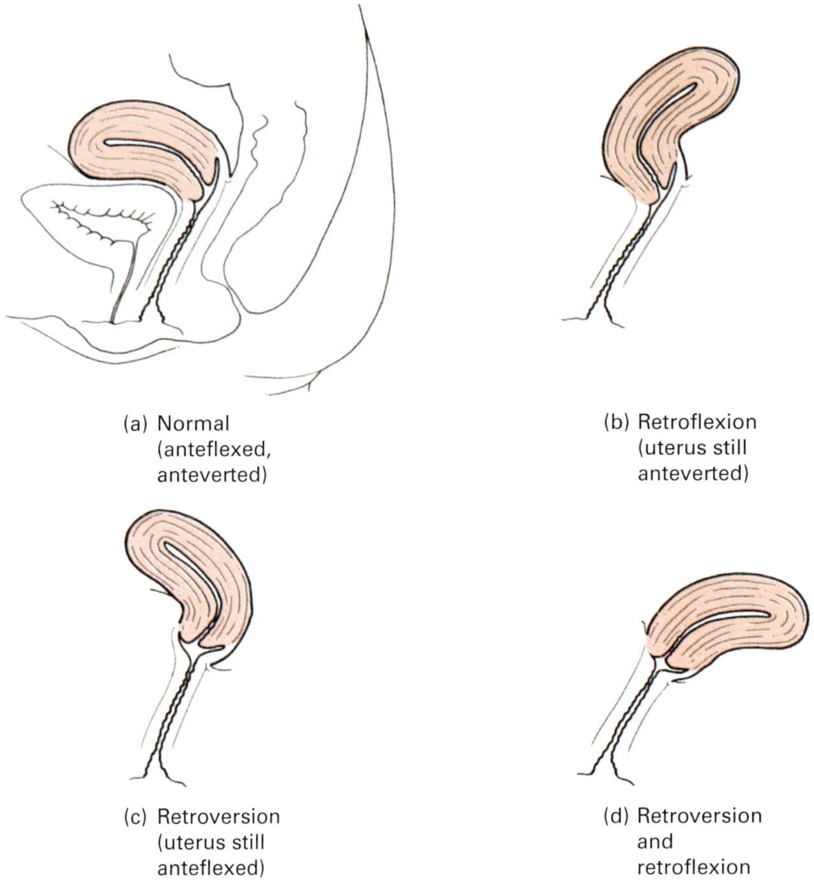

Fig. 101 Variations in uterine position and their terminology.

Frequently these two conditions coexist. They may be mobile and symptomless – as a result of distension of the bladder or purely as a development anomaly. Indeed, mobile retroversion is found in a quarter of the female population and may be regarded as a normal variant. Less commonly, they are fixed, the result of adhesions, previous pelvic infection, endometriosis or the pressure of a tumour in front of the uterus (Fig. 101).

Relations

- *Anteriorly* – the body is related to the uterovesical pouch of peritoneum and lies either on the superior surface of the bladder or on coils of intestine. The supravaginal cervix is related directly to the bladder, separated only by connective tissue. The infravaginal cervix has the anterior fornix immediately in front of it.
- *Posteriorly* – lies the pouch of Douglas, with coils of intestine within it.
- *Laterally* – the broad ligament and its contents; *the ureter lies approximately 1.2 cm (0.5 in) lateral to the supravaginal cervix.*

CLINICAL FEATURES

The most important single practical relationship in this region is that of the ureter to the supravaginal cervix. At this point, the ureter lies just above the level of the lateral fornix, below the uterine vessels as these pass across within the broad ligament (Fig. 102). In performing a hysterectomy, the ureter may be accidentally divided in clamping the uterine vessels, especially when the pelvic anatomy has been distorted by a previous operation, a mass of fibroids, infection or malignant infiltration.

The ureter is readily infiltrated by lateral extension of a carcinoma of the uterus; bilateral hydronephrosis with uraemia is a frequent mode of termination of this disease.

The close relationship of the ureter to the lateral fornix is best appreciated by realizing that a ureteric stone at this site can be palpated on vaginal examination. (This is the answer to the examination question: 'When can a stone in the ureter be felt?')

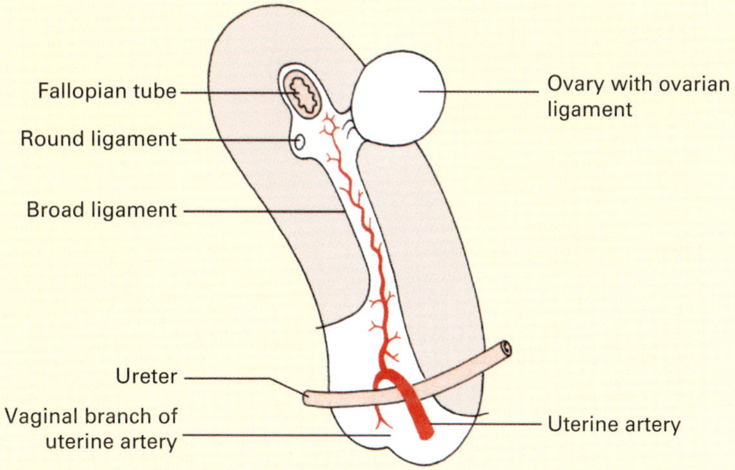

Fig. 102 Lateral view of the uterus (schematic) to show the composition of the broad ligament, the relations of the ureter and uterine artery and the peritoneal covering of the uterus (pink).

Blood supply

The *uterine artery* (from the internal iliac) runs in the base of the broad ligament and crosses above and at right angles to the ureter to reach the uterus at the level of the internal os (Fig. 102). The artery then ascends in a tortuous manner alongside the uterus, supplying the corpus, and then anastomoses with the *ovarian artery*. The uterine artery also gives off a descending branch to the cervix and branches to the upper vagina. The veins accompany the arteries and drain into the internal iliac veins, but they also communicate via the pelvic plexus with the veins of the vagina and bladder.

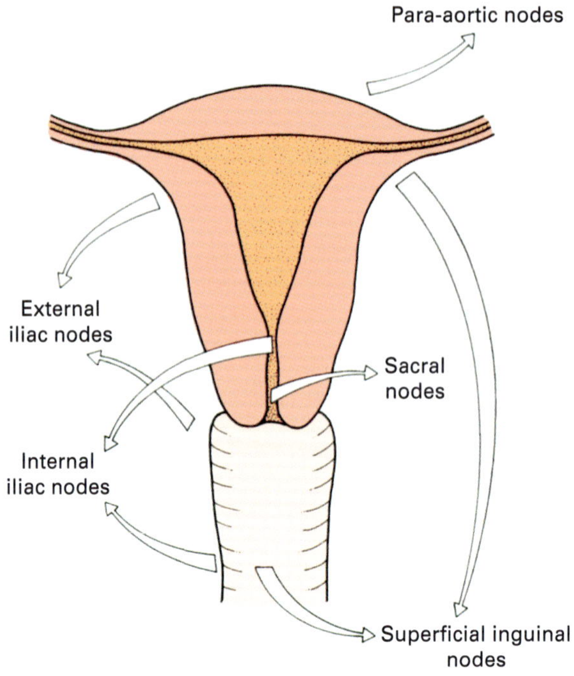

Fig. 103 Lymphatic drainage of the uterus and vagina.

Lymphatic drainage (Fig. 103)

1 The fundus (together with the ovary and Fallopian tube) drains along the ovarian vessels to the aortic nodes – apart from some lymphatics, which pass along the round ligament to the inguinal nodes.
2 The body drains via the broad ligament to nodes lying alongside the external iliac vessels.
3 The cervix drains in three directions – laterally, in the broad ligament, to the external iliac nodes; posterolaterally along the uterine vessels to the internal iliac nodes; and posteriorly along the recto-uterine folds to the sacral nodes.

Always examine the inguinal nodes in a suspected carcinoma of the corpus uteri – they may be involved by lymphatic spread along the round ligament.

Structure

The body of the uterus is covered with peritoneum except where this is reflected off at two sites, anteriorly onto the bladder at the uterine isthmus and laterally at the broad ligaments. Anteriorly, the peritoneum is only loosely adherent to the supravaginal cervix; this allows for bladder distension. The muscle wall is thick and made up of a criss-cross of involuntary fibres mixed with fibroelastic connective tissue.

The *mucosa* is applied directly to muscle with no submucosa intervening. The mucosa of the body of the uterus is the *endometrium*, made up of a single layer of cuboidal ciliated cells forming simple tubular glands which dip down to the underlying muscular wall. Below this epithelium is a stroma of connective tissue containing blood vessels and round cells.

The cervical canal epithelium is made up of tall columnar cells which form a series of complicated branching glands; these secrete an alkaline mucus that forms a protective '*cervical plug*' filling the canal.

The vaginal aspect of the cervix is covered with a stratified squamous epithelium continuous with that of the vagina.

The mucosa of the corpus undergoes extensive changes during the menstrual cycle, which may be briefly summarized thus:

1 first 4 days – desquamation of its superficial two-thirds with bleeding;
2 subsequent 2–3 days – rapid reconstitution of the raw mucosal surface by growth from the remaining epithelial cells in the depths of the glands;
3 by the 14th day the endometrium has reformed; this is the end of the *proliferative phase*;
4 the 14th day until the menstrual flow commences is the *secretory phase*; the endometrium thickens, the glands lengthen and distend with fluid and the stroma becomes oedematous and stuffed with white cells.

At the end of this phase three layers can be defined:

1 a compact superficial zone;
2 a spongy middle zone – with dilated glands and oedematous stroma;
3 a basal zone of inactive non-secreting tubules.

With degeneration of the corpus luteum there is shrinkage of the endometrium, the arteries retract and coil, producing ischaemia of the middle and superficial zones, which then desquamate. It is probable that spasm of the vessels in the basal layer (which remains non-desquamated) prevents the woman bleeding to death.

Only very slight desquamation and bleeding takes place in the mucosa of the cervical canal.

The Fallopian tubes (Fig. 104)

The Fallopian, or uterine, tubes are approximately 10 cm (4 in) long; they lie in the free edge of the broad ligaments and open into the cornu of the uterus. Each comprises four parts.

1 *The infundibulum* – the bugle-shaped extremity extending beyond the broad ligament and opening into the peritoneal cavity by the *ostium*. Its mouth is fimbriated and overlies the ovary, to which one long fimbria actually adheres (*fimbria ovarica*).
2 *The ampulla* – wide, thin-walled and tortuous.
3 *The isthmus* – narrow, straight and thick-walled.
4 *The interstitial part* – which pierces the uterine wall.

Structure

Apart from the interstitial part, the tube is clothed in peritoneum. Beneath this is a muscle of outer longitudinal and inner circular fibres.

The mucosa is formed of columnar, mainly ciliated cells and lies in longitudinal ridges, each of which is thrown into numerous folds.

The ova are propelled to the uterus along this tube, partly by peristalsis and partly by ciliary action.

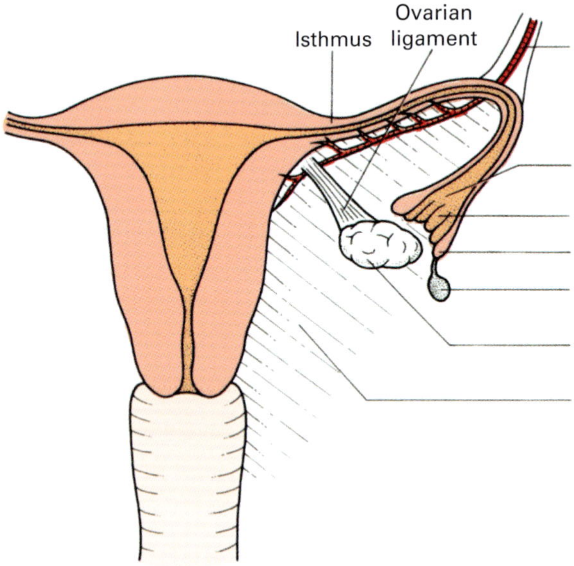

Fig. 104 The Fallopian tube, ovary and broad ligament (viewed from behind).

CLINICAL FEATURES

1 Note that the genital canal in the female is the only direct communication into the peritoneum from the exterior and is a potential pathway for infection (e.g. in gonorrhoea).

2 The fertilized ovum may implant ectopically, i.e. in a site other than the endometrium of the corpus uteri. When this occurs in the Fallopian tube it is called, according to the exact site, fimbrial, ampullary, isthmic or interstitial, of which the ampullary is the commonest and interstitial the rarest.

As the ectopic embryo enlarges, it may abort into the peritoneal cavity (where rarely it continues to grow as a secondary abdominal pregnancy), or else ruptures the tube. This second fate is particularly likely to occur in the narrow and relatively non-distensible isthmus; rupture is usually into the peritoneal cavity but may rarely occur into the broad ligament.

The ovary (Fig. 104)

The ovary is an almond-shaped organ, 4 cm (1.5 in) long, attached to the back of the broad ligament by the *mesovarium*. The ovary has two other attachments: the *infundibulopelvic ligament* (sometimes called the *suspensory ligament of the ovary*), along which pass the ovarian vessels, sympathetic nerves and lymphatics from the side wall of the pelvis, and the *ovarian ligament*, which passes to the cornu of the uterus.

Relations

The ovary is usually described as lying on the side-wall of the pelvis opposite the *ovarian fossa*, which is a depression bounded by the external iliac vessels in front and the ureter and internal iliac vessels behind and which contains the obturator nerve. However, the ovary is extremely variable in its position and is frequently found prolapsed into the pouch of Douglas in perfectly normal women.

The ovary, like the testis, develops from the genital ridge and then descends into the pelvis. In the same way as the testis, it therefore drags its blood supply and lymphatic drainage downwards with it from the posterior abdominal wall.

Blood supply, lymphatic drainage and nerve supply

Blood supply is from the ovarian artery, which arises from the aorta at the level of the renal arteries. The ovarian vein drains, on the right side, to the IVC and, on the left, to the left renal vein, exactly comparable to the venous drainage of the testis.

Lymphatics pass to the aortic nodes at the level of the renal vessels, following the general rule that lymphatic drainage accompanies the venous drainage of an organ.

Nerve supply is from the aortic plexus (T10 and T11); hence, referral of ovarian pain to the loin and groin. These are sympathetic (pain-conducting) afferent fibres.

All these structures pass to the ovary in the infundibulopelvic ligament.

Structure

The ovary has no peritoneal covering; the serosa ends at the mesovarian attachment. It consists of a connective tissue stroma containing *Graafian follicles* at various stages of development, *corpora lutea* and *corpora albicantia* (hyalinized, regressing corpora lutea, which take several months to absorb completely).

The surface of the ovary in young children is covered with a so-called 'germinal epithelium' of cuboidal cells. It is now known, however, that the primordial follicles develop in the ovary in early fetal life and do not differentiate from these cells. In adult life, in fact, the epithelial covering of the ovary disappears, leaving only a fibrous capsule termed the *tunica albuginea*.

After the menopause the ovary becomes small and shrivelled; in old age, the follicles disappear completely.

The endopelvic fascia and the pelvic ligaments (Fig. 105)

Pelvic fascia is the term applied to the connective tissue floor of the pelvis covering levator ani and obturator internus. The *endopelvic fascia* is the extraperitoneal cellular tissue of the uterus (the *parametrium*), vagina, bladder and rectum. Within this endopelvic fascia are three important condensations of connective tissue which sling the pelvic viscera from the pelvic walls.

1 The *cardinal ligaments* (transverse cervical, or Mackenrodt's ligaments), which pass laterally from the cervix and upper vagina to the side-walls of the pelvis along the lines of attachment of levator ani, are composed of white fibrous connective tissue with some involuntary muscle fibres and are pierced in their upper part by the ureters.

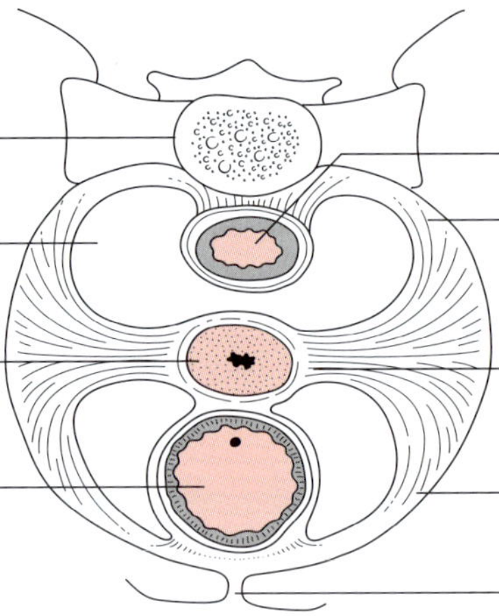

Fig. 105 The pelvic ligaments seen from above.

2 The *uterosacral ligaments*, which pass backwards from the posterolateral aspect of the cervix at the level of the isthmus and from the lateral vaginal fornices deep to the uterosacral folds of peritoneum in the lateral boundaries of the pouch of Douglas, are attached to the periosteum in front of the sacro-iliac joints and the lateral part of the third piece of the sacrum.

3 The *pubocervical fascia* extends forwards from the cardinal ligament to the pubis on either side of the bladder, for which it acts as a sling.

These three ligaments act as supports to the cervix of the uterus and the vault of the vagina, in conjunction with the important elastic muscular foundation provided by levator ani. In prolapse, these ligaments lengthen (in procidentia – complete uterine prolapse – they may be 15 cm [6 in] long) and any repair operation must include their reconstitution.

Two other pairs of ligaments take attachments from the uterus.

1 The *broad ligament* is a fold of peritoneum connecting the lateral margin of the uterus with the side-wall of the pelvis on each side. The uterus and its broad ligaments, therefore, form a partition across the pelvic floor dividing off an anterior compartment, containing the bladder (the *uterovesical pouch*), from a posterior compartment, containing the rectum (the pouch of Douglas or *recto-uterine pouch*).

The broad ligament contains or carries (Figs 102, 104):

- the Fallopian (uterine) tube in its free edge;
- the ovary, attached by the mesovarium to its posterior aspect;
- the round ligament;
- the ovarian ligament, crossing from the ovary to the uterine cornu (see 'The ovary', page 150);
- the uterine vessels and branches of the ovarian vessels;
- lymphatics and nerve fibres.

The ureter passes forwards to the bladder deep to this ligament and lateral to and immediately above the lateral fornix of the vagina.

2 The *round ligament* – a fibromuscular cord – passes from the lateral angle of the uterus in the anterior layer of the broad ligament to the internal inguinal ring; thence along the length of the inguinal canal before emerging at the superficial inguinal ring and fusing

with the labium majus. Taken together with the ovarian ligament, it is equivalent to the male gubernaculum testis and can be thought of as the pathway along which the female gonad might have descended, but in fact did not, to the labium majus (the female homologue of the scrotum). Compare this process with descent of the testis (page 126).

Vaginal examination

The relations of the vagina to the other pelvic organs must be constantly borne in mind when carrying out a vaginal examination.

Inspection (by means of a speculum) enables the vaginal walls and cervix to be examined and a biopsy or cytological smear to be taken. Inspection of the introitus while straining detects prolapse and the presence of stress incontinence.

- *Anteriorly* – the urethra, bladder and symphysis pubis are felt.
- *Posteriorly* – the rectum (invasion of the vagina by a rectal neoplasm must always be kept in mind when examining a woman with a suspected or proven rectal cancer). Collections of fluid, malignant deposits, endometriotic nodules, prolapsed uterine tubes and ovaries or coils of distended bowel may be felt in the pouch of Douglas.
- *Laterally* – the ovary and Fallopian tube, and the side-wall of the pelvis. Rarely, a stone in the ureter may be felt through the lateral fornix. The strength of the perineal muscles can be assessed by asking the patient to tighten up her perineum.
- *Apex* – the cervix is felt projecting back from the anterior wall of the vagina. In the normal anteverted uterus the anterior lip of the cervix presents; in retroversion, either the cervical os or the posterior lip are first to be felt.

Pathological cervical conditions – for example, neoplasms – can be felt, as can physiological softening of the cervix in pregnancy and its dilatation during labour.

Bimanual examination assesses the pelvic size and position of the uterus, enlargements of ovary or uterine tubes and the presence of other pelvic masses.

The obstetrician can assess the pelvic size in both the transverse and anteroposterior diameter. Particularly important is the distance from the lower border of the symphysis pubis to the sacral promontory, which is termed the *diagonal conjugate*. If the pelvis is of normal size, the examiner's fingers should fail to reach the promontory of the sacrum. If it is readily palpable, pelvic narrowing is present (see 'Obstetrical pelvic measurements', page 135).

Embryology of the Fallopian tubes, uterus and vagina (Fig. 106)

The *paramesonephric* (or *Müllerian*) *ducts* develop, one on each side, adjacent to the *mesonephric* (*Wolffian*) *ducts* in the posterior abdominal wall – they are mesodermal in origin. All these four tubes lie close together caudally, projecting into the anterior (urogenital) compartment of the cloaca.

One system disappears in the male, the other in the female, each leaving behind congenital remnants of some interest to the clinician.

In the male, the paramesonephric duct disappears, apart from the appendix testis and the prostatic utricle. In the female, the mesonephric system (which in the male develops into the vas deferens and epididymal ducts) persists as remnants in the broad ligament termed the *epoöphoron*, *paroöphoron* and *ducts of Gärtner*.

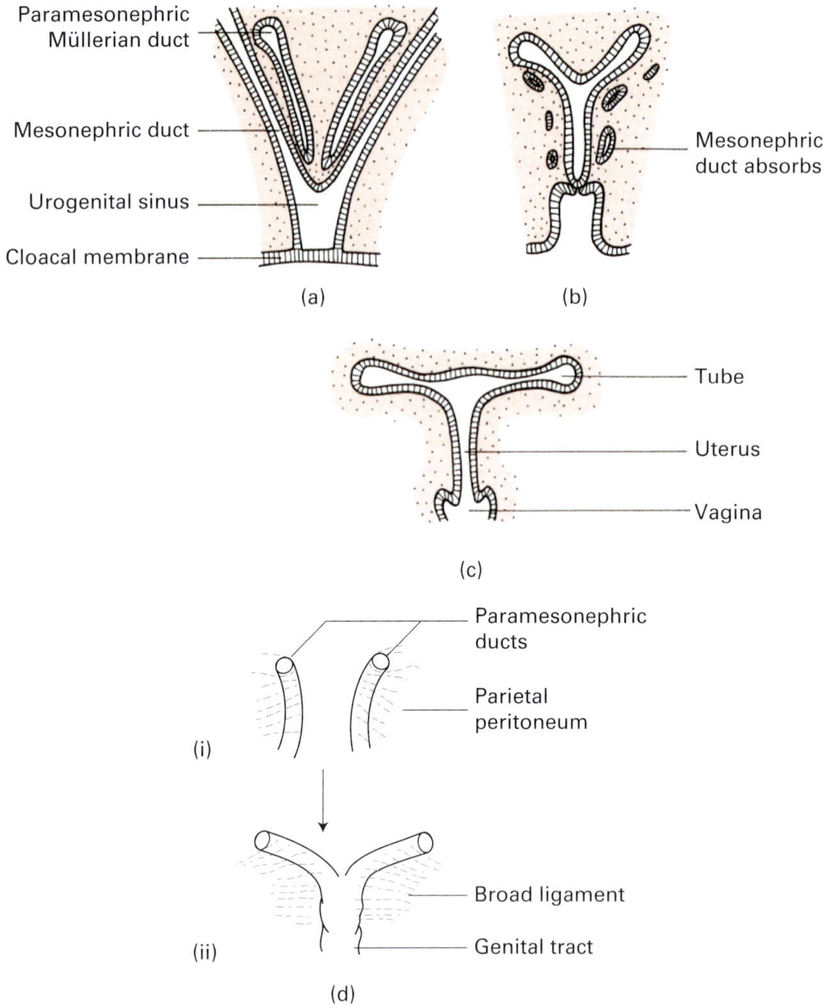

Fig. 106 Development of the Fallopian tubes, uterus and vagina from the paramesonephric (Müllerian) ducts and the urogenital sinus (after Hollinshead) (a–c), and formation of the broad ligament (d).

The paramesonephric ducts in the female form the Fallopian tubes cranially. More caudally, they come together and fuse in the midline (dragging, as they do so, a peritoneal fold from the side-wall of the pelvis which becomes the broad ligament). The median structure so formed differentiates into the epithelium of the uterine body (endometrium), cervical canal and upper one-third of the vagina, which are first solid and later become canalized. The rest of the vaginal epithelium develops by canalization of the solid sinuvaginal node at the back of the urogenital sinus. This accounts for the differences in lymphatic drainage of the upper and lower vagina (Fig. 103). The muscle of the Fallopian tubes, uterine body, cervix and vagina develops from surrounding mesoderm, so that remnants of the mesonephric duct system of the female are found in the myometrium, cervix and vaginal wall.

Developmental abnormalities of this system can easily be deduced. All stages of division of the original double tube may persist from a bicornuate uterus to a complete reduplication of the uterus and vagina. Alternatively, there may be absence, hypoplasia or atresia of the duct system on one or both sides.

Failure of canalization of the originally solid caudal end of the duct results, after puberty, in the accumulation of menstrual blood above the obstruction. First the vagina may distend with blood, then the uterus and then the tubes (haematocolpos, haematometra and haematosalpinx, respectively).

The posterior abdominal wall

The bed of the posterior abdominal wall is made up of three osseous parts and four muscular structures.

The osseous parts are:

- the lumbar vertebral column (comprising the five lumbar vertebrae);
- the sacrum;
- the wings (ala) of the ilium.

The muscles are:

- the diaphragm – posterior part;
- the quadratus lumborum;
- the psoas major;
- the iliacus.

The diaphragm has been considered in the section on the thorax (see page 14).

The psoas must be dealt with in more detail because of the involvement of its sheath in the formation of a psoas abscess.

The *psoas major* arises from the transverse processes of all the lumbar vertebrae and from the sides of the bodies and the intervening discs of the T12 to L5 vertebrae. It passes downwards and laterally at the margin of the brim of the pelvis, narrowing down to a tendon which crosses the front of the hip joint beneath the inguinal ligament to be inserted, with iliacus, into the lesser trochanter of the femur (Fig. 107).

The psoas major, together with iliacus, flexes the hip on the trunk, or, alternatively, the trunk on the hips (e.g. in sitting up from the lying position). *Psoas minor*, absent in 40% of subjects, lies on psoas major and attaches to the iliopubic eminence.

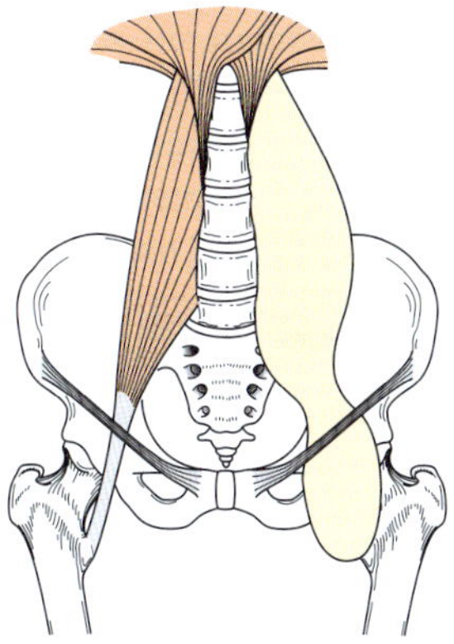

Fig. 107 Psoas sheath and psoas abscess. On the right side is a normal psoas sheath; on the left side it is shown distended with pus, which tracks under the inguinal ligament to present in the groin.

CLINICAL FEATURES

1 The femoral artery lies on the psoas tendon in the groin, and it is this firm posterior relation of the femoral artery at the groin which enables it here to be identified and compressed easily by the finger.
2 The psoas is enclosed in the psoas sheath, which is a compartment of the lumbar fascia. Pus from a tuberculous infection of the lumbar vertebrae is limited in its anterior spread by the anterior longitudinal vertebral ligament, and therefore passes laterally into its sheath (*psoas abscess*), which may also be entered by pus tracking down from the posterior mediastinum in disease of the thoracic vertebrae. Pus may then spread under the inguinal ligament into the femoral triangle, where it produces a soft swelling (Fig. 107). Occasionally, in completely neglected cases, pus tracks along the femoral vessels, along the subsartorial canal and eventually appears in the popliteal fossa.

The retroperitoneal organs are: the pancreas, kidneys and ureters (which have already been considered), the suprarenals, the aorta and IVC and their main branches, the para-aortic lymph nodes and the lumbar sympathetic chain.

The suprarenal glands (Fig. 79)

The suprarenal glands cap the upper poles of the kidneys and lie against the crura of the diaphragm. The left is related anteriorly to the stomach across the lesser sac; the right lies behind the right lobe of the liver and tucks medially behind the IVC.

Each gland, although weighing only 3–4 g, has three arteries supplying it:
1 a direct branch from the aorta;
2 a branch from the ipsilateral inferior phrenic artery;
3 a branch from the ipsilateral renal artery.

The right suprarenal vein is a very short vessel and drains from the hilum of the gland directly into the nearby IVC. The left suprarenal vein drains into the left renal vein and thereby into the IVC.

The suprarenal gland comprises a cortex and medulla, which represent two developmentally and functionally distinct and independent endocrine glands within the same anatomical structure. The medulla is derived from the neural crest (neuroectoderm), whose cells also give rise to the sympathetic ganglia. The cortex, on the other hand, is derived from the mesoderm. The suprarenal medulla receives preganglionic sympathetic fibres from the splanchnic nerves and secretes adrenaline (epinephrine) and noradrenaline (norepinephrine). The cortex secretes the adrenocortical hormones.

Abdominal aorta (Fig. 108)

The aorta enters the abdomen via the aortic hiatus in the diaphragm at the level of the 12th thoracic vertebra and ends at the level of L4 in the supracristal (transcristal) plane (Fig. 40). It lies throughout this course against the vertebral bodies and may be palpable in a slim individual, more or less in the midline. The normal abdominal aorta measures approximately 1–1.5 cm (0.5 in) in diameter. In the elderly it is frequently thickened

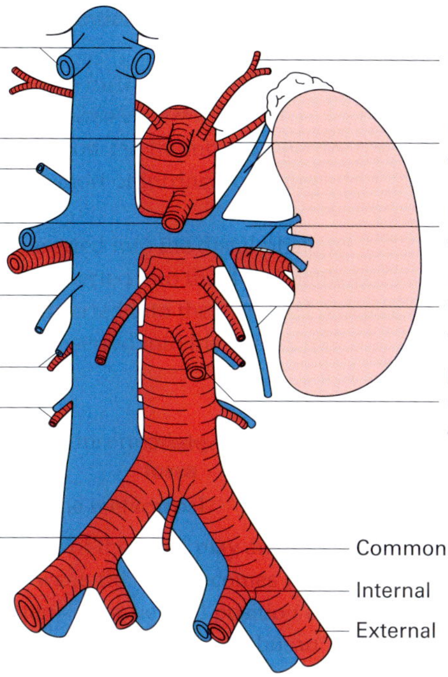

Fig. 108 The abdominal aorta, the inferior vena cava and their main branches.

and dilated. An early aneurysmal dilatation is considered to be present if the diameter reaches 4 cm (1.5 in).

Anteriorly, from above down, it is related to the pancreas which separates the aorta from the stomach), the third part of the duodenum and coils of small intestine. It is crossed anteriorly by the left renal vein, just below the origin of the superior mesenteric artery. A large tumour of pancreas or stomach, a mass of enlarged para-aortic nodes or a large ovarian cyst may transmit the pulsations of the aorta and be mistaken for an aortic aneurysm.

The branches of the abdominal aorta are:

1 three anterior unpaired branches passing to the viscera:
- **a** the *coeliac axis* – giving off the;
  - hepatic artery
  - splenic artery
  - left gastric artery
- **b** the *superior mesenteric artery;*
- **c** the *inferior mesenteric artery.*

2 three laterally directed, paired branches to viscera:
- **a** the *suprarenal artery;*
- **b** the *renal artery;*
- **c** the *testicular or ovarian artery.*

3 five lateral paired branches to the parietes:
- **a** the *inferior phrenic artery;*
- **b** four *lumbar* branches.

4 terminal branches:

a the *right and left common iliacs;*

b the *median sacral artery.*

The *common iliac arteries* pass, one on each side, downwards and outwards to bifurcate into the internal and external iliacs in front of the sacro-iliac joint, at the level of the sacral promontory. They give no other branches.

At the bifurcation, the common iliac artery is crossed anteriorly by the ureter – a convenient site to identify this latter structure in pelvic operations.

The *external iliac artery* runs along the brim of the pelvis on the medial side of psoas major. The artery passes below the inguinal ligament to continue as the (common) femoral artery, giving off, immediately proximal to the inguinal ligament, the *inferior epigastric artery*, which demarcates the medial edge of the internal inguinal ring (Fig. 43) and also the *deep circumflex iliac artery*.

The *internal iliac artery* passes backwards and downwards into the pelvis, sandwiched between the ureter anteriorly and the internal iliac vein posteriorly. At the upper border of the greater sciatic notch it divides into anterior and posterior divisions, which give off numerous branches to supply the pelvic walls, pelvic organs, perineum, gluteal region and sacral canal (Fig. 109). These are:

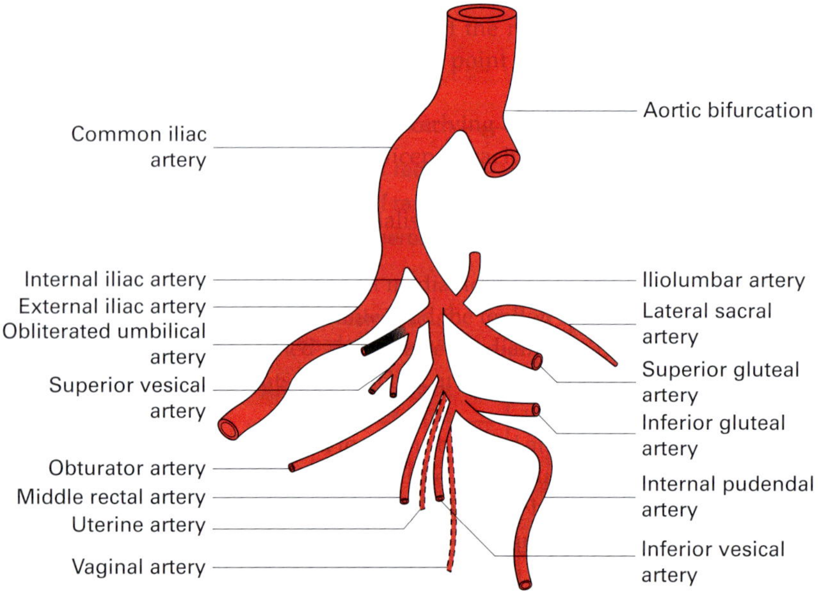

Fig. 109 The aortic bifurcation and the right internal iliac artery. The internal iliac artery divides into anterior and posterior divisions. The latter gives rise to the superior gluteal artery, whereas the former gives off all the visceral branches. (Although the branches of the internal iliac artery are fairly constant, the arrangement of these branches is variable.) Hatching indicates arteries present only in the female.

1 parietal branches to the inner and outer walls of the pelvis, sacrum and sacral canal, the perineum and the gluteal region:
  a iliolumbar;
  b lateral sacral;
  c obturator;
  d superior gluteal;
  e inferior gluteal;
  f internal pudendal.
2 visceral branches to the pelvic organs:
  a superior vesical;
  b inferior vesical (vaginal in the female);
  c middle rectal.

In addition, in the female, the uterine artery, which arises above the vaginal.

These arteries are accompanied by their corresponding veins, which drain to the internal iliac vein.

Inferior vena cava (Fig. 108)

The IVC commences at the level of L5, somewhat to the right of the midline by the confluence of the right and left common iliac veins *behind* the right common iliac artery (unlike the usual arrangement of a vein being superficial to its corresponding artery). It lies to the right of the aorta as it ascends until separated from it by the right crus of the diaphragm. The IVC itself passes through the central tendon of the diaphragm at T8 (Fig. 11), traverses the pericardium and drains into the right atrium.

As the IVC ascends, it is related anteriorly to coils of small intestine, the third part of the duodenum, the head of the pancreas with the common bile duct and the first part of the duodenum. It then passes behind the foramen of Winslow. In front of this foramen, within the free edge of the lesser omentum lies the portal vein along with the common bile duct and hepatic artery. Finally, the IVC lies in a deep groove in the liver before crossing the vena caval hiatus in the diaphragm. Within the liver, the IVC receives the right and left hepatic veins. Occasionally, these veins join to form a single trunk that opens directly into the IVC; on other occasions, the central hepatic vein (which usually enters the left hepatic vein near the latter's termination) drains directly into the IVC (Fig. 72). Awareness of these variations is of considerable practical importance to the surgeon when carrying out hepatic segmental resections.

Lumbar sympathetic chain

The lumbar part of the sympathetic trunk commences deep to the medial arcuate ligament of the diaphragm as a continuation of the thoracic sympathetic chain (see Fig. 270). On each side it lies against the bodies of the lumbar vertebrae, overlapped, on the right side, by the IVC and, on the left, by the aorta.

The lumbar arteries cross posterior to the chain but the lumbar veins may cross in front of the chain and are of importance because they may be damaged when performing a lumbar sympathectomy.

Inferiorly, the lumbar sympathetic trunk passes posterior to the iliac vessels, crosses the pelvic brim and continues as the sacral sympathetic trunk in front of the sacrum. Inferiorly, the chains converge and unite in front of the coccyx at the small *ganglion impar*.

Usually the lumbar trunk features four ganglia, although sometimes, due to fusion of two adjacent ganglia, the trunk may appear to possess only three ganglia. All four ganglia send grey rami communicantes to the lumbar spinal nerves; in addition, the upper two ganglia receive white rami.

Branches from the chain pass to plexuses around the abdominal aorta and its branches, which also receive fibres from the splanchnic nerves and the vagus. Other branches pass in front of the common iliac vessels as the superior hypogastric plexus ('presacral nerve') to supply the pelvic viscera via plexuses of nerves distributed along the branches of the internal iliac artery.

The splanchnic nerves also carry afferent fibres from the abdominal viscera to the spinal cord and thence to the brain. These nerves are stimulated by excessive visceral muscle contraction ('colic'), ischaemia, inflammation, distension and traction and account for the perception of pain from the abdominal and pelvic viscera under pathological conditions (see also pages 422 and 423 and Fig. 270).

The parasympathetic supply to the pelvic viscera arises from the lateral horn cells of the sacral grey matter and the fibres travel in the anterior rami of S2, S3 and S4 and are distributed through the pelvic plexuses (see page 417).

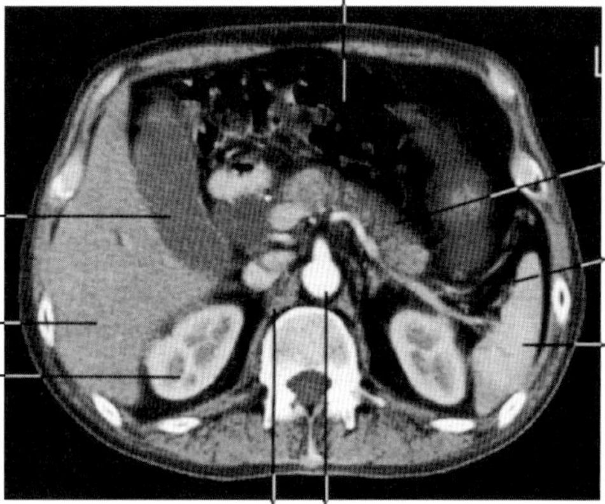

Fig. 110 CT scan at the level of the 1st lumbar vertebra. This demonstrates the liver, gall bladder, aorta with the commencement of the superior mesenteric artery, the inferior vena cava, the crura of the diaphragm, the kidneys, the pancreas and the spleen. The splenic vein can be seen as it passes to the splenic hilum posterior to the body of the pancreas. The vena cava lies on the right crus. The vessels have been enhanced by an intravenous injection of contrast (Dr Sheila Rankin).

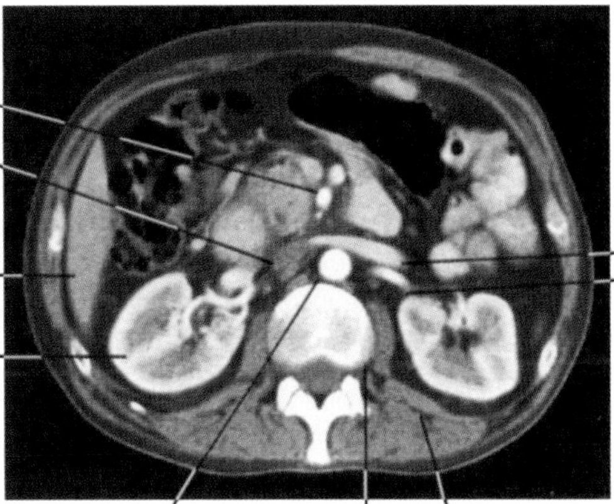

Fig. 111 CT scan at the level of the 2nd lumbar vertebra demonstrating the kidneys, aorta, inferior vena cava, the liver, renal and superior mesenteric vessels and the muscles of the abdominal wall. The blood vessels, again, have been enhanced by an intravenous injection of contrast (Dr Sheila Rankin).

Computed axial tomography

Computed axial tomography (CT scanning) has revealed a fresh dimension to the importance of topographical anatomy. It is now necessary for clinicians to possess a detailed knowledge of the cross-sectional relationships of the body in health so that pathological abnormalities can be appreciated. Figures 110 and 111 demonstrate CT scan cuts of the abdomen at the levels of the 1st and 2nd lumbar vertebral bodies, respectively. Clinical students should take every opportunity of studying normal scans with the help of an experienced radiologist.

Part 3
The Upper Limb

Surface anatomy and surface markings of the upper limb

Much of the surface anatomy of the limbs can be studied on oneself or on an obliging colleague with a suitable body mass index!

Bones and joints (see Figs 117, 119, 120, 122)

The subcutaneous border of the *clavicle* can be palpated along its entire length; the supraclavicular nerves crossing the surface of the clavicle can occasionally be felt against the underlying bone.

The *acromion process* forms a distinct bony edge at the lateral extremity of the *scapular spine*. It lies immediately above the smooth bulge of the *deltoid muscle*, which itself covers the *greater tubercle of the humerus*. Less easily identified is the *coracoid process* of the scapula, lying immediately below the clavicle at the junction of the middle and outer thirds, and covered by the anterior fibres of the deltoid.

The medial border of the scapula can be both seen and felt. Abduction of the arm is a complex affair made up of abduction at the shoulder joint, depression at the sternoclavicular joint and rotation of the scapula; the last two are readily confirmed by self-palpation.

With the shoulder abducted, the *head of the humerus* can be felt at the apex of the axilla; note its movement with rotation of the arm.

At the elbow, the three bony landmarks are the *olecranon process* and the *medial* and *lateral epicondyles*. A supracondylar fracture lies above these points, which therefore remain in their triangular relationship to each other; in dislocation of the elbow, however, the olecranon comes to lie more or less in line with the epicondyles (Fig. 112).

Note a hollow in the posterolateral aspect of the extended elbow distal to the lateral epicondyle; this lies over the *head of the radius*, which can be felt to rotate during pronation and supination of the forearm.

The posterior border of the *ulna* is subcutaneous along its entire length and is not crossed by any named vessels or nerve; it can therefore be exposed surgically from end to end without fear of damaging any important structures.

At the wrist, the *styloid processes* of the radius and ulna can be felt; the former extends more distally. The radial styloid lies in the floor of the 'anatomical snuffbox', while the ulnar styloid can be felt (and usually seen) on the dorsal aspect of the *head* of the ulna (note that it is the distal, not proximal, end of the ulna that is termed the 'head'). The *dorsal tubercle of Lister* is palpable on the posterior aspect of the distal end of the radius.

In the palm of the hand, palpate the *pisiform* at the base of the hypothenar eminence. *Flexor carpi ulnaris* is inserted into it and when this tendon is relaxed by flexing the wrist the pisiform can be moved a little from side to side. The *hook of the hamate* can be felt by deep palpation just disto-radial to the pisiform. The *scaphoid* is felt at the base of the thenar eminence and also within the anatomical snuffbox, where there is characteristic tenderness when this bone is fractured. In a thin subject, the pisiform and the tubercle of the scaphoid can be seen as bulges when the wrist is extended.

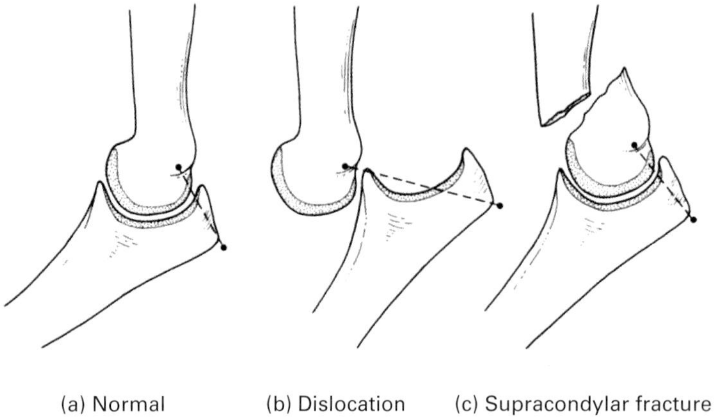

Fig. 112 The relationship of the medial and lateral epicondyles to the olecranon process (a) is disturbed in a dislocation of the elbow (b) but maintained in a supracondylar fracture (c).

Muscles and tendons

The anterior fold of the axilla is formed by the *pectoralis major*, and the posterior fold of the axilla by the *teres major* and *latissimus dorsi*. The digitations of *serratus anterior* can be seen in a muscular subject on the medial axillary wall.

In the upper arm the *deltoid* forms the smooth contour of the shoulder. The *biceps* and *brachialis* constitute the bulk of the anterior aspect of the arm and the *triceps* its posterior aspect. The tendon of biceps is easily felt, and often seen, at the elbow when this is flexed to a right angle. Immediately medial to this, palpate the pulse of the brachial artery. Firm pressure immediately medial to the brachial artery pulsation may, in turn, produce paraesthesia in the hand as the median nerve is palpated (see Fig. 134).

When the semi-pronated forearm is flexed against resistance, the *brachioradialis* presents prominently along its radial border.

At the wrist (Figs 113, 114, 115) it is convenient to commence at the radial pulse. The tendon medial to this is that of the *flexor carpi radialis*. Continuing medially, the next tendon is that of *palmaris longus* (which may be absent in 10–15% of individuals), then the cluster of tendons of *flexor digitorum superficialis*. The tendon of *flexor carpi ulnaris* lies most medially, inserting into the pisiform; the ulnar pulse can be felt just to the radial side of this tendon.

On the dorsal aspect of the wrist (Figs 114, 115) the anatomical snuffbox is bordered by the tendons of *abductor pollicis longus* and *extensor pollicis brevis* laterally and that of *extensor pollicis longus* medially (i.e. towards the ulnar border) – the last can be traced to the base of the terminal phalanx of the extended thumb. The tendons of extensor digitorum are seen in the extended hand passing over the dorsal aspects of the proximal phalanges of the fingers.

Vessels

Feel the pulsations of the *subclavian artery* against the first rib (often difficult), the *brachial artery* against the humerus, the *radial* and *ulnar* arteries at the wrist and the *radial artery* again in the anatomical snuffbox.

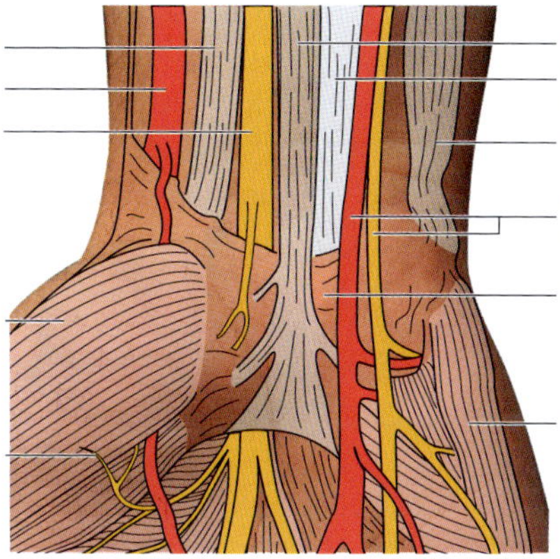

Fig. 113 The structures on the anterior aspect of the right wrist.

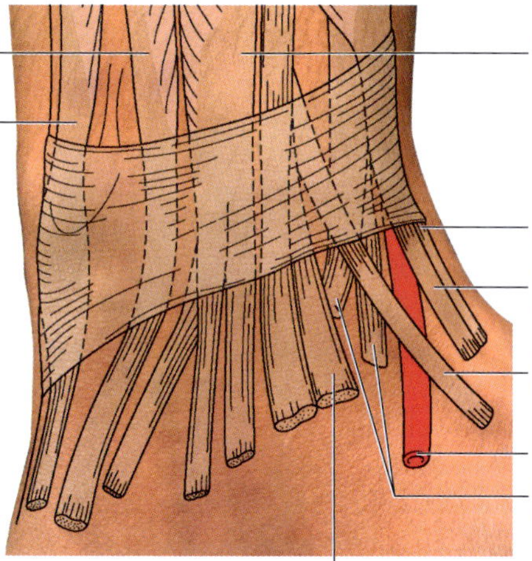

Fig. 114 The structures on the posterior aspect of the right wrist.

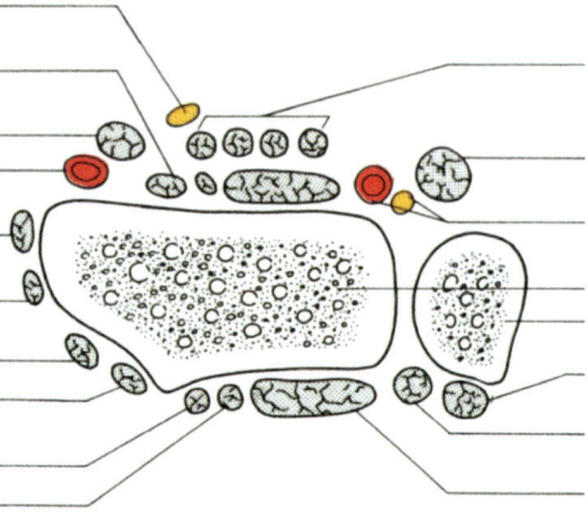

Fig. 115 Section immediately above the wrist joint.

The brachial artery bifurcates into its radial and ulnar branches at the level of the neck of the radius and the line of the radial artery and then corresponds, approximately, to the slight groove which can be seen along the ulnar border of the tensed brachioradialis.

The veins of the upper limb (Fig. 116) comprise the *deep venae comitantes*, which accompany all the main arteries, usually in pairs, and the superficial veins which are of immense value in clinical practice because of the relative ease with which they may be accessed for venepuncture and transfusion.

These superficial veins can be seen as a dorsal venous network on the back of the hand that drains into the *cephalic vein* laterally and into the *basilic vein* on the medial side.

The cephalic vein at its origin lies fairly constantly in the superficial fascia just posterior to the radial styloid; even if not visible it can be reached easily at this site for a venous cut-down. It then runs up the anterior aspect of the forearm and crosses the elbow region to lie in a groove along the lateral border of the biceps in the arm, and then, after piercing the deep fascia, it lies in the groove between pectoralis major and the deltoid, where again it can readily be exposed for an emergency cut-down. It finally penetrates the clavipectoral fascia to enter the axillary vein.

The basilic vein runs along the posteromedial aspect of the forearm, passes on to the anterior aspect just below the elbow and pierces the deep fascia at about the middle of the upper arm. At the edge of the posterior axillary fold, it is joined by the venae comitantes of the brachial artery to form the axillary vein.

Linking the cephalic and basilic veins just distal to the front of the elbow crease is the *median cubital* vein, one of the more prominent superficial veins in the body and often visible or palpable. It usually runs upwards and medially from the cephalic to the basilic vein, often receiving a median forearm vein. A frequent variant is for the median forearm vein to bifurcate just distal to the cubital fossa – one branch passing to the cephalic, the other to the basilic vein – giving an 'M'-shaped pattern, which replaces the median cubital vein (Fig. 116b,c). It was the median cubital vein that was favoured for the operation of bleeding (blood-letting) or phlebotomy, in days gone by; the underlying brachial artery was protected from the barber–surgeon's knife by the *bicipital aponeurosis*, a tough fascial extension from the biceps tendon. This fascia was therefore termed the *'grace a Dieu'* (praise be to God) fascia.

The median cubital vein is best avoided for the injection of intravenous barbiturates and other irritant drugs because of the slight risk of inadvertently entering the brachial artery and also because of the danger of piercing a superficially placed abnormal ulnar artery in occasional instances of high brachial artery bifurcation.

Nerves

A number of nerves in the upper limb are palpable, some more readily than others particularly in a thin subject; these are the *supraclavicular nerves*, as they pass over the clavicle, the cords of the *brachial plexus* against the humeral head (with the arm abducted), the *median nerve* in the mid-upper arm, crossing over the brachial artery, the *ulnar nerve* in the groove behind the medial epicondyle and the *superficial radial nerve* as it passes over the tendon of extensor pollicis longus at the wrist.

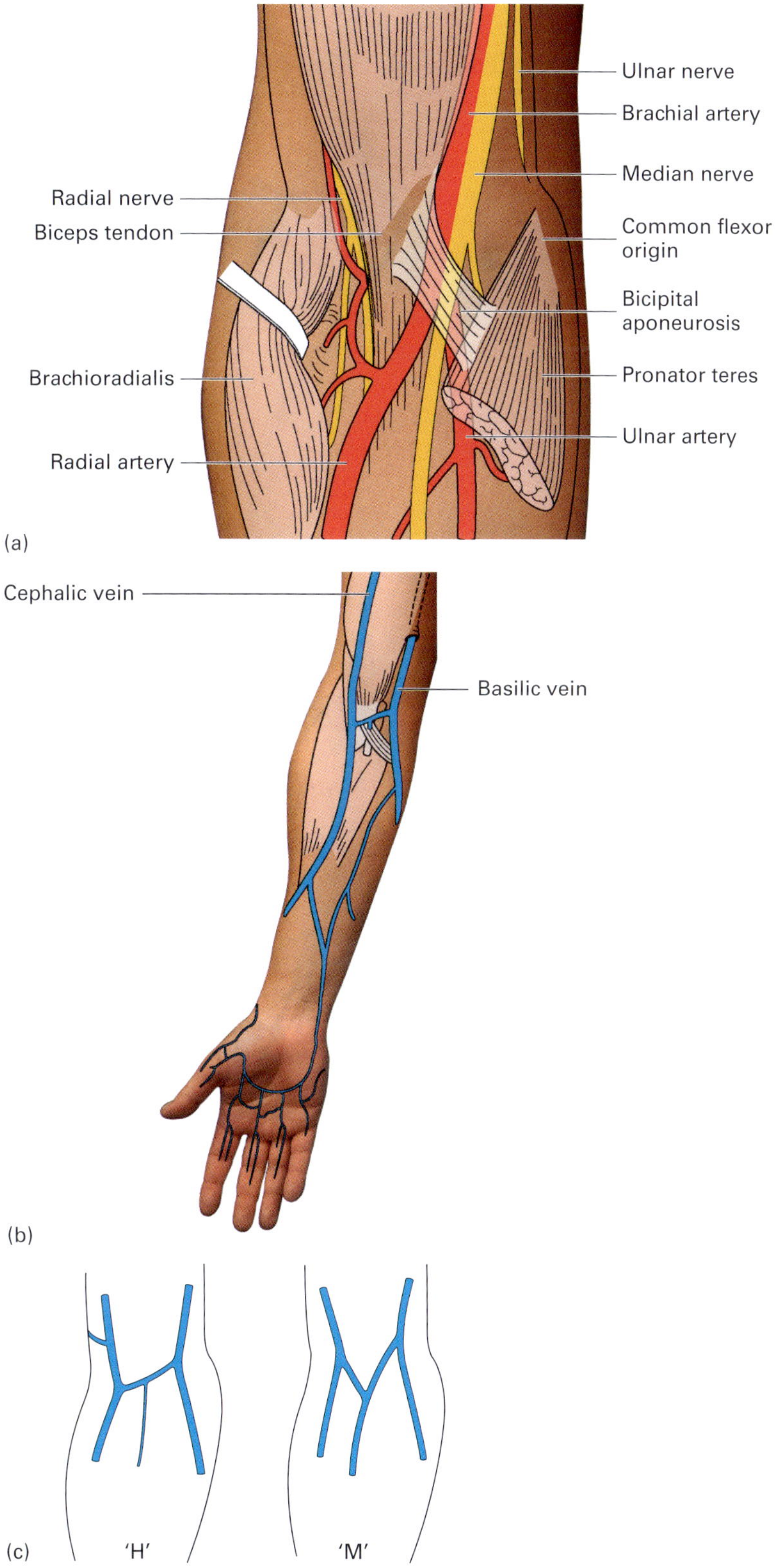

Fig. 116 (a) The right cubital fossa with the bicipital aponeurosis in detail. (b) The superficial veins of the upper limb. (Note the bicipital aponeurosis situated between the median cubital vein and brachial artery.) (c) Two common arrangements in the formation of the median cubital vein.

The median nerve lies first lateral then medial to the brachial artery, crossing it at the mid-upper arm, usually superficially but occasionally deeply. This close relationship is of historical interest: Nelson (Lord [Viscount] Horatio Nelson [1758–1805] one of England's greatest naval heroes) had his median nerve accidentally incorporated in the ligature around the artery when he underwent amputation of his arm above the elbow.

Useful surface markings of other, impalpable, nerves may be listed as follows.

1 The *axillary nerve* is related closely to the surgical neck of the humerus 5 cm (2 in) below the outer edge of the acromion process.
2 The *radial nerve* crosses, obliquely, the posterior aspect of the humeral shaft at its mid-level.
3 The *posterior interosseous branch* of the radial nerve is located by Henry's method as it winds round the radius. Place three fingers along the lateral aspect of the upper end of the radius; the uppermost finger lies on the radial head (feel it rotate on pronation and supination), and the lowermost lies over the nerve.
4 The *median nerve* (Figs 113, 115) in the forearm lies, as its name suggests, in the median plane. Its area of distribution in the hand may be anaesthetized by injecting local anaesthetic in the midline at the flexor aspect of the wrist.
5 The *ulnar nerve* at the wrist lies immediately medial to the ulnar pulse (Figs 113, 115). In the hand, it passes on the radial side of the pisiform and then lies on the hook of the hamate. If you press with your fingernail just lateral to the pisiform bone, you will experience tingling in your ulnar two fingers.

The bones and joints of the upper limb

The scapula (Fig. 117)

This triangular bone bears three prominent features: the *glenoid fossa* laterally (which is the scapula's contribution to the shoulder joint), the *spine* on its posterior aspect, projecting laterally as the *acromion process*, and the *coracoid process* on its anterior aspect.

Its strong muscular coverings protect the scapula and only rarely is it fractured.

The clavicle (Fig. 117)

This long bone has a number of unusual features.

1 It has no medullary cavity.
2 It is the first to ossify in the fetus (5th–6th week).
3 Although a long bone, it develops in membrane and not in cartilage.
4 It is a commonly fractured long bone in young individuals.

The clavicle is made up of a medial two-thirds, which is circular in section and convex anteriorly, and a lateral one-third, which is flattened in section and convex posteriorly.

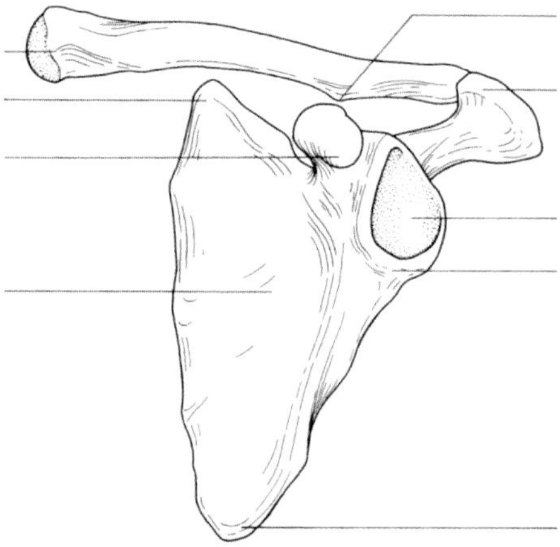

Fig. 117 The left scapula and clavicle (anterior aspect).

Medially it articulates with the manubrium at the *sternoclavicular joint*, which contains a cartilaginous disc (an important, and often overlooked, structure). It is an atypical synovial joint that moves reciprocally with the movements of the shoulder joint, around its fulcrum – the costoclavicular ligament. Put a finger on the medial end of your clavicle; raise your shoulder – the sternoclavicular joint is depressed; retract your shoulder – the sternoclavicular joint protracts and so on. The patient may complain of a 'painful stiff shoulder' when he or she actually has arthritis of the sternoclavicular joint.

Laterally the clavicle articulates with the acromion at the acromioclavicular joint (also an atypical synovial joint containing an incomplete intra-articular disc) and, in addition, is attached to the coracoid process by the tough coracoclavicular ligament.

The subclavian vessels and the trunks of the brachial plexus pass behind the middle third of the shaft of the clavicle, separated only by the thin subclavius muscle. Fractures of the clavicle are common, yet associated injury of the underlying subclavian vessels (except in penetrating gunshot wounds) is extremely rare because of the protection offered by this slip of a muscle. Rarely, these vessels (protected by the subclavius) are torn by the fragments of a fractured clavicle; this was the presumed cause of death of Sir Robert Peel (Prime Minister of the United Kingdom 1834–1835, and again 1841–1846) following a fall from his horse.

The sternal end of the clavicle has important posterior relations; behind the sternoclavicular joints lie the common carotid artery on the left and the bifurcation of the brachiocephalic artery on the right. The internal jugular vein lies a little more laterally on either side. These vessels are separated from bone by the strap muscles – the sternohyoid and sternothyroid.

CLINICAL FEATURES

The clavicle has three principal functions:

1 to transmit forces from the upper limb to the axial skeleton;
2 to act as a strut holding the arm free from the trunk;
3 to provide attachment for muscles.

The weakest point along the clavicle is the junction of the middle and outer third. Transmission of forces to the axial skeleton in falls on the shoulder or hand may prove greater than the strength of the bone at this site, and this indirect force is the usual cause of fracture.

When fracture occurs, the trapezius is unable to support the weight of the arm so that the characteristic picture of the patient with a fractured clavicle is that of a person supporting a sagging upper limb with the opposite hand. The lateral fragment is not only depressed but also drawn medially by the shoulder adductors, principally teres major, subscapularis, latissimus dorsi and pectoralis major (Fig. 118).

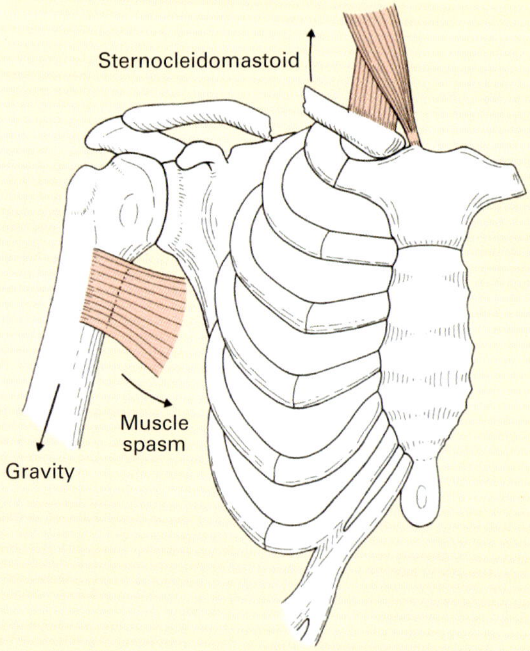

Fig. 118 The deformity of a fractured clavicle – downward displacement and adduction of the outer fragment by gravity and muscle spasm, respectively; slight elevation of the inner fragment by the sternocleidomastoid.

The humerus (Fig. 119)

The upper end of the humerus consists of a *head* (one-third of a sphere) facing medially, upwards and backwards, separated from the *greater* and *lesser tubercles* by the *anatomical neck*. The tubercles, in turn, are separated from each other by the *bicipital groove*

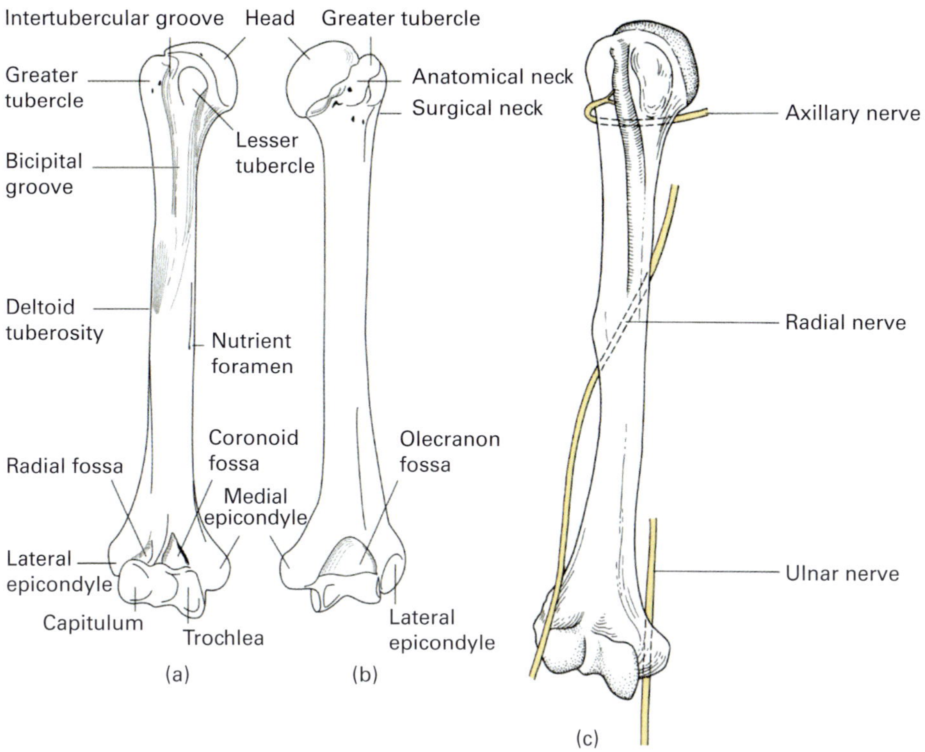

Fig. 119 The (a) anterior and (b) posterior views of the right humerus. (c) The humerus with its three major related nerves – axillary, radial and ulnar – all of which are in danger of injury in humeral fractures.

(*intertubercular sulcus*) along which emerges the long head of biceps from the shoulder joint.

The very upper end of the shaft of the humerus just below the level of the greater and lesser tuberosities is the *surgical* neck, against which lie the axillary nerve and circumflex humeral vessels. The shaft itself is circular in section above and flattened in its lower part. The posterior aspect of the shaft bears the faint *spiral groove* demarcating the origins of the medial and lateral heads of the triceps between which wind the radial nerve and the accompanying profunda vessels.

The lower end of the humerus bears the rounded *capitulum* laterally, for articulation with the radial head, and the spool-shaped *trochlea* medially, articulating with the trochlear notch of the ulna.

The *medial* and *lateral epicondyles*, on either side, are extracapsular; the medial is the larger of the two, extends more distally and bears a groove on its posterior aspect for the ulnar nerve.

Three important nerves thus come into close contact with the humerus – the axillary, the radial and the ulnar; they may be damaged, respectively, in fractures of the humeral neck, midshaft and lower end (Fig. 119).

It is an important practical point to note that the lower end of the humerus is angulated forwards 45° on the shaft. This is easily confirmed by examining a lateral radiograph of the elbow, when it will be seen that a vertical line continued downwards along the front of the shaft bisects the capitulum. Any decrease of this angulation indicates backward displacement of the distal end of the humerus and is good radiographic evidence of a supracondylar fracture.

The radius and ulna (Fig. 120)

The radius consists of the *head*, *neck*, *shaft* (with its *radial tuberosity*) and expanded distal end. The ulna comprises *olecranon*, *trochlear fossa*, *coronoid process* (with its *radial notch* for articulation with the radial head), *shaft* and small distal *head*, which articulates with the medial side of the distal end of the radius at the inferior radio-ulnar joint.

In pronation and supination, the head of the radius rotates against the radial notch of the ulna, the shaft of the radius swings around the relatively fixed ulnar shaft (the two bones being connected by the fibrous interosseous membrane) and the distal end of the radius (carrying with it, the carpus and the rest of the hand) rotates against the head of the ulna. This axis of rotation passes from the radial head proximally to the ulnar head distally.

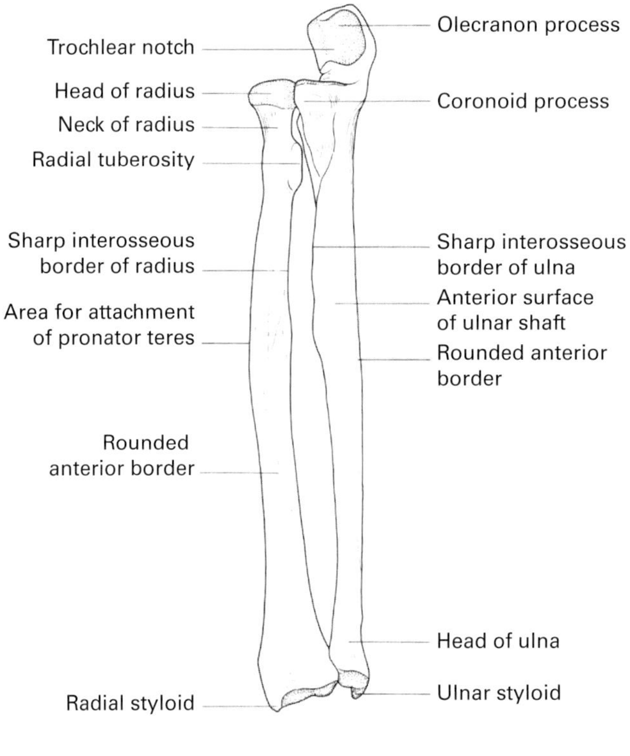

Fig. 120 The right radius and ulna – anterior aspect.

CLINICAL FEATURES

1 The pronator teres is inserted midway along the radial shaft. If the radius is fractured proximal to this, the proximal fragment is supinated (by the action of the biceps) and the distal fragment is pronated by pronator teres. The fracture must, therefore, be splinted with the forearm supinated so that the distal fragment is aligned with the supinated proximal end. If the fracture is distal to the midshaft, the actions of biceps and the pronator muscles more or less balance and the fracture is, therefore, immobilized with the forearm in the neutral position (Fig. 121).

2 The force of a fall on the hand produces different effects in different age groups: in a child it may cause a posterior displacement of the distal radial epiphysis; in the young adult the shafts of the radius and ulna may fracture, or the scaphoid may fracture

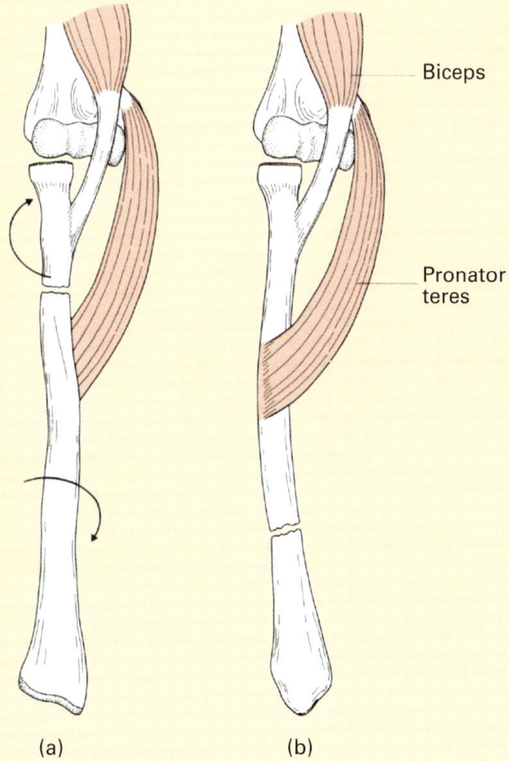

Fig. 121 The important role of pronator teres in radial fractures. (a) In proximal fractures, above the insertion of pronator teres, the distal fragment is pronated. Such a fracture must be splinted in the supinated position. (b) When the fracture is distal to the insertion of pronator teres, the action of this muscle on the proximal fragment is cancelled by the supinator action of biceps. This fracture is, therefore, held reduced in the neutral position, midway between pronation and supination.

(see page 178); in the elderly the most likely result will be a *Colles' fracture*. In the last injury, the radius fractures approximately 2.5 cm (1 in) proximal to the wrist joint; the distal fragment is displaced posteriorly and usually becomes impacted. The shortening which results brings the styloid processes of the radius and ulna more or less in line with each other.

Another forearm injury resulting from a fall on the outstretched hand is fracture of the head of the radius, due to it being crushed against the capitulum of the humerus.

3 The olecranon process may be fractured as a result of a direct blow but more often it is avulsed by forcible contraction of the triceps, which is inserted into its upper aspect. In these circumstances the bone ends are widely displaced and operative repair, to reconstruct the integrity of the elbow joint, becomes essential.

4 A subcutaneous bursa is constantly present over the olecranon and is likely to become inflamed when subjected to repeated trauma. This condition, termed olecranon bursitis goes by the colloquialisms 'student's elbow' and 'miner's elbow' (presumably on account of the tendency of students and miners, in days gone by, to rest their elbows on a hard surface for prolonged periods!).

The bones of the hand (Fig. 122)

The *carpus* is made up of two rows, each containing four bones. In the proximal row, from the lateral to the medial side, are the *scaphoid*, *lunate* and *triquetral*, the last bearing the *pisiform* on its anterior surface, into which sesamoid bone the flexor carpi ulnaris tendon is inserted.

In the distal row, from the lateral to the medial side, are the *trapezium*, *trapezoid*, *capitate* and *hamate*. The interval between the proximal and distal rows of carpal bones, seen in a plain radiograph as a sinuous dark shadow, is the **midcarpal joint**, a synovial joint.

The carpus as a whole is arched transversely, the palmar aspect being concave. This is maintained by:

1 the shapes of the individual bones, which are broader posteriorly than anteriorly (except for the lunate, which is broader anteriorly);

2 the tough *flexor retinaculum* passing from the scaphoid and the ridge of the trapezium laterally to the pisiform and the hook of the hamate medially (Fig. 123);

3 distal to the carpal bones lie the five metacarpals, slender bones apart from the first – that of the thumb, which is stout and set at right angles to the palm of the hand. In front of the head of this metacarpal are two tiny sesamoid bones (in the insertions of the heads of flexor pollicis longus), which are easily visible on a plain radiograph of the hand. Distally, the metacarpals articulate with the phalanges, of which there are two in the thumb and three in each of the other four fingers (Fig. 122). The important articulations between these small bones of the hand are considered on page 186.

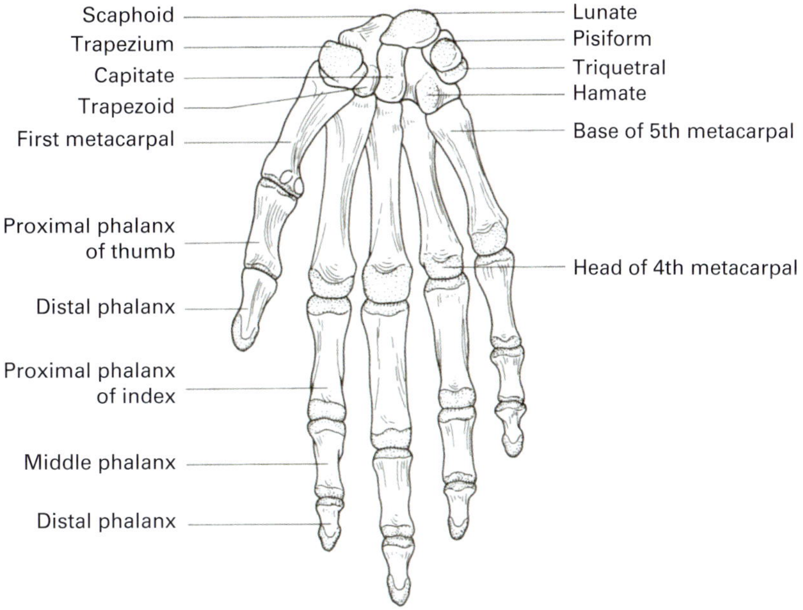

Fig. 122 The right carpus, metacarpus and phalanges (anterior aspect).

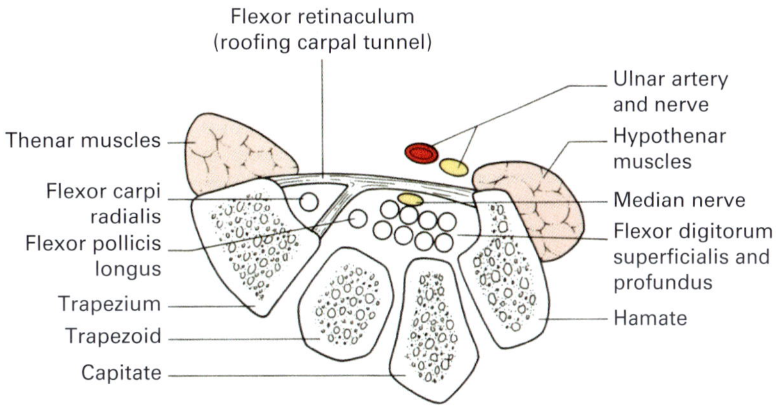

Fig. 123 Transverse section through the distal carpus (right side viewed from the distal end), showing the attachments of the flexor retinaculum. Note the separate osseofascial compartment for the tendon of flexor carpi radialis. Note also that, at this level, the tendon of flexor carpi ulnaris has 'disappeared'. It attaches to the pisiform, in the proximal row of carpal bones.

CLINICAL FEATURES

1 A fall on the hand may dislocate the rest of the carpal arch backwards from the lunate which, as commented on previously, is wide-based anteriorly (perilunate dislocation of the carpus). The dislocated carpus may then reduce spontaneously, only to push the

lunate forwards and tilt it over so that its distal articular surface faces forwards (dislocation of the lunate).

2 The scaphoid may be fractured by a fall on the palm with the hand abducted, in which position the scaphoid lies directly facing the radius. The blood supply of the scaphoid in one-third of cases enters distally along its waist so that, if the fracture is proximal, the blood supply to this small proximal fragment may be completely cut off with resultant avascular necrosis of this portion of bone (Fig. 124).

3 *'The carpal tunnel syndrome'*. The flexor retinaculum forms the roof of a tunnel, the floor and walls of which are made up of the concavity of the carpus. Packed within this tunnel are the long flexor tendons of the fingers and thumb together with the median nerve (Fig. 123). Any lesion diminishing the size of the compartment – for example, an old fracture or arthritic change – may result in compression of the median nerve, resulting in paraesthesiae, numbness and motor weakness in its distribution. Since the superficial palmar branch of the median nerve is given off proximal to the retinaculum, there is usually no sensory impairment over the thenar eminence.

It is interesting that this syndrome also often occurs, especially in elderly women, without any very obvious cause, although symptoms are relieved by dividing the retinaculum longitudinally.

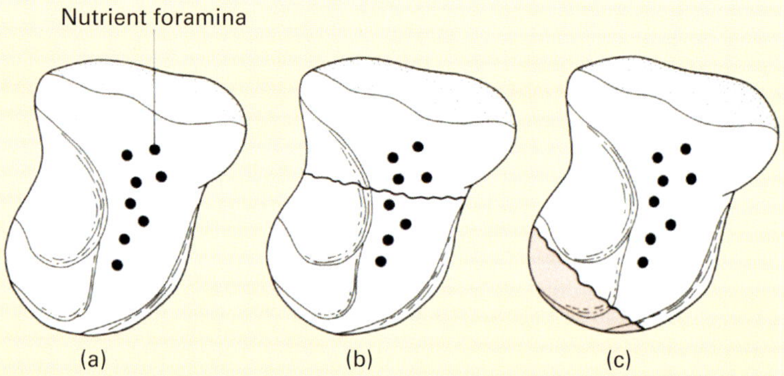

Fig. 124 Blood supply of the scaphoid. (a) Blood vessels enter the bone principally in its distal half. (b) A fracture through the waist of the scaphoid – vessels to the proximal fragment are preserved. (c) A fracture near the proximal pole of the scaphoid – in this case there are no vessels supplying the proximal fragment and aseptic necrosis of bone is therefore inevitable.

The shoulder joint (Figs 125, 126)

The shoulder joint (glenohumeral joint) is a typical synovial joint of the ball-and-socket type, between the relatively large *head of humerus* and the relatively small and shallow *glenoid fossa*, although the latter is widened and deepened somewhat by the fibrocartilaginous ring of the *labrum glenoidale*.

The joint *capsule* is strong but sufficiently lax so as not to impede the impressive mobility of the joint and is attached around the epiphyseal lines of both the glenoid and

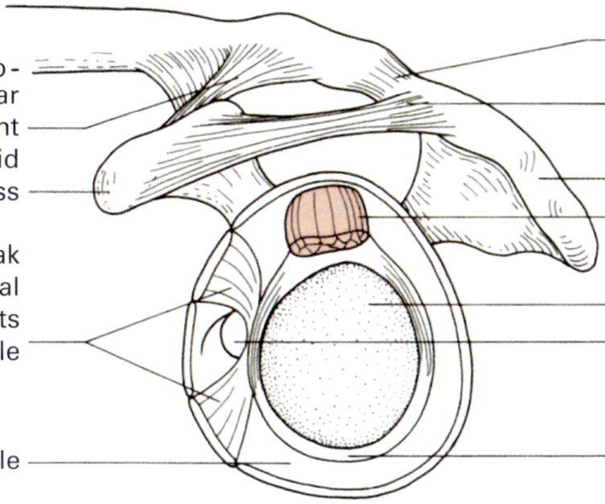

Fig. 125 The left shoulder joint (viewed from the lateral aspect) – its ligaments are shown after removal of the humerus.

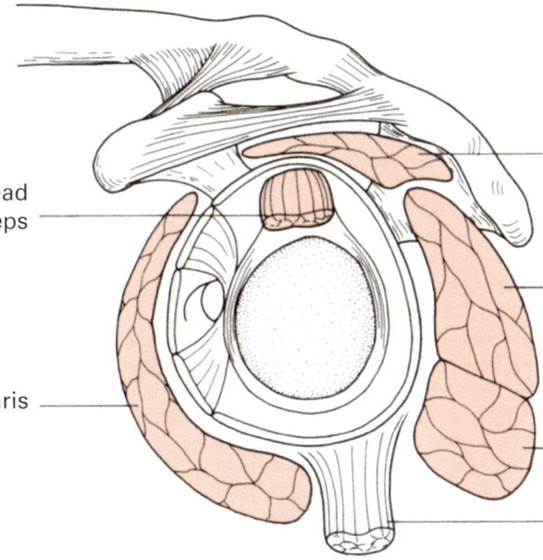

Fig. 126 The shoulder joint – the same view as in Fig. 125, but now with the addition of the surrounding muscles.

the humeral head. However, it does extend down on to the diaphysis on the medial aspect of the neck of the humerus, so that an osteomyelitis of the upper end of the humeral shaft may involve the joint by direct spread.

The capsule is lined on the inside by synovial membrane, which is prolonged along the tendon of the long head of the biceps as this traverses the joint. The synovial cavity of the shoulder joint invariably communicates with the *subscapular bursa* beneath the tendon of subscapularis.

The stability of the shoulder joint depends on a number of restraining factors.

These may be classified as static restraints and dynamic restraints. The former include the glenoid labrum (which serves to deepen and widen the articular surface of the glenoid fossa), the superior, middle and inferior glenohumeral ligaments, the coracohumeral ligament and the negative intra-articular pressure that normally exists within the joint cavity

The dynamic restraints include the rotator cuff muscles (see following section), the deltoid, teres major, the long heads of biceps and triceps and the more peripherally situated powerful muscles arising from the chest wall, namely pectoralis major and latissimus dorsi.

Movements of the shoulder girdle

The movements of the shoulder joint itself cannot be divorced from those of the whole shoulder girdle. Even if the shoulder joint is fused, a wide range of movement is still possible by elevation, depression, rotation and protraction of the scapula, leverage occurring at the sternoclavicular joint, the pivot being the costoclavicular ligament.

Abduction of the shoulder is initiated by the supraspinatus; the deltoid can then abduct to 90°. Further movement to 180° (hyperabduction/elevation) is brought about by rotation of the scapula upwards and outwards by the trapezius and serratus anterior acting synergistically. Shoulder and shoulder girdle movements combine into one smooth action. As soon as abduction commences at the shoulder joint, so rotation of the scapula begins. Test this on yourself or on a colleague by palpating the lower pole of the scapula. This will be felt to swing outwards on initiation of shoulder abduction. Movements of the scapula occur with reciprocal movements at the sternoclavicular joint. Place a finger on this joint; elevate the shoulder and the sternoclavicular joint will be felt to tilt downwards; swing the shoulder forwards and it will be felt to move backwards, and so on.

Rotator cuff (Figs 126, 127) is the name given to the sheath of tendons of the short muscles of the shoulder (short scapular muscles) which covers and blends with all but the inferior aspect of the capsule of the glenohumeral joint. The muscles are the supraspinatus, infraspinatus and teres minor, which are inserted from above down onto the humeral greater tubercle (tuberosity), and the subscapularis, which is inserted onto the lesser tubercle (tuberosity). All originate from the scapula.

Of these muscles, the supraspinatus is of particular practical importance. It passes over the apex of the shoulder beneath the acromion process and coracoacromial ligament, from which it is separated by the *subacromial bursa*. This bursa is continued laterally beneath the deltoid as the *subdeltoid bursa* forming, together, the largest bursa in the body.

The supraspinatus initiates the abduction of the glenohumeral joint; if the tendon is torn as a result of injury, active initiation of abduction becomes impossible and the patient has to develop the trick movement of tilting his body towards the injured side so that gravity passively swings the arm out from the trunk. Once this occurs, the deltoid and the scapular rotators can then come into play.

Inflammation of the supraspinatus tendon ('supraspinatus tendinitis') is characterized by a painful arc of shoulder movement between 60° and 120°; in this range, the tendon impinges against the overlying acromion and the coracoacromial ligament. The investigation of soft-tissue lesions in and around the shoulder has been greatly facilitated, enhanced and improved by magnetic resonance imaging (MRI), which reveals the anatomical structures in exquisite detail (Fig. 127b).

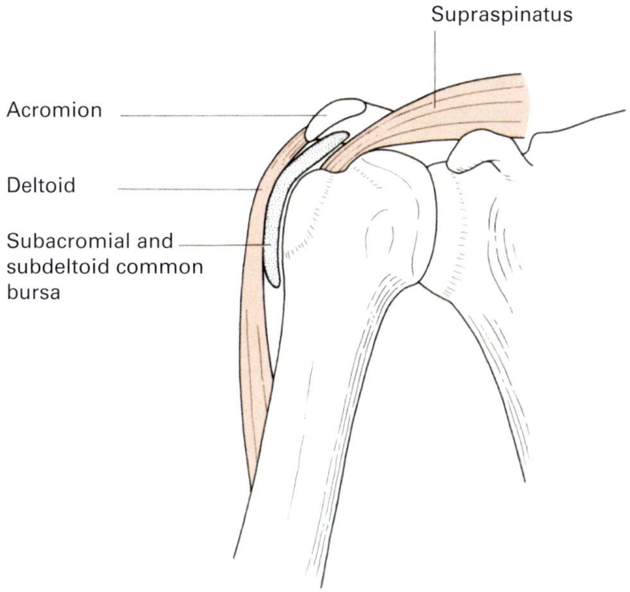

(a)

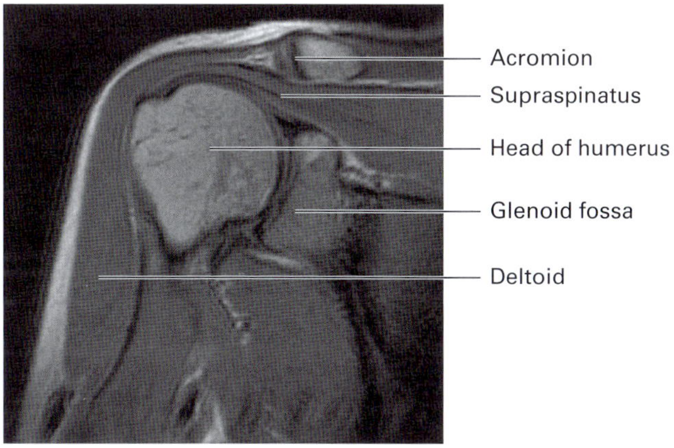

(b)

Fig. 127 (a) Supraspinatus and the subacromial–subdeltoid bursa. Note that the supraspinatus tendon lies close against the acromion – if this tendon is inflamed, there is a painful arc of movement as the shoulder is abducted from 60° to 120°, because, in this range, the inflamed tendon impinges against the acromion. (b) Magnetic resonance imaging of the shoulder showing the detailed anatomy revealed by this technique. Source: Professor Adrian Dixon.

Principal muscles acting on the shoulder joint

Abductors
- supraspinatus (initiates)
- deltoid

Adductors
- pectoralis major
- latissimus dorsi
- subscapularis

Flexors
- biceps brachii
- pectoralis major
- coracobrachialis
- deltoid (anterior fibres)

Extensors
- triceps brachii
- teres major
- latissimus dorsi
- deltoid (posterior fibres)

Medial rotators
- pectoralis major
- latissimus dorsi
- teres major
- deltoid (anterior fibres)
- subscapularis

Lateral rotators
- infraspinatus
- teres minor
- deltoid (posterior fibres)

CLINICAL FEATURES

Dislocation of the shoulder

The wide range of movement possible at the shoulder is achieved only at the cost of stability, and for this reason it is the most commonly dislocated major joint. Its inferior aspect is completely unprotected by muscles and it is here that, in sudden and forceful abduction, the humeral head may slip away from the glenoid fossa to lie in the subglenoid region, whence it usually passes anteriorly into a subcoracoid position (Fig. 128).

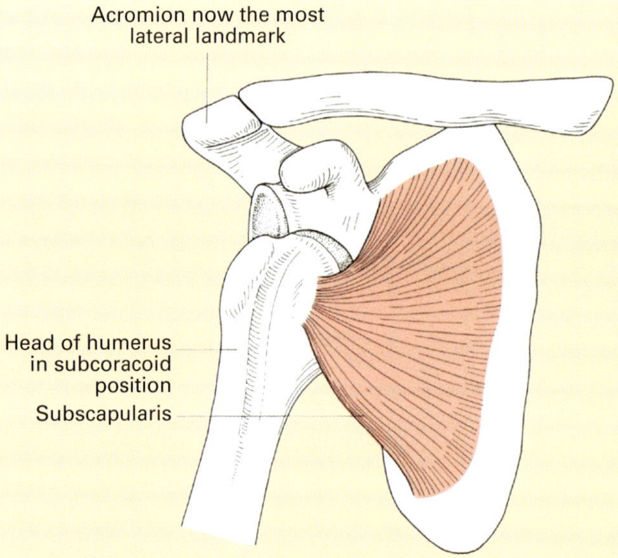

Fig. 128 The deformity of shoulder dislocation. The dislocated head of the humerus is held adducted by the shoulder girdle muscles and internally rotated by subscapularis.

The axillary nerve, lying in relation to the surgical neck of the humerus, may be damaged in this injury. Assess this in the patient before reducing the dislocation by testing for loss of cutaneous sensation over the upper lateral aspect of the arm.

The head of the humerus is drawn medially by the powerful adductors of the shoulder; its greater tubercle, therefore, no longer remains the most lateral bony projection of the shoulder region, being replaced for this honour by the acromion process. The normal bulge of the deltoid over the greater tubercle is lost; instead, there is the characteristic flattening of this muscle.

In reducing the dislocation by *Kocher's method* the elbow is flexed and the forearm rotated outwards; this stretches the subscapularis, which is holding the humeral head internally rotated. The elbow is then swung medially across the trunk, thus levering the head of the humerus laterally so that it slips back into place.

In the *Hippocratic method*, the foot (of the operator) is used to provide counter-traction in the axilla, while traction and adduction are being applied to the arm and forearm; in this way, the humeral head is levered outwards into its normal position.

The elbow joint (Figs 129, 130)

The elbow joint, although a single synovial cavity, is made up of three distinct articulations, which are:

1 the *humero-ulnar*, between the trochlea of the humerus and the trochlear notch of the ulna (a hinge joint);

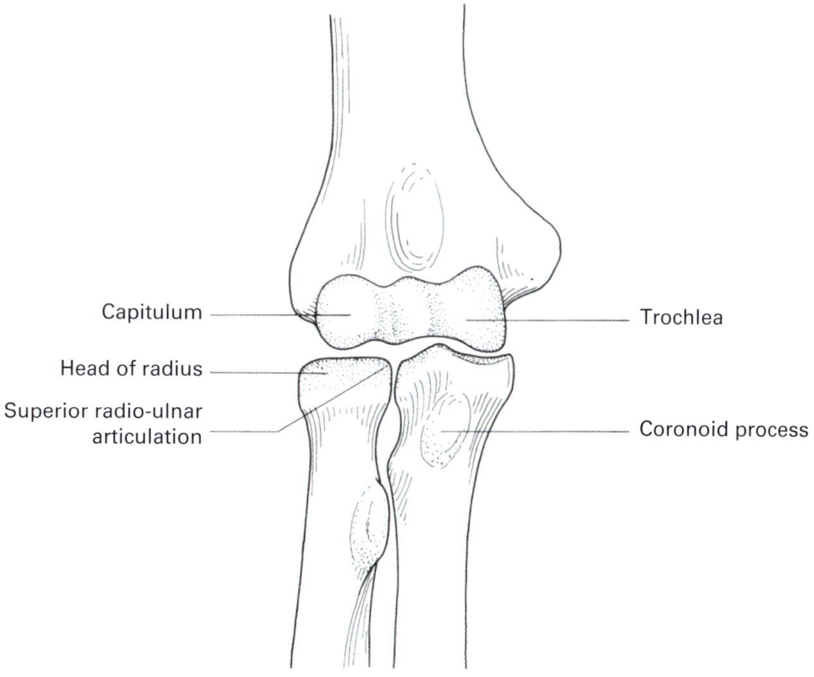

Fig. 129 The bony components of the elbow joint (right side; anterior aspect). Note the three sets of articular surfaces.

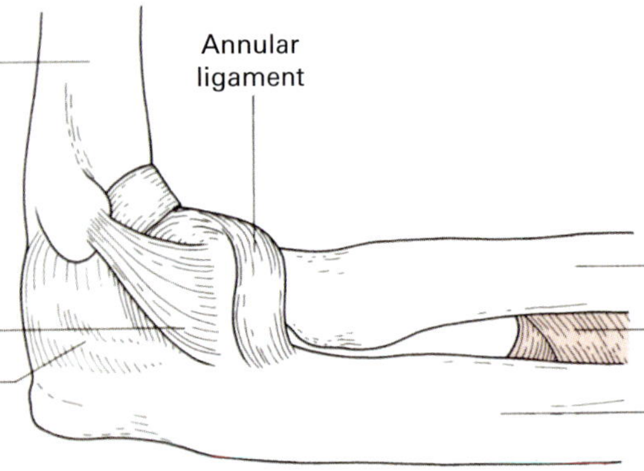

Fig. 130 The joint capsule of the right elbow – lateral aspect.

2 the *humeroradial*, between the capitulum of the humerus and the upper concave surface of the radial head (a shallow ball-and-socket joint, of sorts);
3 the *superior radio-ulnar*, between the circumference of the head of the radius and the radial notch of the ulna, the head being held in place by the tough annular ligament (a pivot joint).

The *capsule* of the elbow joint is closely applied around this complex articular arrangement; the non-articular medial and lateral epicondyles are extracapsular. The capsule is strong but lax anteriorly and posteriorly to allow flexion and extension, while being reinforced on either side by the *medial* and *lateral collateral* ligaments. The lateral ligament is attached distally to the *annular ligament* around the radial head. In order to allow rotation of the radius, the lower margin of the annular ligament is free and, beneath it, the synovium of the elbow bulges downwards onto the neck of the radius.

Two sets of movements take place at the elbow:
1 flexion and extension at the humero-ulnar and humero-radial joints;
2 pronation and supination involving the proximal and distal radio-ulnar joints.

Muscles acting on the elbow

Flexors
- biceps brachii
- brachialis
- brachioradialis
- the forearm flexor muscles

Extensors
- triceps brachii
- anconeus

Pronators
- pronator teres
- pronator quadratus

Supinators
- biceps brachii
- supinator

The supinator action of the biceps is due to its insertion on to the *posterior* aspect of the tuberosity of the radius. When the biceps contracts, not only is the forearm flexed, but the radius 'unwinds' as its tuberosity is rotated anteriorly, i.e. the forearm supinates (Fig. 131). Biceps is a powerful muscle; hence, supination is a more powerful action than

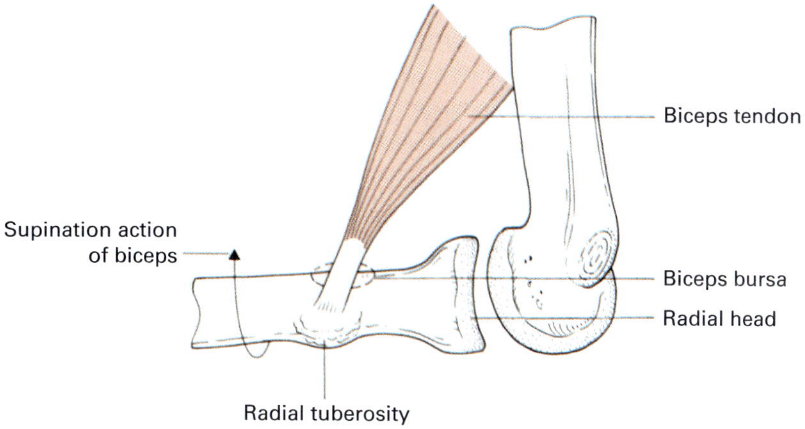

Fig. 131 The supination action of biceps (right elbow viewed from the medial side with the ulna removed).

pronation – try it on yourself. This is reflected in the design of screwdrivers and corkscrews that are screwed in using the supinatory action. As you might imagine, right handed individuals are clearly at an advantage when it comes to using screwdrivers!

CLINICAL FEATURES

1 The elbow joint is safely approached by a vertical posterior incision that divides the triceps expansion.
2 As the capsule is relatively lax anteriorly and posteriorly it will be distended at these sites by an effusion, particularly posteriorly, since the anterior aspect is covered by muscles and dense deep fascia. Aspiration of such an effusion is readily performed posteriorly on one or other side of the olecranon.
3 The annular ligament is funnel-shaped in adults and fits snugly around the radial head and neck, but in young children, the annular ligament is almost cylindrical and, consequently, less snugly applied around the radial head. A sudden jerk on the forearm of a child under the age of 8 years may subluxate the radial head through this ligament (*'pulled elbow'*). Reduction is easily effected by firm supination of the elbow, which 'screws' the radial head back into place.
4 *Posterior dislocation of the elbow* may occur as a result of the indirect thrust of a fall on the hand. Occasionally, the coronoid process of the ulna is fractured in this injury, being snapped off against the trochlea of the humerus. Characteristically, the triangular relationship between the olecranon and the two humeral epicondyles is lost (Fig. 112). Reduction is effected by traction to overcome the protective spasm of the muscles acting on the joint, together with flexion of the elbow, which levers the humero-ulnar joint back into place.

The wrist joint (Fig. 132)

The articular disc of the inferior radio-ulnar joint covers the head of the ulna and is attached to the base of the ulnar styloid process. This disc, together with the distal end

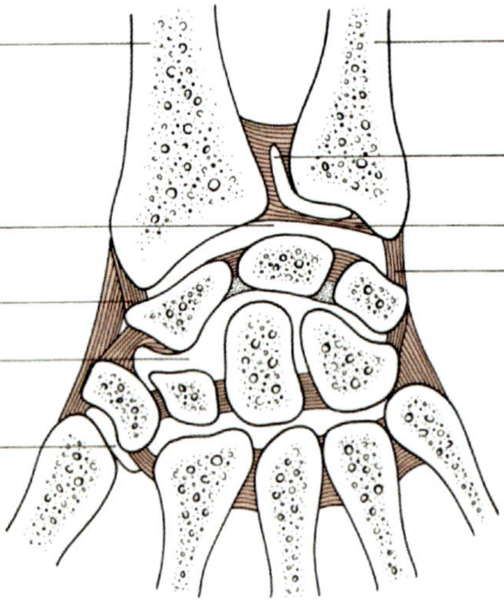

Fig. 132 The wrist, carpal and carpometacarpal joints in section.

of the radius, forms the proximal face of the wrist joint, the distal surface being the proximal articular surfaces of the scaphoid, lunate and triquetral.

The wrist is a condyloid joint – that is to say, it allows flexion, extension, abduction, adduction and circumduction, the last being a combination of the previous four. Flexion and extension are increased by associated sliding movements of the intercarpal joints; although the range of flexion at the wrist is actually less than that of extension, these associated movements make it apparently greater.

Because of the greater distal projection of the radial styloid, the range of abduction at the wrist is considerably less than that of adduction.

Muscles acting on the wrist

Flexors – all the long muscles crossing the anterior aspect of the wrist joint.
Extensors – all the long muscles crossing the posterior aspect of the joint.
Adductors – flexor carpi ulnaris acting in concord with extensor carpi ulnaris.
Abductors – flexor carpi radialis and extensor carpi radialis longus and brevis together with the long abductor and short extensor of the thumb.

The joints of the hand (Fig. 132)

The joints between the individual carpal bones allow gliding movements to occur that increase the range of extension and, more particularly, flexion permitted at the wrist joint.

The *carpometacarpal joint of the thumb* is saddle-shaped and permits flexion and extension (in a plane parallel to the palm of the hand), abduction and adduction (in a plane at a right angle to the palm) and opposition, in which the pulp of the thumb is brought across in contact with the pulps of the fingers. This joint's range contrasts with the limited movements of the other carpometacarpal joints, which allow a few degrees of gliding movement of the 2nd and 3rd metacarpals and a small range of flexion and extension of the 4th and 5th metacarpals.

The opposite state of affairs holds at the *metacarpophalangeal joints*; only a 60° range of flexion and extension is possible at the metacarpophalangeal joint of the thumb, whereas a 90° range of flexion and extension, together with abduction, adduction and circumduction, is possible at the other four metacarpophalangeal joints, which are condyloid in shape.

Note that, when the metacarpophalangeal joints of the fingers are flexed, abduction and adduction become significantly restricted. This is because each metacarpal head, although rounded at its distal extremity, is flattened anteriorly; when the base of the proximal phalanx moves onto this flattened surface, side movements become impossible. Moreover, the collateral ligaments on either side of the metacarpophalangeal joints become taut in flexion and thus limit abduction and adduction.

The metacarpophalangeal joints of the fingers, but not the thumb, are linked by the tough *deep transverse ligaments*, which prevent any spreading of the palm when a firm grip is taken.

All the *interphalangeal joints* have pulley-shaped opposing surfaces and are therefore hinge joints, allowing flexion and extension only. At all the metacarpophalangeal and interphalangeal joints the ligamentous arrangements are similar.

1 *Posteriorly* – the joint capsule is replaced by the expansion of the extensor tendon of the digit concerned.
2 *Anteriorly* – the capsule is formed by a dense plate of fibrocartilage. This *palmar ligament* is the response to the friction of the adjacent flexor tendons.
3 On either side the joints are reinforced by the *collateral ligaments*, which are lax in extension and taut in flexion of the joint.

CLINICAL FEATURES

The *carpometacarpal joint of the thumb* may be regarded a very important anatomical advance in the evolution of the human upper limb. It allows the unique movement, only possible in the human, of opposition of the tip of the thumb to the tip of one or other of the other fingers – for example, in holding a pen or a scalpel. A fracture of the base of the first metacarpal (Bennett's fracture) is therefore a significantly disabling injury. Unless anatomical reduction is achieved by pinning the fragments at open operation, osteoarthritic change will take place in the deformed joint with consequent painful limitation of this important movement.

Muscles acting on the hand

The long flexors of the fingers are:

1 *flexor digitorum profundus*, inserted into the bases of the four distal phalanges;
2 *flexor digitorum superficialis*, inserted into the sides of the bases of the four middle phalanges.

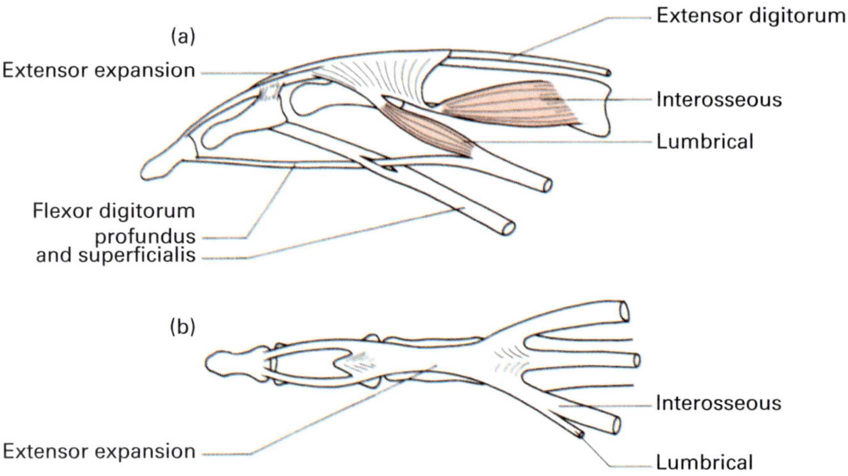

Fig. 133 The tendons of a finger. (a) Lateral view. (b) Dorsal (posterior) view.

The profundus tendon pierces that of superficialis over the proximal phalanx.

The profundus flexes the distal interphalangeal joint; superficialis flexes the proximal interphalangeal joint; acting together they flex the fingers and the wrist (Fig. 133).

The long extensors of the fingers are:

- *extensor digitorum*, reinforced by
- *extensor indicis* } which join the appropriate tendons of extensor digitorum
- *extensor digiti minimi* } longus on their medial (i.e. ulnar) sides.

The tendons of extensor digitorum terminate in each finger by an aponeurotic extensor expansion that covers the dorsum of the metacarpophalangeal joint and proximal phalanx and the sides of the base of the latter. It then attaches by a central slip into the base of the middle phalanx and by two collateral slips to the base of the distal phalanx (Fig. 133).

The margins of the extensor expansion are reinforced by the tendons of the intrinsic muscles of the fingers that originate in the flexor (volar) compartment of the hand:

1 the *dorsal* and *palmar interossei*, arising from the sides and the fronts of the metacarpals, respectively;
2 the *lumbricals*, which arise from the four profundus tendons and run on the radial side of the metacarpophalangeal joints to join the extensor expansion.

These intrinsic muscles, arising from the palmar aspect of the hand and inserting along the dorsal aspects of the fingers, have a unique action in that they *flex* the metacarpophalangeal joints and *extend* the interphalangeal joints.

The interossei, together with *abductor digiti minimi*, are responsible for abduction (dorsal interossei) and adduction (palmar interossei) of the fingers. A weak abduction movement accompanies the action of extensor digitorum and the long flexors adduct the fingers in the movement of full flexion. However, if these movements of extension and flexion are eliminated by laying the hand flat on the table, abduction and adduction of the fingers become purely the actions of the intrinsic muscles. A card gripped between the fingers in this position of the hand is kept there entirely by intrinsic muscle action.

The 5th finger receives two further intrinsic muscles, *opponens digiti minimi* and *flexor digiti minimi*, from the *hypothenar eminence*.

The eight muscles acting on the thumb may be divided into the long (proceeding from the forearm) and the short or intrinsic muscles.

- Long
  flexor pollicis longus – inserted into the distal phalanx;
  extensor pollicis longus – inserted into the distal phalanx;
  extensor pollicis brevis – inserted into the proximal phalanx;
  abductor pollicis longus – inserted into the metacarpal.
- Short
  adductor pollicis, *flexor pollicis brevis*, *abductor pollicis brevis* } inserted into the base of the proximal phalanx;
  opponens pollicis – along the metacarpal.

The flexors and extensors of the wrist play an important synergic role in movements of the hand. Notice how weak the grip becomes when the wrist is fully flexed; it must be held firmly in the extended or neutral position by balanced muscle action in order to allow the long flexors of the fingers and thumb to work at their full stretch and, therefore, at their maximum efficiency.

Three important zones of the upper limb: the axilla, the cubital fossa and the carpal tunnel

The axilla

The axilla (see Figs 139, 142) is a zone of transition between the neck and the upper limb. It is in the shape of an irregular and somewhat tilted pyramid.

The anterior wall of the axilla is two layers thick. The superficial layer is made up of pectoralis major, while the deep layer is made up of pectoralis minor and subclavius and the clavipectoral fascia that stretches between the two muscles, enclosing both.

The posterior wall is considerably longer, and, from above downwards, it is made up successively of subscapularis, teres major and latissimus dorsi.

The medial wall of the axilla is made up of the lateral aspects of the upper four intercostal spaces, covered by digitations of serratus anterior, while its lateral wall is the medial aspect of the upper part of the arm. The base of the axillary pyramid is the deep fascia, which stretches from the lateral aspect of the chest wall to the medial aspect of the arm. Termed the axillary fascia, it is attached to the lower edges of both pectoralis major and latissimus dorsi.

The apex of the axilla is truncated and is, in fact, the gap between the middle third of the clavicle and the outer edge of the first rib. This gap, known as the cervico-axillary opening, transmits the subclavian artery and brachial plexus from the neck into the axilla and the axillary vein from the axilla into the neck. The cervico-axillary opening is also traversed by numerous lymphatic channels.

The *contents* of the axilla are the axillary artery and its branches, the axillary vein and its tributaries, the cords of the brachial plexus and their branches, axillary lymph nodes and the intercostobrachial nerve. All these structures are contained in the axillary fat, which is usually quite substantial.

The organization of the brachial plexus and the course of the axillary artery will be described later (see pages 193 and 192, respectively).

The cubital fossa

The cubital fossa (Fig. 134) is a zone of transition between the arm and forearm. Situated in front of the elbow joint, the cubital fossa is a triangular intermuscular space.

Its boundaries are:

- *proximally* – an imaginary line running between the medial and lateral epicondyles of the humerus (this is the base of the triangle);
- *laterally* – the brachioradialis muscle;
- *medially* – the pronator teres muscle running obliquely from the medial epicondyle of humerus to the lateral aspect of the radial shaft (Fig. 121). The apex of the cubital fossa is, self-evidently, the point where the brachioradialis crosses pronator teres.

The *roof* of the cubital fossa is the overlying deep fascia, which is partially reinforced by an extension from the biceps brachii tendon known as the bicipital aponeurosis.

The *floor* of the fossa is the brachialis muscle, behind which is the capsule of the elbow joint.

The contents of the fossa are, from medial to lateral, the median nerve, the brachial artery flanked by its venae comitantes and the tendon of biceps brachii. If the brachioradialis muscle is undermined and retracted radially, the radial nerve can be brought into view. Of these contents, the brachial artery and the tendon of biceps brachii are readily palpable.

In the distal part of the cubital fossa, the brachial artery divides into its two terminal branches – the radial and ulnar arteries (the latter usually being the larger one).

The contents of the cubital fossa (particularly the brachial artery and median nerve) are vulnerable in supracondylar fractures of the humerus (Fig. 112).

The carpal tunnel

The carpal tunnel (Figs 113, 122, 123) is an osseofibrous space, bounded dorsally by the concave palmar surface of the articulated carpus.

The ventral boundary (i.e. *roof*) of the carpal tunnel is the flexor retinaculum (also known as the transverse carpal ligament).

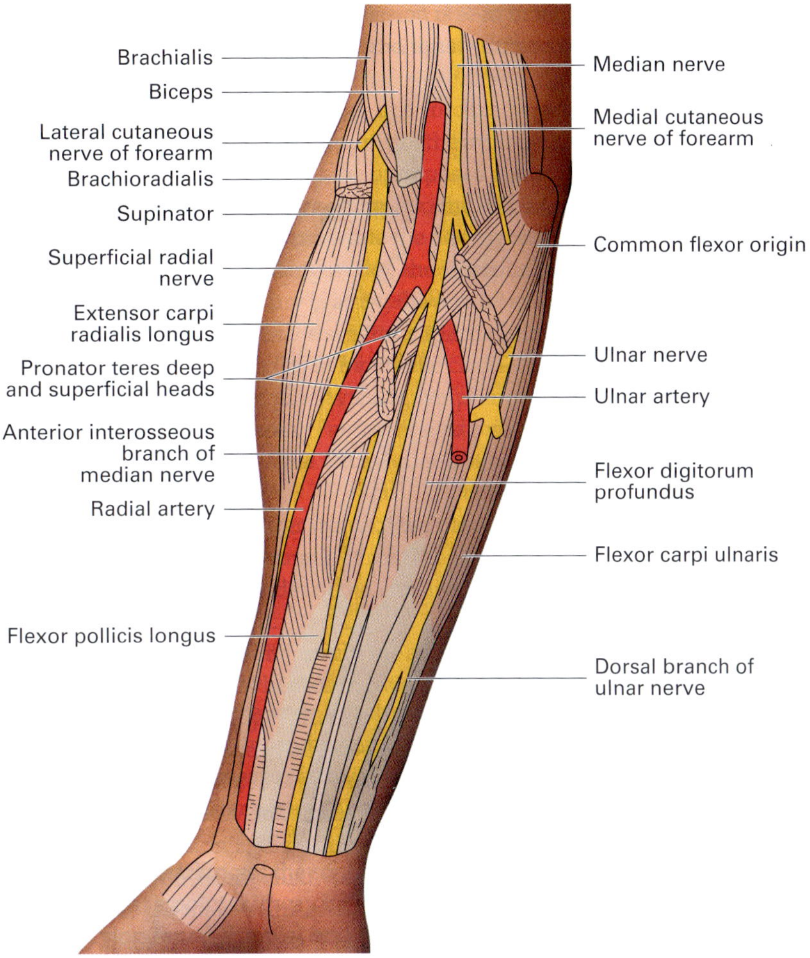

Fig. 134 Dissection of the right forearm (anterior aspect) to show the principal vessels and nerves. The superficial forearm muscles of the common flexor origin have been removed, apart from pronator teres, which has been partly divided.

The flexor retinaculum is a quadrangular sheet of dense fibrous tissue that attaches by its four corners to four carpal bones as follows.

On the radial side it is attached, proximally, to the tubercle of the scaphoid and, distally, to a ridge on the ventral surface of the trapezium. On the ulnar side, it is attached proximally to the pisiform and, distally, to the hook of the hamate. These four bony points are readily palpable in most individuals, enabling the clinician to surface-mark the flexor retinaculum and carpal tunnel with precision.

As has been noted (Fig. 123) the carpal tunnel is traversed longitudinally by the four tendons of flexor digitorum superficialis, the four tendons of flexor digitorum profundus, the tendon of flexor pollicis longus and the tendon of flexor carpi radialis (which runs in its own fibrous compartment within the carpal tunnel). Running within the carpal tunnel, adhering to the deep surface of the flexor retinaculum, is the median nerve. *Carpal tunnel syndrome* (described on page 178) denotes a sustained, pathological and symptomatic compression of the median nerve in the carpal tunnel. *It is by far the most common example of all entrapment neuropathies in human pathology.*

The arteries of the upper limb

The axillary artery

The axillary artery (see Fig. 139) commences at the lateral border of the first rib, as a continuation of the subclavian, and ends at the lower border of the axilla (i.e. the lower border of teres major) to become the brachial artery. For descriptive convenience the axillary artery is divided into three parts by the overlying pectoralis minor muscle as follows: the 1st part is medial to pectoralis minor, the 2nd part is deep to pectoralis minor and the 3rd part is lateral (distal) to pectoralis minor. Except for its very distal extremity, the axillary artery lies covered by pectoralis major.

Medial to pectoralis minor, the brachial plexus lies above and behind the artery, but, deep to pectoralis minor, the cords of the plexus take up their positions around the artery according to their names, i.e. lateral, medial and posterior.

The branches of the axillary artery supply the chest wall and shoulder region. For ease of recall it may be said that the 1st part of the axillary artery gives off one branch, the 2nd part gives two branches and the 3rd part gives three branches, as follows:

1st part: superior thoracic artery
2nd part: acromiothoracic trunk and lateral thoracic artery
3rd part: subscapular artery, anterior circumflex humeral artery and posterior circumflex humeral artery.

All but the circumflex humeral vessels are encountered during the axillary dissection stage of a radical mastectomy.

The brachial artery

The brachial artery is the direct continuation of the axillary artery. It commences in the arm at the level of the lower border of the tendon of latissimus dorsi and ends in the cubital fossa at the level of the neck of the radius by dividing into the radial and ulnar arteries. It is relatively superficial throughout its course, lying immediately deep to the deep fascia except where it is crossed, at the level of the middle of the humerus, by the median nerve, which passes superficially from its lateral to medial side; occasionally, the nerve crosses deep to (behind) the artery. Not infrequently the brachial artery divides into its two terminal branches in the arm.

The named branches of the brachial artery are:

- the *profunda brachii* artery (accompanying the radial nerve);
- the *superior ulnar collateral* artery (accompanying the ulnar nerve);

- the *nutrient* artery (to the humerus);
- the *inferior ulnar collateral* artery.

The radial artery

The radial artery (Fig. 134) commences at the level of the radial neck by lying on the tendon of biceps. In its upper half it lies overlapped by brachioradialis, the surface marking of the artery being the groove which can be seen on the medial side of this tensed muscle in the muscular subject. Distally in the forearm the artery lies superficially between brachioradialis and flexor carpi radialis, and it is between these two tendons that it is palpated at the wrist (Fig. 113).

In the middle third of the forearm the superficial branch of the radial nerve lies to the lateral side of the artery; the nerve, at this site, may inadvertently, be incorporated in a carelessly placed ligature.

Distal to the radial pulse, the artery gives off a branch to assist in forming the superficial palmar arch. It then passes deep to the tendons of abductor pollicis longus and extensor pollicis brevis to enter the anatomical snuffbox (in which it can be felt), pierces the first dorsal interosseous muscle and adductor pollicis, between the 1st and 2nd metacarpals, and goes on to form the deep palmar arch with the deep branch of the ulnar artery.

The ulnar artery

The ulnar artery (Fig. 134) is the larger of the two terminal branches of the brachial artery. Commencing in the cubital fossa at the level of the neck of the radius, it passes beneath the muscles arising from the common flexor origin, lies upon flexor digitorum profundus and is overlapped by flexor carpi ulnaris. The median nerve crosses superficial to the ulnar artery, separated from the latter by the deep head of pronator teres.

In the distal half of the forearm the artery becomes superficial between the tendons of flexor carpi ulnaris and flexor digitorum sublimis; it then crosses the flexor retinaculum to form the superficial palmar arch with the superficial palmar branch of the radial artery.

The ulnar nerve accompanies the artery on its medial side in the distal two-thirds of its course in the forearm and across the flexor retinaculum (Fig. 113).

Note. There is a rich anastomosis of arteries around all major joints. Apart from remembering this fact, the clinical student need not commit to memory the numerous named branches involved.

The brachial plexus

The brachial plexus is of great practical importance to the surgeon. It may be damaged in open, closed or obstetrical injuries, be pressed upon by a cervical rib or be involved in tumour. It is encountered, and hence put in danger, in operations upon the root of the neck.

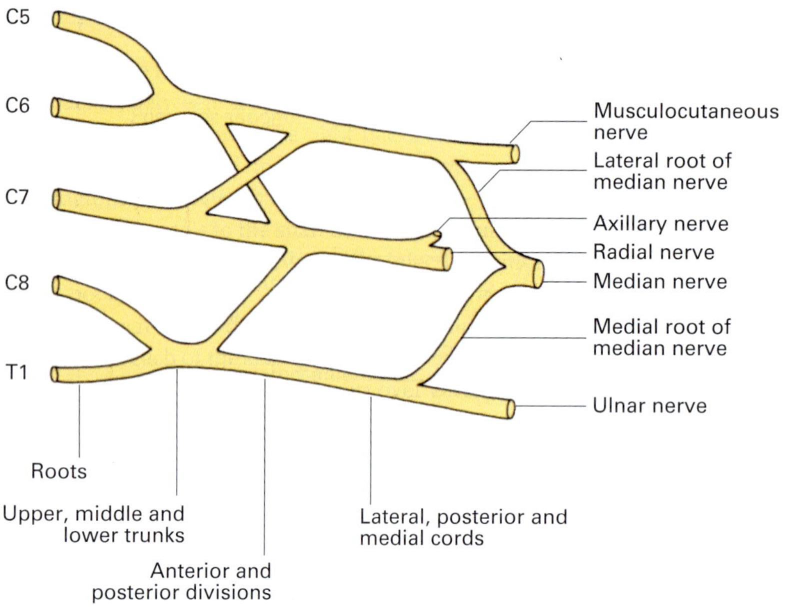

Fig. 135 Scheme of the brachial plexus.

The plexus is formed as follows (Fig. 135):

1 five *roots*, derived from the anterior rami of C5, C6, C7, C8 and T1, link up into:

2 three *trunks*, formed by the union of
- C5 and C6 (upper trunk);
- C7 alone (middle trunk);
- C8 and T1 (lower trunk);

which split into:

3 six divisions, formed by each trunk dividing into an anterior and posterior division, which link up again into:

4 three cords
- lateral cord, from the fused anterior divisions of the upper and middle trunks;
- medial cord, from the anterior division of the lower trunk;
- posterior cord, from the union of all three posterior divisions.

The *roots* lie between the anterior and middle scalene muscles. The *trunks* lie deep to the fascial floor of the posterior triangle of the neck. The *divisions* lie behind the clavicle. The *cords* lie in the axilla.

The cords continue distally to give rise to the main nerve trunks of the upper limb, as follows:

1 the lateral cord bifurcates into the *musculocutaneous nerve* and *the lateral root of the median nerve*;

2 the medial cord bifurcates into the *ulnar nerve* and *the medial root of the median nerve*;

3 the posterior cord bifurcates into the *radial nerve* and the *axillary nerve*;

4 the lateral and medial roots join to form the *median nerve*.

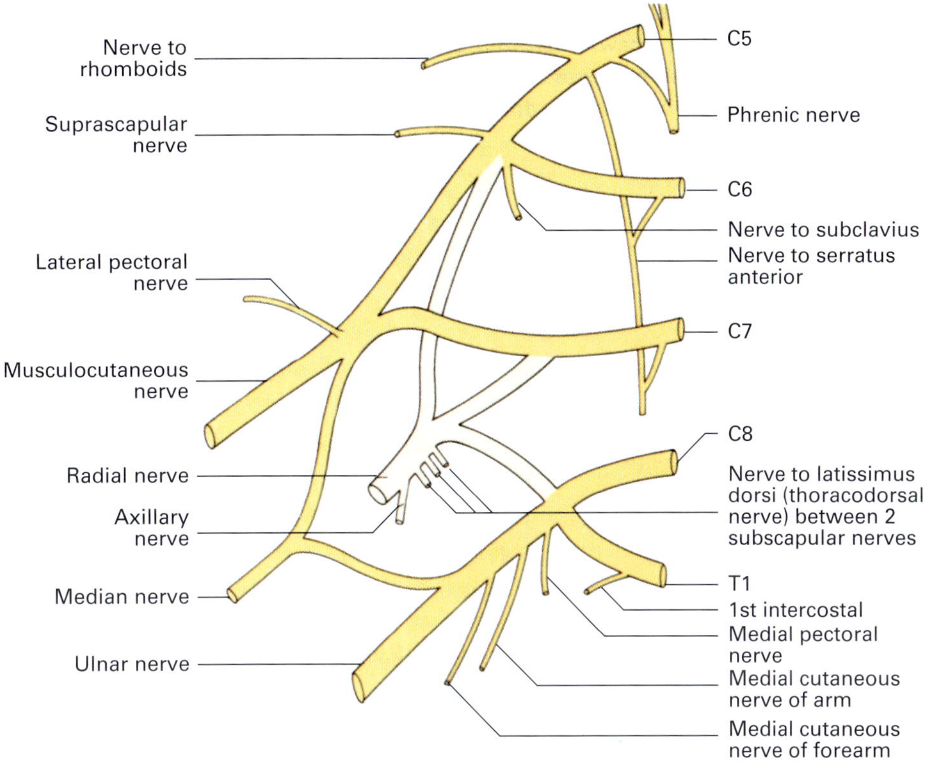

Fig. 136 The derivatives of the brachial plexus. The lightly coloured areas show the posterior divisions.

For reference purposes, the derivatives of the various components of the brachial plexus are as follows (Fig. 136).

- *From the roots*
  - nerve to rhomboids;
  - nerve to subclavius;
  - nerve to serratus anterior (C5, C6, C7).
- *From the trunk*
  - suprascapular nerve – from the upper trunk (supplies supraspinatus and infraspinatus).
- *From the lateral cord*
  - lateral pectoral nerve;
  - musculocutaneous nerve;
  - lateral root of the median nerve.
- *From the medial cord*
  - medial pectoral nerve;
  - medial cutaneous nerves of the arm and forearm;
  - ulnar nerve;
  - medial root of the median nerve.

- *From the posterior cord*
  - subscapular nerves (upper and lower);
  - nerve to latissimus dorsi (thoracodorsal nerve);
  - axillary nerve;
  - radial nerve.

Note that the posterior cord supplies the skin and muscles of the posterior aspect of the limb, whereas the anteriorly placed lateral and medial cords supply the anterior compartment structures.

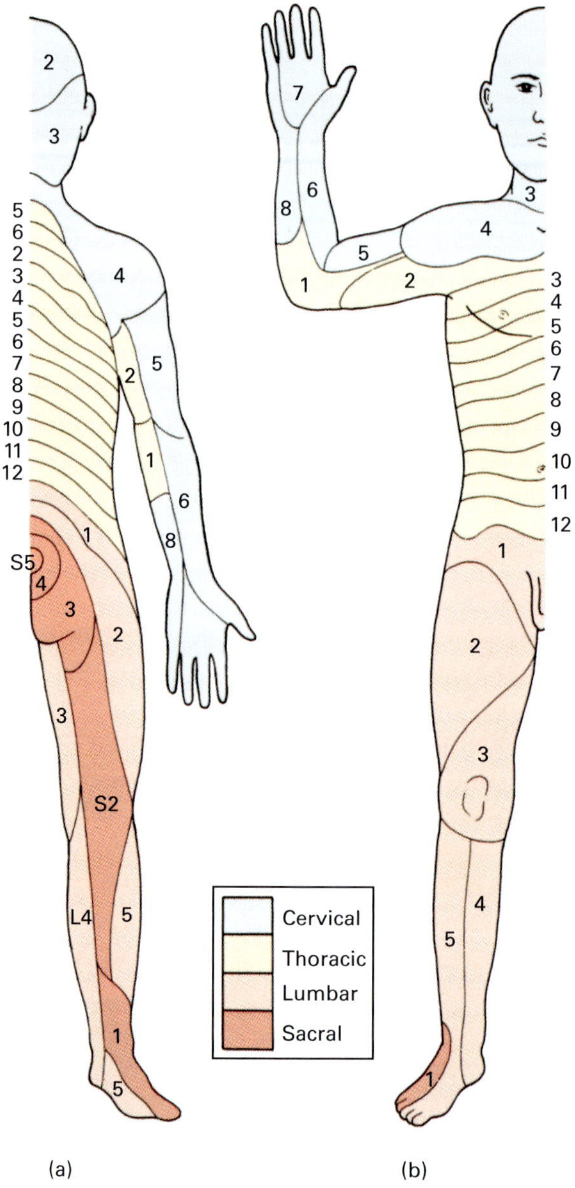

Fig. 137 The segmental cutaneous innervation of the body. (a) Posterior aspect; (b) anterior aspect.

The segmental cutaneous supply of the upper limb (Fig. 137)

In spite of this complex interlacing of the nerves in the brachial plexus, the skin of the upper limb, as with the skin of the rest of the body, has a perfectly regular segmental nerve supply. The cutaneous territory of a specific spinal nerve is called a *dermatome*. The cutaneous distribution of the spinal nerves in the upper limb is as follows:

- *C4* – supplies skin over the shoulder tip;
- *C5* – lateral side of the arm;
- *C6* – radial side of the forearm and hand;
- *C7* – the skin of the hand corresponding to the width of the middle finger;
- *C8* – ulnar side of the hand and forearm;
- *T1* – medial side of the arm;
- *T2* – skin of the axilla (via its intercostobrachial branch).

The course and distribution of the principal nerves of the upper limb

The nerves of the upper limb are derived from the brachial plexus.

The axillary nerve

The axillary (circumflex) nerve (C5, C6) arises from the posterior cord of the plexus and winds round the surgical neck of the humerus in company with the posterior circumflex humeral vessels (Figs 119, 138). Its branches are:

- *muscular* – to deltoid and teres minor;
- *cutaneous* – to a palm-sized area of skin on the lateral aspect of the arm over the deltoid (the so-called 'regimental badge area').

The axillary nerve may be injured in fractures of the humeral neck or in dislocations of the shoulder. This will be followed by weakness of shoulder abduction, wasting of the deltoid and a small patch of anaesthesia overlying this muscle.

The radial nerve

The radial nerve (C5, C6, C7, C8, T1) is the main branch of the posterior cord. Lying first behind the axillary artery, it then passes backwards between the long and medial heads of the triceps to lie in the spiral groove on the back of the humerus between the medial and lateral heads of triceps (Fig. 138). The profunda branch of the brachial artery and its venae comitantes accompany the nerve in this part of its course (Fig. 119).

At the lower third of the humerus, the radial nerve pierces the lateral intermuscular septum to enter the anterior compartment of the arm between brachialis and brachioradialis (a convenient site for surgical exposure; Fig. 134). At the level of the lateral epicondyle its important *posterior interosseous nerve* is given off, which winds round the

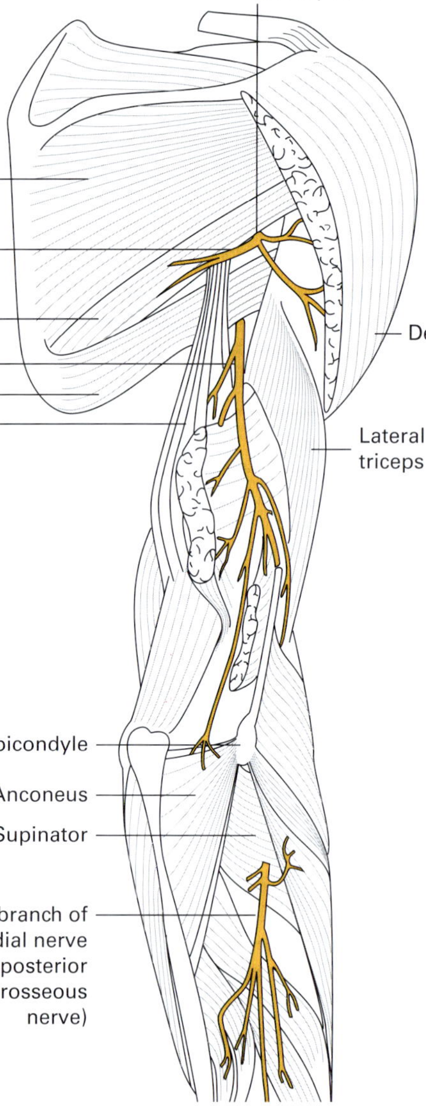

Fig. 138 The distribution of the radial nerve (right upper limb, dorsal aspect).

radius within the supinator muscle then sprays out to be distributed to the extensor muscles of the forearm.

The radial nerve itself continues as the superficial radial nerve, lying deep to brachioradialis (Fig. 134). Above the wrist, it emerges posteriorly from beneath this muscle to end by dividing into cutaneous nerves to the posterior aspects of the radial 3½ digits. Run a fingertip over the extended tendons of extensor pollicis longus (Fig. 114) just distal to the wrist joint. The nerve will be felt as a thin cord flicking over the tendon.

The radial nerve is the nerve of supply to the extensor aspect of the upper limb. The main trunk itself innervates: triceps, anconeus, brachioradialis and extensor carpi radialis longus. It also gives a twig to the lateral part of brachialis.

The posterior interosseous branch of the radial nerve supplies all the remaining extensor muscles of the forearm, including supinator and abductor pollicis longus.

Cutaneous branches are distributed to the back of the arm, forearm and radial side of the dorsum of the hand. So great is the overlap from adjacent nerves, however, that division of the radial nerve results, surprisingly, in only a small area of anaesthesia over the dorsum of the hand, in the web between the thumb and index finger (see Fig. 143a).

The musculocutaneous nerve

The musculocutaneous nerve (C5, C6, C7) continues on from the lateral cord of the plexus. It pierces coracobrachialis then runs between biceps and brachialis (supplying all these three muscles) to innervate, by its terminal cutaneous branch, now termed the lateral cutaneous nerve of the forearm, the skin of the lateral forearm.

The ulnar nerve

The ulnar nerve (C(7), C8, T1; Fig. 139) is formed from the medial cord of the plexus. It lies medial to the axillary and brachial artery as far as the middle of the humerus, then pierces the medial intermuscular septum (in company with the superior ulnar collateral artery) to descend on the anterior face of triceps. It passes behind the medial epicondyle (where it can readily be rolled against the bone), to enter the forearm (Fig. 119). Here, it descends beneath flexor carpi ulnaris until this muscle thins out into its tendon, leaving the nerve to lie superficially on its radial side. In the distal two-thirds of the forearm the nerve is accompanied by the ulnar artery, which lies on the nerve's radial side. Approximately 5 cm (2 in) above the wrist, a dorsal cutaneous branch passes deep to flexor carpi ulnaris to supply the dorsal aspects of the ulnar 1½ fingers and the dorsal aspect or the ulnar side of the hand (Fig. 140).

The ulnar nerve crosses the flexor retinaculum superficially (Figs 113, 115) to break up into a superficial terminal branch, supplying the ulnar 1½ fingers, and a deep terminal branch that supplies the hypothenar muscles and the intrinsic muscles of the hand.

Its branches are:

- *muscular* – to flexor carpi ulnaris, medial half of flexor digitorum profundus, the hypothenar muscles, the interossei, 3rd and 4th lumbricals and adductor pollicis (i.e. it supplies all the intrinsic muscles of the hand apart from those of the thenar eminence and the 1st and 2nd lumbricals, which are innervated by the median nerve);
- *cutaneous* – to the ulnar side of both aspects of the hand and both surfaces of the ulnar 1½ fingers.

The median nerve

The median nerve (C6, C7, C8, T1; Fig. 139) is formed by the union of a branch from the medial cord with another from the lateral cord of the plexus, anterior to the third

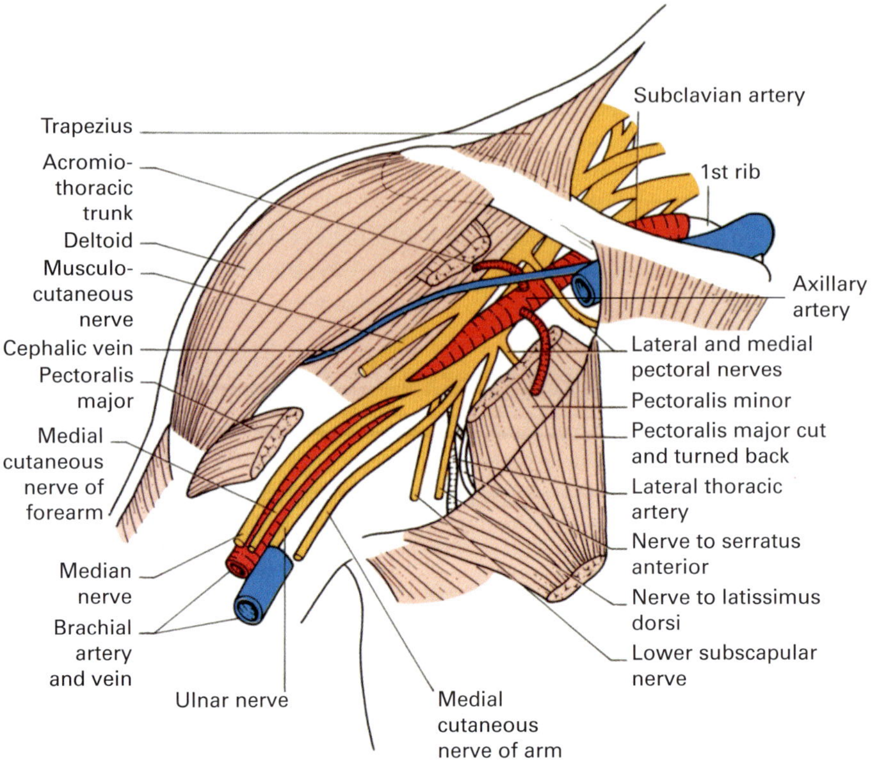

Fig. 139 Dissection of the right axilla and upper arm to show the course of the major nerves.

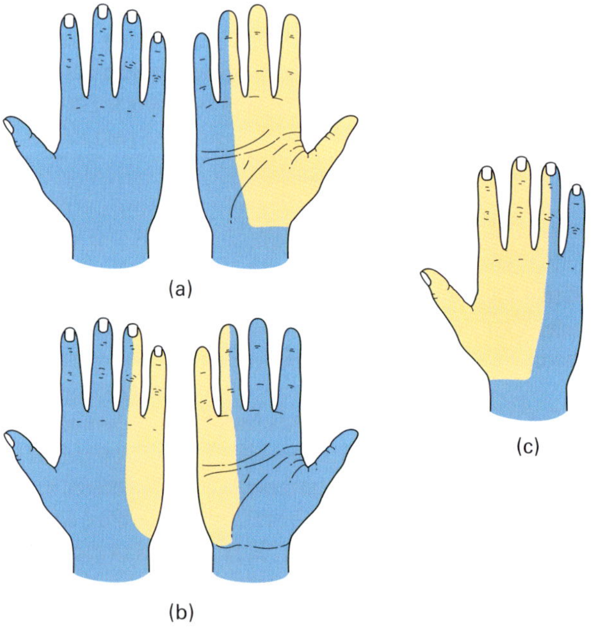

Fig. 140 The usual cutaneous distribution (shown in yellow) of the (a) median, (b) ulnar and (c) radial nerves in the hand (considerable variations and overlap occur).

part of the axillary artery. Continuing along the lateral aspect of the brachial artery, the nerve then crosses superficially (occasionally deep) to the artery at the mid-humerus level to lie on its medial side. The nerve enters the forearm between the heads of pronator teres, the deeper of which separates it from the ulnar artery (Fig. 134). Here the nerve gives off its *anterior interosseous branch* (which supplies flexor pollicis longus, flexor digitorum profundus to the index and middle fingers and pronator quadratus) and then lies on the deep aspect of flexor digitorum superficialis, to which it adheres.

At the wrist, the median nerve becomes superficial on the ulnar side of flexor carpi radialis, exactly in the midline (Fig. 113). Here, it gives off a *palmar cutaneous branch*, which supplies the skin of the thenar eminence. It then passes deep to the flexor retinaculum and gives off an important branch to the thenar muscles, twigs to the radial two lumbricals and cutaneous branches to the palmar aspects of the radial 3½ digits.

Within the carpal tunnel, deep to the flexor retinaculum, the nerve may be compressed – *the carpal tunnel syndrome* (see page 178).

Its branches are:

- *muscular* – to all the muscles of the flexor aspects of the forearm, apart from the flexor carpi ulnaris and the ulnar half of flexor digitorum profundus, and to the thenar eminence muscles and the radial two lumbricals;
- *cutaneous* – to the skin of the radial side of the palm, the palmar aspect and a variable degree of the dorsal aspect of the radial 3½ digits. Note that there is considerable variation in the exact cutaneous distribution of the nerves in the hand; for example, the ulnar nerve may encroach on median territory and supply the whole of the 4th and 5th digits (Fig. 140).

Compartments of the upper limb

In each of the limbs, the skeletal muscles are collectively ensleeved in a layer of deep fascia. From the inner surface of this stocking-like deep fascial envelope, fibrous septa project inwards and attach to the bone(s) lying within a given segment of the limb, thereby separating the muscles of that limb segment into functional groups. Thus, the muscles within each segment of the upper and lower limbs may be pictured as being located in discrete, osseofascial compartments (see Fig. 185). As a general rule, each compartment possesses its own complement of neurovascular structures, with the nerve being responsible for the motor innervation of all the muscles within that compartment. The segments of the upper limb are the arm, forearm and hand.

Compartments in the segments of the upper limb

The arm contains two compartments:

1 anterior (flexor) compartment containing biceps brachii, brachialis and coracobrachialis, all innervated by the musculocutaneous nerve;

2 posterior (extensor) compartment containing triceps brachii, innervated by the radial nerve.

The forearm contains two compartments – the anterior (flexor) compartment and the posterior (extensor) compartment, which are separated from each other by the radius, ulna and interosseous membrane.

1 The muscles of the anterior compartment of the forearm are arranged in two groups:
   - a superficial group comprising pronator teres, flexor carpi radialis, palmaris longus, flexor digitorum superficialis and flexor carpi ulnaris;
   - a deep group comprising flexor pollicis longus, flexor digitorum profundus and pronator quadratus.

2 In the superficial group, all but flexor carpi ulnaris are innervated by the median nerve. Flexor carpi ulnaris is innervated by the ulnar nerve. In the deep group, the median nerve innervates flexor pollicis longus, pronator quadratus and the radial half of flexor digitorum profundus. The medial half of flexor digitorum profundus is innervated by the ulnar nerve.

3 The muscles of the posterior compartment of the forearm (comprising the radial and ulnar extensors of the wrist, the long and short extensors of the thumb, the long abductor of the thumb, the extensors of the digits, supinator and anconeus) are innervated by the radial nerve (chiefly through the posterior interosseous nerve).

Compartment syndrome

The fascial boundaries which limit the osseofascial compartments are inelastic sheets. Any condition that leads to an increase in the volume of the compartmental contents is therefore likely to result in a rise in intracompartmental pressure. Such conditions include haemorrhage following closed fractures, muscle swelling caused by trauma or unaccustomed overuse and local infection. If unrelieved, the increased pressure leads to compression of the vessels in the compartment and secondary ischaemic damage to the nerves and muscles of the compartment. This phenomenon is known as *compartment syndrome*.

Compartment syndrome is a surgical emergency and is treated by performing a *fasciotomy*; this is a procedure in which a generous incision is made in the deep fascia overlying the compartment in order to decompress the compartment.

The female breast

The female breast overlies the 2nd–6th ribs; two-thirds of it rests on pectoralis major, one-third on serratus anterior, while its lower medial edge just overlaps the upper part of the rectus sheath.

Structure

The breast is made up of 15–20 lobules of glandular tissue embedded in fat; the latter accounts for its smooth contour and most of its bulk. These lobules are separated by fibrous septa running from the subcutaneous tissues to the fascia of the chest wall (the *ligaments of Cooper*).

Each lobule drains by its lactiferous duct onto the *nipple*, which is surrounded by the pigmented *areola*. This area is lubricated by the *areolar glands of Montgomery*; these are large, modified sebaceous glands that may form sebaceous cysts, which may, in turn, become infected.

The male breast is rudimentary, comprising small ducts without alveoli and supported by fibrous tissue and fat. Insignificant it may be, but it is still prone to the major diseases that affect the female organ.

Blood supply

1 From the axillary artery, principally via its lateral thoracic and acromiothoracic branches.
2 From the internal thoracic (hence its former name – the internal mammary artery) via its perforating branches; these pierce the 1st–4th fourth intercostal spaces, then traverse pectoralis major to reach the breast along its medial edge. The 1st and 2nd perforators are the largest of these branches.
3 From the intercostal arteries via their lateral perforating branches; a relatively unimportant source.

The venous drainage is to the corresponding veins.

Lymphatic drainage

This is of considerable importance in the spread of breast tumours.

The lymphatic drainage of the breast, as with any other organ, follows the pathway of its blood supply and therefore travels:

1 along tributaries of the axillary vessels to axillary lymph nodes; this accounts for approximately 75% of the total lymphatic drainage of the breast;
2 along the tributaries of the internal thoracic vessels, piercing pectoralis major to traverse each intercostal space to lymph nodes along the internal thoracic chain; these also receive lymphatics penetrating along the lateral perforating branches of the intercostal vessels.

Although the lymph vessels lying between the lobules of the breast communicate freely, there is a tendency for the lateral part of the breast to drain towards the axilla and the medial part to the internal thoracic chain (Fig. 141).

A subareolar plexus of lymphatics below the nipple (the *plexus of Sappey*) and another deep plexus on the pectoral fascia have, in the past, been considered to be the central points to which, respectively, the superficial and deep parts of the breast drain before communicating with the main efferent lymphatics. These plexuses appear, however, to be relatively unimportant; the vessels from these plexuses, in the main, pass directly to the regional lymph nodes.

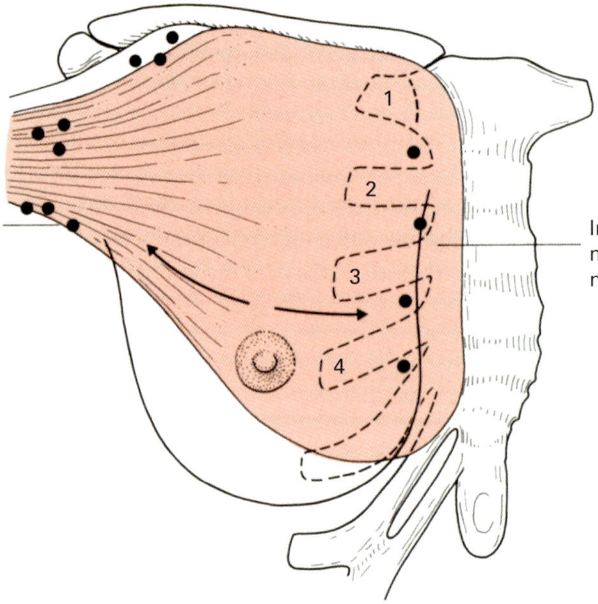

Fig. 141 The principal pathways of lymphatic drainage of the breast. These follow the venous drainage of the breast – to the axilla and to the internal mammary (internal thoracic) chain.

The *axillary lymph nodes* (some 20–30 in number) drain not only the lymphatics of the breast but also those of the pectoral region, upper abdominal wall and the upper limb and are arranged in five groups (Fig. 142):

1 *anterior* – lying deep to pectoralis major along the lower border of pectoralis minor;
2 *posterior* – along the subscapular vessels;
3 *lateral* – along the axillary vein;
4 *central* – in the axillary fat;
5 *apical (through which all the other axillary nodes drain)* – immediately behind the clavicle at the apex of the axilla above pectoralis minor and along the medial side of the axillary vein.

Clinicians and pathologists often classify axillary lymph nodes as belonging to one or other of three levels, as defined below. It is on this basis that clinicians and pathologists define metastatic axillary node spread from breast carcinomas:

- *level I* – nodes distal to pectoralis minor;
- *level II* – nodes deep to pectoralis minor;
- *level III* – nodes proximal to pectoralis minor.

From the apical nodes emerges the subclavian lymph trunk. On the right, this either drains directly into the subclavian vein or else joins the right jugular trunk; on the left, it usually drains directly into the thoracic duct.

The parasternal *internal thoracic (internal mammary) nodes,* lying along the internal thoracic vessels, drain to the mediastinal nodes and thence to the thoracic duct on the left and to the right lymphatic duct on the right. Inferiorly, they communicate distantly with the groin nodes via lymphatics which accompany the superior and inferior epigastric vessels.

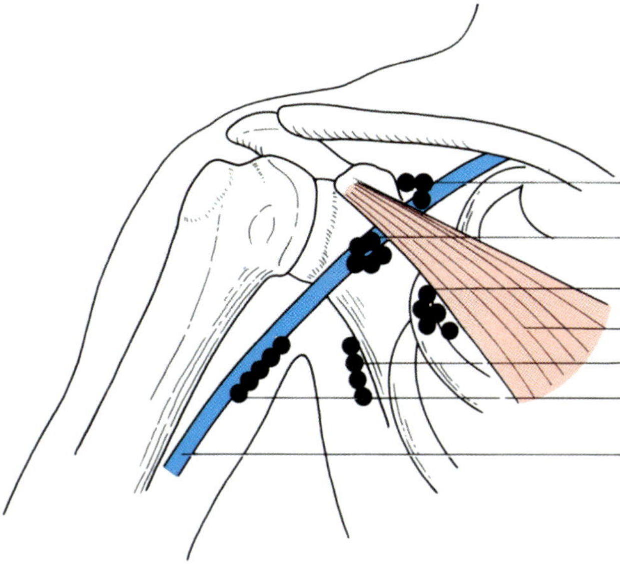

Fig. 142 The lymph nodes of the axilla.

Lymphatic spread of a neoplastic growth of the breast may occur further afield when these normal pathways have become interrupted by malignant deposits, surgery or radiotherapy. Secondaries may then be found in the lymphatics of the opposite breast or in the opposite axillary lymph nodes, the groin lymph nodes (via lymph vessels in the trunk wall), the cervical nodes (as a result of retrograde extension from the blocked thoracic duct or jugular trunk) or in peritoneal lymphatics, spreading there in a retrograde manner from the lower internal thoracic nodes; this is in addition, of course, to spread via the bloodstream.

Development

The breasts develop as an invagination of chest wall ectoderm, which forms a series of branching ducts. Shortly before birth, this site of invagination everts to form the nipple. At puberty, alveoli sprout from the ducts and considerable fatty infiltration of the breast tissue takes place. With pregnancy there is tremendous development of the alveoli which, in lactation, secrete the fatty droplets of milk. At the menopause the gland tissue atrophies.

CLINICAL FEATURES

1 Developmental abnormalities are not uncommon. The nipple may fail to evert, and it is important to find out from the patient whether or not an inverted nipple is a recent event or has been present since birth. Supernumerary nipples or even supernumerary breasts may occur along a vertical 'milk line' – a reminder of the line of mammary glands in more primitive mammals; on the other hand, the breast on one or both sides may be small or even absent (amazia).

2 An abscess of the breast should be opened by a radial incision to avoid cutting across a number of lactiferous ducts. Such an abscess may rupture from one fascial compartment into its neighbours, and it is important at operation to break down any loculi which thus form in order to provide ample drainage.

3 Dimpling of the skin over a carcinoma of the breast results from malignant infiltration and fibrous contraction of Cooper's ligaments – as these pass from breast to skin, their shortening results in tethering of the skin to the underlying tumour. This may also occur, however, in chronic infection, after trauma and, very rarely, in fibroadenosis, so that skin fixation to a breast lump is not necessarily diagnostic of malignancy.

4 Retraction of the nipple, if of recent origin, is suggestive of involvement of the milk ducts in the fibrous contraction of a scirrhous tumour.

5 The excision of a breast carcinoma by *classical radical mastectomy* (almost never performed these days) involved the removal of a wide area of skin around the tumour, all the breast tissue, the pectoralis major (through which the lymphatics pass to the internal mammary chain), the pectoralis minor (which lies as a gateway to the axilla) and the clearance of all axillary fatty tissue and contained lymph nodes. This excision also removed the bulk of the lymphatics from the arm that pass along the anterior and medial aspects of the axillary vein. A few lymph vessels from the upper limb passing above the axillary vein escaped removal.

Most surgeons today perform far less extensive surgery for breast cancer; for example, a *simple mastectomy*, in which the breast alone is removed, or an *extended simple mastectomy*, which combines this with clearance of the axillary fat and its contained nodes. Comparable results are obtained by excision of the lump, followed by radiotherapy to the breast and to the nodal areas of the axilla and the internal thoracic chain.

Oedema of the arm after mastectomy usually occurs only if further damage is done to this precarious lymphatic drainage by infection, malignant infiltration or heavy irradiation, or if additional strain is put on the evacuation of fluid from the limb by ligation or thrombosis of the axillary vein.

The anatomy of upper limb deformities

Now is a good time to revise all the palpable nerves in the upper limb (page 168).

Many deformities of the upper limb, particularly those resulting from nerve injuries, are readily interpreted on an anatomical basis.

Brachial plexus injuries may occur from traction on the arm during birth. The force of downward traction falls upon roots C5 and C6, resulting in paralysis of the deltoid and short muscles of the shoulder, and of brachialis and biceps, both of which flex the elbow. In addition, biceps is also the powerful supinator of the forearm (Fig. 131). The arm, therefore, hangs limply by the side with the forearm pronated and the palm facing backwards, like a porter hinting for a tip (*Erb–Duchenne paralysis*). The sensory loss in this lesion affects the lateral aspect of the upper arm and the radial side of the forearm

(C5 and C6; Fig. 137). In adults, this lesion is seen in violent falls on the side of the head and shoulder, forcing the two apart and thus putting a tearing strain on the upper roots of the plexus.

Upward traction on the arm (e.g. in a forcible breech delivery) may tear the lowest root, T1, which is the segmental supply of the intrinsic hand muscles. The hand assumes a clawed appearance because of the unopposed action of the long flexors and extensors of the fingers; the extensors, inserting into the bases of the proximal phalanges, extend the metacarpophalangeal joints while the flexor profundus and sublimis, inserting into the distal and middle phalanges, flex the interphalangeal joints (*Klumpke's paralysis*). The sensory loss in this injury is along the medial aspect of the arm (T1; Fig. 137). There is often an associated *Horner's syndrome* (partial ptosis and constriction of the pupil), due to traction on the cervical sympathetic chain.

A mass of malignant supraclavicular lymph nodes or the direct invasion of a carcinoma of the pulmonary apex (*Pancoast's syndrome*) may produce a similar neurological picture by involvement of the lowest root of the brachial plexus and cervical sympathetic chain.

Not infrequently, the lower trunk of the plexus (C8, T1) is pressed upon by a cervical rib, or by a fibrous strand running from the extremity of such a rib, resulting in paraesthesiae along the ulnar border of the arm and forearm and weakness and wasting of the small muscles of the hand.

The *radial nerve* may be injured in the axilla by the pressure of a crutch ('crutch palsy') or may be compressed when an individual falls asleep with the arm hanging over the back of a chair ('Saturday night palsy'). Fractures of the humeral shaft may damage the main radial nerve in about 12% of cases, with spontaneous recovery of nerve function occurring in 70%. The posterior interosseous branch of the radial nerve, to the extensor muscles of the forearm, may be injured in fractures or dislocations of the radial head. An ill-placed incision to expose the head of the radius taken more than three fingers' breadth below the head will divide the nerve as it lies in the supinator muscle.

Damage to the main trunk of the radial nerve results in a *wrist drop* owing to paralysis of all the wrist extensors (Fig. 143). Damage to the posterior interosseous nerve, however, leaves extensor carpi radialis longus intact, as it is supplied by the trunk of the radial nerve before the latter gives off the posterior interosseous nerve. This muscle alone may be able to achieve a degree of extension of the wrist.

The disability produced by a wrist drop is inability to grip firmly, since, unless the flexor muscles are stretched by extending the wrist, it is not possible to achieve a strong grip.

Nerve overlap means that division of the radial nerve produces only a small area of anaesthesia of the dorsum of the hand between the 1st and 2nd metacarpals (Fig. 143a).

The *ulnar nerve*, in its vulnerable position behind the medial epicondyle of the humerus, may be damaged in fractures or dislocations of the elbow; it may also be damaged in lacerations of the wrist. In the latter case, all the intrinsic muscles of the fingers (apart from the radial two lumbricals) are paralysed so that the hand assumes the clawed position already described under Klumpke's palsy (Fig. 143d). The clawing is slightly less intense in the 2nd and 3rd digits because of their intact lumbricals, supplied by the median nerve. In late cases, wasting of the interossei is readily seen on inspecting the dorsum of the hand.

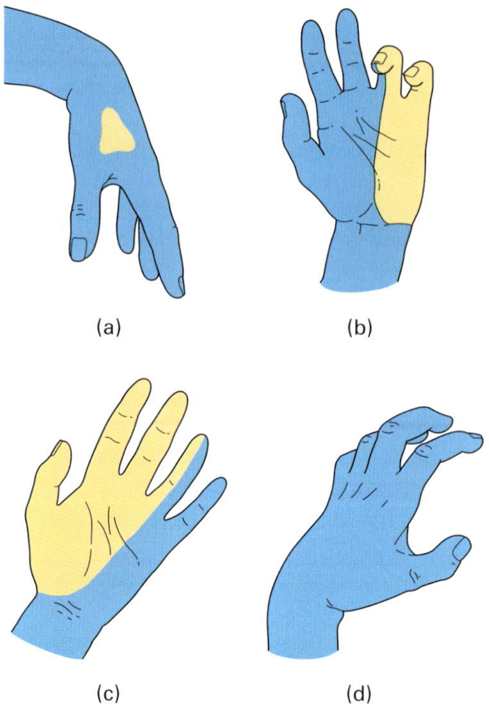

Fig. 143 Deformities of the hand. (a) Radial palsy – wrist drop. (b) Ulnar nerve palsy – 'main en griffe' or claw hand. (c) Median nerve palsy – 'monkey's hand'. (d) Volkmann's contracture – another claw hand deformity. The yellow areas represent the usual distribution of anaesthesia.

If the nerve is injured at the elbow, the flexor digitorum profundus to the 4th and 5th fingers is paralysed so that the clawing of these two fingers is less intense than in division of the nerve at the wrist. Paralysis of the flexor carpi ulnaris results in a tendency to radial deviation of the wrist.

A high division of the ulnar nerve, anywhere above the level of a hand's breadth above the wrist, will be followed by sensory loss over the ulnar side of the hand and the ulnar 1½ fingers on both the palmar and dorsal aspects (Fig. 140). However, if the nerve is divided at, or just above, the wrist, which is the common site for this to occur, the sensory loss is confined to the *palmar* aspect of the ulnar side of the hand and the ulnar 1½ fingers, with sparing of the dorsum of the hand. This is because the dorsal branch of the ulnar nerve, which supplies this area, is given off about a hand's breadth above the level of the wrist (Fig. 134) and is therefore spared from injury.

The *median nerve* is occasionally damaged in supracondylar fractures, but it is in greatest danger in lacerations of the wrist.

If divided at the wrist, only the thenar muscles (excluding adductor pollicis) and the radial two lumbricals are paralysed and wasting of the thenar muscles occurs. The best clinical test for this is to ask the patient, with his hand resting palm upwards on the table, to touch a pencil held above the thumb. Failure to be able to do this (abduction) is diagnostic of paralysis of abductor pollicis brevis. It might be thought that such a lesion is relatively trivial since the only motor defect is loss of accurate opposition movement of the thumb to other fingers. In point of fact, this injury is a serious disability because of the loss of sensation over the thumb, adjacent 2½ fingers and the radial two-thirds of the palm of the hand, which prevents the accurate and delicate adjustments the hand makes in response to tactile stimuli (Fig. 143).

If the median nerve is divided at the elbow, there is significant impairment of muscle function. Pronation of the forearm is lost and is replaced by a trick movement of rotation of the upper arm. Wrist flexion is weak and accompanied by ulnar deviation, since this now depends on the flexor carpi ulnaris and the ulnar half of flexor digitorum profundus.

Volkmann's contracture of the hand follows ischaemia and subsequent fibrosis and contraction of the long flexor and extensor muscles of the forearm (Fig. 143d).

The deformities are readily explained as follows:

1 Since the flexors of the wrist are bulkier than the extensors, their fibrous contraction is greater and the wrist is therefore flexed.

2 The long extensors of the fingers are inserted into the proximal phalanges; their contracture extends the metacarpophalangeal joints.

3 The long flexors are inserted into the distal and middle phalanges and therefore flex the interphalangeal joints.

There is, therefore, flexion at the wrist, extension at the metacarpophalangeal and flexion at the interphalangeal joints.

If the wrist is passively further flexed by the examiner, the tight flexor tendons are somewhat relaxed and therefore the fingers become a little less clawed.

Dupuytren's contracture results from a fibrous contraction of the palmar aponeurosis and palmar fascial structures, particularly of the 4th and 5th fingers.

The palmar aponeurosis is merely part of the deep fascial sheath of the upper limb; it passes from the palm along either side of each finger, blends with the fibrous flexor sheath of the fingers and is attached to the sides of the proximal and middle phalanges. Contracture of this fascia results in a longitudinal thickening in the palm together with flexion of the metacarpophalangeal and proximal interphalangeal joints. However, the distal interphalangeal joints are not involved and, in fact, in an advanced case, are actually *extended* by the distal phalanx being pushed backwards against the palm of the hand.

The spaces of the hand

The spaces of the hand are of practical significance because they may become infected and, in consequence, become distended with pus. The important spaces are:

1 the superficial pulp spaces of the fingers;

2 the synovial tendon sheaths of the 2nd, 3rd and 4th fingers;

3 the ulnar bursa;

4 the radial bursa;

5 the mid-palmar space;

6 the thenar space.

The superficial pulp space of the fingers (Fig. 144)

The tips of the fingers and thumb are composed entirely of subcutaneous fat broken up and packed between fibrous septa, which pass from the skin down to the periosteum of the terminal phalanx. The tight packing of this compartment is responsible for the severe pain of a 'septic finger' – there is little room for the expansion of inflamed and oedematous tissues.

The blood vessels to the shaft of the distal phalanx must traverse this space and may become thrombosed in a severe pulp infection with resulting necrosis of the diaphysis of the bone. The base of the distal phalanx receives its blood supply more proximally from a branch of the digital artery in the middle segment of the finger and therefore survives. At each of the skin creases of the fingers, the skin is bound down to the underlying flexor sheath so that the pulp over each phalanx is in a separate compartment, isolated from the rest of the digit. Infection may, however, track from the pulp space along the neurovascular digital bundles to more proximal regions in the digit and thence to the palm.

Over the palm of the hand there is very little subcutaneous tissue, the skin adhering to the underlying palmar aponeurosis; in contrast, the skin of the dorsum of the fingers and hand is loose and fluid can, therefore, readily collect beneath it. Unless this is remembered, the marked dorsal oedema which may accompany sepsis of the palmar aspect of the fingers or hand may result in the primary site of the infection being overlooked.

The ulnar and radial bursae and the synovial tendon sheaths of the fingers (Fig. 145)

The flexor tendons traverse a fibro-osseous tunnel in each digit. This tunnel is made up posteriorly by the metacarpal head, the phalanges and the fronts of the intervening joints. The anterior fibrous part consists of condensed deep fascia attached to the anterolateral and anteromedial margins of each phalanx and is termed the *fibrous flexor sheath*. This is particularly tough over the phalanges but loose over the front of each joint; it therefore holds the flexor tendons in place without 'bow-stringing' during flexion of the fingers, but does not impede movement of the joints.

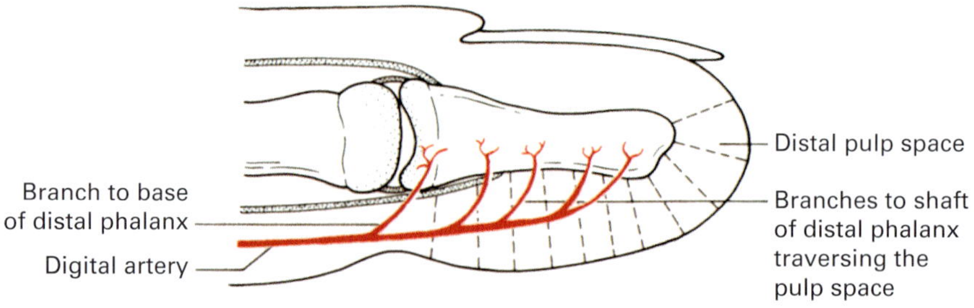

Fig. 144 The distal pulp space of the finger; note the distribution of the arterial supply to the distal phalanx.

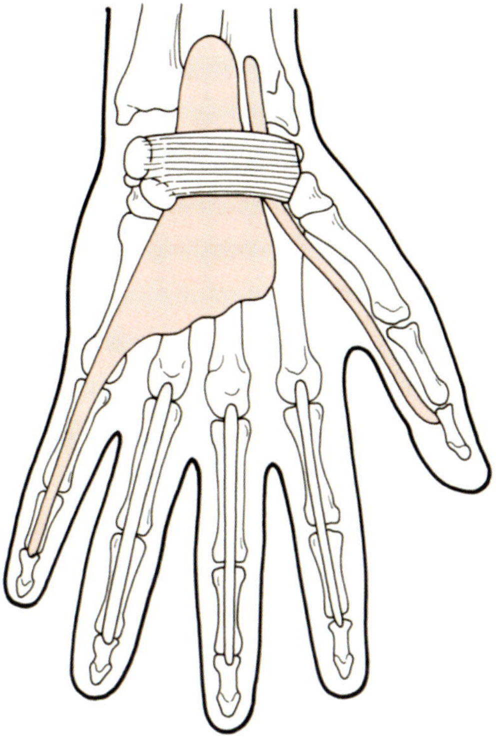

Fig. 145 The synovial sheaths of the flexor tendons of the hand (left) – the radial and ulnar bursae track proximally deep to the flexor retinaculum and provide a potential pathway of infection into the forearm. In many cases, these bursae communicate.

Distally, the fibrous sheath ends at the insertion of the profundus tendon (or flexor pollicis longus tendon in the case of the thumb) at the base of the distal phalanx.

These fibrous sheaths are lined by synovial membrane, which is reflected around each tendon. The tendons of the 2nd, 3rd and 4th fingers have synovial sheaths which are closed off proximally at the metacarpal head, but the synovial sheaths of the thumb and little finger extend proximally into the palm.

That of the long flexor tendon of the thumb extends through the palm, deep to the flexor retinaculum, to approximately 2.5 cm (1 in) proximal to the wrist and is termed the *radial bursa*. The synovial sheath of the 5th finger continues as the *ulnar bursa*, an expanded synovial sheath which encloses all the finger tendons in the palm and which also extends proximally deep to the flexor retinaculum for 2.5 cm (1 in) above the wrist. In approximately 50% of cases the radial and ulnar bursae communicate. These synovial sheaths either may become infected directly – for example, following the entry of a splinter – or may be secondarily involved from a neglected pulp-space infection. Infections of the 2nd, 3rd and 4th sheaths are confined to the finger concerned, but sepsis in the 1st and 5th sheaths may spread proximally into the palm through the radial and ulnar bursa, respectively, and may pass from one bursa to the other via the frequent cross-communications that are present between the two.

Since these bursae both extend proximally beyond the wrist, infection may, on occasion, spread into the forearm.

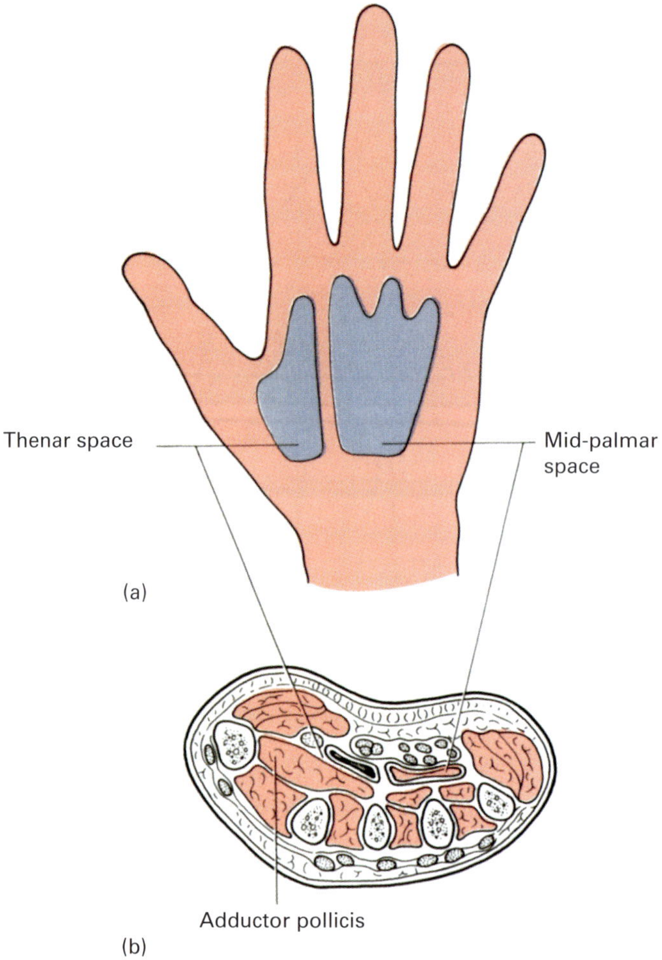

Fig. 146 The mid-palmar and thenar spaces (left hand): (a) projected onto the surface of the hand and (b) in transverse section (viewed from the proximal aspect).

Two spaces deep in the palm of the hand may rarely become distended with pus; these are the mid-palmar and thenar spaces (Fig. 146).

The *mid-palmar space* lies behind the flexor tendons and ulnar bursa in the palm and in front of the 3rd, 4th and 5th metacarpals with their attached interossei. The 1st and 2nd metacarpals are curtained off from this space by the adductor pollicis, which arises from the shaft of the 3rd metacarpal and passes as a triangular sheet to the base of the proximal phalanx of the thumb.

The *thenar space* is the space superficial to the 2nd and 3rd metacarpals and the adductor pollicis. It is separated from the mid-palmar space by a fibrous partition.

Infection of these two spaces sometimes results from penetrating wounds or may be due to secondary involvement from a neglected or inadequately treated tendon sheath infection. Nowadays, they are fortunately extremely rare, thanks to antibiotic treatment and the early surgical drainage of pus collections.

Part 4
The Lower Limb

Surface anatomy and surface markings of the lower limb

Anatomically the upper and lower limbs are comparable to each other as regards the arrangement of the bones, joints, main muscle groups, vessels and nerves. However, compared with the complex movements of the upper limb, designed to place the hand in a multiplicity of positions, together with the intricate and multiple functions of the hand, fingers and thumb, the functions of the lower limb are simple indeed – first, to act as a rigid column in the standing position and, second, to turn into a lever system when the subject walks or runs. In short, the upper limb is designed for prehension, while the lower limb is designed for support and propulsion. As with the upper limb, several aspects of the important clinical anatomy of the lower limb can be examined, reviewed and revised on yourself, your colleagues or on your patients.

Bones and joints

The *anterior superior spine of the ilium* is easily felt and may be visible in the thin subject. The *greater trochanter* of the femur lies a hand's breadth below the iliac crest; it is best palpated with the hip passively abducted so that the overlying hip abductors (tensor fasciae latae and gluteus medius and minimus) are relaxed. In an emaciated patient, the greater trochanter may be seen as a prominent bulge and its overlying skin may be vulnerable to the development of a pressure sore.

The *ischial tuberosity* is covered by gluteus maximus when one stands. In the sitting position, however, the muscle slips away laterally so that weight is taken directly on the bone. To palpate this bony point, therefore, feel for it uncovered by gluteus maximus in the flexed position of the hip.

At the knee, the *patella* forms a prominent landmark anteriorly. When quadriceps femoris is relaxed, this bone is freely mobile from side to side; note that this is so when you stand erect. The *condyles* of the femur and tibia, the *head of the fibula* and the joint line of the knee are all readily palpable; less so is the *adductor tubercle* of the femur, best identified by running the fingers down the medial side of the thigh until they are halted by it, the first bony prominence so to be encountered.

The *tibia* can be felt along the entire length of its anterior subcutaneous border from the *tibial tuberosity* above, which marks the insertion of the quadriceps tendon, to the *medial malleolus* at the ankle. The subcutaneous surface of the tibia, which can be felt immediately medial to its subcutaneous border, is crossed by two structures – the long saphenous vein, which is readily visible immediately in front of the medial malleolus of the tibia, and the adjacent saphenous nerve. The head of the fibula, as noted previously, is easily palpable; note that it lies below and towards the posterior part of the lateral tibial condyle. Distal to its neck, the fibula 'disappears' as it dives into the muscle mass of the peroneal muscles, becoming subcutaneous distally. The *fibula* is subcutaneous for its terminal 7 cm (3 in) above the *lateral malleolus*. The latter extends more distally than the stumpier *medial malleolus* of the tibia.

Immediately in front of the malleoli can be felt a block of bone which is the *head of the talus*. Feel it move up and down in dorsiflexion and plantarflexion of the ankle.

The *tuberosity of the navicular* stands out as a bony prominence 2.5 cm (1 in) in front of the medial malleolus; it is the principal point of insertion of the tibialis posterior tendon. The base of the 5th metatarsal is easily felt on the lateral side of the foot and is the site of insertion of peroneus brevis (fibularis brevis).

If the *calcaneus* (*os calcis*) is carefully palpated, the *peroneal tubercle* can be felt on its lateral surface 2.5 cm (1 in) below the tip of the lateral malleolus. On its medial aspect the *sustentaculum tali* can be felt 2.5 cm (1 in) below the medial malleolus; these represent pulleys for the tendons, respectively, of peroneus longus (fibularis longus) and flexor hallucis longus

Bursae of the lower limb

A number of the bony prominences described in the previous section are associated with overlying bursae, which may become distended and inflamed: the one over the ischial tuberosity may enlarge with too much sitting ('weaver's bottom'); that in front of the patella is affected by prolonged kneeling forwards, as in scrubbing floors or hewing coal ('housemaid's knee', the 'beat knee' of North Country miners or prepatellar bursitis), whereas the bursa over the ligamentum patellae is affected by years of kneeling in a more erect position – as in praying ('clergyman's knee' or infrapatellar bursitis). Individuals who wear fashionable but tight shoes are prone to bursitis over the insertion of the Achilles tendon (calcaneal tendon or tendo calcaneus) into the calcaneus and may also develop bursae over the navicular tuberosity and dorsal aspects of the phalanges.

A 'bunion' is a thickened bursa on the inner aspect of the first metatarsal head, usually associated with hallux valgus deformity. Note that the bursae that may develop (and become inflamed) over the calcaneus, navicular, the phalanges and the head of the first metatarsal are called *adventitial* bursae. They are not found in normal anatomy but occur only in response to the affected part having been subjected to prolonged pressure, stress and friction for several months or years or in the pathological conditions described above. This is in contrast to the pre- and infrapatellar bursae, which are normal anatomical structures and which may become distended with fluid as a result of repeated trauma.

Mensuration in the lower limb

Measurement is an important part of the clinical examination of the lower limb. Unfortunately, students find difficulty in carrying this out accurately and still greater difficulty in explaining and interpreting the results they obtain, yet this is nothing more or less than a simple exercise in applied anatomy.

First note the differences between *real* and *apparent* shortening of the lower limbs. Real shortening is due to actual loss of bone length – for example, when a femoral fracture has united with a good deal of overriding of the two fragments. Apparent shortening is due to a *fixed* deformity of the limb (Fig. 147). Stand up and flex your knee and hip on one side, imagine these are both ankylosed at 90° and note that, although there is no loss of tissue in this limb, it is apparently some 60 cm (2 ft) shorter than its partner.

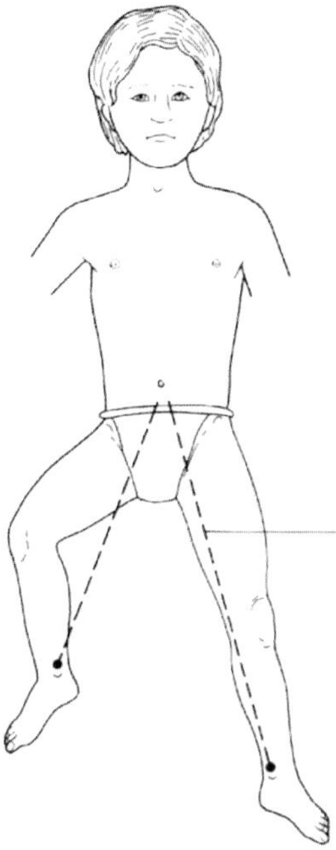

Fig. 147 Apparent shortening – one limb may be apparently shorter than the other because of fixed deformity; the legs in this illustration are actually equal in length but the right is *apparently* considerably shorter because of a gross flexion contracture at the hip. Apparent shortening is measured by comparing the distance from the umbilicus to the medial malleolus on each side.

If there is a fixed pelvic tilt or fixed joint deformity in one limb, there may be this apparent difference between the lengths of the two limbs. By experimenting on yourself you will find that adduction apparently shortens the limb, whereas it is apparently lengthened in abduction.

To measure the real length of the limbs (Fig. 148), overcome any disparity due to fixed deformity by putting both limbs into exactly the same position; where there is no joint fixation, this means that the patient lies with the pelvis 'square', the limbs abducted symmetrically and both limbs lying flat on the couch. If, however, one hip is in 60° of fixed flexion, for example, the other hip must first be put into this identical position. The length of each limb is then measured from the anterior superior iliac spine to the medial malleolus. In order to obtain identical points on each side, slide the finger upwards along the inguinal ligament and mark the bony point first encountered by the finger. Similarly, slide the finger upwards from just distal to the malleolus to determine the apex of this landmark on each side.

To determine apparent shortening, the patient lies with his/her legs parallel (as they would be when standing erect) and the distance from umbilicus to each medial malleolus is measured (Fig. 147).

Now suppose we find 10 cm (4 in) of apparent shortening and 5 cm (2 in) of real shortening of the limb; we interpret this as meaning that 5 cm (2 in) of the shortening is due to true loss of limb length and another 5 cm (2 in) is due to fixed postural deformity.

If the apparent shortening is *less* than the real, this can only mean that the hip has ankylosed in the abducted, and hence apparently elongated, position.

Note this important point: one reason why the orthopaedic surgeon immobilizes a tuberculous hip in the abducted position is that, when the hip becomes ankylosed,

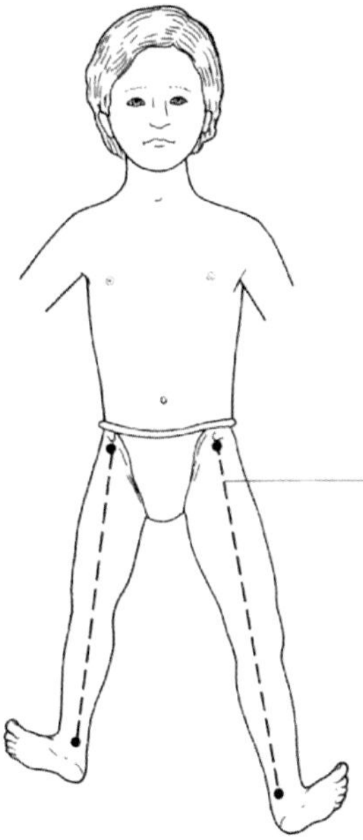

Fig. 148 Measuring real shortening – the patient lies with the pelvis 'square' and the legs placed symmetrically. Measurement is made from the anterior superior spine to the medial malleolus on each side.

shortening due to actual destruction at the hip (i.e. true shortening) will be compensated, to a considerable extent, by the apparent lengthening produced by the fixed abduction.

Having established that there is real shortening present, the examiner must then determine whether this is at the hip, the femur or the tibia, or at a combination of these sites.

At the hip

Place the thumb on the anterior superior spine and the index finger on the upper border of the greater trochanter on each side; a glance is sufficient to tell if there is any difference between the two sides. Nelaton's line and Bryant's triangle (both cumbersome geometrical derivations), once popular, are of no more than historical interest now, having long since been abandoned on account of their limited clinical usefulness.

At the femur

Measure the distance from the anterior superior spine (if hip disease has been excluded) or from the greater trochanter to the line of the knee joint (not to the patella, whose position can be varied by contraction of the quadriceps).

At the tibia

Compare the distance from the line of the knee joint to the medial malleolus on each side.

Muscles and tendons

Quadriceps femoris forms the prominent muscle mass on the anterior aspect of the thigh; its insertion into the medial aspect of the patella can be seen to extend more distally than on the lateral side. In the well-developed subject, *sartorius* can be defined when the hip is flexed and externally rotated against resistance. It extends from the anterior superior iliac spine to the medial side of the upper end of the tibia. It forms the lateral border of the *femoral triangle* and is an important landmark.

Gluteus maximus forms the bulk of the buttock and can be felt to contract in extension of the hip.

Gluteus medius and *minimus* and the *adductors* can be felt to tighten, respectively, in resisted abduction and adduction of the hip.

Define the tendons around the knee joint with the joint comfortably flexed to about 90°:

- posterolaterally – the *biceps* tendon passes to the head of the fibula; the *iliotibial tract* lies approximately 1.25 cm (0.5 in) in front of this tendon and passes to a tubercle on the anterior aspect of the lateral condyle of the tibia;
- posteromedially – the bulge which one feels is the *semimembranosus insertion* on which two tendons, *gracilis* and *semitendinosus*, the former somewhat anteromedial to the latter, are readily palpable. Posteriorly – between the tendons of biceps and semitendinosus can be felt the heads of origin of *gastrocnemius*. This muscle, with soleus, forms the bulk of the posterior bulge of the calf; the two end distally in the *Achilles tendon* (calcaneal tendon).

At the front of the ankle (Fig. 149) the tendon of *tibialis anterior* lies most medially, passing to its insertion at the base of the first metatarsal and the medial cuneiform. More laterally, the tendons of *extensor hallucis longus* and *extensor digitorum longus* are readily visible in the dorsiflexed foot. *Peroneus longus* and *brevis* tendons pass behind the lateral malleolus. The tendon of *peroneus tertius* (fibularis tertius) can be felt on careful palpation on the lateral aspect of the dorsum of the foot, lateral to the tendons of extensor digitorum longus. The peroneus tertius tendon passes to the base of the 5th metatarsal. This is of more than academic interest (Fig. 149). Peroneus tertius is present only in the human. Only humans stand on the whole sole of the foot; lower mammals tend to stand and walk on tiptoe. Presumably peroneus tertius has evolved in humans as a detachment from the lateral aspect of extensor digitorum longus to assist in the development of the plantigrade human foot. Behind the medial malleolus, working from the anteromedial to the posterolateral side, lie the tendons of *tibialis posterior* and *flexor digitorum longus*, the *posterior tibial artery* with its venae comitantes, the *tibial nerve* and, finally, *flexor hallucis longus*, all on their way to the sole of the foot (Fig. 150). All these structures behind the medial malleolus lie against the medial surface of the calcaneus and are roofed over by a dense fascial band called the *flexor retinaculum* of the foot. The interval between the flexor retinaculum and the underlying calcaneus is termed the *tarsal tunnel*. An entrapment neuropathy of the tibial nerve in the tarsal tunnel is called *tarsal tunnel syndrome*. The condition is far less common than carpal tunnel syndrome (median nerve entrapment in the carpal tunnel).

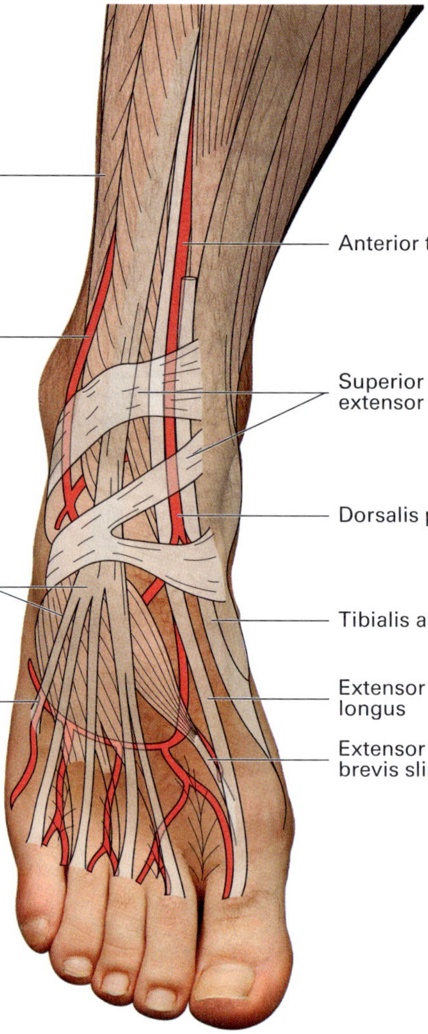

Fig. 149 The structures passing over the dorsum of the ankle (right ankle, anterior aspect).

Vessels

The *femoral artery* (Fig. 151) can be felt pulsating at the mid-inguinal point, halfway between the anterior superior iliac spine and the pubic symphysis. The upper two-thirds of a line joining this point to the adductor tubercle, with the hip somewhat flexed, abducted and externally rotated, accurately indicates the surface marking of this vessel. A finger on the femoral pulse lies directly over the head of the femur, immediately lateral to the femoral vein (and the termination of the great saphenous vein) and a finger's breadth medial to the femoral nerve.

The pulse of the *popliteal artery* is often not easy to detect. It may be felt with the subject prone, the subject's knee flexed and muscles relaxed. The pulse is sought by firm pressure downwards and forwards against the popliteal surface of the femur.

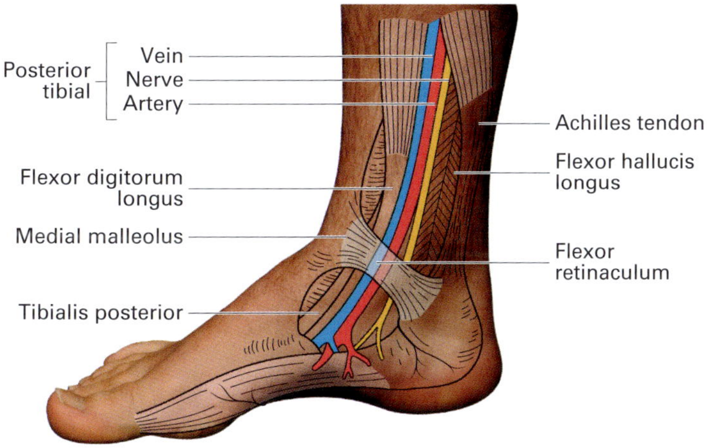

Fig. 150 The structures passing behind the medial malleolus (right ankle, medial aspect).

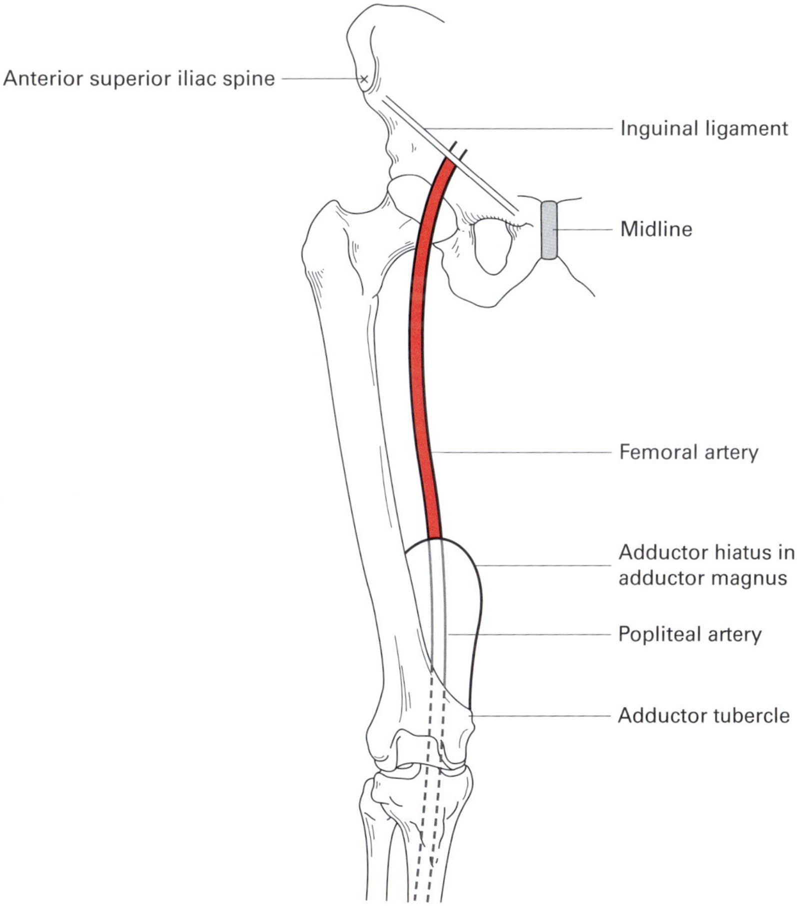

Fig. 151 The surface markings of the femoral artery; the upper two-thirds of a line joining the mid-inguinal point (halfway between the anterior superior iliac spine and the symphysis pubis) to the adductor tubercle.

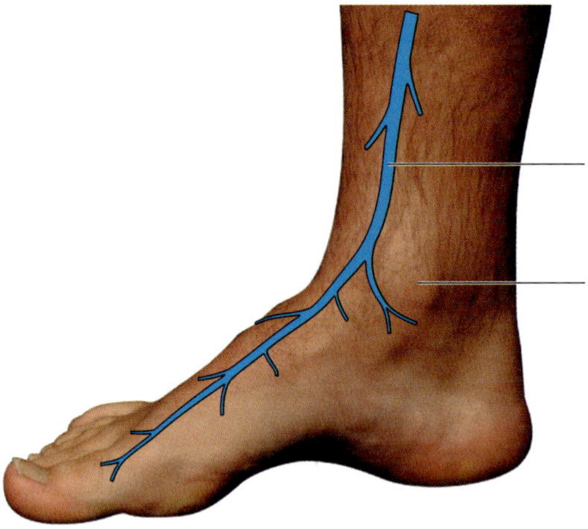

Fig. 152 The relationship of the great (long) saphenous vein to the medial malleolus (right ankle).

The pulse of *dorsalis pedis* (Fig. 149) is felt halfway between the anterior borders of the medial and lateral malleoli. It is situated between the tendons of extensor hallucis longus and extensor digitorum longus on the dorsum of the foot. It is absent in approximately 2% of normal subjects. The *posterior tibial artery* (Fig. 150) may be felt a finger's breadth below and behind the posterior border of the medial malleolus. In approximately 1% of healthy subjects, this artery is replaced by the peroneal (fibular) artery.

The absence of one or both pulses at the ankle is not, therefore, in itself indicative of vascular disease.

The *small (or short) saphenous vein* commences as a continuation of the lateral limb of the subcutaneous venous network on the dorsum of the foot, runs proximally *behind* the lateral malleolus and terminates by draining into the popliteal vein behind the knee. The *great (or long) saphenous vein* arises as a continuation of the medial limb of the dorsal network of veins and passes proximally *in front* of the medial malleolus, with the saphenous nerve anterior to it, eventually joining the femoral vein in the groin, 2.5 cm (1 in) below the inguinal ligament and immediately medial to the femoral pulse.

These veins are readily studied in any patient with extensive varicose veins and are usually visible, in their lower part, in the thin normal subject on standing. (The word 'saphenous' is derived from the Greek for 'clear'.)

From the practical point of view, the constancy of the position of the long saphenous vein immediately in front of the medial malleolus is an important anatomical relationship in clinical practice; no matter how collapsed or obese, or how young and tiny the patient, the vein can be relied upon to be available at this site when urgently required for transfusion purposes (Fig. 152).

Nerves

Only one nerve is easily felt in the lower limb; this is the *common peroneal (fibular) nerve*, which can be rolled against the underlying bone as the nerve winds around the neck of the fibula (Fig. 153). As can be imagined, the nerve may be injured at this site in

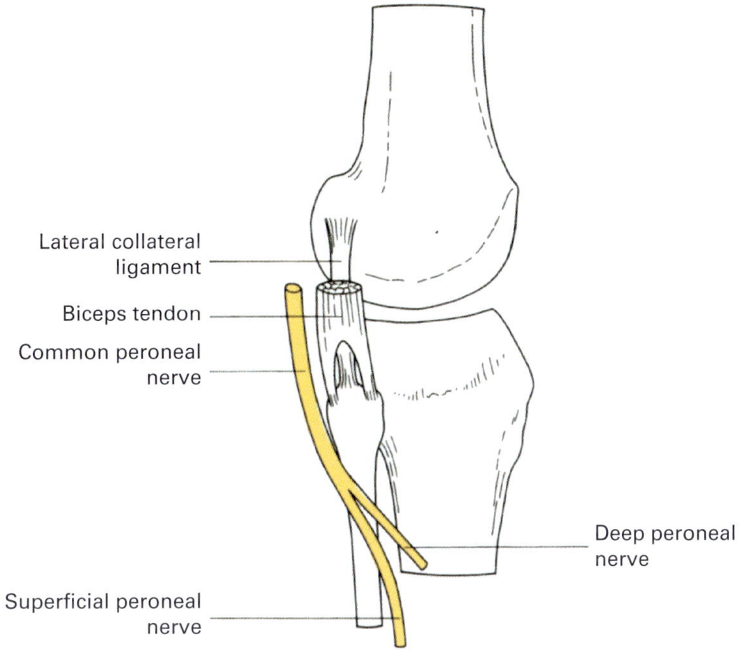

Fig. 153 The close relationship of the common peroneal nerve to the neck of the fibula; at this site it may be compressed by a tight bandage or plaster cast (right knee, lateral aspect).

adduction injuries to the knee or compressed by a tight plaster cast or firm bandage, with a resultant foot drop and inversion (talipes equinovarus; see page 271).

The *femoral nerve* emerges from under the inguinal ligament 1.25 cm (0.5 in) lateral to the femoral pulse. After a very short course, the nerve breaks up into multiple terminal branches.

The surface marking of the *sciatic nerve* (Fig. 154) can be represented by a line which commences at a point midway between the posterior superior iliac spine (identified by the overlying sacral dimple) and the ischial tuberosity, curves outwards and downwards through a point midway between the greater trochanter and ischial tuberosity

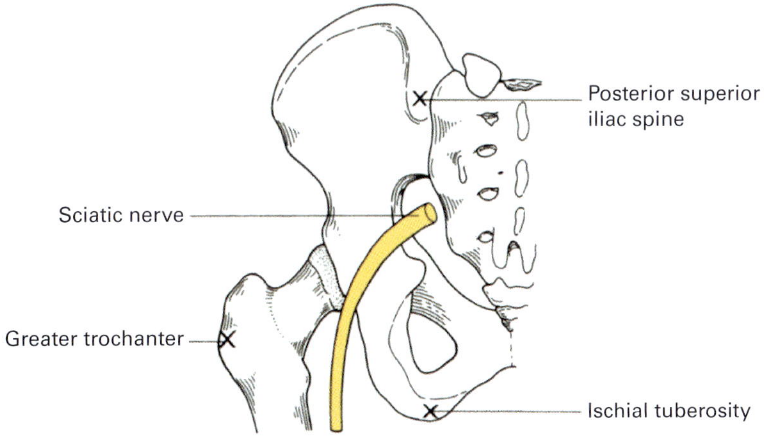

Fig. 154 The surface markings of the sciatic nerve (left gluteal region). Join the midpoint between the ischial tuberosity and posterior superior iliac spine to the midpoint between the ischial tuberosity and the greater trochanter by a curved line; continue this line vertically down the leg – it represents the course of the sciatic nerve.

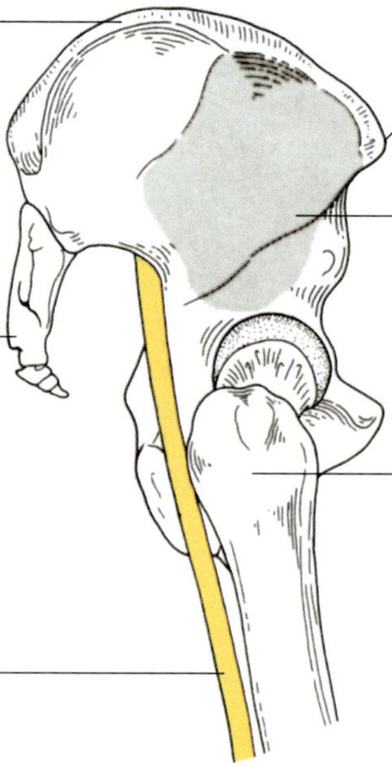

Fig. 155 The 'safe area' for injections in the buttock.

and then continues vertically downwards in the midline of the posterior aspect of the thigh. The nerve ends at a variable point above the popliteal fossa by dividing into its two terminal branches: the *tibial nerve* and *the common peroneal nerves*. The latter is the lateral of the two.

It would seem inconceivable that a nerve with such a constant relationship to well-defined landmarks could be damaged by intramuscular injections, yet this has happened so frequently that it has even been proposed that, in the interests of patient safety, this site be avoided altogether for the administration of intramuscular injections.

A better surface marking for the 'safe area' of buttock injections can be defined as that area which lies under the outstretched hand when the thumb and thenar eminence are placed along the iliac crest with the tip of the thumb touching the anterior superior iliac spine (Fig. 155).

The bones and joints of the lower limb

The os innominatum (os coxae, hip bone)

See 'the pelvis', pages 129–133.

The femur (Figs 156, 157)

The femur is the longest and strongest bone in the body. It is 45 cm (18 in) in length.

The femoral *head* is two-thirds of a sphere and faces upwards, medially and forwards. It is covered with articular hyaline cartilage except for its central *fovea*, where the ligamentum teres is attached.

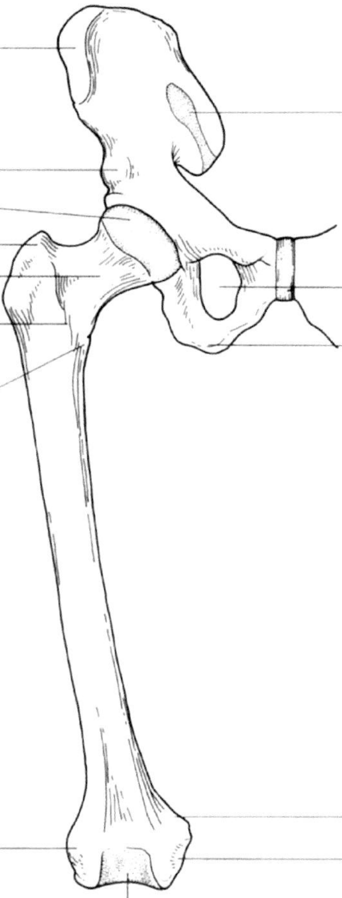

Fig. 156 The anterior aspect of the right femur.

The *neck* is 5 cm (2 in) long and is set at an angle of 135° to the shaft. In the female, with her wider pelvis, the angle is smaller.

The junction between the neck and the shaft is marked anteriorly by the *trochanteric line*, laterally by the *greater trochanter*, medially and somewhat posteriorly by the *lesser trochanter* and posteriorly by the prominent *trochanteric crest*, which extends from the lesser trochanter to the greater trochanter.

The blood supply to the femoral head is derived from vessels travelling up from the diaphysis along the cancellous bone, from vessels in the capsule of the hip joint, where this is reflected onto the neck in longitudinal bands or retinacula, and from the artery in the ligamentum teres; this third source is negligible in adults, but of great importance in children, when the femoral head is separated from the neck by the cartilage of the epiphyseal line (Fig. 158).

The femoral *shaft* is roughly circular in section at its middle but is flattened posteriorly at each extremity. Posteriorly the shaft is characterized by a prominent crest, the

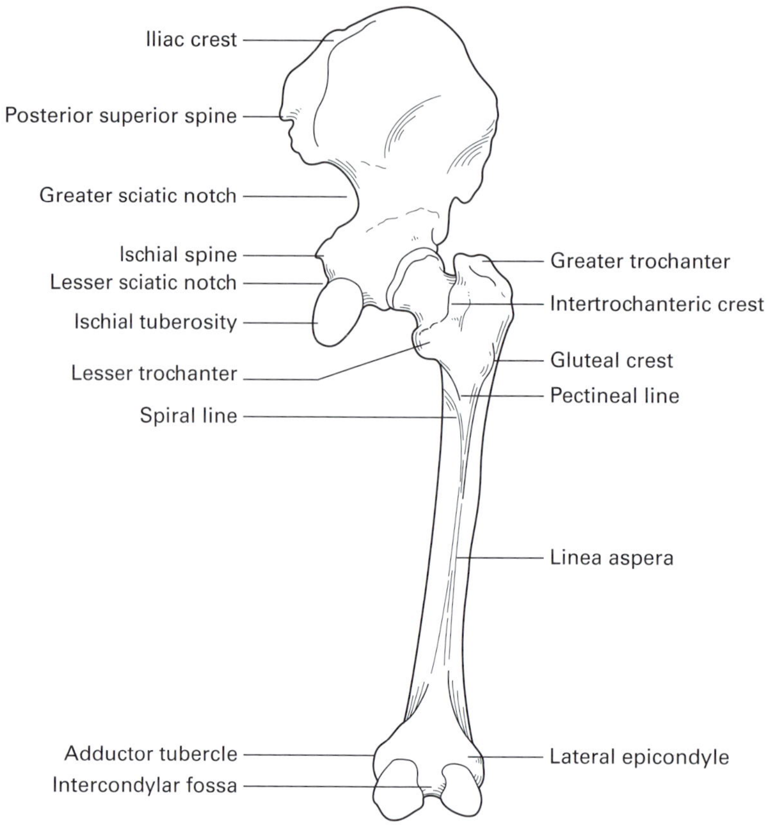

Fig. 157 The posterior aspect of the right femur.

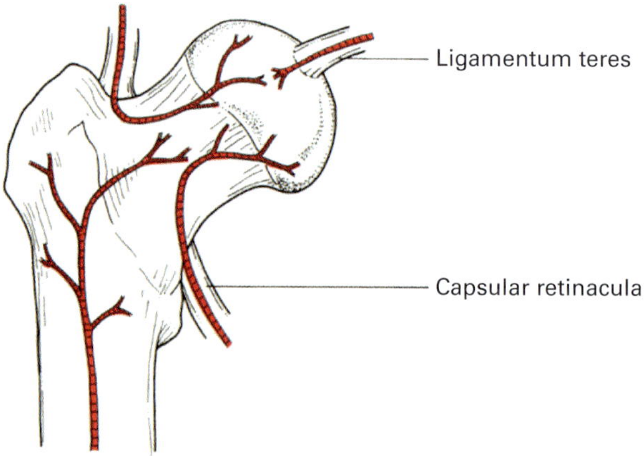

Fig. 158 The sources of blood supply to the femoral head – along the ligamentum teres, through the diaphysis and via the retinacula.

linea aspera. Inferiorly, this crest splits into the medial and lateral *supracondylar lines (ridges)*, leaving a flat *popliteal surface* between them. The medial supracondylar line (ridge) ends distally at the *adductor tubercle*.

The lower end of the femur bears the prominent *condyles*, which are separated by a deep *intercondylar notch* (fossa) posteriorly but which blend anteriorly to form an articular surface for the patella. Viewed from the front, the lateral condyle is the more prominent of the two and is seen to project further forwards than the medial condyle. This feature allows the lateral femoral condyle to resist the tendency for the patella to be displaced laterally when the quadriceps contracts.

CLINICAL FEATURES

1 The upper end of the femur is a common site for fracture in the elderly. The neck may break immediately beneath the head (*subcapital*), near its midpoint (*midcervical*) or adjacent to the trochanters (*basicervical*), or the fracture line may pass between, along or just below the trochanters (Fig. 159).

Fractures of the femoral neck will interrupt completely the blood supply from the diaphysis and, should the retinacula also be torn, avascular necrosis of the femoral head is very likely to ensue. The nearer the fracture to the femoral head, the more tenuous the retinacular blood supply and the more likely it is to be disrupted.

Avascular necrosis of the femoral head in children is seen in Perthes disease and in severe slipped femoral epiphysis, both situations resulting from thrombosis of the artery of the ligamentum teres.

In contrast, pertrochanteric fractures, being outside the joint capsule, leave the retinacula undisturbed; avascular necrosis, therefore, does not follow such injuries (Fig. 160).

There is a curious age pattern of hip injuries: children may sustain greenstick fractures of the femoral neck; schoolboys may displace the epiphysis of the femoral head; in adult life the hip dislocates; in old age fracture of the neck of the femur again becomes the usual lesion.

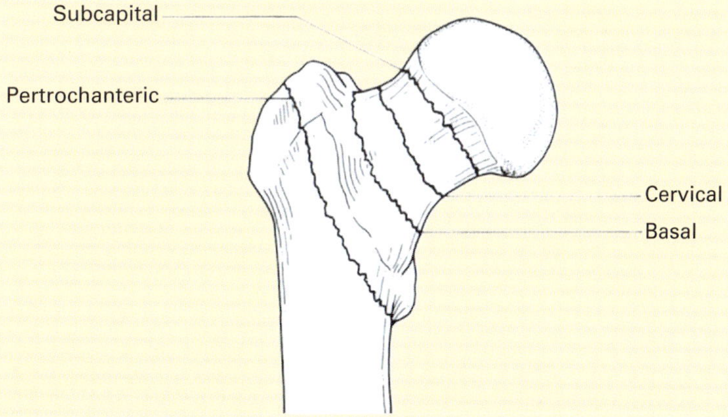

Fig. 159 The head and neck of the femur, showing the terminology of the common fracture sites.

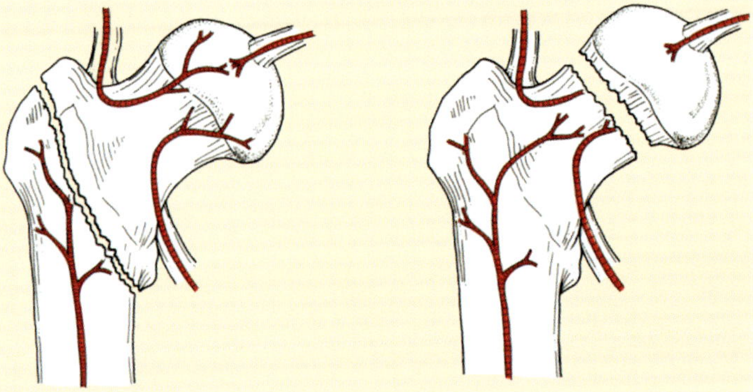

Fig. 160 (a) A pertrochanteric fracture does not damage the retinacular blood supply – aseptic bone necrosis does not occur. (b) A subcapital fracture cuts off most of the retinacular supply to the head – aseptic bone necrosis is common. Note that the blood supply via the ligamentum teres is negligible in adult life.

2 Fractures of the femoral shaft are accompanied by considerable shortening as a result of the longitudinal contraction of the extremely strong surrounding muscles.

The proximal segment is flexed by iliacus and psoas and abducted by gluteus medius and minimus, whereas the distal segment is pulled medially by the adductor muscles. Reduction requires powerful traction, to overcome the shortening, and then manipulation of the distal fragment into line with the proximal segment; the limb must therefore be abducted and also pushed forwards by using a large pad behind the knee.

Fractures of the lower end of the shaft, immediately above the condyles, are relatively rare; fortunately so, because they can be extremely difficult to treat since the small distal fragment is tilted backwards by gastrocnemius, the only muscle which is attached to it. The sharp proximal edge of this distal fragment may also tear the popliteal artery, which lies directly behind it (Fig. 161).

3 The angle subtended by the femoral neck to the shaft may be decreased, producing a *coxa vara* deformity. This may result from adduction fractures, slipped femoral epiphysis or bone-softening diseases. *Coxa valga*, in which the angle is increased, is much rarer but occurs in impacted abduction fractures. Note, however, that in children the normal angle between the neck and shaft is approximately 160°.

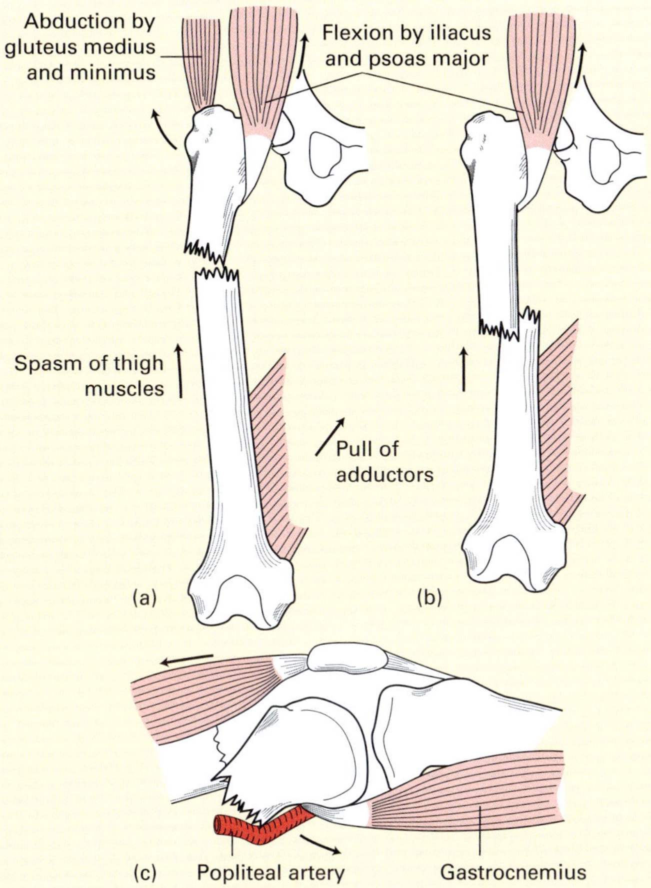

Fig. 161 The deformities of femoral shaft fractures. (a) Fracture of the proximal shaft – the proximal fragment is flexed by iliacus and psoas and abducted by gluteus medius and minimus. (b) Fracture of the mid-shaft – flexion of the proximal fragment by iliacus and psoas. (c) Fracture of the distal shaft – the distal fragment is angulated backwards by gastrocnemius; the popliteal artery may be torn in this injury. (In all these fractures overriding of the bone ends is produced by muscle spasm.)

The patella

The patella is a sesamoid bone, the largest such bone in the body. It is located in the expansion of the quadriceps tendon. The tendon continues from the apex of the bone as the ligamentum patellae (termed 'patellar tendon' by orthopaedic surgeons).

The posterior surface of the patella is covered with cartilage and articulates with the two femoral condyles by means of a larger lateral and smaller medial facet.

Occasionally the patella is *bipartite,* with a small, separate superolateral portion. Usually this anomaly is bilateral. This radiological feature may be mistaken by the inexperienced observer as a fracture.

CLINICAL FEATURES

1 Lateral dislocation of the patella is resisted by the prominent, anteriorly projecting articular surface of the lateral femoral condyle and by the medial pull of the lowermost fibres of vastus medialis, which insert almost horizontally along the medial margin of the patella. If the lateral condyle of the femur is underdeveloped or if there is a considerable *genu valgum* (knock-knee deformity), recurrent dislocations of the patella may occur (Fig. 162).

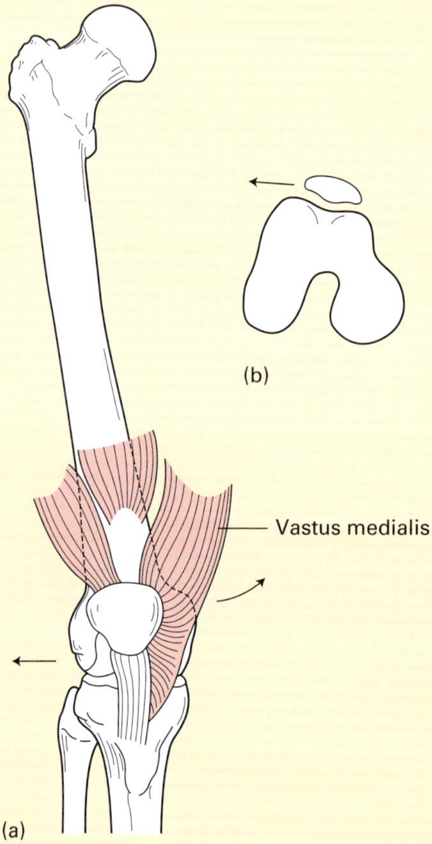

Fig. 162 Factors in the stability of the patella: (a) the medial pull of vastus medialis and (b) the high patellar articular surface and ventral projection of the lateral femoral condyle. These resist the tendency for lateral displacement of the patella, which results from the valgus angulation between the femur and the tibia.

2 A direct blow on the patella may split or shatter it, but the fragments are not avulsed because the quadriceps expansion remains intact.

The patella may also be fractured transversely by a sudden and excessively forceful contraction of the quadriceps – for example, in trying to stop a backwards fall. In this case, the tear extends outwards into the quadriceps expansion, allowing the upper bone fragment to be pulled proximally; there may be a gap of over 5 cm (2 in) between the bone ends. Reduction is impossible by closed manipulation, and operative repair of the extensor expansion is imperative.

Occasionally, this same mechanism of sudden forcible quadriceps contraction tears the quadriceps expansion above the patella, ruptures the ligamentum patellae or avulses the tibial tubercle.

It is interesting that, following complete excision of the patella for a comminuted fracture, knee function and movement may return to near-100% efficiency; it is difficult, then, to ascribe any particular function to this bone other than protection of the soft tissues of the knee joint anteriorly.

The tibia (Fig. 163)

The upper end of the tibia is expanded into the *medial* and *lateral condyles*, the former having the greater surface area of the two. Between the condyles on the upper surface of the tibia (tibial plateau) is the *intercondylar area*, which bears, at its waist, the *intercondylar eminence*, projecting upwards slightly on either side as the *medial* and *lateral intercondylar tubercles*.

The *tuberosity* of the tibia is at the upper end of the anterior border of the shaft and gives attachment to the ligamentum patellae.

The anterior aspect of this tuberosity is subcutaneous, only excepting the infrapatellar bursa immediately in front of it.

The shaft of the tibia is triangular in cross section, its anterior border and anteromedial surface being subcutaneous throughout their whole extent. The subcutaneous surface is crossed only by the easily visible *great saphenous vein*, accompanied by the *saphenous nerve*, immediately in front of the medial malleolus (Fig. 152).

The posterior surface of the shaft bears a prominent oblique line at its upper end termed the *soleal line*, which not only marks the tibial origin of the soleus but also delimits an area above, into which is inserted the popliteus.

The lower end of the tibia is expanded and quadrilateral in section, bearing an additional surface, the *fibular notch*, for the lower tibiofibular joint.

The *medial malleolus* projects from the medial extremity of the bone and is grooved posteriorly by the tendon of tibialis posterior.

The inferior surface of the lower end of the tibia is smooth, cartilage-covered and forms, with the malleoli, the upper articular surface of the ankle (talocrural) joint.

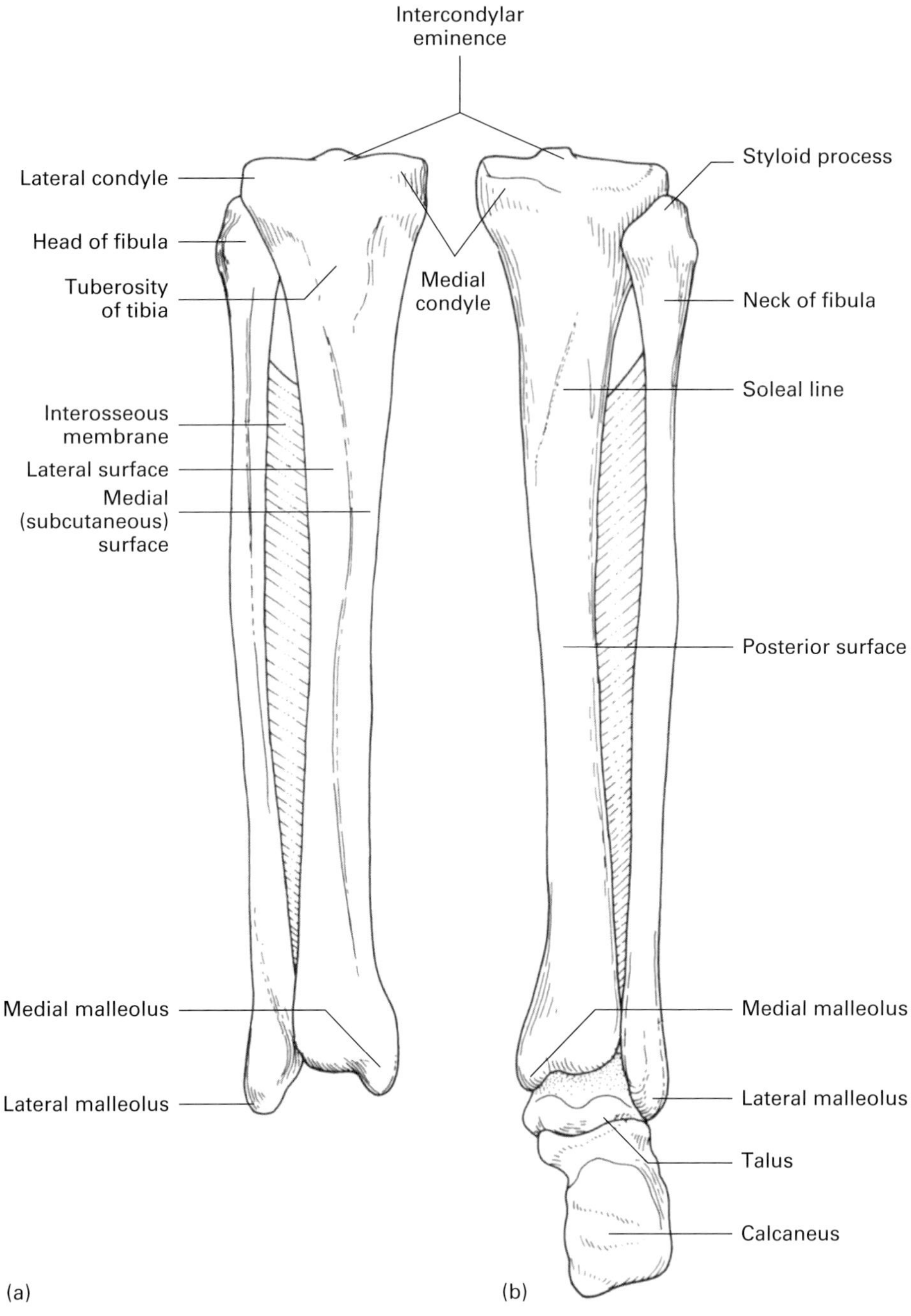

Fig. 163 The tibia and fibula of the right side. (a) Anterior aspect. (b) Posterior aspect.

CLINICAL FEATURES

1 The upper end of the tibial shaft is one of the more common sites for acute osteomyelitis. Fortunately, the capsule of the knee joint is attached closely around the articular surfaces so that the upper extremity of the tibial diaphysis is extracapsular; involvement of the knee joint therefore occurs only in the late and neglected case.
2 The medial surface of the shaft of the tibia is subcutaneous throughout its length and unprotected by muscle. Also it is particularly slender in its lower third. It is not surprising that tibial fractures are common injuries, as are compound tibial fractures.
3 The extensive subcutaneous surface of the tibia makes it a readily accessible donor site for bone grafts.

The fibula (Fig. 163)

The fibula serves three important functions:
1 It gives origin to several muscles.
2 It forms part of the ankle (talocrural) joint.
3 It serves as a pulley for the tendons of peroneus longus and brevis.

From its proximal to distal end, the fibula comprises a *head* with a *styloid process*, *neck* (around which passes the common peroneal nerve; Fig. 153), *shaft* and *lateral malleolus*. The head of the fibula receives the attachments of the lateral collateral ligament of the knee joint, the arcuate popliteal ligament and the tendon of biceps femoris. The distal end of the shaft just proximal to the lateral malleolus bears a roughened surface on its medial aspect for the inferior tibiofibular joint, below which is the articular facet for the talus. A groove on the posterior aspect of the lateral malleolus lodges the tendons of peroneus longus and brevis (brevis anterior to longus).

A note on growing ends and nutrient foramina in the long bones

The shaft of every long bone bears one or more *nutrient foramina,* which are obliquely placed; this obliquity is the result of unequal growth at the upper and lower epiphyses. The artery is obviously dragged in the direction of more rapid growth, and the direction of slope of entry of the nutrient foramen therefore points *away* from the more rapid growing end of the bone.

Growth of the long bones of the lower limb takes place principally at the epiphyses at the lower end of the femur and at the upper end of the tibia. This is in contrast to the upper limb where bone growth occurs mainly at the upper end of the humerus and at the lower ends of the radius and ulna.

The site of the growing end is of considerable practical significance; for example, if a child has to undergo an above-elbow amputation, the humeral upper epiphyseal line continues to grow and the elongating bone may well push its way through the stump end, requiring reamputation.

The bones of the foot

These are best considered as a functional unit and are therefore dealt with together under 'the arches of the foot' (see pages 249–251).

The hip joint (Figs 164, 165)

The hip joint is the largest synovial joint in the body.

It is a perfect example of a ball-and-socket joint (or multi-axial spheroidal joint). Its articular surfaces are the femoral head and the horseshoe-shaped articular surface of the acetabulum, which is deepened by the fibrocartilaginous *labrum acetabular* attached to the outer rim of the acetabulum. The non-articular lower part of the acetabulum, the *acetabular notch*, is closed off below by the *transverse acetabular ligament*. The ligamentum teres arises from the latter and passes to its attachment at the fovea on the femoral head.

The *capsule* of the hip joint is attached proximally to the margins of the acetabulum and to the transverse acetabular ligament. Distally, it is attached along the trochanteric line, the bases of the greater and lesser trochanters and, posteriorly, to the femoral neck approximately 1.25 cm (0.5 in) medial to the trochanteric crest. From this distal attachment, capsular fibres are reflected onto the femoral neck as *retinacula* and provide one pathway for the blood supply to the femoral head (see 'The femur', Fig. 158).

Note that acute osteomyelitis of the upper femoral metaphysis will involve the neck, which is intracapsular and which will therefore rapidly produce a secondary pyogenic arthritis of the hip joint.

Three ligaments reinforce the capsule:

1 the *iliofemoral* (Y-shaped ligament of Bigelow) – which arises from the anterior inferior iliac spine, bifurcates and is inserted at each end of the trochanteric line (Fig. 165);
2 the *pubofemoral* – arising from the iliopubic junction to blend with the inferomedial aspect of the capsule;
3 the *ischiofemoral* – arising from the ischium to be inserted into the posterior aspect of the capsule and to the base of the greater trochanter.

Of these, the iliofemoral is by far the strongest and resists hyperextension strains on the hip. In posterior dislocation it usually remains intact.

The *synovium* of the hip joint lines the inner surface of the capsule, covers the non-articular surfaces of the joint and occasionally bulges out anteriorly to form a bursa beneath the psoas tendon where the latter crosses the front of the joint.

Movements

The hip (a ball-and-socket joint) is capable of a wide range of movements – flexion, extension, abduction, adduction, medial and lateral rotation and circumduction.

The principal muscles acting on the joint are:

- flexors – iliacus and psoas major assisted by rectus femoris, sartorius and pectineus;
- extensors – gluteus maximus and the hamstrings;
- adductors – adductor longus, brevis and magnus assisted by gracilis and pectineus;
- abductors – gluteus medius and minimus and tensor fasciae latae;

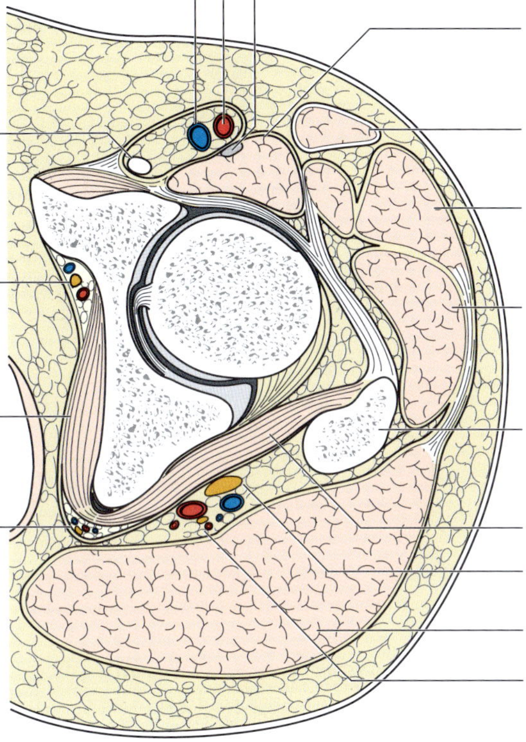

(a)

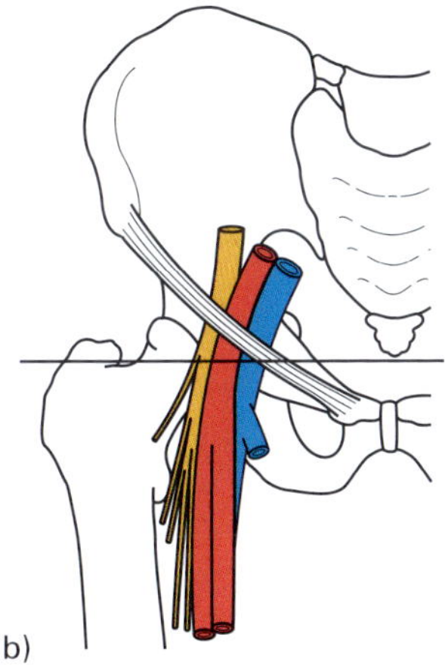

(b)

Fig. 164 (a) The immediate relations of the hip joint (in diagrammatic horizontal section; right hip, viewed from proximal aspect). (b) Scout diagram indicating the level of the section.

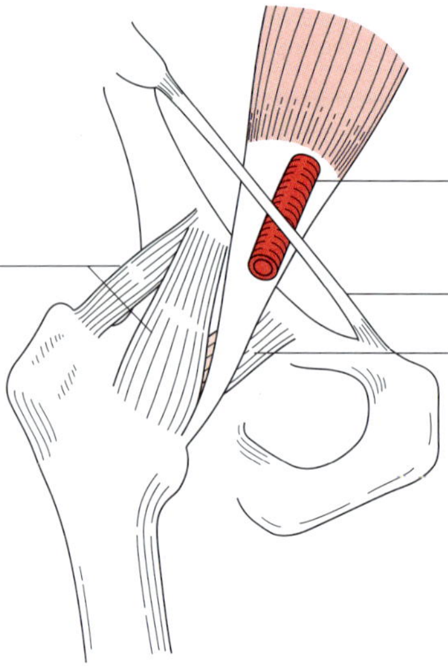

Fig. 165 The anterior aspect of the right hip. Note that the psoas tendon and the femoral artery are intimate anterior relations of the joint.

- lateral rotators – principally gluteus maximus assisted by the obturators, gemelli and quadratus femoris;
- medial rotators – tensor fasciae latae and anterior fibres of gluteus medius and minimus. Medial rotation is therefore a much weaker movement than lateral rotation.

The body is an amazingly economical machine. Walk across the room with your hand on one buttock – gluteus maximus does not contract in quiet walking and extension of the hip is carried out entirely by the hamstrings. Now, forcibly extend your hip and feel your gluteus maximus on that side being called into action in vigorous extension of the hip joint.

Relations (Fig. 164)

The hip joint is surrounded by muscles:
- anteriorly – iliacus, psoas major and pectineus, together with the femoral artery, vein and nerve;
- laterally – tensor fasciae latae and gluteus medius and minimus;
- posteriorly – the tendons of piriformis, obturator internus with the gemelli, quadratus femoris, the sciatic nerve and, more superficially, gluteus maximus;
- superiorly – the reflected head of rectus femoris lying in contact with the joint capsule;
- inferiorly – the obturator externus, passing back to be inserted into the trochanteric fossa.

Surgical exposure of the hip joint therefore inevitably involves considerable and deep dissection.

The *lateral approach* comprises splitting down through the thick fascia behind the tensor fasciae latae and then through the proximal part of vastus lateralis. On a deeper plane gluteus medius and minimus are incised longitudinally to reach the femoral neck. Further access may be obtained by detaching the greater trochanter with the gluteal insertions.

The *anterior approach* passes between sartorius medially and tensor fasciae latae laterally and, on a deeper plane, between the rectus femoris medially and the glutei medius and minimus laterally. The reflected head of rectus femoris is then divided to expose the anterior aspect of the hip joint. More room may be obtained by detaching these glutei from the external aspect of the ilium.

The *posterior approach* is through an angled incision commencing at the posterior superior iliac spine, passing to the greater trochanter and then dropping vertically downwards from this point. Gluteus maximus is split in the line of its fibres and then incised along its tendinous insertion. Deep to gluteus maximus, the short lateral rotators are divided a few centimetres medial to their attachments on the greater trochanter. The medial stumps of the divided short lateral rotators are retracted medially to protect the sciatic nerve. An excellent view of the posterior aspect of the hip joint is thus obtained.

Nerve supply

Hilton's law states that the nerves crossing a joint supply the muscles acting on it, the skin over the joint and the joint itself. The hip is no exception and receives fibres from the femoral, sciatic and obturator nerves. It is important to note that these nerves also supply the knee joint, and, for this reason, it is not uncommon for a patient, particularly a child, to complain bitterly of pain in the knee and for the real cause of the mischief, the diseased hip, to be overlooked.

CLINICAL FEATURES

Trendelenburg test

The stability of the hip in the standing position depends on two factors: the strength of the surrounding muscles and the integrity of the lever system of the femoral neck and head within the intact hip joint. When standing on one leg, the abductors of the hip on this side (gluteus medius and minimus and tensor fasciae latae) come into powerful action to maintain fixation at the hip joint, so much so that the pelvis actually rises slightly on the opposite side. If, however, there is any defect in these muscles or lever mechanism of the hip joint, the weight of the body in these circumstances forces the pelvis to tilt downwards on the opposite (unsupported) side.

This positive Trendelenburg test is seen if the hip abductors are paralysed (e.g. poliomyelitis), if there is an old unreduced or congenital dislocation of the hip, if the head of the femur has been destroyed by disease or removed operatively (pseudarthrosis), if there is an un-united fracture of the femoral neck or if there is a very severe degree of coxa vara.

The test may be said to indicate 'a defect in the osseomuscular stability of the hip joint'.

A patient with any of the conditions enumerated above walks with a characteristic 'dipping gait'.

Dislocation of the hip (Fig. 166)

The hip is usually dislocated backwards, and this is produced by a force applied along the femoral shaft with the hip in the flexed position (e.g. the knee striking against the opposite seat when a train runs into the buffers or in a head-on car collision when the knee hits the dashboard of the car). If the hip is also in the adducted position, the head of the femur is less well accommodated in the acetabulum and dislocation can occur without an associated acetabular fracture. If the hip is abducted, for dislocation to occur, there must be an associated fracture of the posterior acetabular lip.

The sciatic nerve, a close posterior relation of the hip joint, is in danger of damage in these injuries, as will be appreciated by a glance at Fig. 154.

Reduction of a dislocated hip is quite simple providing that a deep anaesthetic is administered to relax the surrounding muscles; the hip is flexed, rotated into the neutral position and lifted back into the acetabulum. Occasionally, forcible abduction

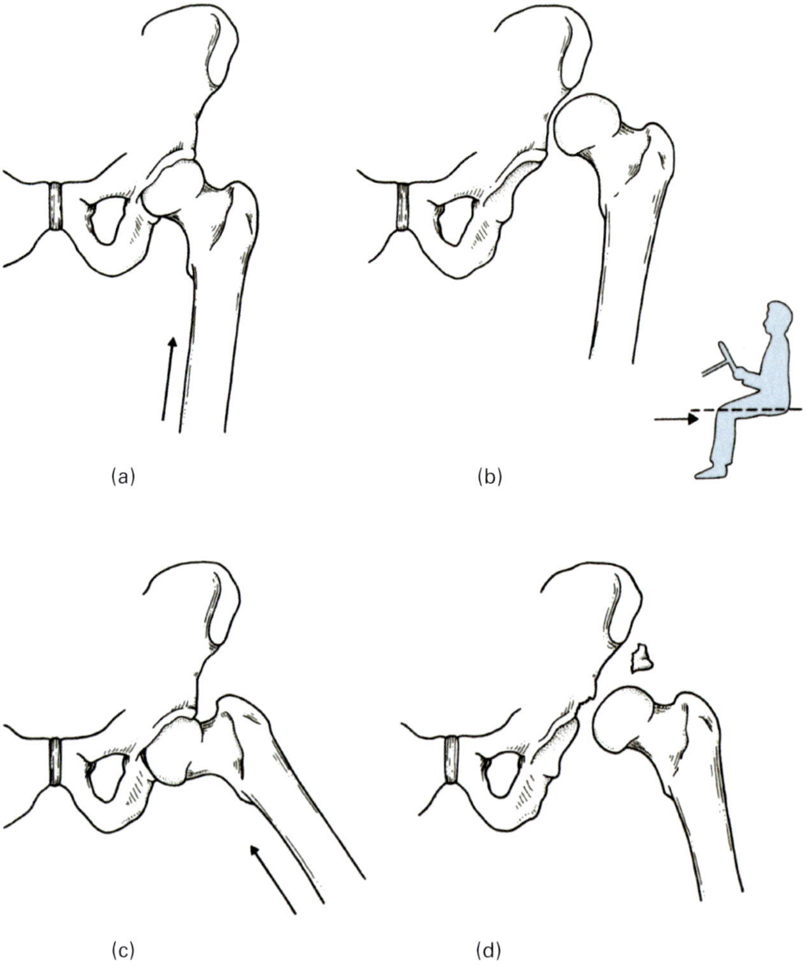

Fig. 166 Dislocation of the hip. If the hip is forced into posterior dislocation while adducted (a), there is no associated fracture of the posterior acetabular lip (b). Dislocation in the abducted position (c) can occur only with a concomitant acetabular fracture (d). (The inset figure indicates the plane of these diagrams.)

of the hip will dislocate the hip forwards. Excessive force along the shaft (e.g. resulting from a fall from a height) may thrust the femoral head through the floor of the acetabulum, producing a central dislocation of the hip.

The knee joint (Figs 167, 168)

The knee is a hinge joint made up of the articulations between the femoral and tibial condyles and between the patella and the patellar surface of the femur.

The *capsule* is attached to the margins of these articular surfaces but communicates above with the *suprapatellar bursa* (between the lower femoral shaft and the quadriceps), posteriorly with the bursa under the medial head of gastrocnemius and often, through it, with the bursa under semimembranosus. It may also communicate with the bursa under the lateral head of gastrocnemius. The capsule is also perforated posterolaterally by the tendon of popliteus, which emerges from it in much the same way that the tendon of the long head of biceps emerges from within the shoulder joint capsule.

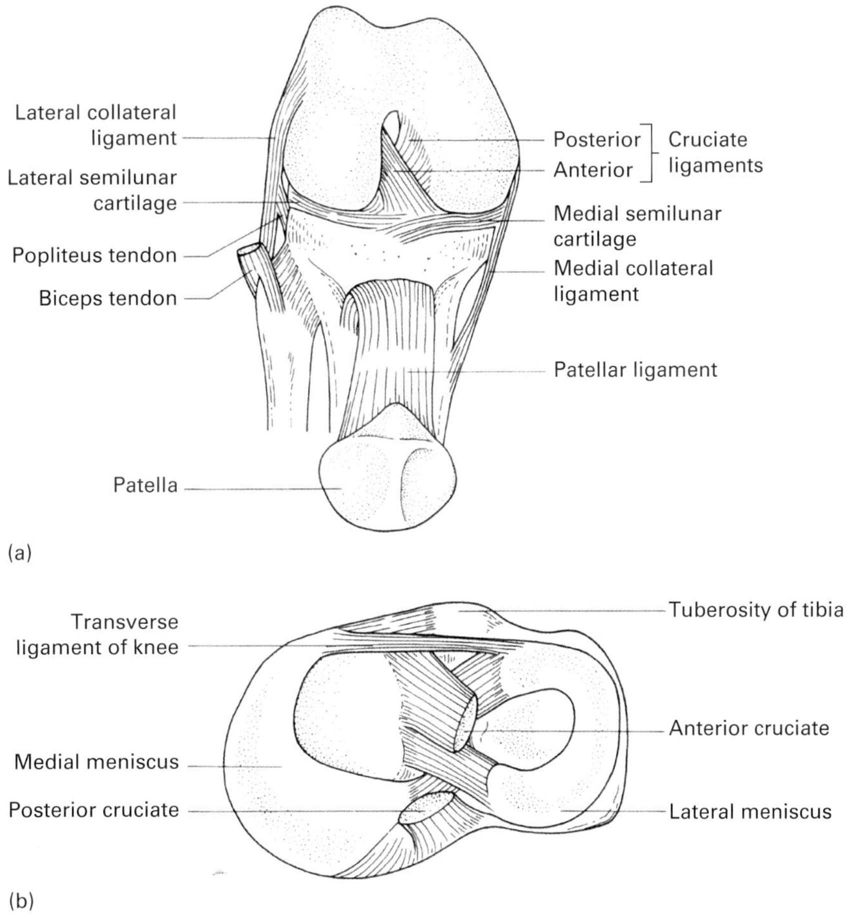

Fig. 167 (a) The right knee – anterior view; the knee is flexed and the patella has been turned downwards. (b) The right knee in transverse section.

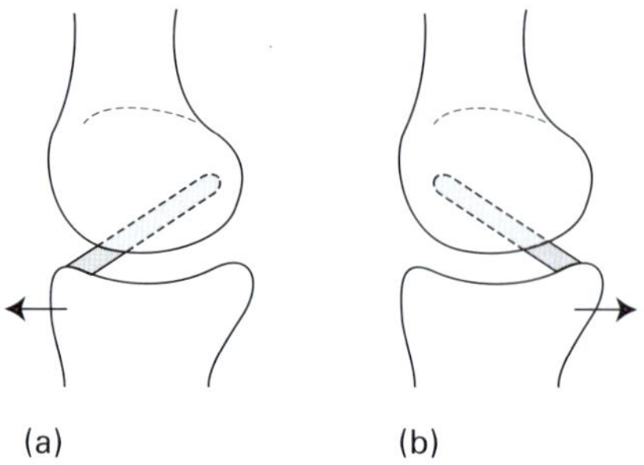

(a) Anterior cruciate ligament – resists forward movement of tibia on femur

(b) Posterior cruciate ligament – resists backward movement of tibia on femur

Fig. 168 The actions of the cruciate ligaments.

The capsule of the knee joint is reinforced on each side by the *medial* and *lateral collateral ligaments*, the latter passing to the head of the fibula and lying free from the capsule. The medial collateral ligament is in two parts: the superficial component extends from the medial epicondyle of the femur to the medial surface of the tibial shaft under cover of the tendons of sartorius, gracilis and semitendinosus. The deep component blends with the medial aspect of the capsule of the knee joint and with the medial edge of the medial meniscus.

Anteriorly, the capsule is considerably strengthened by the *ligamentum patellae*, and, on each side of the patella, by the *medial* and *lateral patellar retinacula*, which are expansions from vastus medialis and lateralis, respectively.

Posteriorly, the tough *oblique popliteal ligament* (of Winslow) arises as an expansion from the insertion of semimembranosus and blends with the joint capsule.

CLINICAL FEATURES

The suprapatellar bursa between the lower femoral shaft and the quadriceps facilitates the contraction of quadriceps in extension of the knee. The bursa extends a hand's breadth above the upper rim of the patella. In injuries of the knee, when there is an effusion of blood (haemarthrosis) or a serous effusion, the diagnosis is easily made by inspection, as on the affected side there is an obvious bulge superior to the patella.

Internal structures (Figs 167, 168)

Within the joint are a number of important structures.

The *cruciate ligaments* are extremely strong connections between the tibia and femur. They arise from the anterior and posterior intercondylar areas of the superior aspect of the tibia, taking their names from their tibial origins, and pass obliquely upwards to attach to the intercondylar notch of the femur.

The anterior cruciate ligament resists forward displacement of the tibia on the femur and becomes taut in hyperextension of the knee; it also resists rotation. The posterior cruciate ligament resists backward displacement of the tibia and becomes taut in hyperflexion.

The menisci (formerly known as *semilunar cartilages*) are crescent-shaped fibrocartilaginous structures that are wedge-shaped in vertical section. The medial meniscus is longer and less curved than the lateral meniscus. They are attached by their extremities to the tibial intercondylar area and by their periphery to the capsule of the joint, although the lateral meniscus is less firmly adherent to the capsule; furthermore the popliteus tendon intervenes between the lateral meniscus and the lateral collateral ligament.

The menisci serve to deepen and widen, the articular area on the tibial plateau available to the femoral condyles and act as effective shock absorbers. If both menisci are removed, the knee can regain satisfactory functional efficiency, although at the cost of a predisposition to premature osteoarthritic degenerative changes.

An *infrapatellar pad of fat* fills the space between the ligamentum patellae and the femoral intercondylar notch. The synovium covering this pad projects into the joint as twofolds termed the *alar folds*.

Movements of the knee

The principal knee movements are flexion and extension, but note on yourself that some degree of rotation of the knee is possible when this joint is in the flexed position. In full extension, i.e. in the standing position, the knee is quite rigid because the medial condyle of the tibia, being rather larger than the lateral condyle, rides forwards on the medial femoral condyle, thus 'screwing' the joint firmly together. The first step in flexion of the fully extended knee is 'unscrewing' or internal rotation. This is brought about by *popliteus*, which arises from the lateral side of the lateral condyle of the femur, emerges from the joint capsule posteriorly and is inserted into the back of the upper end of the tibia.

The principal muscles acting on the knee are:

- extensor – quadriceps femoris;
- flexors – hamstrings assisted by gracilis, gastrocnemius and sartorius;
- medial rotator – popliteus ('unscrews the knee').

CLINICAL FEATURES

1 The stability of the knee depends upon the strength of its surrounding muscles and the integrity of its ligaments. Of the two, the muscles are by far the more important. Providing quadriceps femoris is powerfully developed, the knee will function satisfactorily even in the face of considerable ligamentous damage. Conversely, the most skilful surgical repair of torn ligaments is doomed to failure unless the muscles are functioning strongly; without their support, reconstructed ligaments will merely stretch once more.

2 When considering soft-tissue injuries of the knee joint, think of the three Cs that may be damaged – the collateral ligaments, the cruciates and the cartilages (i.e. menisci).

The *collateral ligaments* are taut in full extension of the knee and are, therefore, liable to injury only in this position. The medial ligament may be partly or completely torn when a violent abduction strain is applied, whereas an adduction force may damage the lateral ligament. If one or other collateral ligament is completely torn, the extended knee can be rocked away from the affected side.

The *cruciate ligaments* may both be torn (along with the collateral ligaments) in severe abduction or adduction injuries. The anterior cruciate, which is taut in extension, may be torn by forceful hyperextension of the knee or in anterior dislocation of the tibia on the femur. Since it resists rotation, it may also be torn in a violent twisting injury to the knee. The posterior cruciate tears in a posterior dislocation (Fig. 168).

If both the cruciate ligaments are torn, unnatural anteroposterior mobility of the knee can be demonstrated.

If there is only increased forward mobility, the anterior cruciate ligament has been divided or is lax. Increased backward mobility implies a rupture or laxity of the posterior cruciate.

The menisci (*semilunar cartilage*) can tear only when the knee is flexed and is thus able to rotate. If you place a finger on either side of the ligamentum patellae on the joint line and then rotate your flexed knee first internally and then externally, you will note how the lateral and medial menisci are respectively sucked into the knee joint. If the flexed knee is forcibly abducted and externally rotated, the medial meniscus will be drawn between, and then split by, the grinding surfaces of the medial condyles of the femur and tibia. This occurs when a footballer twists his/her flexed knee while running. A severe adduction and internal rotation strain may similarly tear the lateral meniscus, but this injury is less common.

The knee 'locks' in this type of injury because the torn and displaced segment of meniscus lodges between the condyles and prevents full extension of the knee.

The tibiofibular joints

The tibia and fibula are connected by:

1 the *superior tibiofibular joint*, which is a synovial joint between the head of the fibula and the lateral condyle of the tibia;
2 the *interosseous membrane*, which is crossed by the anterior tibial vessels above and pierced by the perforating branch of the peroneal artery below;
3 the *inferior tibiofibular joint*, which is a fibrous joint between the triangular areas of each bone immediately above the ankle joint. It represents, in fact, the reinforced distal end of the fibrous tissue of the tibiofibular interosseous membrane.

The ankle joint (Fig. 169)

The ankle joint (talocrural joint) is a hinge joint between a mortice formed by the malleoli and lower end of the tibia and the body of the talus.

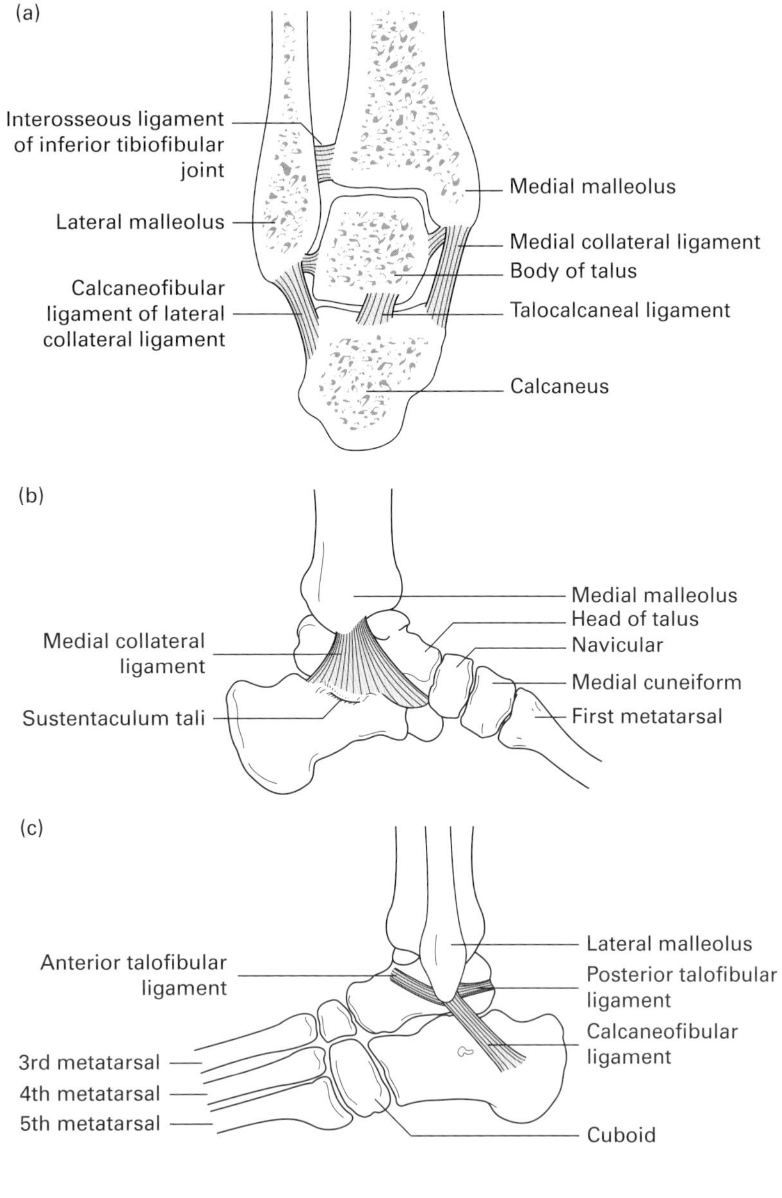

Fig. 169 The left ankle. (a) In coronal section (viewed from behind). (b) Medial aspect. (c) Lateral aspect.

The *capsule* of the joint fits closely around its articular surfaces, and, as in every hinge joint, it is lax anteriorly and posteriorly but reinforced laterally and medially by *collateral ligaments*.

The *medial collateral ligament* (or deltoid ligament) is the stronger of the two. It radiates from its attachment at the tip of the medial malleolus to attach, from before backwards, to the tuberosity of the navicular, the spring ligament, the sustentaculum tali and the medial tuberosity of the talus (Fig. 169b). The *lateral collateral ligament* is a complex of three bands (or ligaments) which radiate from the fibular malleolus. These are the anterior talofibular band, running forwards to the neck of the talus, the calcaneofibular band, passing downwards and backwards to the lateral surface of the calcaneus, and the posterior talofibular band, passing backwards and medially to the talus (Fig. 169c). At first glance, the direction of the anterior talofibular ligament seems illogical! However, put your foot, or the bones of an articulated skeleton, into the plantarflexed position and invert it – you will note that in this position the ligament lies directly in the line of strain.

Movements of the ankle

The ankle joint is a hinge joint capable of being flexed and extended (plantar- and dorsiflexion).

The body of the talus is slightly wider anteriorly and, in full extension (i.e. dorsiflexion), becomes firmly wedged between the malleoli. Conversely, in flexion (i.e. plantarflexion), there is slight laxity at the joint and some degree of side-to-side tilting is possible: test this fact on yourself.

The principal muscles acting on the ankle are:

- dorsiflexors – Tibialis anterior assisted by extensor digitorum longus, extensor hallucis longus and peroneus tertius;
- plantarflexors – gastrocnemius and soleus assisted by tibialis posterior, flexor hallucis longus and flexor digitorum longus.

CLINICAL FEATURES

1 The collateral ligaments of the ankle can be sprained or completely torn by forcible abduction or adduction, the lateral ligament being far the more frequently affected. This is because, first, the medial collateral ligament is more powerful than the lateral and, second – and you can test this on yourself – you are more likely to twist your ankle into forcible inversion than eversion. The first part of the lateral collateral ligament to come under strain is the anterior talofibular ligament, and it is this strand that tears in partial rupture of the lateral ligament. If the ligament is completely disrupted the talus can be tilted in its mortice; this is difficult to demonstrate clinically and is best confirmed by taking an anteroposterior radiograph of the ankle while forcibly inverting the foot.

2 The most usual ankle fracture is that produced by an abduction–external rotation injury; the patient catches his foot in a rabbit hole, his body and his tibia internally rotate while the foot is rigidly held. First, there is a torsional spiral fracture of the lateral malleolus, then avulsion of the medial collateral ligament, with or without avulsion of a flake of the medial malleolus, and finally, as the tibia is carried forward, the posterior margin of the lower end of the tibia shears off against the talus. These stages are termed *1st, 2nd* and *3rd degree Pott's fractures*. Notice that, with widening of the joint, there is forward dislocation of the tibia on the talus, producing characteristic prominence of the heel in this injury.

The joints of the foot

The movements of *inversion* and *eversion* of the foot involve three articulations in the foot; the (subtalar) talocalcaneal joint, the (midtarsal) calcaneocuboid joint and the talocalcaneonavicular joint (a complex, single synovial articulation which is partly subtalar and partly midtarsal). Of these, the talocalcaneonavicular joint is by far the most important. Test this on yourself – immobilize your calcaneus between your finger and thumb; inversion and eversion of the foot are greatly restricted.

Loss of these rotatory movements of the foot, for example after injury or due to arthritis, results in quite severe disability because the foot cannot adapt itself to walking on uneven, rough or sloping ground.

Inversion is brought about by TA and TP assisted by the long extensor and flexor tendons of the hallux; eversion is the function of PL and brevis (assisted by peroneus tertius, which is a member of the extensor muscles).

The other tarsal joints allow slight gliding movements only and, individually, are not of clinical importance. The arrangement of the metatarsophalangeal and interphalangeal joints is on the same basic plan as in the upper limb.

The arches of the foot (Fig. 170)

On standing, the heel and the metatarsal heads are the principal weight-bearing points, but a moment's study of wet footprints on the bathroom floor will show that the lateral margin of the foot and the tips of the phalanges also touch the ground.

The bones of the foot are arranged in the form of two longitudinal arches. The *medial arch* comprises calcaneus, talus, navicular, the three cuneiforms and the three medial metatarsals; the apex of this arch is the talus. The *lateral arch*, which is lower, comprises the calcaneus, cuboid and the lateral two metatarsals; the apex of this arch is the cuboid.

The foot plays a double role; it functions as a rigid support for the weight of the body in the standing position and as a mobile springboard during walking and running.

When one stands, the arches sink somewhat under the body's weight, the individual bones lock together, the ligaments linking them are at maximum tension and the foot becomes an immobile pedestal. When one walks, the weight is released from the arches, which unlock and become a mobile lever system in the spring-like actions of locomotion.

The arches are maintained by:

1 the shape of the interlocking bones;
2 the ligaments of the foot;
3 muscle action.

The ligaments concerned are (Fig. 171):

1 the dorsal, plantar and interosseous ligaments between the small bones of the forefoot;
2 the *spring ligament*, which passes from the *sustentaculum tali* of the calcaneus forwards to the *tuberosity of the navicular* and which supports the inferior aspect of the head of the talus;

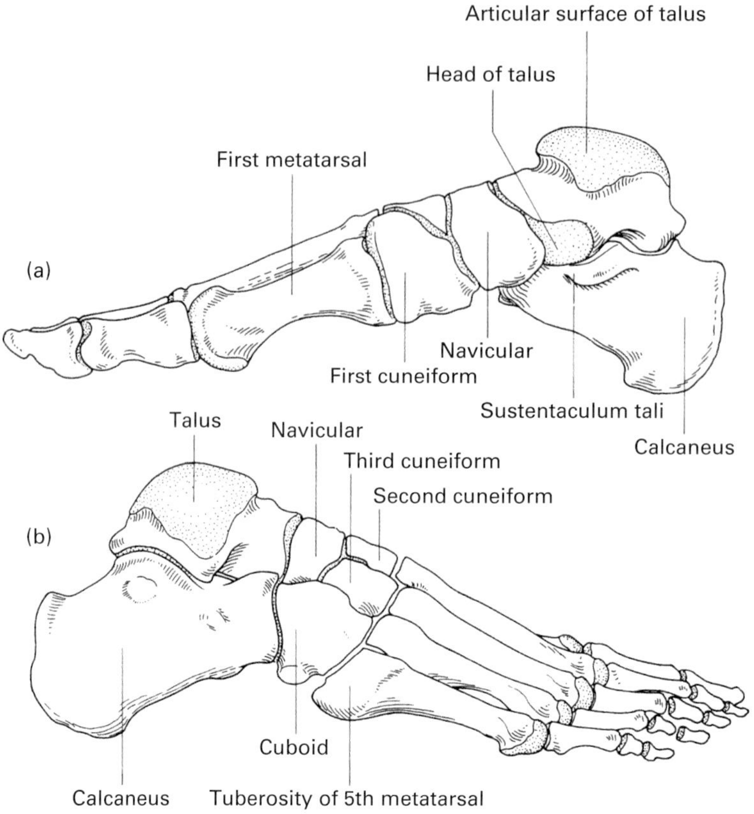

Fig. 170 The longitudinal arches of the right foot. (a) Medial view. (b) Lateral view.

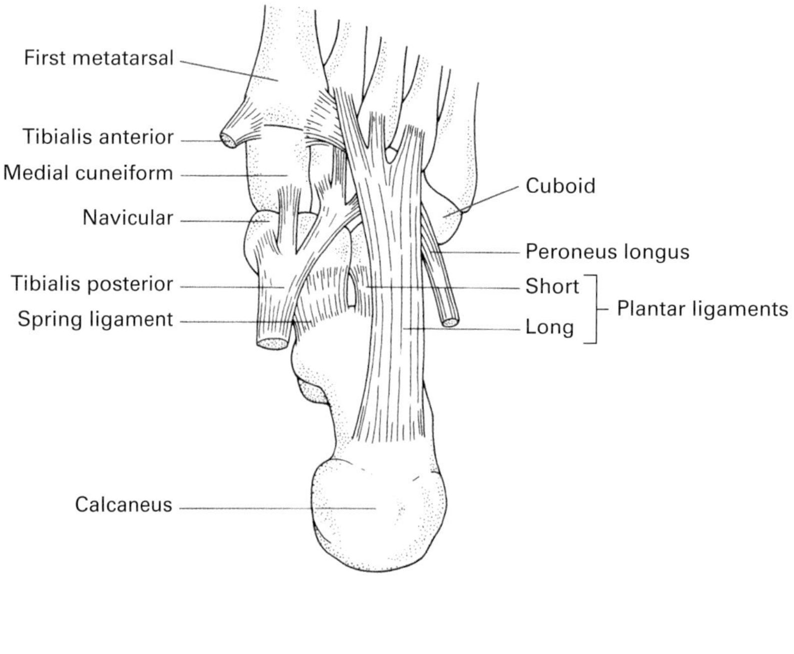

Fig. 171 Plantar aspect of the left foot to show the attachments of the important ligaments and long tendons. (The head of the talus is hidden, deep to the spring ligament.)

3 the *short plantar ligament*, which stretches from the plantar surface of the calcaneus to the cuboid;

4 the *long plantar ligament*, which arises from the posterior tuberosity on the plantar surface of the calcaneus, covers the short plantar ligament, forms a tunnel for the peroneus longus tendon with the cuboid and is inserted into the bases of the 2nd, 3rd and 4th metatarsals.

These ligaments are reinforced in their action by the *plantar aponeurosis*, which is the condensed deep fascia of the sole of the foot. This arises from the plantar aspect of the calcaneus and is attached to the deep transverse ligaments linking the heads of the metatarsals; it also continues forwards into each toe to blend with the fibrous flexor sheaths, in a similar arrangement to that of the palmar fascia of the hand. Indeed, like the palmar fascia, it may be subject to Dupuytren's contracture (page 209).

The principal muscles concerned in the mechanism of the arches of the foot are peroneus longus (aided by brevis and tertius), tibialis anterior and posterior, flexor hallucis longus and the intrinsic muscles of the foot.

Peroneus longus tendon passes obliquely across the sole in a groove on the undersurface of the cuboid bone and is inserted into the lateral side of the base of the 1st metatarsal and the medial cuneiform. Into the medial aspect of these two bones is inserted the tendon of *tibialis anterior* so that these muscles form, in effect, a stirrup between them that supports the arches of the foot.

The medial arch is further reinforced by flexor hallucis longus, whose tendon passes under the sustentaculum tali of the calcaneus, and by *tibialis posterior*, two-thirds of whose fibres are inserted into the tuberosity of the navicular and support the spring ligament.

The longitudinally running intrinsic muscles of the foot also act as ties to the longitudinal arches.

The anatomy of walking

In the process of walking, the heel is raised from the ground, the metatarsophalangeal joints flex to give a 'push-off' movement; the foot then leaves the ground completely and is dorsiflexed to clear the toes.

Just before the toes of one foot leave the ground, the heel of the other makes contact.

Forward progression is produced partly by the 'push-off' of the toes, partly by powerful plantarflexion of the ankle and partly by the forward swing of the hips accentuated by swinging movements of the pelvis. Paraplegics can be taught to walk purely by this pelvic swing action, even though paralysed from the waist downwards.

When one foot is off the ground, tilting of the pelvis to the unsupported side is prevented by the contralateral hip abductors (gluteus medius and minimus and tensor fasciae latae) contracting to steady the pelvis. Their paralysis is one cause of a 'dipping gait' and of a positive Trendelenburg sign (see page 241).

Three important zones of the lower limb: the femoral triangle, adductor canal and popliteal fossa

The femoral triangle (Fig. 172)

The femoral triangle is a triangular intermuscular space situated in the anteromedial aspect of the proximal thigh. It has the outline of an inverted triangle.

This triangle is bounded:

- superiorly – by the inguinal ligament (base of the femoral triangle);
- medially – by the medial border of adductor longus;
- laterally – by the medial border of sartorius.

Its *floor* is gutter-shaped and is made up, from lateral to medial, of iliacus, the tendon of psoas, pectineus and adductor longus.

The *roof* is formed by the deep fascia (fascia lata), which is pierced by the great saphenous vein at the saphenous opening. Overlying the deep fascial roof of the femoral triangle is the superficial fascia, containing the superficial inguinal lymph nodes embedded in subcutaneous fat, the great saphenous vein with its tributaries and the superficial branches of the femoral artery. The *apex* is the point where sartorius overlaps adductor longus.

The contents of the femoral triangle are the femoral nerve and its branches, femoral sheath (containing the femoral vessels and femoral canal) and lymph nodes.

Some of these structures may now be considered in greater detail.

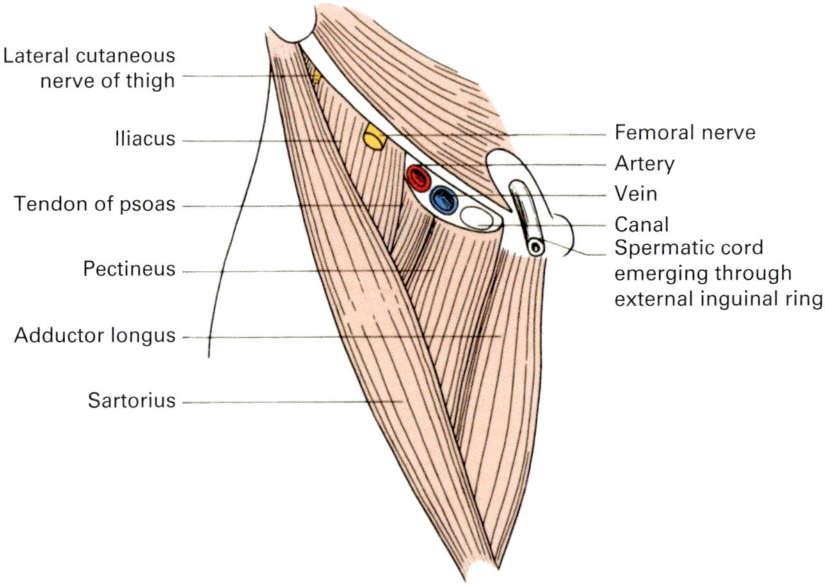

Fig. 172 The right femoral triangle and its contents.

The fascia lata

The deep fascia of the thigh, or fascia lata, extends downwards to ensheath the whole lower limb except over the subcutaneous surface of the tibia (to whose margins it adheres) and at the saphenous opening. Above, it is attached all around to the root of the lower limb – that is to say, to the inguinal ligament, pubis, ischium, sacrotuberous ligament, sacrum and coccyx and the iliac crest. The fascia of the thigh is particularly dense laterally (the *iliotibial tract*), where it receives tensor fasciae latae, and posteriorly, where the greater part of gluteus maximus is inserted into it. The iliotibial tract, when tensed by its attached muscles, assists in the stabilization of the hip and the extended knee when standing.

The fact that a considerable part of the largest muscle of the lower limb, gluteus maximus, inserts into it shows the importance of this tract. Note that when you stand for a long period of time, for example in the operating theatre, you shift from one leg to the other and maintain the leg you are standing on by tension of the iliotibial tract.

The tough lateral fascia of the thigh is an available source of material that can be used for hernial and dural repairs.

The femoral sheath and femoral canal (Fig. 173)

The femoral artery and vein enter the femoral triangle from beneath the inguinal ligament within a fascial sleeve termed the *femoral sheath*. The sheath is derived from the extraperitoneal intra-abdominal fascia. Its anterior wall arises from the transver-

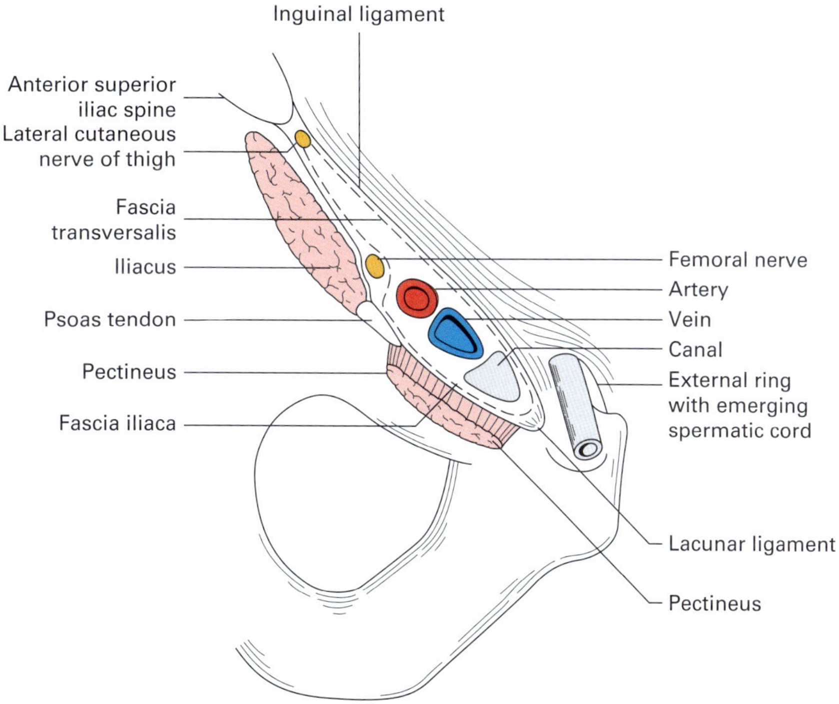

Fig. 173 The femoral canal and its surrounds (right inguinal region).

salis fascia and its posterior wall from the fascia covering the iliacus. Within the sheath the femoral artery lies lateral to the vein. Medial to the vein within the sheath is a space termed the *femoral canal*, which is approximately 1.25 cm (0.5 in) in length and 1 cm in width. A femoral hernia is, by definition, an abnormal protrusion of peritoneum into the femoral canal (and therefore into the femoral sheath). The greater width of the female pelvis means that the canal is somewhat wider in the female. This may be a possible reason for the somewhat greater incidence of femoral hernia in women.

The boundaries of the femoral canal are:

- anteriorly – the inguinal ligament;
- medially – the sharp free edge of the pectineal part of the inguinal ligament, termed the *lacunar ligament (Gimbernat's ligament)*;
- laterally – the femoral vein;
- posteriorly – the pectineal ligament (of Astley Cooper), which is the thickened periosteum along the pectineal border of the superior pubic ramus and which continues medially with the pectineal part of the inguinal ligament.

The canal contains a plug of fat and an inconstant lymph node – the *node of the femoral canal* or *Cloquet's gland*.

The canal has two functions: first, as a dead space for expansion of the distended femoral vein and, second, as a lymphatic pathway from the lower limb to the external iliac nodes.

Femoral hernia

The great importance of the femoral canal is, of course, that it is a potential point of weakness in the abdominal wall through which may develop a femoral hernia. Unlike the indirect inguinal hernia, this is never due to a congenital sac and, although cases do occur rarely in children, it is never found in the newborn.

As the hernial sac enlarges, it emerges through the saphenous opening then turns upwards along the pathway presented by the superficial epigastric and superficial circumflex iliac vessels so that it may come to project above the inguinal ligament. There should not, however, be any difficulty in differentiating between an irreducible femoral and inguinal hernia; the neck of the former must always lie below and lateral to the pubic tubercle, whereas the sac of the latter extends above and medial to this landmark (Fig. 174).

The neck of the femoral canal is narrow and bears a particular sharp medial border; for this reason, irreducibility and strangulation occur more commonly at this site than at any other. In order to enlarge the opening of the canal at operation for a strangulated femoral hernia, this sharp edge of Gimbernat's lacunar ligament may require incision. There is, however, a slight risk of damage to the abnormal obturator artery in this manoeuvre, and it is safer to enlarge the opening by making several small nicks into the ligament. The safer alternative is to divide the inguinal ligament, which can then be repaired.

Note. Normally there is an anastomosis between the pubic branch of the inferior epigastric artery and the pubic branch of the obturator artery. Occasionally, the obturator artery is entirely replaced by this branch from the inferior epigastric – the *abnormal*

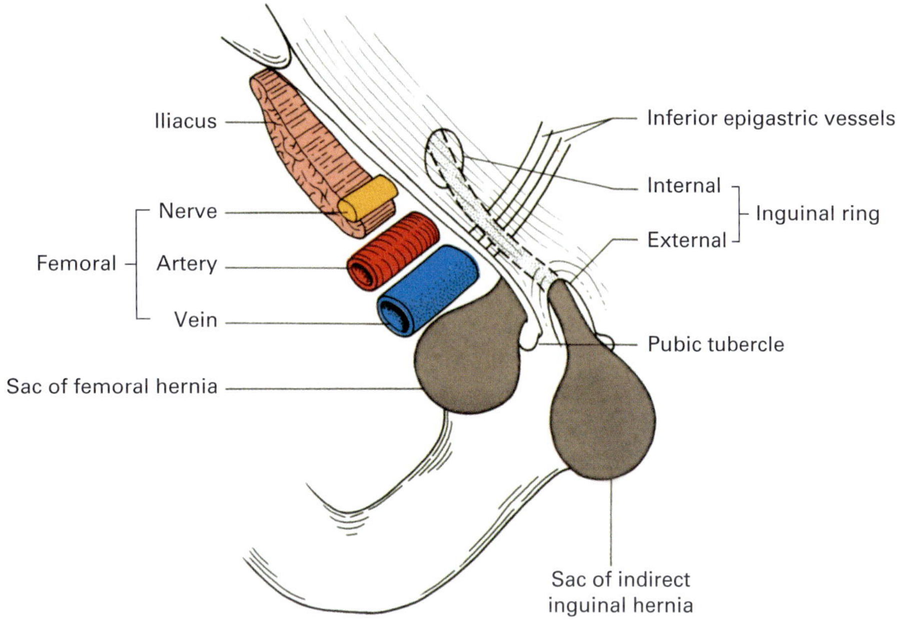

Fig. 174 The relationship of an indirect inguinal and a femoral hernia to the pubic tubercle; the inguinal hernia emerges above and medial to the tubercle and the femoral hernia lies below and lateral to it (right inguinal region).

obturator artery. This aberrant vessel usually passes lateral to the femoral canal and is out of harm's way; more rarely, it passes behind Gimbernat's ligament, and it is then at risk of being accidentally severed.

The lymph nodes of the groin and the lymphatic drainage of the lower limb

The lymph nodes of the groin are arranged in a superficial and a deep group. The *superficial nodes* lie in two chains, a *longitudinal chain* along the great saphenous vein, receiving the bulk of the superficial lymphatic drainage of the lower limb, and a *horizontal chain*, just distal to the inguinal ligament. These horizontal nodes receive lymphatics from the skin and superficial tissues of:

1 the lower trunk and back, below the level of the umbilicus;
2 the buttock;
3 the perineum, scrotum and penis (or lower vagina and vulva) and the anus below its mucocutaneous junction.

In addition, some lymphatics drain via the round ligament to these nodes from the fundus of the uterus.

(All these sites, as well as the whole leg, must be examined carefully when a patient presents with an inguinal lymphadenopathy.)

The two groups of superficial nodes drain through the saphenous opening in the fascia lata into the *deep nodes* lying medial to the femoral vein, which also receive the lymphatic drainage from the tissues of the lower limb beneath the deep fascia. In addition, a small area of skin over the heel and lateral side of the foot drains by lymphatics along the small saphenous vein to nodes in the popliteal fossa and then along the femoral vessels directly to the deep nodes at the groin.

The deep groin nodes drain to the external iliac nodes by lymphatics that travel partly in front of the femoral artery and vein and partly through the femoral canal.

CLINICAL FEATURES

1 Minor sepsis and abrasions of the leg are so common that it is usual to find that the inguinal nodes are palpable in perfectly healthy people.
2 Secondary involvement of the inguinal nodes by malignant deposits may be dealt with by *block dissection of the groin*. This involves removal (*as a single block of tissue*) of the superficial and deep fascial roof of the femoral triangle, the long saphenous vein and its tributaries and the fatty and lymphatic contents of the triangle, leaving only the femoral artery, vein and nerve. The inguinal ligament is detached so that, in addition, an extraperitoneal removal of the external iliac nodes can be carried out.
3 In making a differential diagnosis of a lump in the femoral triangle, think of each anatomical structure that may be involved and of the pathological conditions to which it may give rise, thus:
   - skin and soft tissues – lipoma, sebaceous cyst and sarcoma;
   - artery – aneurysm of the femoral artery;
   - vein – varix of the great saphenous vein;
   - nerve – neuroma of the femoral nerve or its branches;
   - femoral canal – femoral hernia;
   - psoas sheath – psoas abscess;
   - lymph nodes – any of the causes of lymphadenopathy.

The adductor canal (of Hunter) or subsartorial canal (Fig. 175)

The adductor canal is a trough-shaped intermuscular tunnel located in the medial aspect of the distal two-thirds of the thigh. Proximally, it communicates with the femoral triangle through the apex of the latter. The boundaries of the adductor canal are as follows:

- posteromedially – adductor longus and magnus (which form the floor of the adductor canal);
- anterolaterally – vastus medialis;
- anteromedially – sartorius, beneath which lies the dense, subsartorial fascia running from the vastus medialis across to the medial edge of adductor longus and magnus. It is this fascial sheet that forms the roof of the canal.

The contents of the canal are the (superficial) femoral artery, the (superficial) femoral vein (which lies behind the artery), the saphenous nerve and, in its upper part, the nerve to vastus medialis from the femoral nerve.

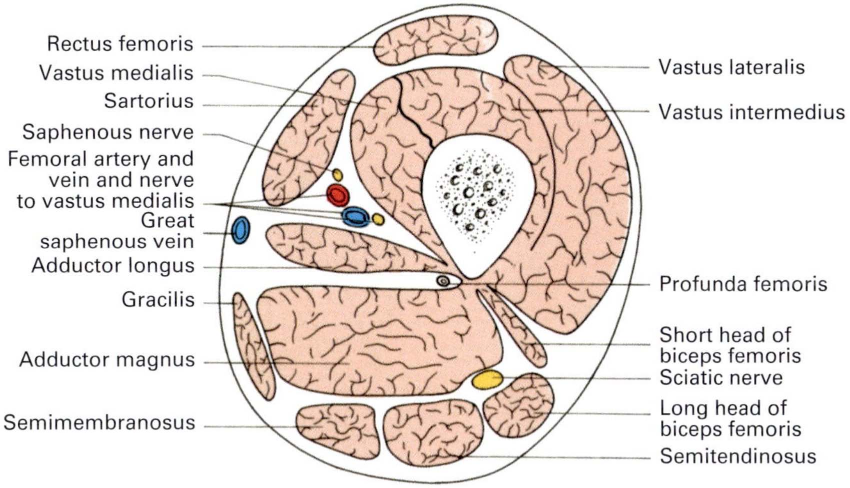

Fig. 175 Cross section through the right thigh in the region of the adductor, or subsartorial, canal of Hunter (viewed from the proximal aspect).

The *adductor hiatus* is a natural gap in the distal part of the tendon of adductor magnus, which leads into the popliteal fossa. It is through this opening that the superficial femoral artery and vein leave the adductor canal to enter the popliteal fossa, as the popliteal artery and vein.

John Hunter described the exposure and ligation of the femoral artery in this canal for aneurysm of the popliteal artery; this method has the advantage that the artery at this site is healthy and will not tear when tied, as may happen if ligation is attempted immediately above the aneurysm.

The popliteal fossa (Fig. 176)

The popliteal fossa is located in the distal part of the posterior compartment of the thigh and communicates through the hiatus in the adductor magnus tendon, with the adductor canal. This 'fossa' is, in fact, a closely packed compartment which becomes the rhomboid-shaped space of anatomical diagrams only when opened up at operation or by dissection.

Its boundaries are:

- superolaterally – biceps femoris tendon;
- superomedially – semimembranosus overlain by semitendinosus;
- inferomedially and inferolaterally – the medial and lateral heads of gastrocnemius, respectively.

The *roof* of the fossa is deep fascia, which is pierced by the small saphenous vein as this enters the popliteal vein.

Its *floor*, from above down, is formed by:

- the popliteal surface of the femur;
- the posterior aspect of the knee joint;
- the popliteus muscle covering the upper posterior surface of the tibia.

From without in, the popliteal fossa contains nerves, vein and artery.

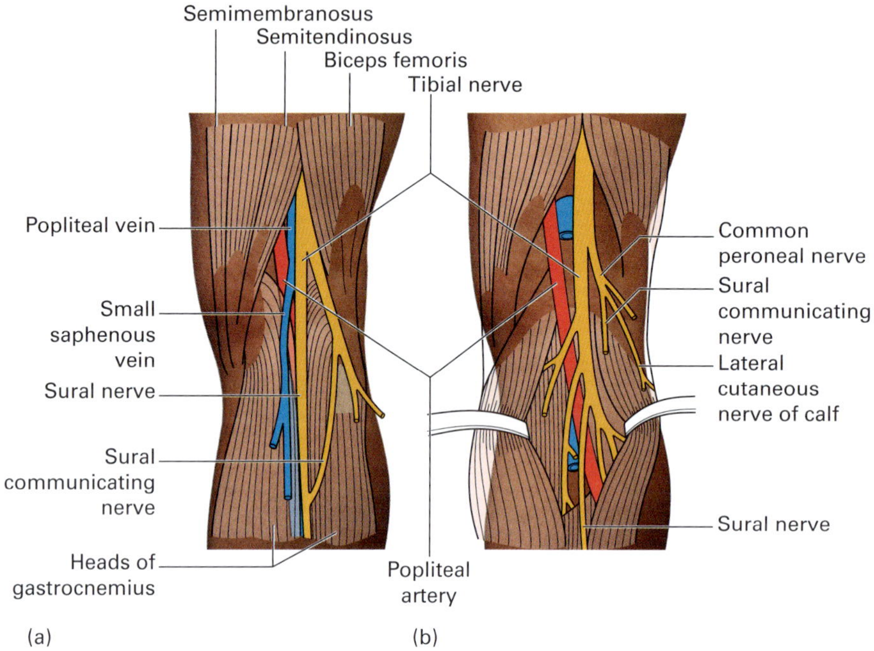

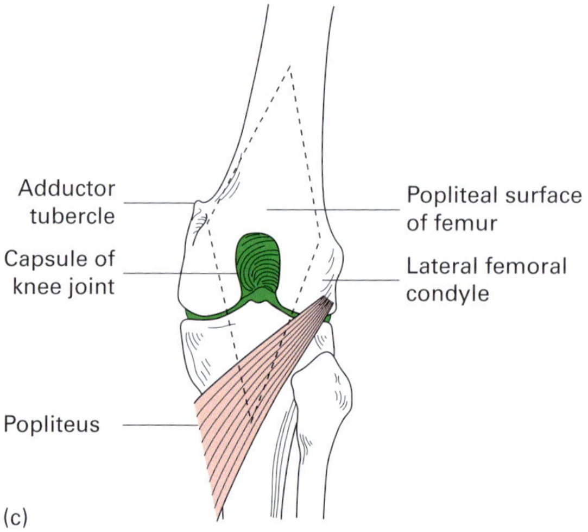

Fig. 176 The right popliteal fossa.
(a) Superficial dissection.
(b) Deep dissection.
(c) Floor.

The *common peroneal nerve* passes out of the fossa along the medial border of the biceps tendon; the *tibial nerve* is first lateral to the popliteal vessels and then crosses superficial to these vessels to lie on their medial side.

The *popliteal vein* lies immediately superficial to the artery; the *popliteal artery* itself lies deepest of all in the fossa.

As well as these important structures, the fossa contains fat, popliteal lymph nodes and a variable number of thin-walled sacs termed bursae.

CLINICAL FEATURES

The popliteal fossa is another good example of the value of thinking anatomically when considering the differential diagnosis of a mass situated in a particular anatomical area.

When examining a lump in the popliteal region, let these possibilities pass through your mind:

- skin and soft tissues – sebaceous cyst, lipoma and sarcoma;
- vein – varicosities of the short saphenous vein in the roof of the fossa;
- artery – popliteal aneurysm;
- lymph nodes – infection secondary to suppuration in the foot;
- knee joint – joint effusion;
- tendons – enlarged bursae, especially those beneath semimembranosus and the heads of gastrocnemius;
- bones – a tumour of the lower end of the femur or upper end of the tibia.

The arteries of the lower limb

Femoral artery

The femoral artery is the distal continuation of the external iliac artery beyond the inguinal ligament. It traverses the femoral triangle and the adductor canal of Hunter, then terminates a hand's breadth above the adductor tubercle by passing through the hiatus in adductor magnus to become the popliteal artery (Fig. 151).

Throughout its course, the femoral artery is accompanied by its vein, which lies first on the medial side of the artery and then passes posterior to it at the apex of the femoral triangle.

Branches

In the groin, the femoral artery gives off:

1 the superficial circumflex iliac artery;
2 the superficial epigastric artery;
3 the superficial external pudendal artery;
4 the deep external pudendal artery.

The first three of these vessels are encountered in the groin incision for repair of an inguinal hernia. Their corresponding veins drain into the great saphenous vein (see Fig. 178).

The *profunda femoris* arises posterolaterally from the femoral artery 5 cm (2 in) distal to the inguinal ligament. It is conventional among vascular surgeons and vascular radiologists to call the femoral artery above this branch the *common femoral artery*, and, below it, the *superficial femoral artery*.

The profunda femoris passes deep to adductor longus and gives off *medial* and *lateral circumflex branches* and four *perforating branches*. These are important both as the source of blood supply to the great muscles of the thigh and as collateral channels that link the rich arterial anastomoses around the hip and the knee.

CLINICAL FEATURES

1 Recapitulate the surface markings of the femoral artery – the upper two-thirds of a line connecting the mid-inguinal point with the adductor tubercle, the hip being held somewhat flexed and externally rotated (Fig. 151).

The femoral artery in the upper 10 cm (4 in) of its course lies in the femoral triangle, where it is relatively superficial and, in consequence, easily injured. A laceration of the femoral artery at this site is an occupational hazard of butchers and bullfighters.

2 The femoral artery at the groin is readily punctured by a hypodermic needle and is the most convenient site from which to obtain arterial blood samples. Arteriography of the peripheral leg vessels is also easily performed at this point. A Seldinger catheter can be passed proximally through a femoral artery puncture in order to carry out aortography or selective renal, coeliac and mesenteric angiography or even coronary angiography.

3 Arteriosclerotic changes, with consequent thrombotic arterial occlusion, frequently commence at the lower end of the femoral artery, perhaps as a result of compression of the diseased vessel by the margins of the hiatus in adductor magnus. Collateral circulation is maintained via anastomoses between the branches of profunda femoris and the popliteal artery. If arteriography demonstrates a patent arterial tree distal to the block, it is possible to bypass the occluded segment by means of a graft between the common femoral and popliteal arteries (femoro-popliteal bypass).

Popliteal artery

The popliteal artery continues on from the femoral artery at the adductor hiatus and terminates at the lower border of the popliteus muscle. It lies deep within the popliteal fossa (see 'The popliteal fossa'), being covered superficially by the popliteal vein and, more superficially still, by the tibial nerve.

The popliteal artery gives off muscular branches, geniculate branches (to the knee joint) and terminal branches – the anterior and posterior tibial arteries.

CLINICAL FEATURES

1 Aneurysm of the popliteal artery, once common, is now rare. Its frequency in former days was presumed to be associated with the repeated friction and traumata of horse riding and the wearing of high riding boots. Pressure of the aneurysm on the adjacent vein may cause venous thrombosis and peripheral oedema; pressure on the tibial nerve may cause severe pain in the leg.

2 The popliteal artery is exposed by deep dissection in the midline within the popliteal fossa, care being taken not to injure the more superficial vein and nerve. It can also be exposed by a medial approach, which divides the insertion of adductor magnus and partially detaches the origin of the medial head of gastrocnemius from the femur.

Posterior tibial artery

The posterior tibial artery is the larger of the two terminal branches of the popliteal artery. It descends deep to soleus, where it can be exposed by splitting gastrocnemius and soleus in the midline, then becomes relatively superficial in the lower third of the leg and passes behind the medial malleolus between the tendons of flexor digitorum longus and flexor hallucis longus. It is accompanied by its venae comitantes and by the tibial nerve (Fig. 177).

Below the ankle, the posterior tibial artery divides into the *medial* and *lateral plantar arteries*, which constitute the principal blood supply to the sole of the foot.

As well as branches to muscles and skin and a large nutrient branch to the tibia, the posterior tibial artery gives off the *peroneal artery* approximately 4 cm (1.5 in) from its origin. The peroneal artery runs down the posterior aspect of the fibula, close to the medial margin of the bone, supplying adjacent muscles and giving a nutrient branch to the fibula. Above the ankle it gives off its *perforating branch*, which pierces the interosseous membrane, descends over the lateral malleolus and anastomoses with the arteries of the dorsum of the foot.

Anterior tibial artery

The anterior tibial artery arises at the bifurcation of the popliteal artery. It passes forwards between the tibia and fibula, under the lower border of popliteus, over the upper margin of the interosseous membrane and descends on this structure in the anterior compartment of the leg.

At first deeply buried, it becomes superficial just above the ankle between the tendons of extensor hallucis longus and tibialis anterior, being crossed superficially by the former immediately proximal to the line of the ankle joint.

The artery continues over the dorsum of the foot as the *dorsalis pedis* (where its pulse may be palpated); this gives off the *arcuate artery*, which, in turn, supplies cutaneous branches to the dorsal aspects of the toes. Dorsalis pedis itself plunges through the

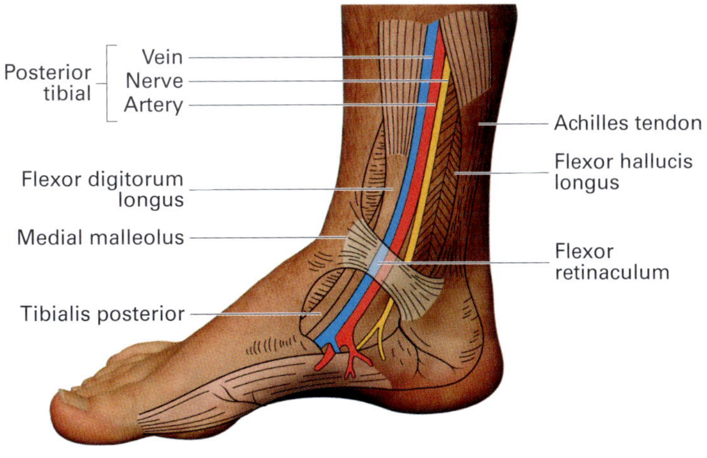

Fig. 177 The relations of the posterior tibial artery as it passes behind the medial malleolus (right ankle region).

proximal part of the first intermetatarsal space (between the 1st and 2nd metatarsals) to join the lateral plantar artery in the formation of the *plantar arch*, from which branches run forwards to supply the plantar aspects of the toes.

The veins of the lower limb

The veins of the lower limb are divided into the deep and superficial groups according to their relationship to the deep fascia of the limb. The *deep veins* accompany the corresponding major arteries. The *superficial veins* are the *great* and *small* (or *long* and *short*) *saphenous veins* and their tributaries (Fig. 178).

The *small (short) saphenous vein* commences at the ankle behind the lateral malleolus where it drains the lateral side of the dorsal venous plexus of the foot. It courses over the back of the calf, perforates the deep fascia over the popliteal fossa and terminates in the popliteal vein. One or more branches run upwards and medially from it to join the great saphenous vein. The small saphenous vein is accompanied by the sural

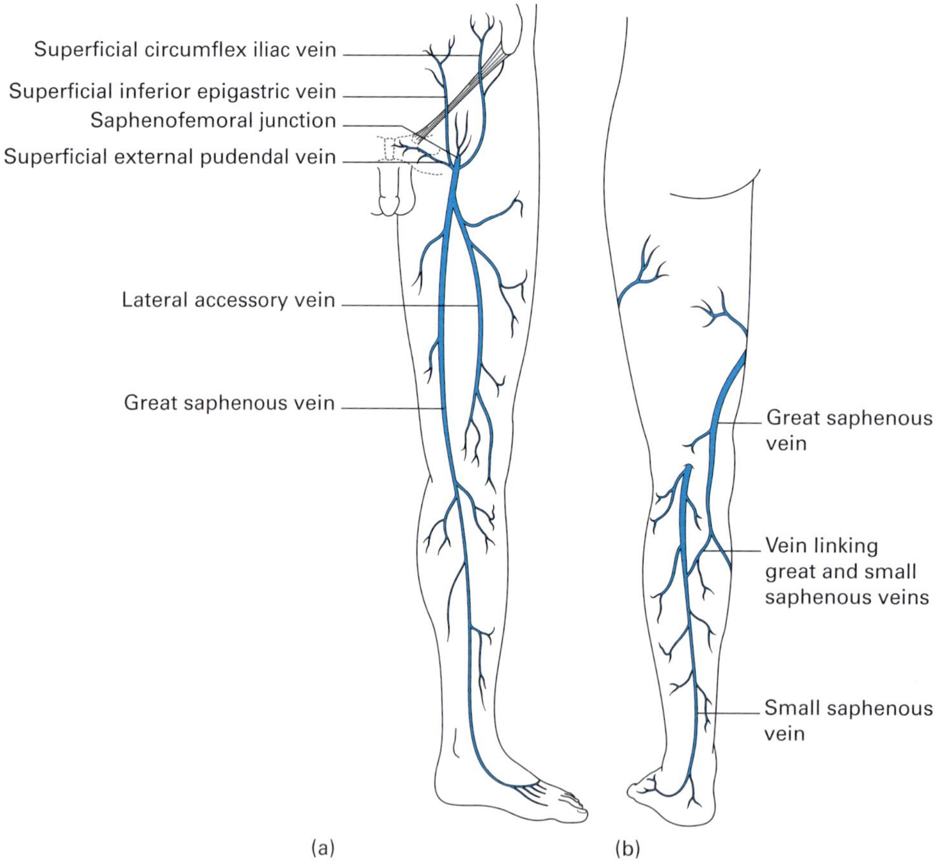

Fig. 178 The superficial veins of the left lower limb. (a) Anteromedial. (b) Posterior view.

nerve – a sensory branch of the tibial nerve (Fig. 176a), which may be damaged when operating on varices of this vein.

The *great (long) saphenous vein* drains the medial part of the venous plexus on the dorsum of the foot and passes upwards immediately in front of the medial malleolus (Fig. 152); here, branches of the saphenous nerve lie in front of and behind the vein. The vein then ascends over the posterior parts of the medial condyles of the tibia and femur to the groin, where it pierces the deep fascia at the saphenous opening 2.5 cm (1 in) below the inguinal ligament, to enter the femoral vein, medial to the femoral pulse.

The great saphenous vein is joined by one or more branches from the small saphenous vein and by the *lateral accessory vein*, which usually enters the main vein at the mid-thigh, although it may not do so until the saphenous opening is reached.

At the groin a number of tributaries from the lower abdominal wall, thigh and scrotum enter the great saphenous vein; these tributaries are variable in number and arrangement but usually comprise (Fig. 178):

1 the superficial epigastric vein;
2 the superficial circumflex iliac vein;
3 the superficial external pudendal vein.

The superficial epigastric vein communicates with the lateral thoracic tributary of the axillary vein via the *thoraco-epigastric vein*. This dilates (and may become readily visible coursing over the trunk) following obstruction of the inferior vena cava. The great saphenous vein communicates with the deep venous system not only at the groin but also at a number of points along its course through *perforating veins*; one is usually present a hand's breadth above the knee and another a hand's breadth below.

The skin of the medial aspect of the leg is drained to the deep veins by two or three *direct perforating veins* that pierce the deep fascia behind the great saphenous vein.

CLINICAL FEATURES

1 We have already noted (under 'Surface anatomy and surface markings of the lower limb') the great importance of the constant position of the great saphenous vein lying immediately in front of the medial malleolus (Fig. 152). Knowledge that a vein *must* be present at this site, even if not visible in an obese or collapsed patient, may be life-saving when urgent transfusion is required. Occasionally, the adjacent saphenous nerve may, inadvertently, be caught in a ligature during a venous cut-down procedure. The patient, if conscious, will complain of sharp and acute pain, should this happen.
2 The saphenous veins frequently become dilated, their valves become incompetent and the veins become varicose. Usually this condition is idiopathic but may result from the increased venous pressure caused by more proximal venous obstruction (a pelvic tumour or the pregnant uterus, for example) or may be secondary to obstruction of the deep venous pathway of the leg by thrombosis.
3 Stagnation of blood in the skin of the lower limb may result from venous thrombosis or valve incompetence; the skin, in consequence, is poorly nourished and may, in the course of time, break down and form a *varicose ulcer*. This is especially liable to occur

over the subcutaneous anteromedial surface of the tibia where the cutaneous blood supply may be tenuous.

4 In operating upon varicose veins it is important that all tributaries of the long saphenous vein in the groin are ligated, *prior* to ligation of the long saphenous vein just distal to the saphenofemoral junction. Failure to ligate one or other tributary may well result in recurrence of varices. The proximal termination of the great saphenous vein at the groin is found by palpating the femoral pulse. The femoral vein lies a finger's breadth medial to this pulse, so that a vertical or transverse incision at this site will come down upon the great saphenous vein as it lies in the superficial fascia immediately before it plunges through the hiatus in the deep fascia to join the femoral vein. The great saphenous vein is distinguished from the femoral vein in that (1) it lies in the superficial fascia, whereas the femoral vein lies deep to the deep facia, and (2) the great saphenous vein bears a number of tributaries, whereas the femoral vein receives only one at that level; the great saphenous vein itself! It is important to be mindful of this to avoid inadvertent injury to the femoral vein during surgery for varicose veins.

The course and distribution of the principal nerves of the lower limb

The nerves of the lower limb are derived from the lumbar and sacral plexuses.

The lumbar plexus (Fig. 179)

The lumbar plexus is made up of the anterior rami of L1–L4.

These rami enter the psoas major muscle and make connections within the substance of the muscle before emerging from the muscle as the various named nerves of the lumbar plexus. All but two of the branches of the lumbar plexus emerge from under cover of the lateral border of psoas major. The two exceptions are: the obturator nerve which appears at the medial border of psoas major and the genitofemoral nerve which emerges on the anterior aspect of the muscle. The nerves that emerge from the lateral aspect of psoas major are the iliohypogastric nerve, the ilioinguinal nerve, the lateral cutaneous nerve of thigh and the femoral nerve, in that order, from above downwards.

The principal branches of the plexus are the femoral nerve and the obturator nerve.

The *femoral nerve* (L2–L4) emerges from the substance of psoas major and then passes under the inguinal ligament a finger's breadth lateral to the femoral artery, to break up into its terminal branches after a course in the lower limb of just a few centimetres.

Its branches are:

- muscular – to the anterior compartment of the thigh (quadriceps, sartorius and pectineus);

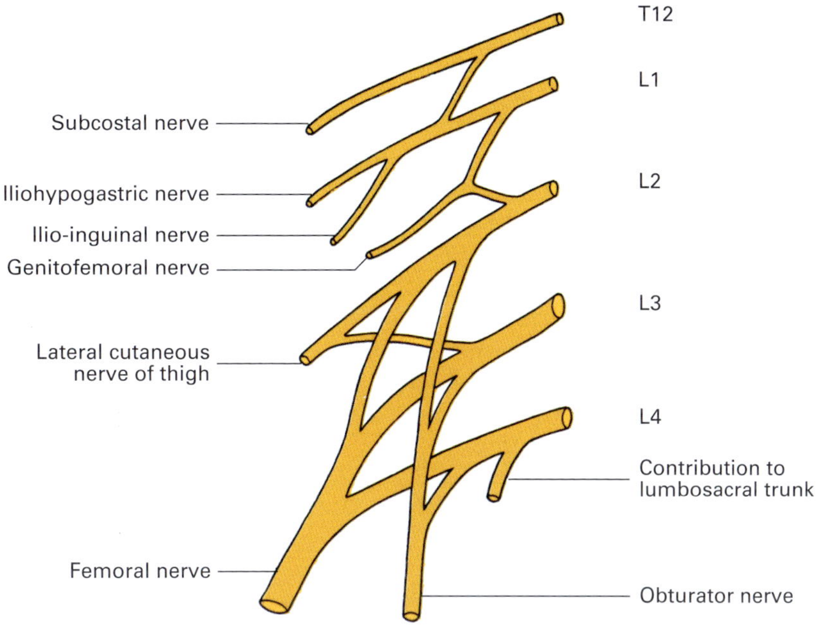

Fig. 179 Plan of the lumbar plexus (muscular branches have been omitted for clarity).

- cutaneous – the medial and intermediate cutaneous nerves of the thigh and the saphenous nerve, which traverses the adductor canal to supply the skin of the medial side of the knee, leg, ankle and foot as far as the great toe;
- articular – to the hip and knee joints.

The femoral nerve supplies the skin of the medial and anterior aspects of the thigh via its medial and intermediate cutaneous branches, but the lateral aspect is supplied by the *lateral cutaneous nerve of the thigh* (L2–L3). This arises directly from the lumbar plexus and enters the thigh usually by passing deep to the inguinal ligament. Occasionally, the nerve pierces the ligament and may then be pressed upon by it with resultant pain, paraesthesia and/or anaesthesia over the upper outer thigh (*meralgia paraesthetica*). This is relieved by dividing the deeper fasciculus of the inguinal ligament where the nerve is trapped.

The *obturator nerve* (L2–L4) emerges from the medial aspect of the psoas and runs downwards and forwards, crosses the pelvic brim deep to the internal iliac vessels, to reach the superior part of the obturator foramen. This the nerve traverses, in company with the obturator vessels, to enter the thigh.

Its branches are:

- muscular – to obturator externus, the adductor muscles (brevis, longus and magnus) and gracilis;
- cutaneous – to an area of skin over the medial aspect of the thigh;
- articular – to the hip and knee joints.

CLINICAL FEATURES

1 Spasm of the adductor muscles of the thigh in spastic paraplegia can be relieved by division of the obturator nerve (*obturator neurectomy*). This can be performed through a midline lower abdominal incision exposing the nerve trunk extraperitoneally on each side as it passes towards the obturator foramen.
2 Rarely, an *obturator hernia* develops through the canal where the obturator nerve and vessels traverse the membrane covering the obturator foramen. Pressure of a strangulated obturator hernia upon the nerve causes referred pain in its area of cutaneous distribution, so that intestinal obstruction associated with pain along the medial side of the thigh should suggest this diagnosis.
3 The femoral and obturator nerves, as well as the sciatic nerve and its branches, supply sensory fibres to both the hip and the knee; it is not uncommon for hip disease to present disguised as pain in the knee.

The sacral plexus (Fig. 180)

This plexus originates from the anterior primary rami of L4–L5 and S1–S4.

Note that L4 is shared by both the lumbar and sacral plexuses. Indeed about half of the fibres of L4 join the whole of L5 to form the *lumbosacral trunk*, which carries its important contribution, roughly half the total nerve fibre input, to the sacral plexus. The plexus might therefore be better named the lumbosacral plexus.

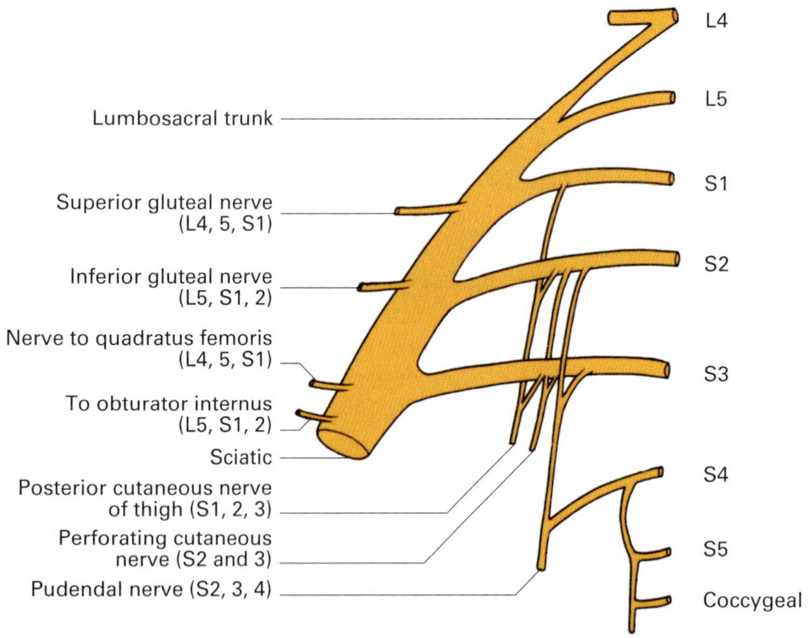

Fig. 180 Plan of the sacral plexus.

The sacral nerves emerge from the anterior sacral foramina and unite in front of piriformis, where they are joined by the lumbosacral trunk.

Branches from the plexus supply:

- the pelvic muscles;
- the muscles of the hip;
- the skin of the buttock and the back of the thigh.

The plexus itself terminates as the pudendal nerve and the sciatic nerve.

The *pudendal nerve* (S2–S4) provides the principal innervation of the perineum. It has a complex course, passing from the pelvis, briefly through the gluteal region, along the side-wall of the ischioanal (ischiorectal) fossa and through the deep perineal pouch to end by supplying the skin of the external genitalia (Fig. 181).

It arises as the lower main division of the sacral plexus, although it is dwarfed by the giant sciatic nerve. It leaves the pelvis through the greater foramen below the

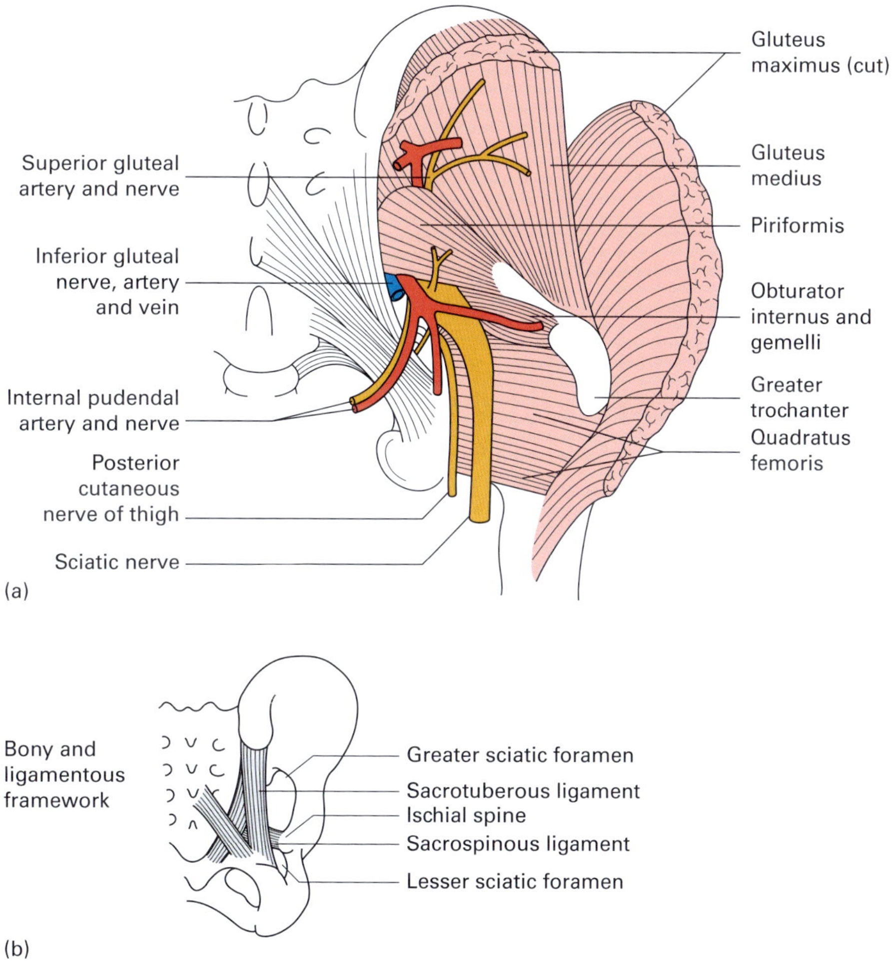

Fig. 181 The sciatic foramina (right side). (a) Contents and related muscles. (b) Boundaries and ligamentous framework.

piriformis muscle. It crosses the dorsum of the ischial spine and immediately disappears through the lesser sciatic foramen into the perineum. The nerve now runs in the lateral wall of the ischioanal fossa in company with the internal pudendal vessels and lies within a distinct fascial compartment on the medial aspect of obturator internus termed the pudendal canal (Alcock's canal; Fig. 97). Within the canal it first gives off the *inferior rectal nerve*, which crosses the fossa to innervate the external anal sphincter and the perianal skin. The pudendal nerve then divides into its terminal branches; the perineal nerve and the dorsal nerve of the penis (or clitoris).

The *perineal nerve* is the larger of the two. It bifurcates almost at once; its deeper branch supplies the sphincter urethrae and the other muscles of the anterior perineum (the ischiocavernosus, bulbospongiosus and the superficial and deep transverse perinei). Its more superficial branch innervates the skin of the posterior aspect of the scrotum or vulva.

The *dorsal nerve of the penis* (or *clitoris*) traverses the deep perineal pouch, pierces the perineal membrane and then penetrates the suspensory ligament of the penis to supply the dorsal aspect of this structure.

CLINICAL FEATURES

In obstetric practice the pudendal nerve can be blocked with local anaesthetic prior to forceps delivery by inserting a long needle through the vaginal wall and, guided by a finger, to the ischial spine, which can be palpated per vaginam. Alternatively, the needle can be introduced just medial to the ischial tuberosity to a depth of 2.5 cm (1 in). When the procedure is carried out bilaterally, there is loss of the anal reflex (which is a useful test that a successful block has been achieved), relaxation of the pelvic floor muscles and loss of sensation to the vulva and lower one-third of the vagina (Fig. 97b).

The sciatic nerve

The sciatic nerve (L4, L5, S1–S3) is the largest nerve in the body (Fig. 182). It is broad and flat at its origin, although distally it becomes rounded.

The nerve emerges from the greater sciatic foramen below piriformis and under cover of gluteus maximus, crosses the posterior surface of the ischium, crosses obturator internus, with its gemelli and quadratus femoris, and descends on adductor magnus (Figs 181, 182). Here, it lies deep to the hamstrings and is crossed only by the long head of biceps.

The sciatic nerve terminates by dividing into the *tibial* and *common peroneal nerves* (Fig. 176). The level of this division is variable – usually it is at the mid-thigh, but the two nerves may be separate even at their origins from the sacral plexus. Alternatively, the nerve may divide in the popliteal fossa.

Branches

The trunk of the sciatic nerve supplies the hamstring muscles (biceps, semimembranosus and semitendinosus) and also part of the adductor magnus, the latter being innervated, principally, by the obturator nerve.

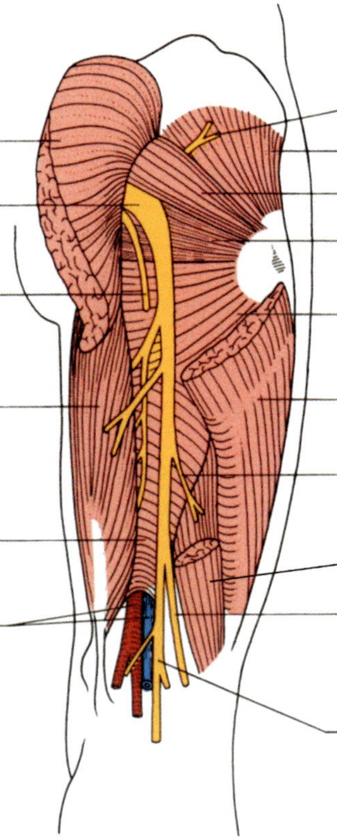

Fig. 182 Dissection of the sciatic nerve in the thigh and popliteal fossa (right side). Note that gluteus medius has been removed to show the otherwise completely hidden gluteus minimus.

All the muscle branches apart from the one to the short head of biceps arise on the medial side of the nerve from its tibial component; its lateral border is therefore the side of relative safety in surgical exposures.

CLINICAL FEATURES

1 The sciatic nerve may be wounded in penetrating injuries or in posterior dislocation of the hip associated with fracture of the posterior lip of the acetabulum, to which the nerve is closely related (Fig. 166).

Damage to the sciatic nerve is followed by paralysis of the hamstrings and all the muscles of the leg and foot (supplied by its distributing branches); there is loss of all movements in the lower limb below the knee joint with foot drop deformity. Sensory loss is complete below the knee, except for an area along the medial side of the leg, over the medial malleolus and down to the hallux, which is innervated by the saphenous branch of the femoral nerve.

2 The sciatic nerve is accompanied by a companion artery (derived from the inferior gluteal artery), which bleeds quite considerably when the nerve is divided during an above-knee amputation. The artery must be neatly isolated from the surrounding neural tissue by dissection and tied separately without any nerve fibres being incorporated in the ligature, as otherwise, a stump neuroma may develop, causing severe pain in the stump.

The tibial nerve (Fig. 176a,b)

The tibial nerve (L4, L5, S1–S3) is the larger of the two terminal branches of the sciatic nerve; it traverses the popliteal fossa superficial to the popliteal vein and artery, which it crosses from the lateral to the medial side.

Branches

1 In the popliteal fossa:
   - muscular – to gastrocnemius, soleus and popliteus;
   - cutaneous – the *sural nerve*, which descends over the back of the calf, behind the lateral malleolus to the 5th toe; it receives a communicating branch from the common peroneal nerve and supplies the lateral side of the leg, foot and 5th toe;
   - articular – to the knee joint.

   It then descends deep to soleus, in company with the posterior tibial vessels, passes on their lateral side behind the medial malleolus to end by dividing into the *medial* and *lateral plantar* nerves.
2 In the leg – the tibial nerve supplies flexor hallucis longus, flexor digitorum longus and tibialis posterior. Its terminal plantar branches supply the intrinsic muscles and skin of the sole of the foot; the medial plantar nerve having an equivalent distribution to that of the median nerve in the hand, the lateral plantar nerve being comparable to the ulnar nerve.

The common peroneal (fibular) nerve

The common peroneal nerve (L4, L5, S1, S2) is the smaller of the two terminal branches of the sciatic nerve. It enters the upper part of the popliteal fossa, passes along the medial border of the biceps tendon, then curves around the neck of the fibula where it lies in the substance of PL and divides into its terminal branches, the *deep peroneal* and *superficial peroneal nerves* (Fig. 153).

Branches

While still in the popliteal fossa, the common peroneal nerve gives off the *lateral cutaneous nerve of the calf*, a *peroneal (sural) communicating branch* and twigs to the knee joint, but has no muscular branches at this level.

The deep peroneal (fibular) nerve

The deep peroneal nerve pierces extensor digitorum longus, then descends, in company with the anterior tibial vessels, over the interosseous membrane and then across the ankle joint. Medially lies tibialis anterior, whereas laterally lies first extensor digitorum longus and then extensor hallucis longus. Its branches are:

- muscular – to the muscles of the anterior compartment of the leg – extensor digitorum longus, extensor hallucis longus, tibialis anterior and peroneus tertius – and extensor digitorum brevis on the dorsum of the foot;
- cutaneous – to a small area of skin in the web between the 1st and 2nd toes.

The superficial peroneal (fibular) nerve

The superficial peroneal nerve runs in the lateral compartment of the leg.

Its branches are:

- muscular – to the lateral compartment muscles (peroneus longus and brevis);
- cutaneous – to the skin of the distal two-thirds of the anterolateral aspect of the leg and to the dorsum of the foot (apart from the small area between the 1st and 2nd toes supplied by the deep peroneal nerve).

CLINICAL FEATURES

The common peroneal nerve is in a particularly vulnerable position as it winds around the neck of the fibula. It may be damaged at this site by the pressure of a tight bandage or plaster cast or it may be compressed if the leg is placed *within*, rather than outside, the supporting poles when the patient is put into the 'lithotomy' position, for example when undergoing an operation in the perineal region. It may also be damaged in severe adduction injuries to the knee. Damage to this nerve is followed by foot drop (due to paralysis of the ankle and foot extensors) and inversion of the foot (due to paralysis of the peroneal muscles with unopposed action of the foot flexors and invertors). This deformity is termed *talipes equinovarus* (*talipes* refers to the foot; *equino*, the foot is held plantar flexed, as in the horse; and *varus* means the foot is adducted, i.e. internally rotated). There is also anaesthesia over the anterior and lateral aspects of the leg and dorsum of the foot, although the medial side escapes since this is innervated by the saphenous branch of the femoral nerve.

Segmental cutaneous supply of the lower limb (Fig. 183)

The *cutaneous distribution of the spinal nerves* supplying the lower limb is as follows:

- L1, L2 and L3 – supply the anterior aspect of the thigh from above down, in that order;
- L4 – supplies the anteromedial aspect of the leg;
- L5 – supplies the anterolateral aspect of the leg but also extends onto the dorsum of the foot;
- S1 – supplies the lateral side of the foot and the sole;
- S2 – supplies the posterior surface of the leg and thigh;
- S3 and S4 – supply the buttocks and perianal region.

A little aid to memory is that '5' supplies the 1st toe and '1' supplies the 5th toe.

Note that, although S3 supplies the posterior part of the scrotum (or vulva), L1 supplies the anterior part of these structures via the ilioinguinal nerve.

Compartments of the lower limb

In each of the limbs, the skeletal muscles are collectively ensleeved in a layer of deep fascia. From the inner surface of this stocking-like deep fascial envelope, fibrous septa project inwards and attach to the bone(s) lying within a given segment of the

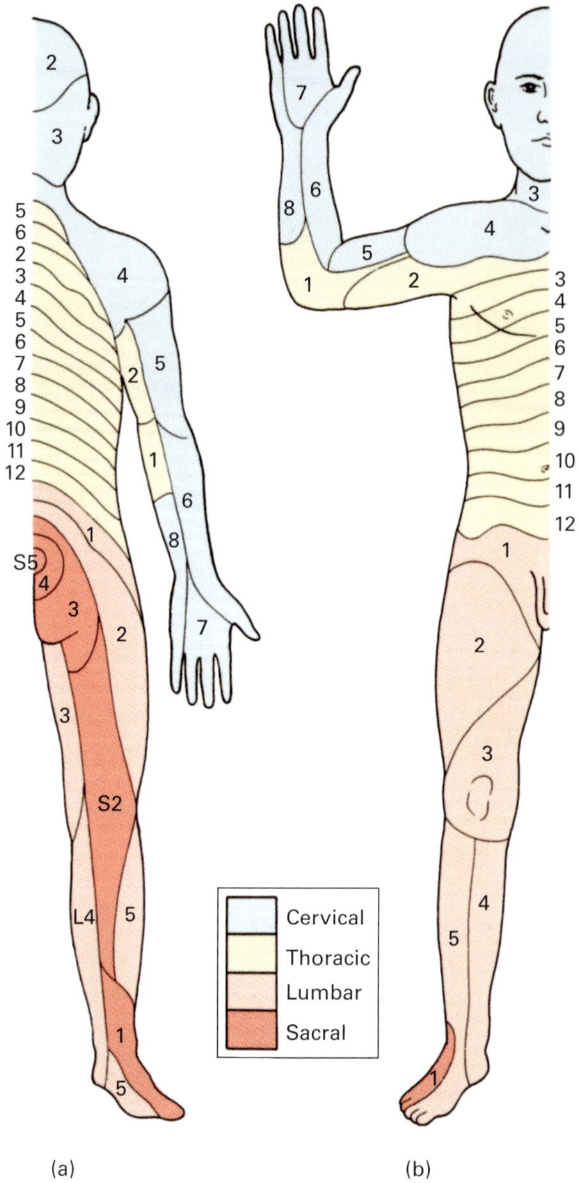

Fig. 183 The segmental cutaneous nerve supply of the skin. (a) Posterior aspect. (b) Anterior aspect.

limb, thereby separating the muscles of that limb segment into functional groups. Thus, the muscles within each segment of the upper and lower limbs may be pictured as being located in discrete, osseofascial compartments (Fig. 184). As a general rule, each compartment possesses its own complement of neurovascular structures, with the nerve being responsible for the motor innervation of all the muscles of the compartment. The segments of the lower limb are the thigh, leg and foot.

Compartments in the segments of the lower limb

Thigh

The thigh contains two distinct and physically separate compartments:

1 The anterior (extensor) compartment comprises quadriceps femoris and sartorius. The nerve of this compartment is the femoral nerve.
2 The posterior compartment of the thigh contains two groups of muscles that are functionally distinct – the hamstrings, which are innervated by the sciatic nerve, and the adductors, which are innervated by the obturator nerve.

Leg

A very definite fascial separation into anterior (extensor), posterior (flexor) and lateral (evertor) compartments exists in the leg (Fig. 184). Furthermore, the posterior compartment is divided by a fascial layer into superficial and deep subdivisions. Thus, the leg contains four distinct compartments. The anterior compartment contains tibialis anterior, extensor digitorum longus, extensor hallucis longus and peroneus tertius, all of which are innervated by the deep peroneal nerve and supplied by the anterior tibial artery. The lateral compartment contains the peroneus longus and brevis muscles, which are innervated by the superficial peroneal nerve. The superficial group of posterior compartment muscles comprises gastrocnemius, soleus and plantaris, whereas the deep group is made up of flexor digitorum longus, flexor hallucis longus, tibialis posterior and popliteus. All the muscles of the posterior compartment (superficial and deep groups) are innervated by the tibial nerve. (In the view of some authorities, the posterior compartment of the leg has three, rather than two, subdivisions. According to this view, tibialis posterior occupies a compartment of its own.)

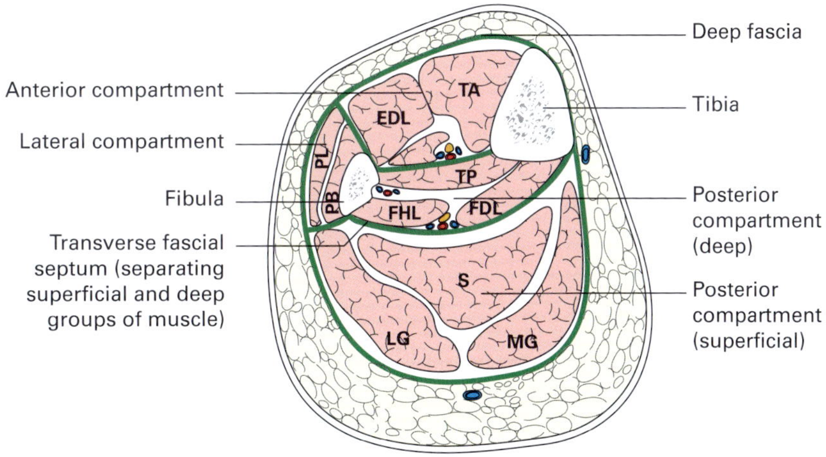

Fig. 184 Cross-sectional representation of the compartments of the right leg. EDL, extensor digitorum longus; FDL, flexor digitorum longus; FHL, flexor hallucis longus; LG, lateral head of gastrocnemius; MG, medial head of gastrocnemius; PB, peroneus brevis; PL, peroneus longus; S, soleus; TA, tibialis anterior; TP, tibialis posterior.

Compartment syndrome

The fascial boundaries that limit the osseofascial compartments are inelastic sheets. Any condition that leads to an increase in the volume of the compartmental contents is therefore likely to result in a rise in intracompartmental pressure. Such conditions include haemorrhage following closed fractures, muscle swelling caused by trauma or unaccustomed overuse and local infection. If unrelieved, the increased pressure leads to compression of the vessels in the compartment and secondary ischaemic damage to the nerves and muscles of the compartment. This phenomenon is known as *compartment syndrome* and involves, most commonly, the compartments of the leg (especially, the anterior compartment of leg).

Compartment syndrome is a surgical emergency and is treated by performing a fasciotomy; a procedure in which a generous incision is made in the deep fascia overlying the compartment in order to decompress the compartment. Closure of the incision is deferred until the clinical condition has improved and it is safe to repair the wound.

Part 5
The Head and Neck

Surface anatomy of the neck

Introduction

The differential diagnosis of lumps in the neck and the effective clinical and surgical management of pathological lesions in the neck require a sound knowledge of the surgical anatomy of the head and neck. From a practical viewpoint, it is helpful to picture the neck as being made up of two parts:

1 a posterior part – comprising the cervical vertebral column (including the contained spinal cord) and the postvertebral musculature;
2 an anterior part – which includes the prevertebral musculature covered by prevertebral fascia, in front of which lies the centrally located visceral region; this region includes the right and left carotid sheaths, the submandibular glands and the anterior cervical musculature.

In the anterior midline, from above down, can be felt (Fig. 185):

1 the *hyoid bone* – at the level of C3;
2 the notch of the *thyroid cartilage* – at the level of C4;
3 the isthmus of the thyroid cartilage – at levels C4 and C5;
4 the (median) *cricothyroid* ligament – important in cricothyroid puncture;
5 the *cricoid cartilage* – continuous inferiorly, with the trachea. The lower border of the *cricoid cartilage* corresponds to the level of C6 (or upper part of C7);
6 the rings of the *trachea* – overlying the 2nd and 3rd rings is the *isthmus of the thyroid gland* (sometimes palpable);
7 *the suprasternal notch* (also known as the *sternal notch* or *jugular notch*).

Note that the lower border of the cricoid is an important level in the neck; it corresponds not only to the level of the 6th cervical vertebra but also to:

1 the junction of the larynx with the trachea;
2 the junction of the pharynx with the oesophagus;
3 the level at which the inferior thyroid artery enters, and the middle thyroid vein leaves the thyroid gland;
4 the level at which the vertebral artery enters the transverse foramen in the 6th cervical vertebra;
5 the level at which the superior belly of the omohyoid crosses the carotid sheath;
6 the level at which the middle cervical sympathetic ganglion is located;
7 the level at which the carotid artery can be compressed against the transverse process of C6 (the carotid tubercle).

Pressing the jaw laterally to one side, against the resistance of one's hand causes the contralateral *sternocleidomastoid* to become tense. This muscle demarcates the posterior triangle of the neck (bounded by sternocleidomastoid, trapezius and the clavicle) from the anterior triangle (bounded by the right and left sternocleidomastoids on either side and by the mandible superiorly) (Fig. 186).

Clench the jaws and, simultaneously, widen your mouth; the platysma then comes into view as a sheet of muscle, passing from the mandible down over the clavicles, lying in the superficial fascia of the neck. The *external jugular vein* lies immediately deep to the platysma, crosses the surface of the sternocleidomastoid into the posterior triangle, perforates the deep fascia just above the clavicle and enters the subclavian vein.

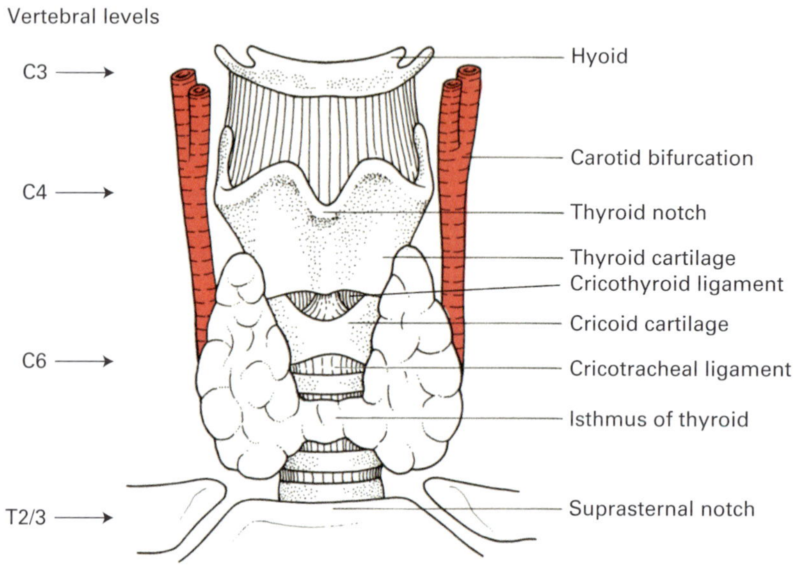

Fig. 185 Structures palpable on the anterior aspect of the neck, together with their corresponding vertebral levels.

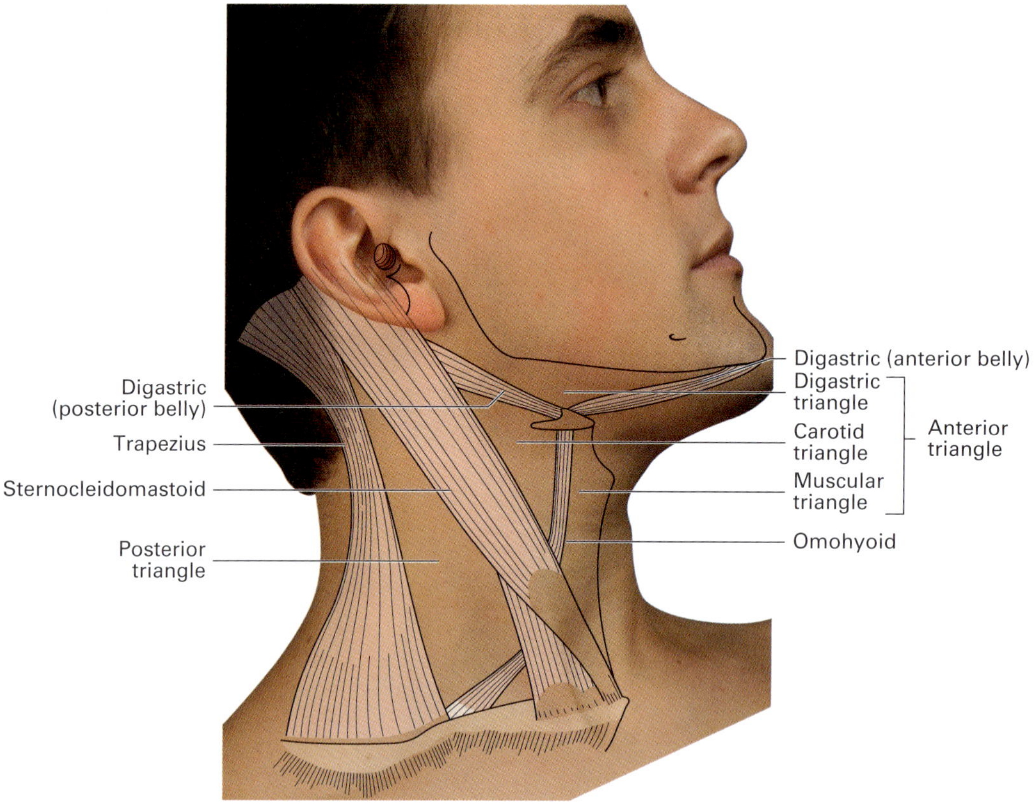

Fig. 186 The triangles of the neck.

It is readily visible in a thin subject when the latter is straining and is often seen from the audience on a singer's neck when the singer hits a sustained high note or on the neck of an orthopaedic surgeon when the latter strains to reduce a difficult fracture!

The *common carotid artery* pulse can be felt by pressing backwards against the prominent anterior tubercle of the transverse process of C6. The line of the carotid sheath can be marked out by a line joining a point midway between the tip of the mastoid process and the angle of the jaw to the ipsilateral sternoclavicular joint. Along this line, the common carotid bifurcates into the *external* and *internal carotid arteries* at the level of the upper border of the thyroid cartilage; at this level, the vessels lie within the carotid sheath beneath the investing layer of the deep cervical fascia, where their pulsation is palpable and, occasionally, visible.

The fascial compartments of the neck (Fig. 187)

A thorough appreciation of the topographical arrangement of the fascial and muscular planes in the anterior aspect of the neck is fundamental to accuracy in the clinical diagnosis of neck lumps, besides being an essential prerequisite to safety and precision in neck surgery.

Tissue planes and fascial layers in the anterior part of the neck

Deep to the skin of the neck is the superficial fascia or panniculus adiposus, which is essentially a layer of subcutaneous fat, more or less homogeneous. The degree of adiposity in this layer varies between individuals; it also varies, to some extent, between the anterior and posterior aspects of the neck in the same individual, being generally somewhat thinner in the front of the neck than at the back. Lying immediately deep to the subcutaneous fat, on either side of the anterior midline, is the platysma, a relatively thin but wide sheet of muscle. The platysma is a feature of the anterolateral part of the neck and does not extend to the back of the neck. Above the level of the hyoid, the medial borders of the right and left platysma muscles are contiguous, whereas, below the hyoid level, they are separated from each other by an interval of 2.5 cm (1 in) or so. The *deep fascia* can be classified into four parts: investing layer of deep cervical fascia, pretracheal fascia, prevertebral fascia and carotid sheaths (right and left).

Immediately deep to the platysma is the *investing layer of deep cervical fascia*, the most superficial of the multiple layers of the deep cervical fascia. It invests the neck like a collar. Superiorly, its attachment may be traced circumferentially along the entire length of the lower border of the mandible, the mastoid processes and superior nuchal lines on either side and to the external occipital protuberance in the posterior midline. In the interval between the angle of the mandible and the mastoid process, the investing layer of deep cervical fascia encloses the parotid salivary gland as the *parotid fascia*.

Inferiorly, the circumferential attachment of the investing layer of deep cervical fascia is to the sternal notch (i.e. the notched, thick upper border of the manubrium sterni) and, in continuity, on each side, to the upper surface of the clavicle, the acromion and the corresponding spine of the scapula and thus to the posterior midline. Traced laterally

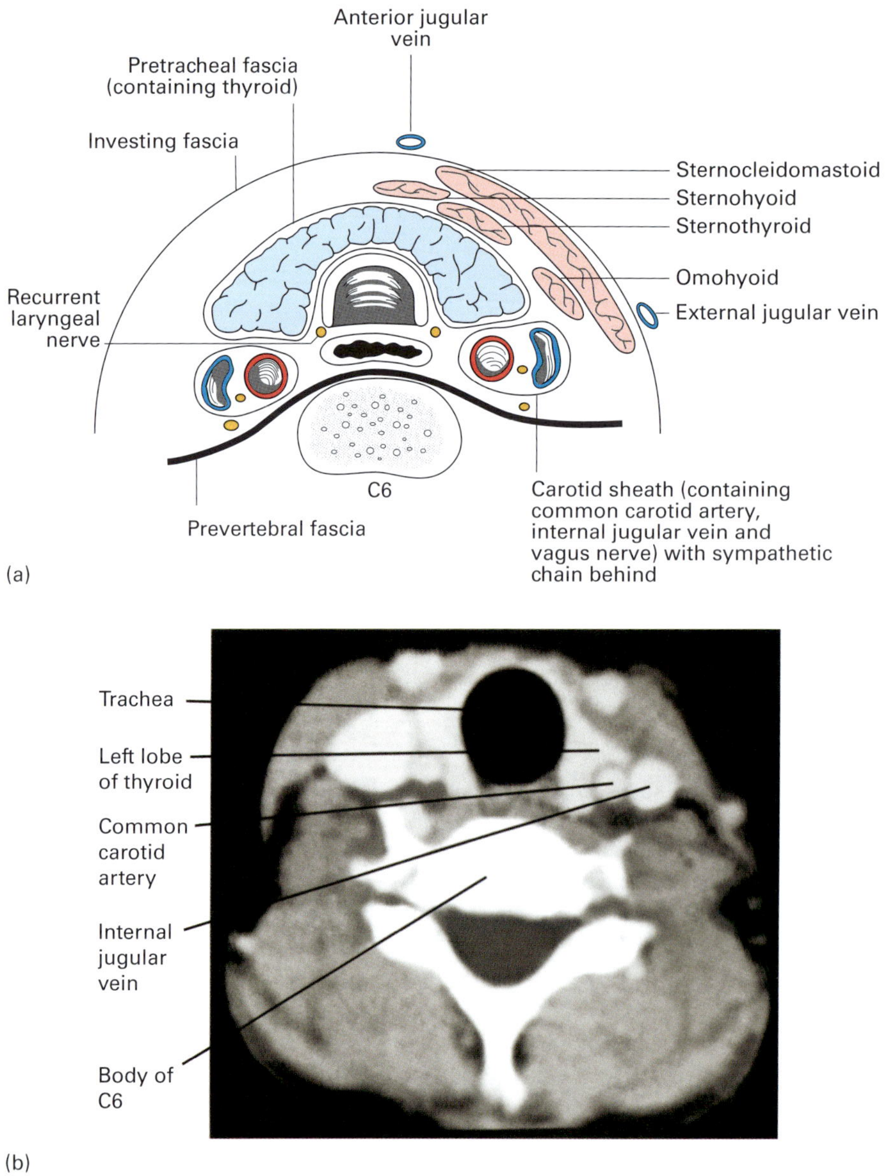

Fig. 187 (a) Transverse section of the neck through C6, showing the fascial planes and also the 'visceral compartment of the neck'. (b) Computed tomography (CT) scan through the C6 level; compare this with (a). Source: Dr Jeremy Rabouhans.

from the anterior midline, between its upper and lower attachments, the investing layer of deep cervical fascia meets, on each side, the medial border of the corresponding sternocleidomastoid muscle and splits to enclose the muscle. Thereafter, it continues posterolaterally as the fascial roof of the posterior triangle of the neck, and, upon reaching the anterior edge of the trapezius muscle, it splits to enclose the trapezius.

In its descent from the lower border of the mandible, the investing layer of deep cervical fascia is firmly adherent to the front of the hyoid body and to the lateral aspects of the greater horns of the hyoid. Thus, all the cervical viscera, major blood vessels and nerves of the neck and all the cervical muscles (with the sole exception of the platysma) come to lie within the embrace of the investing layer of deep cervical fascia.

The external jugular vein runs in the plane between the platysma and the underlying investing layer of deep fascia. It pierces the latter above the clavicle. If the vein is divided here, it is held open by the deep fascia that is attached to its margins, air is sucked into the venous lumen during inspiration and a fatal air embolism may ensue.

Lying immediately deep to the investing layer of deep cervical fascia and running longitudinally on either side of the anterior midline of the neck are the infrahyoid anterior cervical muscles, also known as the strap muscles. On each side of the vertical midline, the strap muscles are disposed in two planes. The superficial plane consists of the sternohyoid and omohyoid muscles lying side by side (sternohyoid medial to omohyoid), and the deep plane consists of the sternothyroid muscle, which extends vertically from the posterior surface of the manubrium sterni to the oblique line of the thyroid cartilage. Extending upwards from the oblique line of the thyroid cartilage to the greater horn of the hyoid is the thyrohyoid muscle, which may be regarded as the upward continuation of the sternothyroid muscle.

The deepest layer of the deep cervical fascia is the prevertebral fascia, a relatively dense layer that covers the anterior aspects of the prevertebral musculature and the cervical vertebral column. The *prevertebral fascia* passes across the vertebrae and prevertebral muscles behind the oesophagus, the pharynx and the great vessels. Above, it is attached to the base of the skull. Laterally, the fascia covers the scalene muscles, the phrenic nerve as the nerve lies on scalenus anterior, the emerging brachial plexus and subclavian artery. In this location the prevertebral fascia forms the fascial floor of the posterior triangle. The brachial plexus and subclavian artery, on their way to the axilla, carry with them a covering layer of prevertebral fascia. This prolongation of prevertebral fascia into the axilla surrounding the brachial plexus and axillary artery is termed the *axillary sheath*. A few centimetres into the axilla, the axillary sheath ends by fusing with the adventitia of the artery and the epineurium of the brachial plexus.

Inferiorly, the prevertebral fascia blends with the anterior longitudinal ligament of the upper thoracic vertebrae in the posterior mediastinum.

Caseous, necrotic pus from a tuberculous cervical vertebra bulges behind this dense fascial layer and may form a midline swelling causing the posterior wall of the pharynx to bulge anteriorly. The abscess may also track laterally, deep to the prevertebral fascia, to a point behind the sternocleidomastoid.

Deep to the strap muscles and anterior to the prevertebral fascial layer is the centrally located visceral column of the neck.

Lying lateral to the cervical visceral column and in front of the prevertebral fascia are the right and left carotid sheaths. Situated posteromedial to each carotid sheath and anterior to the prevertebral fascia is the ganglionated, cervical sympathetic chain.

The cervical visceral column flanked by the right and left carotid sheaths comprises, most posteriorly, the pharynx and its distal continuation – the oesophagus. The pharyngo-oesophageal junction, as has been noted, is typically at the level of the lower border of the cricoid cartilage (corresponding to the level of the lower border of the 6th cervical vertebra).

Situated in front of the pharynx and oesophagus are, respectively, the larynx and trachea; the laryngotracheal junction being at the same horizontal level as the pharyngo-oesophageal junction. Lying astride the anterior aspect of the upper trachea is the thyroid isthmus, which on either side of the midline is continuous with the corresponding thyroid lobe. The entire thyroid gland is enveloped in a further layer of deep cervical fascia termed the *pretracheal fascia*. The pretracheal fascia is itself firmly adherent to the front of the upper trachea behind the isthmus and, elsewhere, to the sides of the cricoid and thyroid cartilages. Indeed, the encasement of the thyroid by the pretracheal fascia and the attachment of the latter to the trachea and laryngeal cartilages account for the clinical observation that all thyroid swellings move upwards during the second phase of swallowing. During this phase of swallowing, the larynx and trachea ascend. The thyroid gland contained within the pretracheal fascia thus moves upwards obligatorily.

Inferiorly, the *pretracheal fascia* continues as a thin layer to fuse with the anterior surface of the fibrous pericardium.

The cervical lymph nodes may be broadly categorized into two sets:

1 superficial cervical lymph nodes (i.e. those that are superficial to the investing layer of deep cervical fascia);
2 deep cervical lymph nodes (i.e. those that are deep to the investing layer of deep cervical fascia).

Each of these categories is further subdivided into groups based on location and territory of drainage.

The fascial planes of the neck are of considerable importance to the surgeon; they form convenient lines of cleavage through which the surgeon may separate the tissues in operative dissections. Also the fascial layers may serve to contain the spread of pus in neck infections.

(Additional points of clinical significance concerning the deep cervical fascia are to be found on page 281.)

To facilitate the description of the topographical anatomy of the neck, the anterior and lateral aspects of the neck are collectively divided into three large triangular regions by the obliquely placed right and left sternocleidomastoid muscles. These three triangles are the centrally placed anterior triangle flanked by the right and left posterior triangles (Fig. 186).

The anterior triangle has the outline of an inverted triangle. The base of the anterior triangle is the lower border of the mandible, the apex is the sternal notch and the two sides (lateral boundaries) of the triangle are the medial (anterior) borders of the right and left sternocleidomastoid muscles.

The posterior triangle on each side has the outline of an upright, somewhat spiralized triangle. The base of the triangle is the upper surface of the middle third of the clavicle. The anterior boundary of the triangle is the lateral (posterior) border of the sternocleidomastoid muscle, while the posterior boundary is the anterior edge of the ipsilateral trapezius muscle. The apex of the triangle is on the superior nuchal line, a few centimetres medial to the base of the mastoid process where the posterior border of sternocleidomastoid and the anterior edge of trapezius are practically contiguous.

Note that the anterior border of sternocleidomastoid forms the lateral boundary of the anterior triangle, and the posterior border of sternocleidomastoid forms the anterior boundary of the posterior triangle. The width of the muscle between its anterior and posterior borders thus belongs neither to the anterior nor the posterior triangle. For the most part, it overlaps the carotid sheath.

The anterior triangle can be divided into two symmetrical and equal halves by an imaginary vertical line in the anterior midline running from the symphysis menti above to the midpoint of the sternal notch, below (Fig. 186). Each of these halves may be further subdivided into the digastric (or submandibular) triangle, carotid triangle and muscular triangle (Fig. 186).

The thyroid gland

The thyroid gland is made up of (Fig. 188):

1 the *isthmus* – overlying the 2nd and 3rd rings of the trachea;
2 the right and left *lateral lobes* – each extending from the side of the thyroid cartilage down to the level of the 6th tracheal ring;
3 an inconstant *pyramidal lobe* projecting upwards from the isthmus, usually on the left side, which represents a remnant of the embryological descent of the thyroid.

Relations (Fig. 187)

The gland is enclosed in the pretracheal fascia, in turn covered by the strap muscles and overlapped by the sternocleidomastoids. The anterior jugular veins course over the isthmus. When the thyroid enlarges, the strap muscles stretch and adhere to the

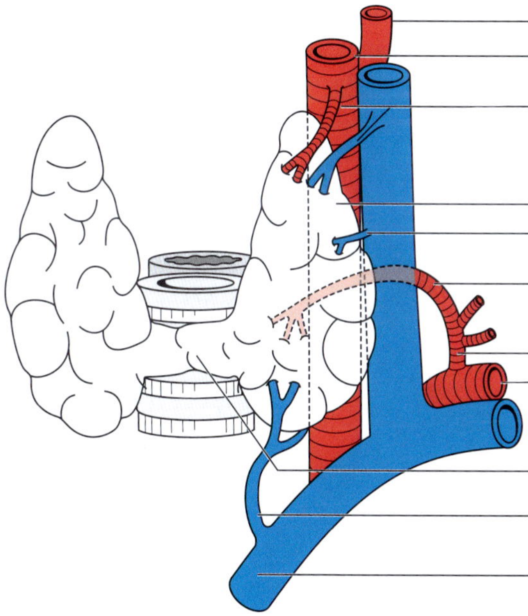

Fig. 188 The thyroid and its blood vessels.

pretracheal fascia covering of the gland so that, at operation, they often appear to be thin layers of fascia.

On the deep aspect of the thyroid lie the larynx and trachea, with the pharynx and oesophagus behind the larynx and trachea and the carotid sheath on either side. Two nerves lie in close relationship to the gland; in the groove between the trachea and oesophagus lies the *recurrent laryngeal nerve*, and deep to the upper pole of the thyroid lies the *external branch* of the *superior laryngeal nerve* passing to the cricothyroid muscle.

Blood supply

The endocrine glands, gram for gram, have the richest blood supply of any tissue in the body; the thyroid gland is no exception to this rule.

Three arteries supply and three veins drain the thyroid gland (Fig. 188):

- the *superior thyroid artery* – arises from the external carotid and passes to the upper pole;
- the *inferior thyroid artery* – arises from the thyrocervical trunk of the 1st part of the subclavian artery and passes behind the carotid sheath to the back of the gland;
- the *thyroidea ima artery* – is inconstant; when present, it arises from the aortic arch or the brachiocephalic artery and runs upwards to the inferior aspect of the gland;
- the *superior thyroid vein* – drains the upper pole to the internal jugular vein;
- the *middle thyroid vein* – drains from the lateral side of the gland to the internal jugular;
- the *inferior thyroid veins* – often several; drain the lower poles and isthmus of the thyroid to the brachiocephalic veins.

As well as these named branches, numerous small vessels pass to the thyroid from the pharynx and trachea so that, even when all the main vessels are tied, the gland still bleeds when cut across during a partial or subtotal thyroidectomy.

Development

The thyroid develops from a bud, which pushes downwards from the fetal tongue (see Fig. 198). This outgrowth, termed the thyroglossal duct, then descends to its definitive position in the neck. The lower end of the thyroglossal duct proliferates to become the thyroid gland, while the rest of the thyroglossal duct disintegrates and disappears. The site of origin of the thyroglossal duct is, however, indicated by the *foramen caecum*, the midline punctum at the junction of the middle and posterior thirds of the tongue. The inconstant *pyramidal lobe* on the isthmus is a remnant of the distal end of the thyroglossal duct (Fig. 189).

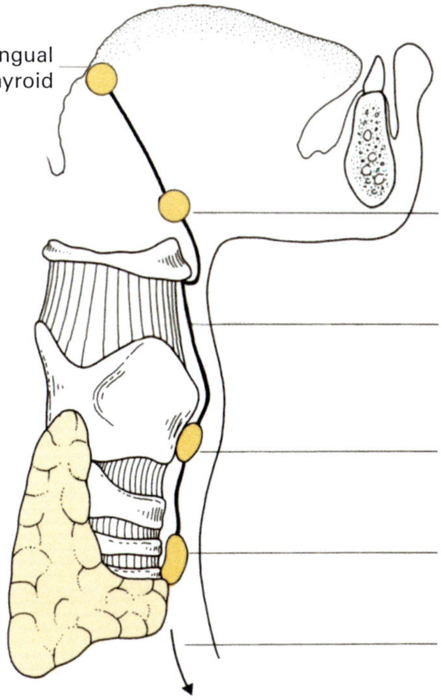

Fig. 189 The descent of the thyroid, showing possible sites of ectopic thyroid tissue or thyroglossal cysts, and also the course of a thyroglossal fistula. (The arrow shows the further descent of the thyroid that may take place retrosternally into the superior mediastinum.)

CLINICAL FEATURES

1 The embryological development of the thyroid accounts for the rare occurrence of the whole or a part of the gland remaining as a swelling at the tongue base (*lingual thyroid*) and for the much commoner occurrence of a *thyroglossal cyst* or *sinus* along the pathway of descent. Such a sinus can be dissected from the midline of the neck along the front of the hyoid (in such intimate contact with the hyoid that the centre of the hyoid must be excised during the dissection) then backwards through the muscles of the tongue to the foramen caecum (Fig. 189).

Descent of the thyroid may go beyond the normal position in the neck down into the superior mediastinum (*retrosternal goitre*).

2 A benign enlargement of the thyroid may compress or displace any of the structures in its immediate vicinity. Thus, the trachea and oesophagus may be narrowed, with resulting difficulty in breathing and swallowing, and the carotid sheath may be displaced posteriorly. A carcinoma of the thyroid tends to invade its neighbours rather than displace them – thereby infiltrating the trachea or oesophagus or invading the carotid sheath and occasionally causing severe haemorrhage therefrom. The recurrent

laryngeal nerve and the cervical sympathetic chain may be involved, resulting in dysphonia and Horner's syndrome, respectively.

3 We have already noted, in dealing with the fasciae of the neck, that the thyroid gland is enclosed in the pretracheal fascia. This thyroid capsule is much denser in front than behind and the enlarging gland therefore tends to push backwards, burying itself round the sides and even the back of the trachea and oesophagus. Because of the attachments of the pretracheal fascia that envelops the thyroid, a large goitre may also extend downwards into the superior mediastinum ('plunging goitre').

As stated earlier, the pretracheal fascia's attachment to the larynx accounts for the upward movement of the thyroid gland with each act of swallowing.

4 *Thyroidectomy* is carried out through a transverse 'collar' incision, two fingers' breadth above the suprasternal notch. This lies in the line of the natural skin folds of the neck. Skin flaps are reflected, together with platysma, and the investing fascia is opened longitudinally between the strap muscles and between the anterior jugular veins.

If more room is required in the case of a large goitre, the strap muscles are divided; this is carried out at their upper extremity because their nerve supply (the ansa cervicalis) enters the lower part of the muscles and is hence preserved.

The pretracheal fascia is then divided, exposing the thyroid gland; unless this tissue plane deep to the fascia is found, dissection is a difficult and bloody procedure.

The thyroid is then mobilized and its vessels ligated seriatim. Both the recurrent and superior laryngeal nerves are at risk during this procedure and must be carefully avoided (Fig. 190).

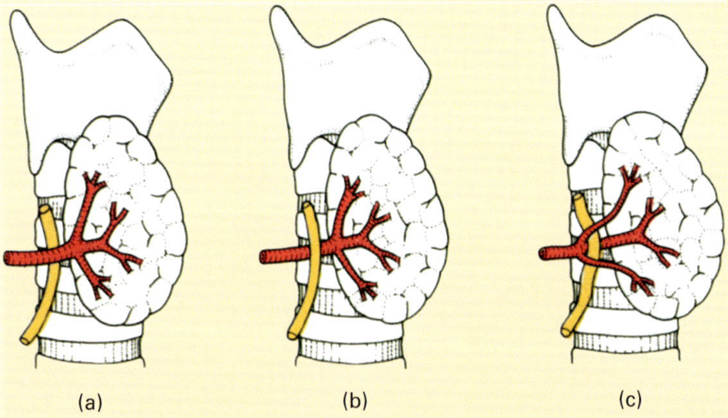

Fig. 190 The relationship of the recurrent laryngeal nerve to the thyroid gland and the inferior thyroid artery. (a) The nerve is usually deep to the artery but may be (b) superficial to it or (c) pass through its branches. In these diagrams the lateral lobe of the thyroid is pulled forwards, as it would be in a thyroidectomy.

The parathyroid glands (Fig. 191)

These are usually four in number, a superior and inferior on either side; however, the numbers vary from two to six. Ninety per cent are in close relationship to the thyroid, 10% are aberrantly located, the latter most commonly being the inferior glands.

Each gland is about the size of a split pea and is of a yellowish-brown colour. The superior parathyroid is more constant in position than the inferior gland. It usually lies a third of the way up from the lower pole on the posterior border of the thyroid lobe, just above the level at which the inferior thyroid artery crosses the recurrent laryngeal nerve. The inferior parathyroid is usually situated below the inferior thyroid artery near the lower pole of the thyroid gland. The next most common site, however, is within 1.25 cm (0.5 in) inferior to the lower pole of the thyroid gland. Aberrant inferior parathyroids may descend along the inferior thyroid veins in front of the trachea and may even track into the superior mediastinum in company with thymic tissues, for which there is an embryological explanation (see next section). Less commonly, the inferior gland may lie behind and outside the fascial sheath of the thyroid and be found behind the oesophagus or even in the posterior mediastinum. Only on extremely rare occasions are the glands actually completely buried within thyroid tissue (Fig. 192). All four parathyroid glands receive their blood supply, principally, from the pair of *inferior thyroid arteries*. The superior thyroid arteries play a much smaller role in the supply of the parathyroids. The venous drainage of the parathyroids is to the inferior and middle thyroid veins.

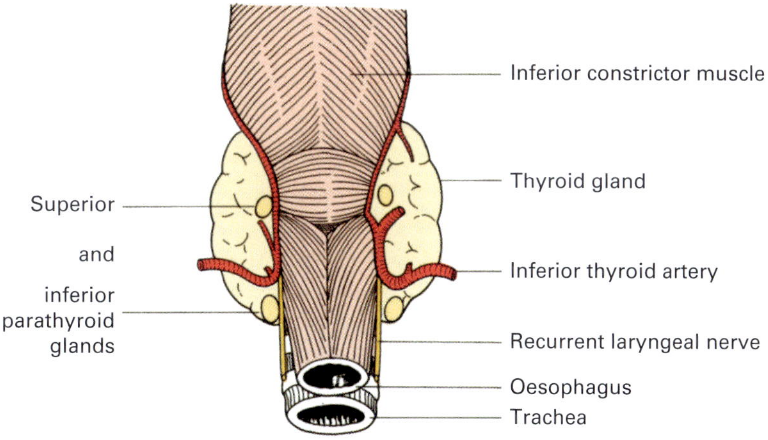

Fig. 191 The normal sites of the parathyroid glands (posterior aspect).

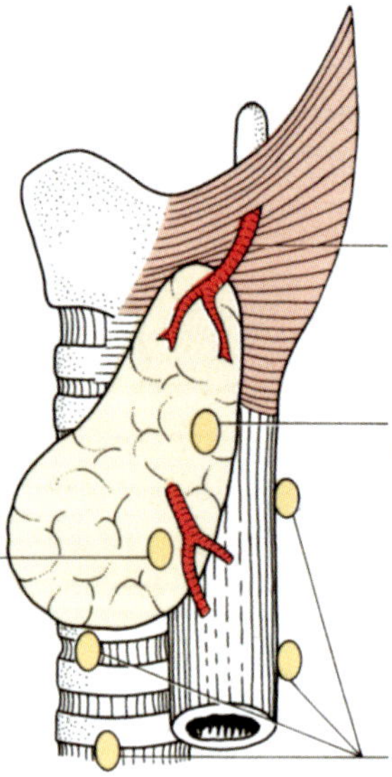

Fig. 192 Normal and abnormal sites of the parathyroid glands (lateral view).

Development

The superior parathyroids differentiate from the 4th pharyngeal (branchial) pouch. The inferior glands develop from the 3rd pouch in company with the thymus (Fig. 193; see Table 4, page 332). As the latter descends, the inferior parathyroids are dragged down with it.

It is thus easily understood that the inferior parathyroid may be dragged beyond the thyroid into the mediastinum and explains why, although very rarely, parathyroid tissue is found actually within the thymus.

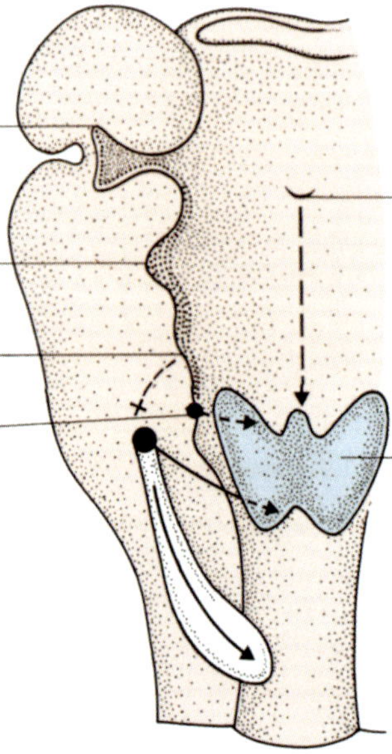

Fig. 193 The derivatives of the branchial pouches. Note that the inferior parathyroid migrates downwards from the 3rd pouch, whereas the superior parathyroid (derived from the 4th pouch) has a much shorter course of travel.

CLINICAL FEATURES

1 These possible aberrant sites are, of course, of great importance when searching for a 'hidden' parathyroid adenoma in hyperparathyroidism.
2 The parathyroids are usually safe in subtotal thyroidectomy because the posterior rim of the thyroid is preserved in this operation. However, they may be inadvertently removed or damaged, with resultant tetany due to the lowered serum calcium.

The palate

The palate separates the nasal and buccal cavities and comprises:

1 the *hard palate* – which is vault-shaped and made up of the palatine plate of the maxilla and the horizontal plate of the palatine bone; it is bounded by the alveolar margin anteriorly and laterally, and merges posteriorly with;
2 the *soft palate* – hanging as a curtain between the naso- and oropharynx; centrally, it bears the *uvula* on its free posterior edge; laterally, it blends into the palatoglossal and palatopharyngeal arches (respectively, the anterior and posterior pillars of the fauces).

The hard palate is made up of bone, periosteum and a squamous mucosa in which are embedded tiny accessory salivary glands.

The framework of the soft palate is formed by the aponeurosis of the tensor palati muscle, which adheres to the posterior border of the hard palate. To this fibrous sheet are attached the palatine muscles covered by a mucous membrane, whose epithelial lining is stratified squamous on its inferior (oral) aspect and ciliated columnar on its superior (nasopharyngeal) surface.

The sensory supply of the palate is largely from the maxillary division of V, but fibres of IX supply its most posterior part.

Motor innervation to the palatine muscles is from vagus (X) fibres in the pharyngeal plexus (with the qualification that the vagus derives these motor nerve fibres from XI, the cranial accessory nerve). The tensor palati is the exception to this rule and is supplied by the mandibular division of V.

In speaking, swallowing and blowing, the soft palate closes off the nasopharynx from the buccal cavity. If the palate is paralysed, as may occur in brainstem lesions or after diphtheria, the voice is impaired and swallowed fluids may be directed, in part, to the nasopharynx and thereby into the nasal cavity.

The development of the face, lips and palate with special reference to their congenital deformities

(Fig. 194)

Around the primitive mouth, or stomodaeum, develop the following:

1 the *frontonasal process*, which projects down from the cranium. Two olfactory pits develop in it and rupture into the pharynx to form the nostrils. Definitively, this process forms the nose, the nasal septum, nostrils, the philtrum of the upper lip

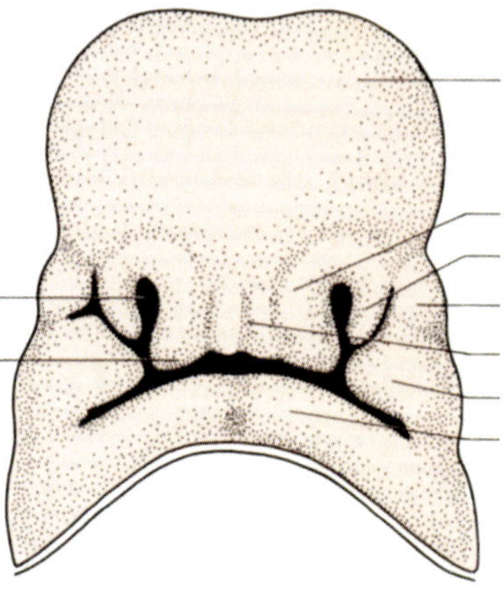

Fig. 194 The ventral aspect of a fetal head showing the three processes, frontonasal, maxillary and mandibular, from which the face, nose and jaws are derived.

(the small midline depression) and the premaxilla – the V-shaped anterior portion of the upper jaw which usually bears the four incisor teeth;

2 the *maxillary processes* on each side, which fuse with the frontonasal process and become the cheeks, upper lip (excluding the philtrum), upper jaw and palate (apart from the premaxilla);

3 the *mandibular processes*, which meet in the midline to form the lower jaw.

Abnormalities of this complex fusion process are numerous and constitute one of the commonest groups of congenital deformities. It is estimated that one child in 600 in England is born with some degree of either cleft lip or cleft palate (Fig. 195).

Frequently, these anomalies are associated with other congenital conditions such as spina bifida or syndactyly (fusion of fingers or toes). Indeed, it is always sound clinical practice to search for additional anomalies elsewhere in the body, when faced with a patient presenting with a congenital defect.

The following anomalies are associated with defects of fusion of the face:

1 *Macrostoma* and *microstoma* are conditions in which either too little or too great a closure of the stomodaeum occurs.

2 *Cleft upper lip* (or 'hare lip') – this is only very rarely like the upper lip of a hare, i.e. a median cleft, although this may occur as a failure of development of the philtrum from the frontonasal process. Much more commonly, the cleft is on one or both sides of the philtrum, occurring as failure of fusion of the maxillary and frontonasal processes. The cleft may be a small defect in the lip or may extend into the nostril, split the alveolus or even extend along the side of the nose as far as the orbit. There may be an associated cleft palate.

3 *Cleft lower lip* – occurs very rarely but may be associated with a cleft tongue and cleft mandible.

4 *Cleft palate* is a failure of fusion of the segments of the palate. The following stages may occur (Fig. 195):

a bifid uvula, of no clinical importance;

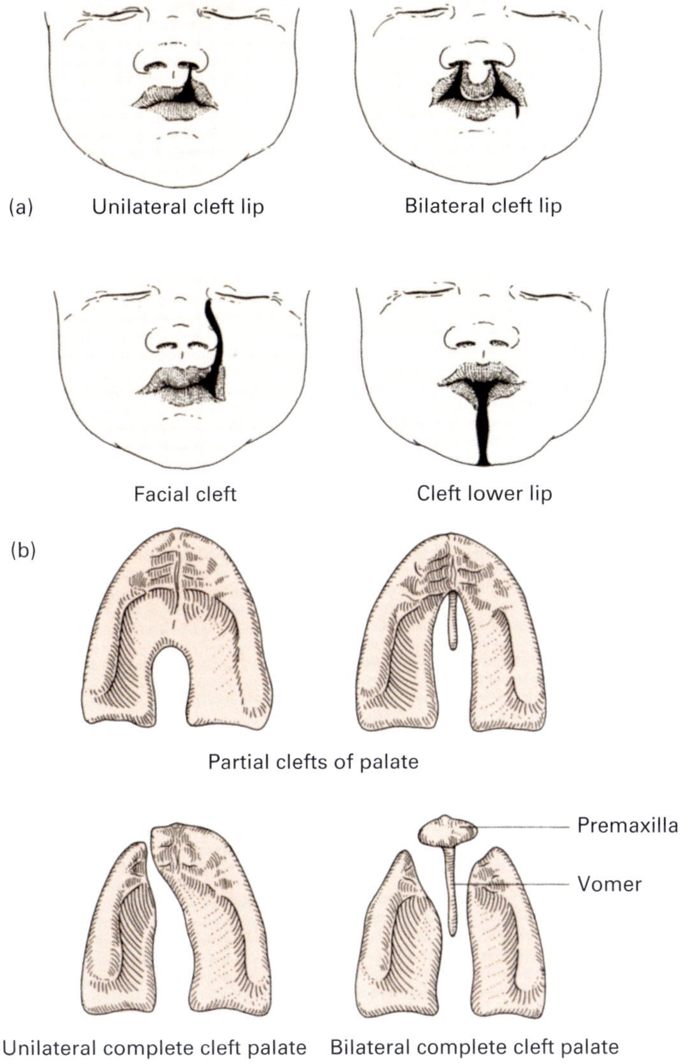

Fig. 195 Types of (a) cleft lip and (b) cleft palate.

b partial cleft, which may involve the soft palate only or the posterior part of the hard palate also;

c complete cleft, which may be unilateral, running the full length of the maxilla and then alongside one edge of the premaxilla, or bilateral, in which the palate is cleft with an anterior V separating the premaxilla completely.

5 *Inclusion dermoids* may form along the lines of fusion of the face. The most common of these is the *external angular dermoid* at the lateral extremity of the upper eyebrow. Occasionally, this dermoid extends through the skull to attach to the underlying dura.

The oral cavity, tongue and floor of the mouth

The oral cavity

The oral cavity extends from the lips to the oropharyngeal isthmus (the interval between the right and left palatoglossal arches). It is conventionally described as having an outer part, *the vestibule*, which lies outside the alveolar processes of the upper and lower jaws but inside the lips and cheek, and a larger part inside the alveolar processes, *the oral cavity proper*. The entire oral cavity is lined with stratified squamous epithelium. Opening into the oral cavity are the ducts of the three paired, major salivary glands; the parotid, submandibular and sublingual glands. The parotid ducts open into the vestibule, the parotid duct orifice being located in the cheek mucosa opposite the crown of the ipsilateral upper second molar tooth. The submandibular and sublingual ducts have their openings in the floor of the mouth within the oral cavity proper. Scattered within the mucosa of the entire oral cavity are numerous islands of glandular tissue, the minor salivary glands. The entire mucosa of the oral cavity (vestibule and oral cavity proper) derives its sensory innervation from the mandibular and maxillary divisions of the trigeminal nerve.

The tongue

The tongue is a thick, mobile mass of skeletal (voluntary) muscle covered all over by stratified squamous epithelium. It lies partly in the oral cavity and partly in the oropharynx. The tongue is the principal organ of taste, besides being a most useful aid in the act of chewing and swallowing food. It is also indispensable to articulate speech; a function that is not sufficiently appreciated. In shape the tongue has an approximately elliptical outline and may be described as having a tip or apex as its anterior extremity. The apex is the most mobile part of the tongue. The posterior extremity of the tongue is termed the *root of the tongue,* which is the least mobile part, being anchored to the upper aspect of the hyoid bone. Between the root and apex are the right and left lateral margins of the tongue which meet at the apex and which demarcate the dorsal surface of the tongue from the ventral surface. The former faces the roof of the oral cavity, while the latter faces the floor. The dorsal surface of the tongue features a V-shaped groove, the *sulcus terminalis*, the apex of the 'V' being located posteriorly. At the apex of the sulcus terminalis is a shallow depression, the *foramen caecum*, marking the embryological origin of the thyroid (see page 288; Fig. 193). Immediately in front of and parallel to the V-shaped sulcus lies a row of large vallate (circumvallate) papillae. The row of vallate papillae demarcates the anterior two-thirds of the tongue (oral part of the tongue) from the posterior one-third (pharyngeal part of the tongue). Interestingly, these two parts have different embryological derivations. They also have different sensory innervations with practically no overlap. Also, the lymphatic drainage from these two parts is to different destinations (lymph node stations). The row of vallate papillae, lying in the presulcal area, belongs to the posterior third of the tongue (based on sensory innervation and lymphatic drainage).

The inferior (ventral) aspect of the tongue bears a median fold, the *frenulum linguae*; the mucosa is thin on this surface and the lingual veins can thus be seen on either side of the frenulum. The lingual nerve and the lingual artery are medial to the vein but not visible. More laterally can be seen a fringed fold of mucous membrane termed the *plica fimbriata*. On either side of the base of the frenulum can be seen the orifice of the submandibular duct surmounting a papilla. Inspect this in a mirror and note the discharge of saliva when you press on your submandibular gland just below the angle of the jaw.

Structure

The thick stratified squamous mucosa of the dorsum of the tongue bears papillae over the anterior two-thirds back as far as the sulcus terminalis. These papillae (particularly the vallate) bear the taste buds. The posterior one-third of the tongue behind the sulcus terminalis has no papillae but carries numerous lymphoid nodules which, with the palatine tonsils and adenoids, make up the *lymphoid ring of Waldeyer*.

Small glands are scattered throughout the submucosa of the dorsum; these are predominantly serous anteriorly and mucous posteriorly.

The tongue is divided by a median vertical fibrous septum, indicated on the dorsal surface by a shallow longitudinal groove. On each side of this septum are the intrinsic and extrinsic muscles of the tongue (Fig. 196).

The *intrinsic muscles* are disposed in vertical, longitudinal and transverse bundles; they serve to alter the shape of the tongue.

The *extrinsic muscles* move the tongue as a whole. They pass to the tongue from the symphysis of the mandible, the hyoid, styloid process and the soft palate; respectively, the *genioglossus*, *hyoglossus*, *styloglossus* and *palatoglossus*. The functions of the individual extrinsic muscles can be deduced from their relative positions (Fig. 196). Genioglossus protrudes the tongue, styloglossus retracts it and hyoglossus depresses

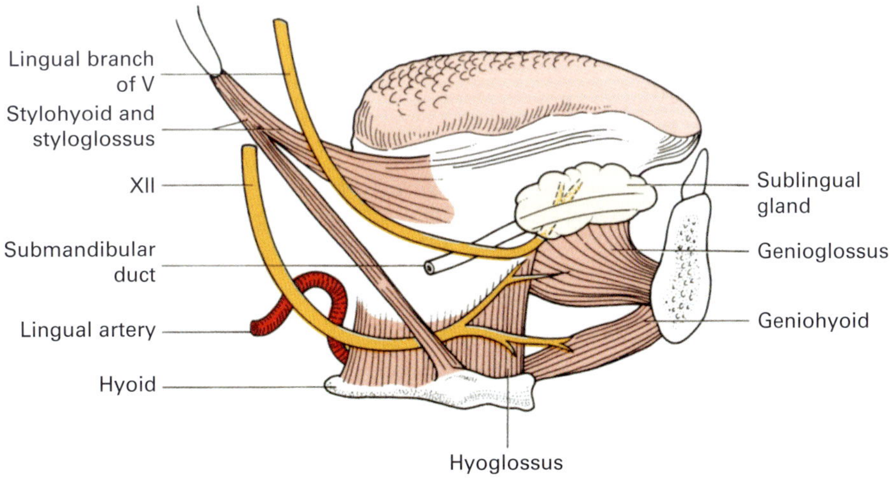

Fig. 196 Lateral view of the tongue, its extrinsic muscles and its nerves.

it. Palatoglossus is, in fact, a palatal muscle and helps to narrow the oropharyngeal isthmus during swallowing.

Blood supply

Blood supply to the tongue is principally from the lingual branch of the external carotid artery. There is minimal crossover of blood supply from one side to the other, across the median raphe (septum), which is therefore a relatively avascular plane.

Lymphatic drainage (Fig. 197)

The drainage zones of the mucosa of the tongue can be grouped into three:

1 the tip of the tongue drains to the submental nodes;

2 the anterior two-thirds of the tongue drains to the submental and submandibular nodes and thence to the *lower* nodes of the deep cervical chain (jugular lymph nodes) along the carotid sheath;

3 the posterior one-third of the tongue drains to the *upper* nodes of the deep cervical chain and also to the deeply situated parapharyngeal and retropharyngeal nodes.

Within the posterior one-third of the tongue, there is a rich anastomosis of lymphatic channels across the midline between the two sides so that a tumour on one side readily metastasizes to contralateral nodes. In contrast, there is little crossover of lymphatic channels from one side to the other, in the anterior two-thirds, where growths more than 1.25 cm (0.5 in) from the midline do not metastasize to the opposite side of the neck until late in the disease.

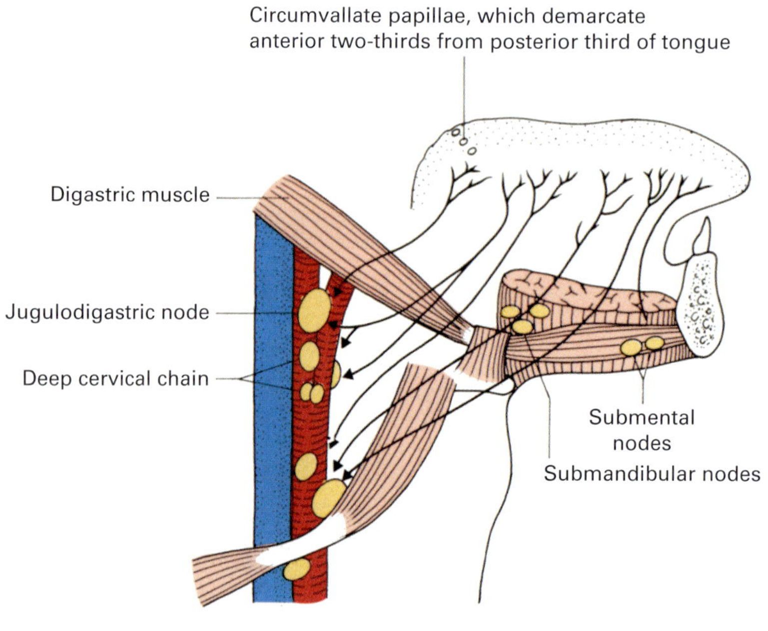

Fig. 197 The lymphatic drainage of the tongue. Note two points. (i) The anterior part of the tongue tends to drain to the nodes farthest down the deep cervical chain, whereas the posterior part drains to the upper chain. (ii) The anterior two-thirds of the tongue drain unilaterally, the posterior one-third bilaterally.

Nerve supply

The anterior two-thirds of the tongue receives its sensory supply from the lingual branch of V (subserving common sensation); the lingual nerve also conveys the gustatory fibres of the chorda tympani (VII) to the gustatory receptors on the anterior two-thirds of the tongue.

The sensory innervation of the posterior one-third of the tongue, including the region of the vallate papillae, both for common sensation and taste perception, is derived from the glossopharyngeal nerve (IX). A few fibres of the internal laryngeal branch of the superior laryngeal nerve (branch of X) carry sensory fibres from the very posterior part of the tongue.

On each side of the midline, all the intrinsic and extrinsic muscles of the tongue except palatoglossus are supplied by the ipsilateral hypoglossal nerve (XII); palatoglossus, a muscle of the soft palate, is innervated by the pharyngeal branch of the vagus (X).

Development (Fig. 198)

A small nodule, the *tuberculum impar*, is the first evidence of the developing tongue in the floor of the primitive pharynx. This is soon covered over by the *lingual swellings*, one on each side, derived from the first branchial arch. These fuse in the midline to form the definitive anterior two-thirds of the tongue supplied by the lingual nerve (V) and reinforced by the chorda tympani (a branch of VII).

Posteriorly, this mass meets the *copula* (or *hypobranchial eminence*), a central swelling in the pharyngeal floor that represents the conjunction of the 2nd, 3rd and 4th arches and which forms the posterior one-third of the tongue (nerve supply glossopharyngeal (IX) and vagus (X)).

The tongue muscles develop from the occipital myotomes, which migrate forwards, dragging with them their nerve supply (XII, the hypoglossal nerve).

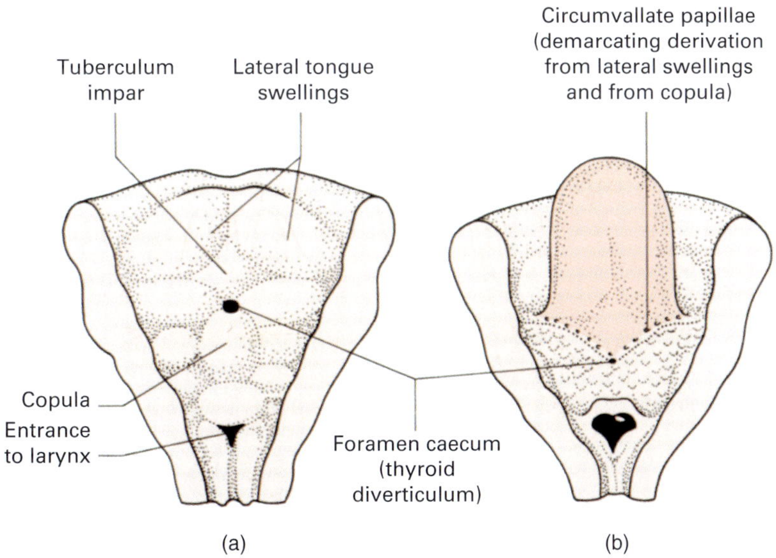

Fig. 198 Stages in the development of the tongue.

CLINICAL FEATURES

1 Damage to the hypoglossal nerve is manifested clinically by eventual hemiatrophy of the ipsilateral side of the tongue, loss of rugosity of the overlying dorsal mucosa and muscle fasciculation. When asked, the patient will find it impossible to protrude the tongue without the tongue deviating to the paralysed side. In terms of function, while the patient may have a degree of difficulty in swallowing, the interference with articulate speech is the far greater disability experienced by the patient.
2 If the unconscious or deeply anaesthetized patient is laid supine, the posterior aspect of the tongue may drop back to produce a laryngeal obstruction. This can be prevented either by lying the patient in the lateral decubitus position with the head down ('the tonsil position'), when the tongue flops forwards with the weight of gravity, or by pushing the mandible forwards by pressure on the angle of the jaw on each side; this is effective because genioglossus, attached to the symphysis menti, drags the tongue forwards along with the lower jaw.
3 Although lymphatics pierce the floor of the mouth (i.e. the mylohyoid muscle) to reach the submental and submandibular lymph nodes, it is an interesting fact that these tissues are not affected by lymphatic spread of malignant cells (although they may be invaded by direct extension of growth). It seems that the nodes are involved by lymphatic emboli and not by a permeation of the lymphatic channels.

   The bilateral lymphatic spread of growths of the posterior one-third of the tongue is one factor contributing to the poor prognosis of tumours at this site.

The floor of the mouth

The floor of the mouth is formed principally by the mylohyoid muscles. These stretch as a diaphragm from their origin along the mylohyoid line on the medial aspect of the body of the mandible on each side, to their insertion along a median raphe and into the hyoid bone. Thus, together, the right and left mylohyoid muscles form a curved, sheet-like sling that supports the tongue (Fig. 199). The mylohyoid muscle is an important surgical landmark insofar as it constitutes the boundary between the neck and oral region.

On the lower (superficial) aspect of this diaphragm, on each side, are the anterior and posterior bellies of the digastric muscle, the superficial part of the submandibular gland and the submandibular lymph nodes, all covered by the investing layer of deep cervical fascia and platysma.

Lying above mylohyoid are the tongue muscles, as a central mass, with the sublingual salivary gland and the deep part of the submandibular gland and its duct lying beneath the mucosa of the mouth floor on either side.

CLINICAL FEATURES

Ludwig's angina is a cellulitis of the floor of the mouth, usually originating from a carious molar tooth. The infection spreads above the mylohyoid; oedema forces the tongue upwards; and the mylohyoid itself is pushed downwards so that there is swelling both below the chin and within the mouth. There is considerable danger of spread of infection backwards with oedema of the glottis and asphyxia.

Drainage is carried out by a deep incision below the mandible that must divide the mylohyoid muscle.

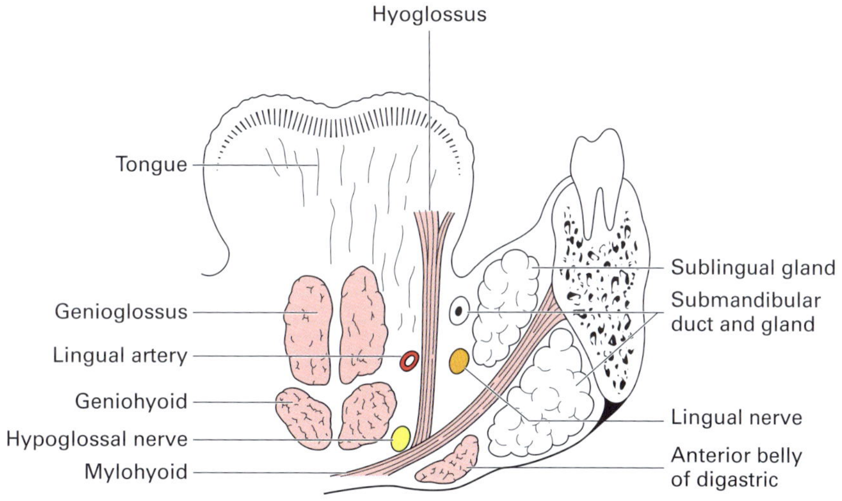

Fig. 199 Coronal section of the floor of the mouth.

The pharynx

The pharynx is a funnel-shaped musculofascial tube, extending from the skull base, superiorly, to the pharyngo-oesophageal junction, inferiorly. It is widely patent anteriorly and acts as a common entrance to the respiratory and alimentary tracts. From above downwards, the pharynx lies successively behind the nasal cavity, the oral cavity and the larynx and communicates with the nasal cavity through the right and left posterior nasal apertures, with the oral cavity through the oropharyngeal isthmus and with the larynx through the laryngeal aditus.

Based on this topographical relationship, the pharynx is described as being made up of three parts (Fig. 200). From above downwards these are:

1 the *nasopharynx* – lying behind the posterior nasal apertures and above the soft palate, its vertical extent being from the basiocciput above to the uvula below;

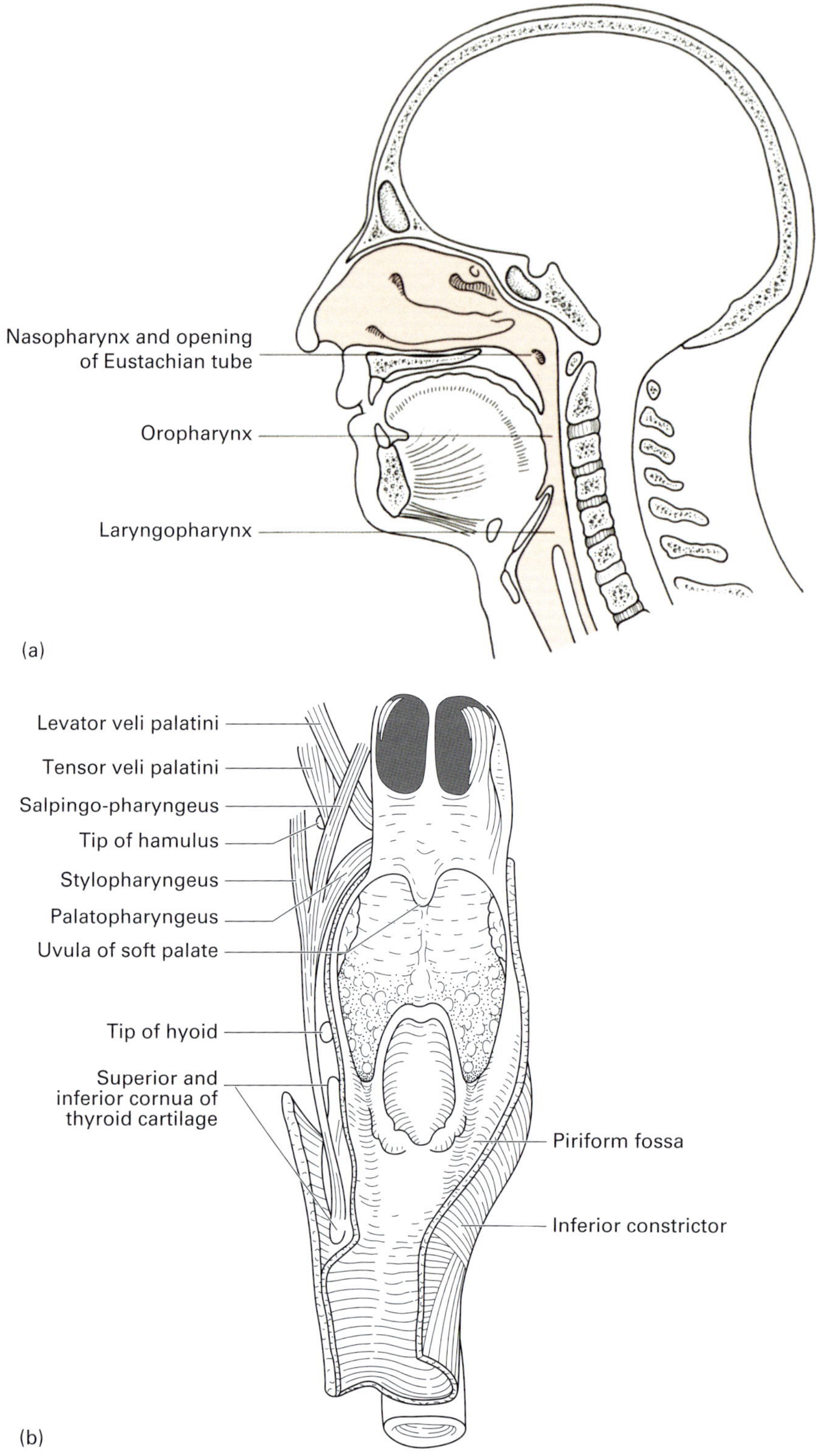

Fig. 200 (a) Schematic sagittal section through the head and neck to show the subdivisions of the pharynx. (b) Interior of the pharynx viewed from behind after removing the posterior wall of the pharynx.

2 the *oropharynx* – lying behind the palatoglossal folds (anterior pillars of the fauces). The vertical extent of the oropharynx is from the tip of the uvula above to the upper margin of the epiglottis below.
3 the *laryngopharynx* – lying behind the larynx, from the level of the upper margin of the epiglottis above to the commencement of the oesophagus below.

The nasopharynx

The nasopharynx (commonly referred to, by ENT surgeons, as the *postnasal space*) lies above the soft palate. The latter temporarily shuts off the nasopharynx from the rest of the pharynx during deglutition and thereby prevents regurgitation of food and drink into the nose.

Two important structures lie in the nasopharynx.

The *nasopharyngeal tonsil* ('the *adenoids*') consists of a collection of lymphoid tissue beneath the epithelium of the roof and posterior wall of this region. It helps to form a continuous lymphoid ring (*Waldeyer's ring*) with the palatine tonsils and the lymphoid nodules on the dorsum of the tongue (the so-called lingual tonsil).

The *orifice of the pharyngotympanic or auditory tube* (*Eustachian canal*) lies on the side-wall of the nasopharynx level with the inferior concha of the nasal cavity. The posterior lip of this opening is prominent, due to the underlying cartilage of the Eustachian tube, and is termed the *Eustachian* or *pharyngeal cushion*, behind which lies the slit-like *nasopharyngeal recess*.

CLINICAL FEATURES

1 The nasopharynx may be inspected indirectly by a mirror passed through the mouth (posterior rhino-pharyngoscopy). These days, however, excellent and detailed views of the nasal cavity and the entire pharynx may be obtained by fibreoptic naso-endoscopy, done as a relatively simple and straightforward outpatient procedure, without anaesthesia.
2 The nasopharyngeal tonsils (adenoids) are prominent in children but usually undergo atrophy after puberty. When chronically inflamed they may all but fill the nasopharynx, causing mouth-breathing and also, by blocking the opening of the auditory tube, deafness and middle ear infection.
3 The Eustachian tube provides a ready pathway of sepsis from the pharynx to the middle ear and accounts for the frequency with which otitis media is the result of throat infections.
4 The middle ear can be intubated through a catheter passed into the Eustachian tube. The catheter is passed along the nasal floor to the posterior wall of the nasopharynx. Its curved tip is then rotated laterally so that it lies in the pharyngeal recess; it is then withdrawn over the Eustachian cushion to slip into the orifice of the auditory tube.

The oropharynx

This part of the pharynx lies behind the mouth and tongue. Its anterior boundaries are the right and left palatoglossal arches (anterior pillars of the fauces), and it extends from the uvula of the soft palate above to the tip of the epiglottis below. Its most important contents are the palatine tonsils, situated in the lateral wall on either side. The interval between the right and left palatoglossal arches is termed the *oropharyngeal isthmus* and marks the junction between the oral cavity in front and the oropharynx behind. The posterior third of the tongue and the pre-epiglottic space thus belong to the oropharynx.

The palatine tonsils

The palatine tonsil lies in the *tonsillar fossa* between the palatoglossal and palatopharyngeal arches (anterior and posterior pillars of the fauces, respectively). The anterior pillar, or *palatoglossal arch*, forms the boundary between the buccal cavity and the oropharynx; it fuses with the lateral wall of the tongue and contains the palatoglossus muscle. The posterior pillar, or *palatopharyngeal arch*, blends with the wall of the pharynx and contains the palatopharyngeus muscle (Fig. 201).

The floor of the tonsillar fossa is formed by the superior constrictor of the pharynx separated from the tonsil by the *tonsillar capsule*, which is a thick condensation of the pharyngeal submucosa (the pharyngobasilar fascia). This capsule is itself separated from the superior constrictor by a film of loose areolar tissue.

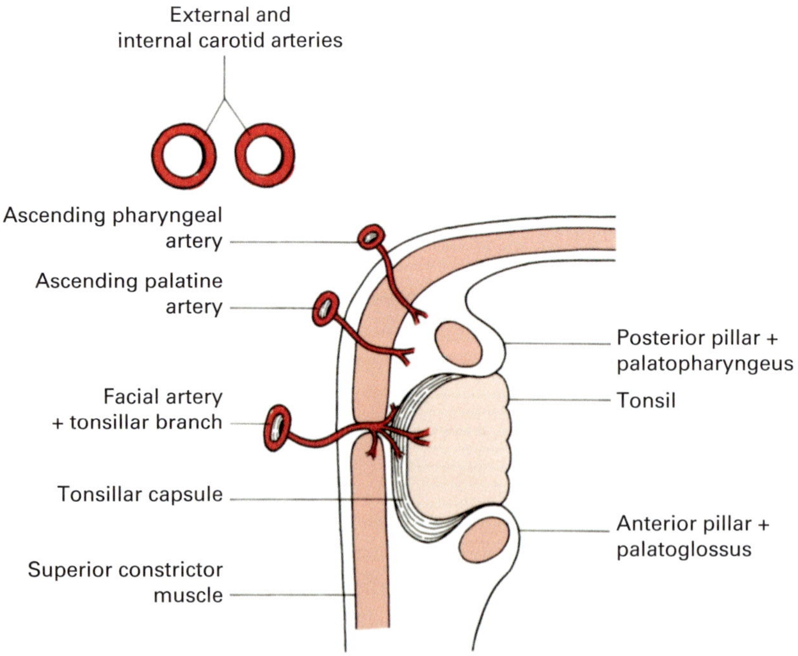

Fig. 201 Diagram of the palatine tonsil and its relations – in horizontal section.

The palatine tonsil consists of a collection of lymphoid tissue covered medially by stratified squamous epithelium. This epithelium is pitted by *crypts*, up to twenty in number, and often bears a deep *intratonsillar cleft* in its upper part.

The lymphoid material may extend up to the soft palate, down to the tongue or into the anterior faucial pillar. From late puberty onwards this lymphoid tissue undergoes progressive atrophy.

Blood supply is principally from the tonsillar branch of the facial artery entering at the lower pole of the tonsil, although twigs are also derived from the lingual, ascending palatine and ascending pharyngeal arteries.

The venous drainage passes to the pharyngeal plexus. An important constant vein, the *paratonsillar vein*, descends from the soft palate across the lateral aspect of the tonsillar capsule. It is nearly always divided in tonsillectomy and may give rise to troublesome intraoperative, or even post-operative, haemorrhage.

Lymphatic drainage is via lymphatics that pierce the superior constrictor muscle and pass to the nodes along the internal jugular vein, especially the *tonsillar or jugulodigastric node* at the angle of the jaw. This node is often affected in tonsillitis, and tonsillitis being a very common affliction, the jugulodigastric lymph node is among the commoner nodes to undergo pathological enlargement.

Embryologically, the tonsil is derived from the second branchial pouch (Fig. 193).

CLINICAL FEATURES

1 *Tonsillectomy* may be carried out by dissection or by the guillotine method; both depend on removing the lymphoid tissue and underlying fascial capsule from the loose areolar tissue clothing the inside of the superior constrictor in the floor of the tonsillar fossa. In dissection, an incision is made in the mucosa of the anterior pillar immediately in front of the tonsil; the gland is then freed by blunt dissection until it remains attached only by its pedicle of vessels near its lower pole. This pedicle is then crushed and divided by means of a wire snare.

   In the second method, the guillotine is applied so that the tonsil bulges through the ring in the instrument. The tonsil is then removed by closing the blade of the guillotine.

   Unless there have been repeated infections, the superior constrictor lies separated from the palatine tonsil and its capsule by loose areolar tissue that prevents the pharyngeal wall being dragged into danger during tonsillectomy.

   Similarly, the internal carotid artery, although only 2.5 cm (1 in) postero-lateral to the tonsil, is safe from injury in this operation since it lies separated from the pharyngeal wall by a layer of fatty tissue surrounding the carotid sheath.

2 A *quinsy* is suppuration in the peritonsillar tissue secondary to tonsillitis. It is drained by an incision in the most prominent part of the abscess where softening can be felt.

The laryngopharynx

The laryngopharynx extends from the level of the tip of the epiglottis to the junction of the pharynx with the oesophagus at the level of C6.

The inlet of the larynx, defined by the epiglottis, aryepiglottic folds and the arytenoids, lies anteriorly. The larynx itself bulges into this part of the pharynx leaving a deep recess anterolaterally on either side, the *piriform fossa*, in which ingested sharp foreign bodies (for example, fish bones) may lodge.

The structure of the pharynx

From inside out, the pharynx is made up of mucosa, containing mucus-secreting goblet cells, submucosa, muscle and a loose areolar sheath. The mucosa is lined by pseudostratified, ciliated columnar epithelium in the nasopharynx, but elsewhere, the lining is one of stratified squamous epithelium. Beneath this, the submucosa is thick and fibrous (the *pharyngobasilar fascia*), and it is this layer which forms the capsule of the tonsil.

The three *pharyngeal constrictor muscles* (superior, middle and inferior) are arranged like flower pots stacked one inside the other, but are open in front at the entries of the nasal, buccal and laryngeal cavities.

Each constrictor muscle is attached anteriorly to the side-wall of these cavities and fans out to insert into a median raphe along the posterior aspect of the pharynx, extending from the base of the skull to the oesophagus (Fig. 202).

Covering these muscles is a thin areolar layer continuous with that covering the buccinator and hence is termed the *buccopharyngeal fascia*.

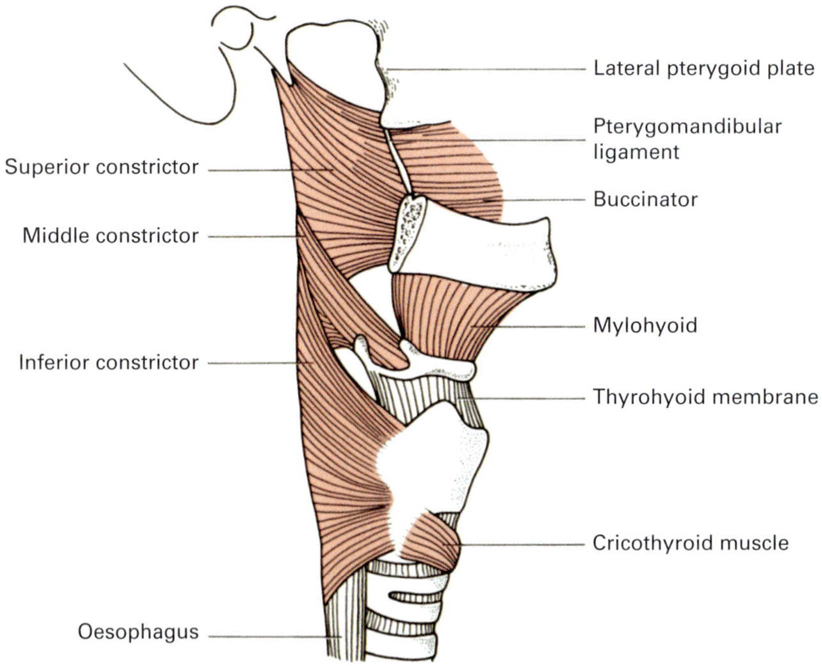

Fig. 202 The constrictor muscles of the pharynx.

Blood supply

The pharynx receives its arterial supply mainly from the superior thyroid and ascending pharyngeal branches of the external carotid.

A pharyngeal venous plexus lies in the areolar tissue that covers the pharynx and drains bilaterally into the internal jugular veins.

Nerve supply

The pharyngeal branches of IX and X constitute the principal sensory and motor supply of the pharynx, respectively. The maxillary division of V supplies the sensory innervation of the nasopharynx.

The mechanism of deglutition

The act of swallowing not only conveys food down the oesophagus but also disposes of mucus with entrapped dust, bacteria and debris from the respiratory passages. Moreover, during deglutition, the Eustachian auditory tube is opened, thus equalizing the pressure on either side of the ear drum.

Deglutition is a complex, orderly series of reflexes. It is initiated voluntarily but is completed by involuntary reflex actions set up by stimulation of the pharynx. If the pharynx is anaesthetized then normal swallowing cannot take place. The reflexes are co-ordinated by the deglutition centre in the medulla, which lies near the vagal nucleus and the respiratory centres.

The food is first crushed by mastication and lubricated by saliva. It is a common experience that it is well-nigh impossible to swallow a pill when the throat is dry. The bolus is then pushed back through the oropharyngeal isthmus by the pressure of the tongue against the palate, assisted by the muscles in the floor of the mouth.

During swallowing, the oral, nasal and laryngeal openings must be closed off to prevent regurgitation of food or fluid through the openings; each of these openings is guarded by a highly effective sphincter mechanism.

The nasopharynx is closed by elevation of the soft palate, which shuts against a contracted ridge of superior pharyngeal constrictor, the *ridge of Passavant*. At the same time, the tensor palati opens the ostium of the Eustachian tube. The oropharyngeal isthmus is partially blocked by contraction of palatoglossus on each side, which narrows the space between the anterior faucial pillars. The residual gap is closed by the dorsum of the tongue wedging into it.

The protection of the larynx is a complex affair, brought about not only by closure of the sphincter mechanism of the larynx but also by tucking the larynx behind the overhanging mass of the tongue and by utilizing the epiglottis to guide the bolus away from the laryngeal entrance. The central nervous component of the swallowing reflex is depressed by narcotics, anaesthesia and cerebral and brainstem trauma. In these circumstances aspiration of foreign material into the tracheobronchial tree is a constant hazard, particularly if the patient is lying supine or in a head-up position.

The laryngeal sphincters are at three levels:

1 the aryepiglottic folds, defining the laryngeal inlet, which are apposed by the aryepiglottic and oblique arytenoid muscles;
2 the walls of the vestibule of the larynx, which are approximated by the thyroepiglottic muscles;
3 the vocal folds, which are closed by the lateral cricoarytenoid and interarytenoid muscles.

The larynx is elevated and pulled forwards by the action of the thyrohyoid, stylohyoid, stylopharyngeus, digastric and mylohyoid muscles so that it comes into apposition with the base of the tongue, which is projecting backwards at this phase. While the larynx is raised and its entrance closed there is reflex inhibition of respiration.

The action of the epiglottis has been the subject of much speculation. As the head of the bolus reaches the epiglottis, the latter is first tipped backwards against the pharyngeal wall and momentarily holds up the onward passage of the food. The larynx is then elevated and pulled forwards, drawing with it the epiglottis so that it now stands erect, guiding the food bolus into streams along both piriform fossae and away from the laryngeal orifice, like a rock sticking up into a waterfall. Finally, the epiglottis is seen indeed to flap backwards as a cover over the laryngeal inlet, but this occurs only after the main bolus has passed beyond it. The epiglottis acts as a laryngeal lid at this stage to prevent deposition of fragments of food debris over the inlet of the larynx during re-establishment of the airway.

The cricopharyngeus then relaxes, allowing the bolus to cross the pharyngo-oesophageal junction. Fluids may shoot down the oesophagus passively under the initial impetus of the tongue action; semi-solid or solid material is carried down by peristalsis. The oesophageal transit time is about 15 seconds, relaxation of the cardia occurring just before the peristaltic wave reaches it. Gravity has little effect on the transit of the bolus, which occurs just as rapidly in the lying as in the erect position. It is, of course, quite easy to swallow fluid or solids while standing on one's head, a well-known party trick; here, oesophageal transit is inevitably an active muscular process.

CLINICAL FEATURES

Pharyngeal pouch

The inferior constrictor muscle is made up of an upper oblique and a lower transverse part, the former arising from the side of the thyroid cartilage (the thyropharyngeus) and the latter from the cricoid (the cricopharyngeus).

Posteriorly, in the midline, there is a potential gap between these two components termed the *pharyngeal dimple* or *Killian's dehiscence*. The mucosa and submucosa of the pharynx may bulge through this weak area to form a pharyngeal pouch (Fig. 203), possibly as a result of muscle incoordination or of spasm of the cricopharyngeus. This diverticulum first protrudes posteriorly; as it enlarges, backward extension is prevented by the prevertebral fascia and it therefore has to project to one or other side of the pharynx – usually to the left.

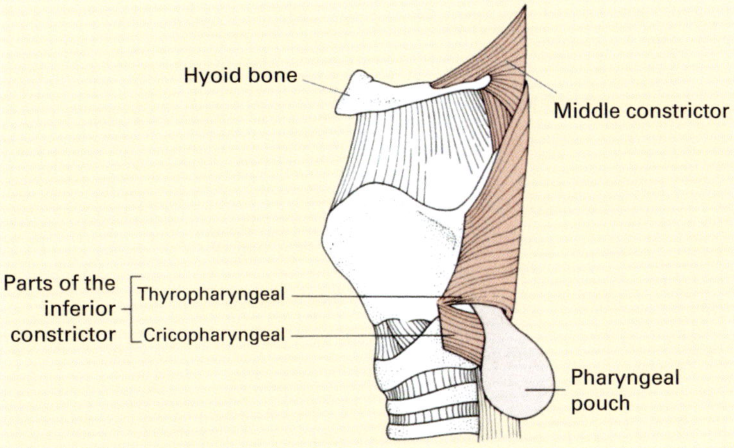

Fig. 203 A pharyngeal pouch emerging between the two components of the inferior constrictor muscle.

With further enlargement, the pouch pushes the oesophagus aside and lies directly in line with the pharynx; most food then passes into the pouch with resultant dysphagia. Spillage of the pouch contents into the larynx is liable to cause inhalation of food material into the bronchi with respiratory infection and lung abscess as possible consequences.

The larynx

The larynx has a triple function: that of an open valve in respiration, that of a partially closed valve whose orifice can be modulated in phonation and that of a closed valve, protecting the trachea and bronchial tree during deglutition. Coughing is possible only when the larynx can be closed effectively.

The structures which form its framework are the epiglottis, thyroid cartilage, cricoid and the arytenoids (Fig. 204).

The larynx is slung from the U-shaped hyoid bone by the *thyrohyoid membrane* and *thyrohyoid muscle*. The hyoid bone itself is attached to the mandible and tongue by the hyoglossus, the mylohyoid, geniohyoid and digastric muscles, to the styloid process by the stylohyoid ligament and muscle and to the pharynx by the middle constrictor. Three of the four strap muscles of the neck, the omohyoid, sternohyoid and thyrohyoid, find attachment to it, only the sternothyroid failing to gain it.

The *epiglottis* is a leaf-shaped elastic cartilage lying behind the root of the tongue. It is attached anteriorly to the body of the hyoid by the hyoepiglottic ligament and below to the back of the thyroid cartilage by the thyroepiglottic ligament immediately above the vocal cords. The sides of the epiglottis are connected to the arytenoids by the

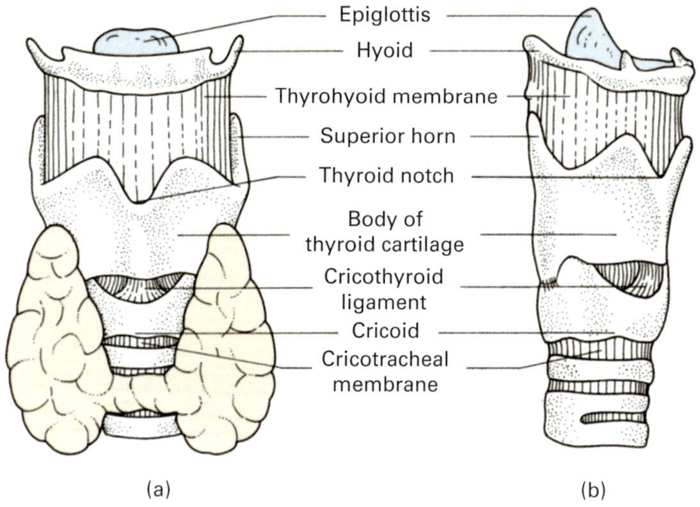

Fig. 204 External view of the larynx. (a) Anterior aspect. (b) Anterolateral aspect (with the thyroid gland removed).

aryepiglottic folds that run backwards to form the margins of the entrance, or *aditus*, of the larynx.

The upper anterior surface of the epiglottis projects above the hyoid bone; the epiglottic mucosa is reflected forwards to the base of the tongue and is raised up into a median glossoepiglottic fold and a pair of lateral pharyngoepiglottic folds. The two depressions, one on either side of the median glossoepiglottic fold, are termed the *valleculae* (see Fig. 206). This pre-epiglottic area including the valleculae is part of the oropharynx.

The *thyroid cartilage* is shield-like, being made up of two lateral plates meeting in the midline in the prominent 'V' of the 'Adam's apple', the laryngeal prominence that is readily visible in most, and palpable in all. It tends to be more prominent in the adult male.

The *cricoid* is signet-ring shaped, deepest behind. It is the only complete ring of cartilage throughout the respiratory tract. Inferiorly, it is attached to the trachea by the *cricotracheal membrane*.

The *arytenoids* sit one on each side of the posterior 'signet' of the cricoid cartilage.

In addition, there are two small nodules of cartilage at the inlet of the larynx; the *corniculate cartilage*, a nodule lying at the apex of the arytenoid, and the *cuneiform cartilage*, a flake of cartilage within the margin of the aryepiglottic fold. These are of no functional importance. They are, however, seen when the larynx is inspected through a laryngoscope (see Fig. 206) and, to the uninitiated, might mimic pathological nodules.

The *cricothyroid membrane* (cricovocal membrane) connects the thyroid, cricoid and arytenoid cartilages. It is composed mainly of yellow elastic tissue. Its upper edge is attached anteriorly to the posterior surface of the thyroid cartilage and behind to the vocal process of the arytenoid. Between these two structures, the upper edge of the membrane is thickened slightly to form the *vocal ligament*. Anteriorly, the membrane thickens, as the *cricothyroid ligament*; this is subcutaneous, easily felt and is used in emergency cricothyroid puncture for laryngeal obstruction.

Passing forwards from the arytenoid to the back of the thyroid cartilage, just below the epiglottic attachment, are two folds of mucosa. The upper is the *vestibular fold*, containing a small amount of fibrous tissue and forming on each side the so-called *false vocal cord*. The lower fold (the *vocal fold* or *cord*) contains the vocal ligament (Fig. 205).

The mucosa is firmly adherent to the vocal ligament without there being any intervening submucosa. This accounts for the pearly white, avascular appearance of the vocal cords as seen on laryngoscopy. Oedema of the larynx cannot involve the true cords since there is no submucous tissue in which fluid can collect. The interval between the right and left vocal cords is the *rima glottidis*. These folds divide the larynx into three zones, as follows:

1 the supraglottic compartment (*vestibule*) lies between the laryngeal inlet and the vestibular folds;
2 the cleft-like interval, on either side, between the vestibular fold and vocal fold is termed the ventricle of the larynx;
3 the subglottic (infraglottic) compartment lies between the vocal folds and the first ring of the trachea.

On either side of the larynx the pharynx forms a recess, the *piriform fossa (piriform recess)* (Fig. 200b).

The muscles of the larynx function to open the glottis in inspiration, close the vestibule and glottis in deglutition and alter the tone of the true vocal cords in phonation.

The cricothyroid (Fig. 202) is the only *intrinsic* laryngeal muscle that lies on the external surface of the thyroid and cricoid cartilages. By its contraction it tenses the vocal cord (the only muscle to do so) by a slight tilting action on the cricoid. It is supplied by the external branch of the superior laryngeal nerve.

The remaining muscles constitute a single encircling sheet whose various attachments are denoted by the names of its separate parts: the thyroarytenoid, posterior and lateral cricoarytenoid, the aryepiglottic, thyroepiglottic and interarytenoid muscles. These are all supplied by the ipsilateral recurrent laryngeal nerve.

All these muscles except one have a sphincter action; the exception is the posterior cricoarytenoid on each side which, by rotating the arytenoids outwards, separates the vocal cords.

Blood supply

The larynx receives a superior and inferior laryngeal artery from the superior and inferior thyroid artery, respectively. These vessels accompany the superior and recurrent laryngeal nerves.

Lymphatic drainage

Above the vocal cords the larynx drains to the upper deep cervical and then to the mediastinal lymph nodes, some lymphatics passing via small nodes lying on the thyrohyoid membrane.

Below the cords, drainage is to the lower deep cervical nodes, partially via nodes on the front of the larynx and trachea.

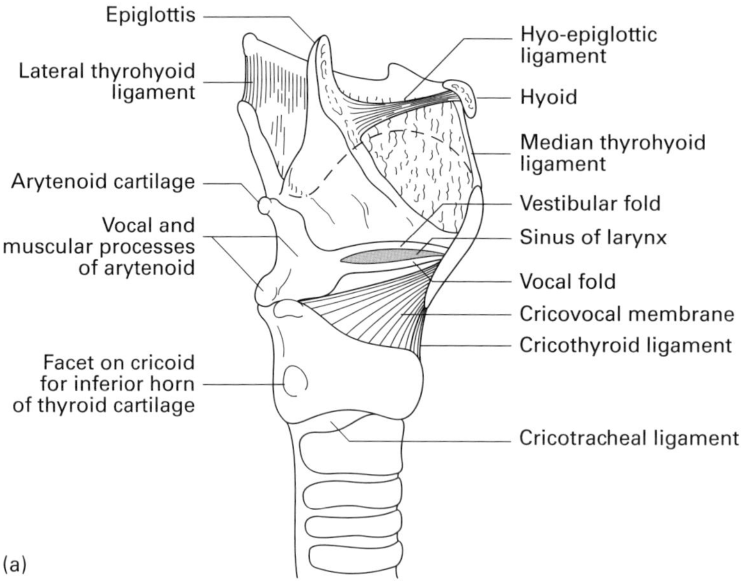

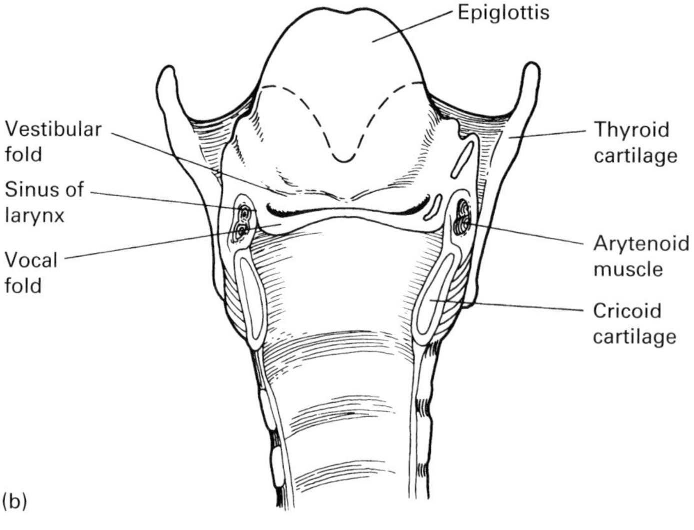

Fig. 205 (a) The internal structure of the larynx – the lamina of the thyroid cartilage has been cut away. (b) The larynx dissected from behind, with cricoid cartilage divided, to show the true and false vocal cords with the sinus of the larynx between. (c) The cartilages and ligaments of the larynx seen from behind (see facing page).

The vocal cords themselves act as a complete barrier separating the two lymphatic areas, but posteriorly there is free communication between them; a laryngeal carcinoma may thus seed throughout the lymphatic drainage area of the larynx.

Nerve supply

The nerve supply of the larynx is of great practical importance and comprises the superior laryngeal nerve and the recurrent laryngeal nerve, both being branches of the vagus nerve (X).

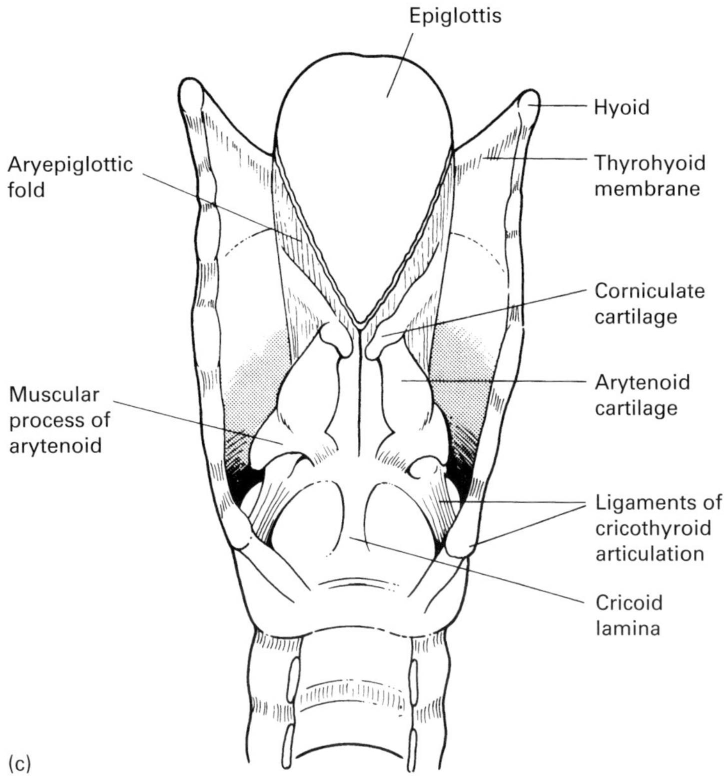

Fig. 205 (*Continued*)

The *superior laryngeal nerve* passes deep to the internal and external carotid arteries where it divides; its internal branch pierces the thyrohyoid membrane together with the superior laryngeal vessels to supply the mucosa of the larynx down to the vocal cords. The external branch passes deep to the superior thyroid artery to supply the cricothyroid muscle.

The *recurrent laryngeal nerve* has a different course on each side. The right arises from the vagus as this crosses the front of the subclavian artery, passes deep to and behind this vessel, then ascends behind the common carotid to lie in the tracheo-oesophageal groove accompanied by the inferior laryngeal vessels. The nerve then passes deep to the inferior constrictor muscle of the pharynx to enter the larynx behind the cricothyroid articulation.

The left nerve arises on the arch of the aorta, winds below and behind it, deep to the ligamentum arteriosum, and ascends to the trachea. It then lies in the tracheo-oesophageal groove and is distributed as on the right side.

The recurrent laryngeal nerves supply all the intrinsic laryngeal muscles, apart from the cricothyroid (supplied by the external branch of the superior laryngeal nerve), and provide the sensory innervation to the mucosa below the vocal cords.

CLINICAL FEATURES

1 The laryngeal nerves bear relationships to the thyroid arteries, which are of considerable practical importance in thyroidectomy. The external branch of the superior laryngeal nerve lies immediately deep to the superior thyroid artery and may be injured when ligating this vessel.

The recurrent laryngeal nerve, lying in the tracheo-oesophageal groove, is usually behind the terminal branches of the inferior thyroid artery. Occasionally, however, the nerve lies in front of these vessels or passes between them (Fig. 190). Moreover, when a large thyroid is pulled forwards during thyroidectomy, the nerve is dragged forwards with it and is therefore placed in further jeopardy. For all these reasons, meticulous care is necessary to avoid injury to the recurrent laryngeal nerve in thyroid surgery.

2 Damage to the superior nerve causes some weakness of phonation owing to the loss of the tightening effect of the cricothyroid muscle on the cord.

3 Complete division of a recurrent laryngeal nerve causes the cord on the affected side to take up the neutral (or paramedian) position between abduction and adduction. Usually the other cord is able to compensate in a remarkable way and speech is not greatly affected; if both nerves are divided, however, the voice is completely lost and breathing becomes difficult through the only partially opened glottis.

4 If the recurrent nerve is only bruised or partially damaged, the abductors (posterior cricoarytenoids) are affected more than the adductors; this is known as *Semon's law*. The affected cord adopts the midline adducted position. In bilateral incomplete paralysis, therefore, the cords come together, stridor is intense and tracheotomy may become essential.

5 The left recurrent laryngeal nerve, in its thoracic course, may become involved in a bronchial or oesophageal carcinoma, or in a mass of enlarged mediastinal nodes, or may become stretched over an aneurysm of the aortic arch. The enlarged left atrium in advanced mitral stenosis may produce a recurrent laryngeal palsy by pushing up the left pulmonary artery which compresses the nerve against the aortic arch.

Either nerve, in the neck, may be damaged by an invasive, expanding thyroid carcinoma or malignant lymph nodes. For these reasons, loss of voice must always be regarded as an ominous symptom requiring careful investigation.

6 The larynx can be inspected either directly, by means of the rigid or fibreoptic laryngoscope, or indirectly through a laryngeal mirror. The base of the tongue, valleculae, epiglottis, aryepiglottic folds and piriform fossae are viewed; then the false cords, which are red and widely apart; then, between these, the pearly white true cords (Fig. 206).

For the passage of the rigid laryngoscope, endotracheal tube or bronchoscope it is essential to know the position which brings the axes of the mouth, oropharynx and laryngeal inlet into line; this is achieved by bringing the neck forwards and at the same time extending the head fully at the atlanto-occipital joint – it is the position in which one sniffs at the fresh air after a long day in the operating theatre.

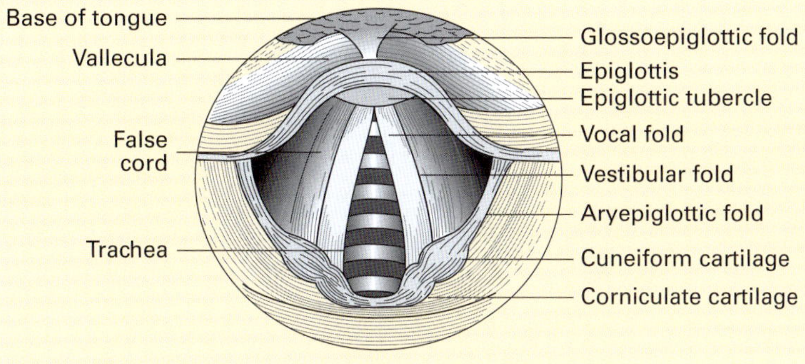

Fig. 206 The larynx as seen at laryngoscopy.

The salivary glands

The salivary glands comprise three pairs of major salivary glands; parotid, submandibular and sublingual. In addition, numerous islands of glandular tissue, the so-called minor, accessory salivary glands are scattered throughout the mucosa of the oral cavity. Secretion of saliva by the major salivary glands is under parasympathetic neural control in response to physical, chemical and psychological stimuli.

The parotid gland

This is the largest of the salivary glands, lying wedged between the ramus of the mandible and mastoid process, and spreading over both of these structures and their attachments (Fig. 207).

Relations

- Above – lie the external auditory meatus and temporomandibular joint.
- Below – it overlaps the posterior belly of digastric.
- Anteriorly – it overlaps the mandibular ramus with the overlying masseter.
- Posteriorly – it overlaps the mastoid process with the overlying sternocleidomastoid.
- Medially – lies the styloid process and its muscles separating the parotid from the internal jugular vein, internal carotid artery, last four cranial nerves and the lateral wall of the pharynx.

The gland itself is enveloped by the investing layer of deep cervical fascia, which splits to enclose the parotid. This fascial envelope is called the parotid fascia or parotid capsule, lying both outside and within which are the parotid lymph nodes. Antero-inferiorly, this parotid fascia is thickened to form the stylomandibular ligament, which is interposed between the parotid and the submandibular gland

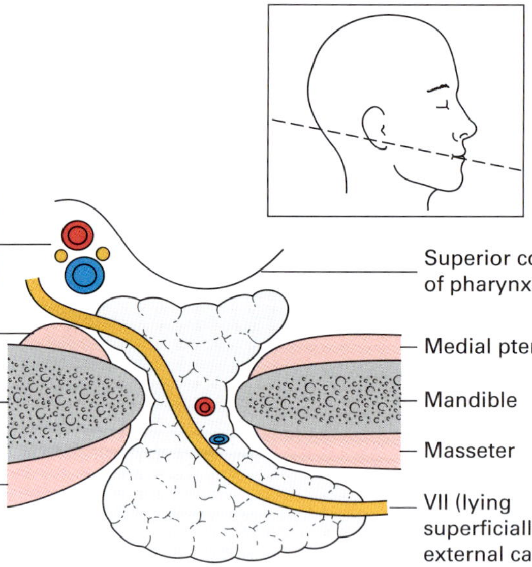

Fig. 207 The parotid and its surrounds in a schematic horizontal section – the facial nerve is the most superficial of the structures traversing the gland. (The line of section is shown in the inset head.)

Coursing through the gland are the following:

1 the facial nerve (see next section);

2 the retromandibular (posterior facial) vein, formed by the confluence of the superficial temporal and maxillary veins (see Fig. 215);

3 the external carotid artery, dividing at the level of the neck of the mandible into its two terminal branches; superficial temporal artery and maxillary artery.

Of these three structures lying in the parotid, the facial nerve lies most superficially, the external carotid artery most deeply and the retromandibular vein, between the two.

The *parotid duct* (*of Stensen*) is 5 cm (2 in) long. It arises from the anterior part of the gland, runs over the masseter a finger's breadth below the zygomatic arch, dips inwards to pierce the buccinator and opens in the cheek mucosa opposite the second upper molar tooth. Inspect this in the mirror in your own mouth. The duct can easily be felt by a finger rolled over the masseter if this muscle is tensed by clenching the teeth.

The relations of the facial nerve to the parotid

The facial nerve is unique in traversing the substance of a gland, a fact of considerable importance to the surgeon. This coexistence is explained embryologically; the parotid gland develops in the crotch formed by the two major branches of the facial nerve. As the gland enlarges it overlaps these nerve trunks, the superficial and deep parts fuse and the nerve comes to lie buried within the gland. The fanciful comparison between the nerve and the two parotid lobes and a sandwich-filling between two slices of bread is not valid because the two lobes of the parotid come to fuse intimately with each other both around and between the branches of the nerve.

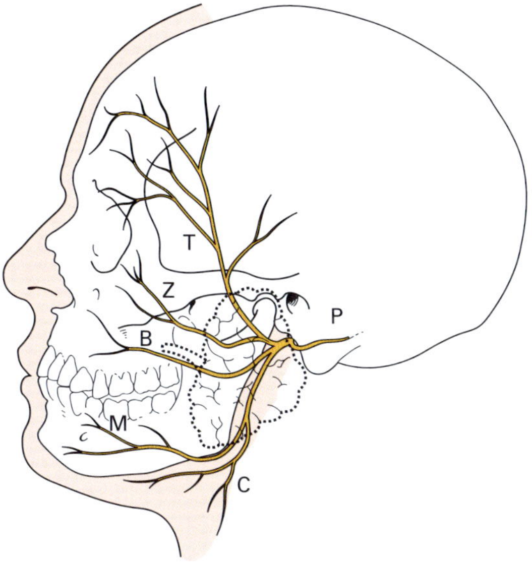

Fig. 208 The named branches of the facial nerve which traverse the parotid gland. B, buccal; C, cervical; M, mandibular; P, posterior auricular; T, temporal; Z, zygomatic.

The facial nerve emerges from the stylomastoid foramen and winds lateral to the styloid process before entering the deep surface of the parotid gland. The nerve can be exposed surgically, at this point, in the inverted 'V' between the bony part of the external auditory meatus and the mastoid process.

Within a centimetre of its entry into the parotid gland, the facial nerve bifurcates into its two main divisions (very occasionally it may bifurcate before entering the gland). The upper division divides into *temporal* and *zygomatic* branches; the lower division gives the *buccal*, *mandibular* and *cervical* branches (Fig. 208).

These two divisions may remain completely separate within the parotid or, most usually, display a number of cross-communications, resembling a plexus.

The five branches of the facial nerve then emerge from the peripheral margin of the parotid to lie on the masseter, usually as five groups of nerve filaments, before passing to the muscles of the face. No branches emerge from the superficial (lateral) aspect of the gland, which can therefore be completely exposed with impunity.

CLINICAL FEATURES

1 The parotid gland is the commonest site for salivary gland tumours. Most salivary gland tumours, however, are benign (pleomorphic adenomas).

A malignant tumour of the parotid gland, unlike benign lesions, may invade the facial nerve and produce a facial palsy. Indeed a facial palsy associated with a parotid tumour is practically pathognomonic of malignancy.

2 In removing a benign mixed salivary tumour (pleomorphic adenoma) of the parotid, the facial nerve is exposed posteriorly in the wedge-shaped space between the bony

canal of the external auditory meatus and the mastoid process. It is then traced into the gland, its main divisions defined and the tumour excised with a wide margin of normal gland, carefully preserving the exposed nerves.

It is interesting that giant mixed tumours 'extrude' clear away from the facial nerve and can be excised with an adequate margin without even seeing the nerve.

3 The parotid duct and its ramifications can be demonstrated radiologically by injecting radio-opaque contrast through a cannula placed in the mouth of the duct (a parotid sialogram).

The submandibular gland

The submandibular salivary gland is made up of a large superficial and a small deep lobe that connect with each other around the free posterior border of the mylohyoid.

The superficial lobe of the gland lies near the angle of the jaw, wedged between the inner surface of the body of the mandible and the mylohyoid, within the boundaries of the submandibular triangle (Fig. 199). Posteriorly, it almost abuts the parotid gland, separated only by a condensation of the fascial sheath of the latter (the stylomandibular ligament).

Superficially, the submandibular gland is covered by the investing layer of deep cervical fascia which, in turn, is overlain by the platysma muscle. The plane between the two is traversed by the cervical and marginal mandibular branches of the facial nerve (VII) and by the facial vein. The deep aspect of the submandibular gland lies against the mylohyoid for the most part, but posteriorly the gland rests against the hyoglossus muscle and here comes into contact with the lingual (V) and the hypoglossal (XII) nerves, both of which lie on hyoglossus as they pass forwards to the tongue (see Fig. 196).

The facial artery also comes into close relationship with the gland, approaching it posteriorly, then arching over its superior aspect (which it grooves), to reach the inferior border of the mandible, thence to ascend to the face in front of the masseter.

From the medial aspect of the superficial part of the gland projects its deep prolongation (deep lobe) along the cleft-like interval between the mylohyoid and hyoglossus.

The *submandibular duct* (*Wharton's duct*) arises from this deep part of the gland and runs forwards, beneath the mucosa of the floor of the mouth along the side of the tongue, to open immediately lateral to the frenulum linguae (Fig. 196). Here, its orifice is readily visible on the summit of a papilla termed the sublingual papilla and saliva can be seen trickling through this orifice.

The sublingual gland (see next section) lies immediately lateral to the submandibular duct.

The lingual nerve reaches the tongue by passing from the lateral side of the duct below and then medial to it – thus 'double-crossing' it.

The *submandibular lymph nodes* lie within the submandibular triangle, mainly outside the gland although an occasional node may lie embedded within the gland.

CLINICAL FEATURES

1 Submandibular gland excision (submandibular adenectomy) is a surgical procedure that may be undertaken for chronic calculus disease or for a submandibular adenocarcinoma. This operation is carried out through a skin crease incision sited below and parallel to the lower border of the mandible, level with the hyoid bone. The reason for placing the skin incision at this distance from the lower border of the mandible is to avoid the risk of damaging the marginal mandibular branch of the facial nerve (VII).

The marginal mandibular branch of VII emerges from the lower margin of the parotid and crosses the lower border of the mandible to enter the upper part of the neck. After an oblique course of 2 to 3 cms in the neck, it turns upwards to cross the lower border of the mandible to re-enter the face where it supplies the depressor muscles of the lower lip. The incision for submandibular gland excision must therefore be placed rather more than 2.5 cm (1 in) below the lower border of the mandible in order to preserve this nerve. Other nerves that are at risk of inadvertent injury during the procedure are the lingual nerve and the hypoglossal nerve.

2 The presence of small lymph nodes within the substance of the gland makes removal of the gland an imperative part of radical block dissection of the neck.

3 In differentiating between an enlarged submandibular gland and a mass of submandibular lymph nodes, one remembers that the gland not only lies below the mandible but also extends into the floor of the mouth; it can therefore be palpated bimanually between a finger in the mouth and a finger below the angle of the jaw. Try this on yourself. Enlarged lymph nodes are felt only at the latter site.

4 A stone in Wharton's duct can be felt bimanually in the floor of the mouth and can be seen if sufficiently large.

The sublingual gland

This is an almond-shaped salivary gland lying immediately beneath the mucosa of the floor of the mouth and immediately in front of the deep part of the submandibular gland. Laterally, it rests against the sublingual groove of the mandible while medially it is separated from the base of the tongue by the submandibular duct and its close companion, the lingual nerve (Fig. 196).

The gland opens by a series of ducts into the floor of the mouth and also in the submandibular duct.

The sublingual gland produces a mucus secretion; the parotid a serous secretion; and the submandibular gland a mixture of the two.

As well as these main salivary glands, small accessory glands are found scattered within the mucosa over the palate, lips, cheek, tonsil and tongue. These glands are very rare sites for development of a mixed salivary tumour.

The major arteries of the head and neck

The common carotid arteries

The *left common carotid artery* arises directly from the aortic arch in front and to the right of the origin of the left subclavian artery. It passes behind the left sternoclavicular joint, lying in its thoracic course at first in front and then to the left side of the trachea, with the left lung and pleura, the left vagus nerve and left phrenic nerve as its lateral relations.

The *right common carotid artery* begins behind the right sternoclavicular joint at the bifurcation of the brachiocephalic artery.

In the neck, both common carotids have essentially similar courses and relationships; they ascend in the carotid fascial sheath, which contains also the internal jugular vein laterally and the vagus nerve between the two somewhat posteriorly but within the carotid sheath. Embedded in the anterior wall of the carotid sheath and to be regarded as a content of the carotid sheath is the ansa cervicalis, which provides the motor innervation for the strap muscles.

The cervical sympathetic chain ascends posteromedial to the carotid sheath, outside the sheath. These five structures form a quintet which should always be considered in this inseparable manner; the relations of any one are those of the other four (Figs 187, 209).

In the neck, each common carotid artery lies on the cervical transverse processes, separated from them by the prevertebral (scalene) muscles. Medially are the larynx and trachea, with the recurrent laryngeal nerve, pharynx and oesophagus, together with the thyroid gland, which partially overlaps the anterior aspect of the carotid sheath. Superficially, the carotid sheath is covered by the sternocleidomastoid muscle and, in its lower part, by the strap muscles and is crossed by the intermediate tendon of omohyoid.

The common carotid artery usually gives off no side branches but terminates at the level of the upper border of the thyroid cartilage (at the vertebral level C4) into the external and internal carotids, which are more or less equal in size in the adult. In the neonate and infant however, the internal carotid artery is significantly larger than the external carotid artery.

The external carotid artery

This artery lies first deep to the anterior border of the sternocleidomastoid and then quite superficially in the anterior triangle of the neck, where its pulsations may be palpable. At first it is slightly deep to the internal carotid, then passes anterior and lateral to it. The internal jugular vein is first lateral to the external carotid then posterior to it, coming into lateral relationship to the internal carotid artery. The pharynx lies medially.

The external carotid artery ascends deep to the XII nerve and the posterior belly of the digastric to enter the parotid gland, within which it lies deep to the facial nerve and the retromandibular vein (Figs 197, 207, 209).

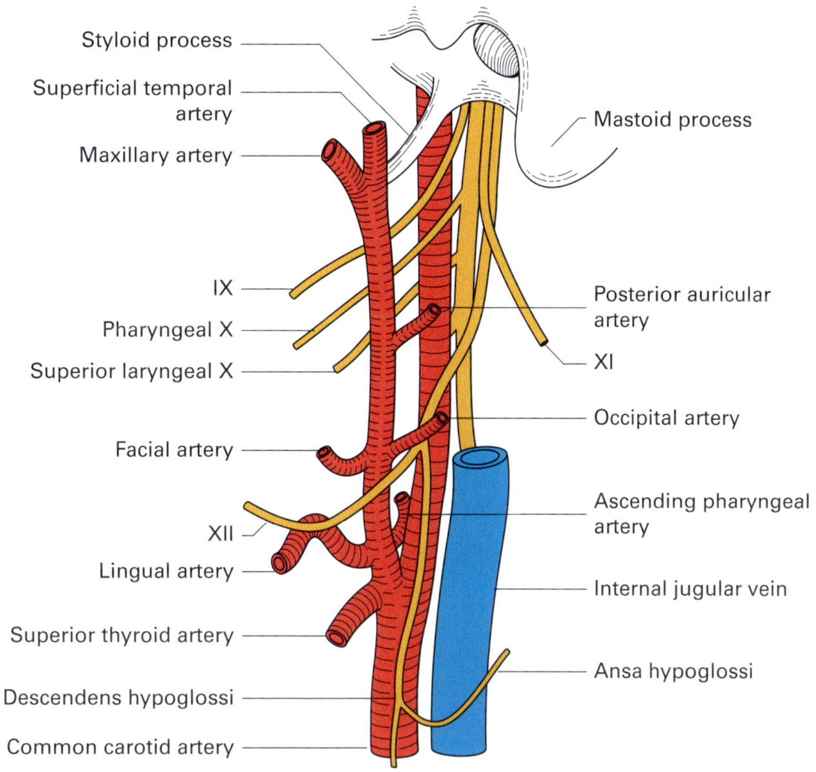

Fig. 209 The carotid arteries, their branches and their related nerves.

The artery ends within the parotid gland at the level of the neck of the mandible by dividing into the superficial temporal and maxillary arteries.

Branches (Fig. 209)

Arising from the anterior aspect of the external carotid artery, in succession, are:

1 The *superior thyroid artery* (giving off the superior laryngeal artery).

2 The *lingual artery*, passing deep to the hyoglossus to supply the tongue.

3 The *facial artery*, which gives off its important branch to the palatine tonsil, loops over the submandibular gland, hooks around the lower border of the mandible (against which it can be felt pulsating) and ascends on to the face.

Arising from the posterior aspect of the external carotid artery, in succession, are:

4 The *occipital artery*, which runs along the inferior border of the digastric muscle's posterior belly, grooving the inferior aspect of the temporal bone, to the back of the scalp, where its pulse is often palpable.

5 The *posterior auricular artery*, which supplies the skin of the back of the ear and behind the ear.

Arising from the inner aspect of the external carotid artery is:

6 The *ascending pharyngeal artery*, the smallest branch, which ascends between the internal carotid and the pharynx, supplying the latter.

The terminal branches of the external carotid artery are:

- the *superficial temporal artery*, which is palpable on the zygomatic process;
- the *maxillary artery*, which supplies the upper and lower jaws, nasal cavity and the muscles of mastication, accompanying the various branches of the maxillary and mandibular divisions of the trigeminal nerve, and also gives off the all-important middle meningeal artery. This small vessel ascends through the foramen spinosum to enter the cranial cavity, where it helps to supply the meninges. Its importance in surgical practice lies in the fact that it may be torn in a skull fracture, resulting in the formation of an extradural haematoma.

The internal carotid artery

This artery commences at the bifurcation of the common carotid and, at its origin, is dilated to form the *carotid sinus*. This area receives a rich nerve supply from the glossopharyngeal nerve (IX) and acts as a *baroreceptor*; through this mechanism a rise of blood pressure brings about reflex slowing of the heart and peripheral vasodilatation. Situated in, or deep to, the crotch of the common carotid bifurcation is the small, yellowish *carotid body*, which is also supplied by IX. This is a *chemoreceptor* that produces a reflex increase in the rate and depth of respiration in response to any rise in carbon dioxide tension or fall in the oxygen tension of the blood.

The internal carotid lies at first, posterolateral to the external carotid but rapidly passes medial and posterior to it, to ascend along the side-wall of the pharynx. It does so with the internal jugular vein, vagus and cervical sympathetic chain in the same relationship to it that they bear to the common carotid artery. At first the artery is covered superficially only by the sternocleidomastoid, the hypoglossal nerve (XII) and the common facial vein; it then passes under the posterior belly of the digastric muscle and parotid gland to the base of the skull. It is separated from the external carotid artery not only by the parotid but also by the styloid process and the muscles arising from it, by IX and by the pharyngeal branches of the vagus nerve (X) (Figs 207, 209).

At the base of the skull, the internal carotid artery enters the carotid canal in the petrous temporal bone. Only at the skull base does the internal jugular vein lose its close lateral relation to the internal carotid, passing posterior to the artery into the jugular foramen. At this point the two vessels are separated by the emerging last four cranial nerves.

Usually the internal carotid artery gives off no significant branches in the neck.

The internal carotid, on entering the skull, commences an extraordinary twisted course. It passes forwards and medially within the petrous temporal bone, upwards into the cavernous sinus, forwards in the sinus, upwards through the roof of the sinus to lie medial to the anterior clinoid process, turns back on itself above the cavernous sinus and then passes up once more, lateral to the optic chiasma, to end by dividing into the *anterior* and *middle cerebral arteries*. There are thus six bends in the intracranial course of this artery (readily appreciated by studying a lateral carotid arteriogram). These bends are referred to as the *carotid siphon* and are believed to lessen the impact of the pulsating force of the arterial systolic blood pressure on the delicate cerebral tissues.

The *ophthalmic artery* originates from the internal carotid immediately after its emergence from the cavernous sinus, enters the orbit through the optic foramen below and lateral to the optic nerve and supplies the orbital contents and the skin above the eyebrow (via the supratrochlear and supra-orbital branches). Its most important branch, however, is the *central artery of the retina*, which is an end-artery and is the sole blood supply to the delicate and precious retina.

The two terminal branches of the internal carotid are distributed as follows (Fig. 210).

The *anterior cerebral artery* winds around the genu of the corpus callosum to supply the medial and superolateral aspects of the cerebral hemisphere.

The *middle cerebral artery* enters the lateral cerebral sulcus, gives off central branches to supply the internal capsule ('the *artery of cerebral haemorrhage*') and feeds most of the lateral aspect of the cerebral cortex.

The *arterial circle of Willis* (Fig. 211) is completed in front by the *anterior communicating artery*, which links the two anterior cerebral arteries, and behind by a *posterior communicating artery* on each side, passing backwards from the internal carotid to anastomose with the ipsilateral posterior cerebral artery, a terminal branch of the *basilar artery*, the latter being formed by the union of the two *vertebral arteries*, in front of the pontomedullary junction.

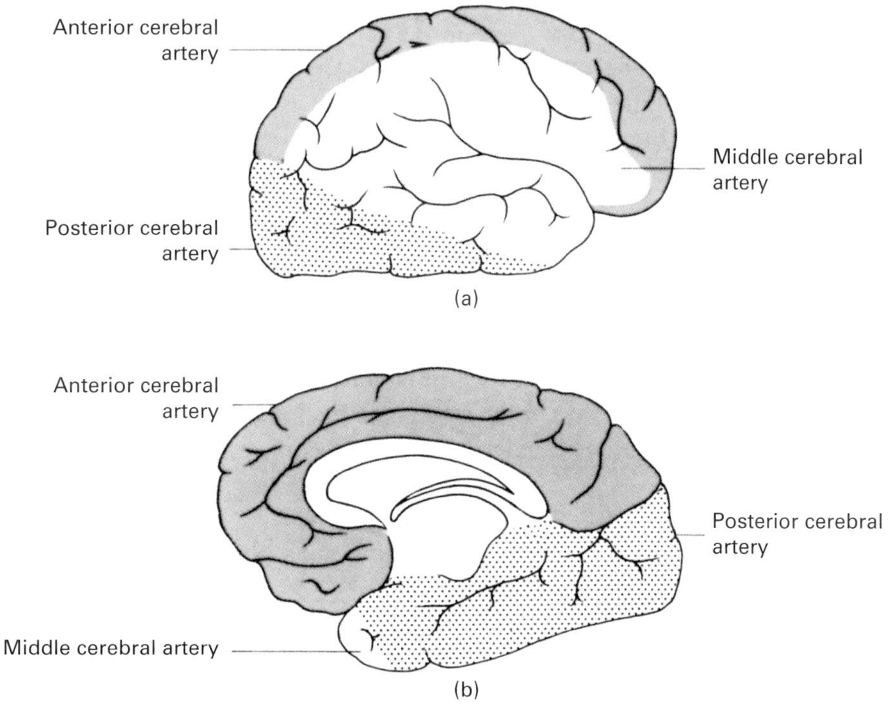

Fig. 210 The arterial supply of the cerebral cortex. Right cerebral hemisphere. (a) Lateral aspect. (b) Medial aspect.

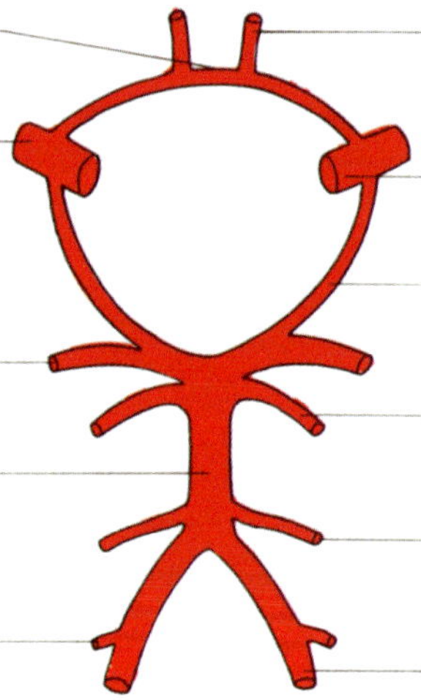

Fig. 211 The circle of Willis.

CLINICAL FEATURES

The internal and external carotids, as well as the terminal part of the common carotid artery, can be exposed through an incision along the anterior border of the sternocleidomastoid, centred at the level of the hyoid. After incising the skin, platysma and investing layer of deep cervical fascia, all in the line of the skin incision, the sternocleidomastoid is retracted, the common facial vein is divided, but the hypoglossal nerve, crossing the external and internal carotids just below the posterior belly of the digastric, is carefully sought and preserved.

It may, at times, be difficult to differentiate between the external and internal carotid arteries at operation; the former is the more anteriorly placed structure at the common carotid bifurcation and, moreover, is the one which gives off branches in the neck.

The subclavian arteries (Fig. 212)

The *left subclavian artery* arises from the arch of the aorta, immediately behind the commencement of the left common carotid artery. It ascends against the mediastinal surface of the left lung and pleura laterally and the trachea and oesophagus medially, to lie behind the sternoclavicular joint.

The *right subclavian artery* is formed behind the right sternoclavicular joint by the bifurcation of the brachiocephalic artery; beyond this point, the course of the two arteries is much the same.

The cervical course of the subclavian arteries is conveniently divided by the scalenus anterior muscle into three parts.

The first part lies medial to scalenus anterior and arches over the dome of the pleura and lies deep to the sternocleidomastoid and the strap muscles. It is crossed at its origin by the carotid sheath and, more laterally, by the phrenic and vagus nerves. At this site,

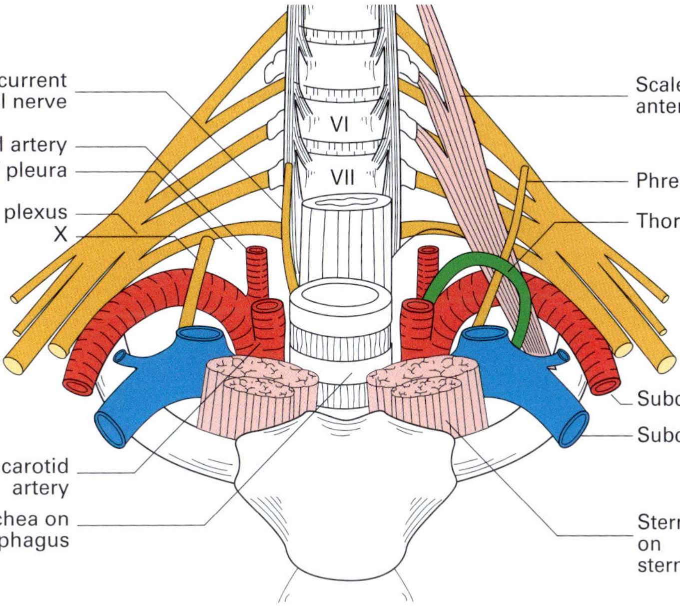

Fig. 212 The root of the neck. For clarity, only the vagus nerve is shown on the right and only the phrenic nerve on the left, as this lies on scalenus anterior.

on the right side, the vagus gives off its recurrent laryngeal branch, which hooks around the artery before reaching the tracheo-oesophageal groove.

On the left side, the thoracic duct crosses the first part of the artery before opening into the commencement of the left branchiocephalic vein.

The second part of the artery lies behind scalenus anterior, which separates it from the subclavian vein in front. Behind the artery lie scalenus medius and also the trunks of the brachial plexus.

The *third* part lies lateral to scalenus anterior and extends up to the lateral border of the first rib, against which it can be compressed and its pulse sometimes felt in a thin neck. Immediately behind the artery is the lower trunk of the brachial plexus, which is, in fact, responsible for the 'subclavian groove' on the upper surface of the first rib. At the outer border of the first rib, the subclavian artery changes its name to the axillary artery.

The branches of the subclavian artery are as follows:

- From the 1st part
  1 The vertebral artery
  2 The thyrocervical trunk:
    a inferior thyroid artery
    b transverse cervical artery
    c suprascapular artery
  3 The internal thoracic artery (internal mammary artery).
- From the 2nd part – the costocervical trunk (supplying deep structures of the neck via its deep cervical branch, and the superior intercostal artery, which gives off the 1st and 2nd posterior intercostal arteries).
- From the 3rd part – no constant branch is given.

The vertebral artery

This is the most important of the branches of the subclavian artery. It crosses the dome of the pleura, traverses the transverse foramina of the upper six cervical vertebrae and then turns posteriorly and medially over the posterior arch of the atlas to enter the cranial cavity at the foramen magnum by piercing the dura mater. It then runs on the anterolateral aspect of the medulla to join its fellow in front of the ponto-medullary junction to form the *basilar artery* (Fig. 211).

The following are the important branches of the vertebral artery:

1 anterior and posterior spinal arteries;
2 posterior inferior cerebellar artery.

From the basilar:

3 anterior inferior cerebellar artery;
4 pontine branches;
5 superior cerebellar artery;
6 posterior cerebral artery (supplying the occipital lobe and medial aspect of the temporal lobe; Fig. 210).

In addition, in the neck, the vertebral artery gives off spinal branches to the cervical spinal cord and vertebrae and muscular branches. Within the foramina transversaria it is accompanied by vertebral veins and a sympathetic plexus which, together with the carotid plexus, provides sympathetic fibres to the cranial contents.

CLINICAL FEATURES

1 The right subclavian artery is grafted end-to-side into the right pulmonary artery to short-circuit the pulmonary stenosis of the tetralogy of Fallot (Blalock's operation) (Fig. 33). It is important to note, therefore, that variations may occur in the origin of the right subclavian artery. The vessel may arise directly from the aortic arch either as its first or as its last branch. In the latter case, the right subclavian artery passes behind the trachea and oesophagus to reach the right side of the neck; this vessel may then compress the oesophagus and produce difficulty in swallowing (*dysphagia lusoria*). Occasionally, the left subclavian artery has a common origin with the left common carotid from the aortic arch.
2 An aneurysm of the subclavian artery is a recognized and well-documented condition; when present it tends to involve the third part of the artery. The proximity of the subclavian artery to the brachial plexus accounts for the pain, weakness and numbness in the arm which accompany this condition. Oedema of the arm may result from compression of the nearby subclavian vein.
3 A cervical rib may elevate the subclavian artery and render it unduly palpable; under these circumstances it may closely simulate an aneurysm and, in fact, there may be aneurysmal dilation of the artery distal to the edge of the cervical rib (post-stenotic dilatation). Vascular changes in the arm associated with a cervical rib are probably due to peripheral emboli thrown off from thrombi forming on the walls of the compressed subclavian artery.

The veins of the head and neck

The cerebral venous system

The venous drainage of the brain follows two pathways:

1 the superficial structures, e.g. the cerebral and cerebellar cortices, drain to the nearest available dural venous sinus (see next section) by thin-walled veins;

2 the deep structures drain through the *internal cerebral vein* on each side, which is formed at the interventricular foramen by the confluence of the *choroid vein* (draining the choroid plexus of the lateral ventricle) and the *thalamostriate vein* (draining the basal ganglia).

The two internal cerebral veins unite to form the *great cerebral vein* (*the vein of Galen*), which emerges from under the splenium of the corpus callosum to join the inferior sagittal sinus in the formation of the straight sinus.

The intracranial dural venous sinuses (Fig. 213)

The intracranial venous sinuses lie between the layers of the dura. They receive the venous drainage of the brain and of the skull (the *diploic veins*) and ultimately drain chiefly into the right and left internal jugular veins. They also communicate with the veins of the scalp, face and neck via *emissary veins* that pass through a number of foramina in the skull. The intracranial venous sinuses lack valves and form an interconnected network.

The *superior sagittal sinus* lies along the attached edge of the falx cerebri and ends posteriorly (usually) in the right transverse sinus. Connecting with it are a number of venous lakes (*lacunae laterales*) into which project the *Pacchionian bodies* of arachnoid, filtering cerebrospinal fluid (CSF) back into the blood.

The *inferior sagittal sinus* lies in the free margin of the falx cerebri and opens into the straight sinus.

The *straight sinus* lies along the line of attachment of the tentorium cerebelli with the falx cerebri. It is formed by the union of the great cerebral vein of Galen with the inferior sagittal sinus and runs backwards to open (usually) into the left transverse sinus.

The *transverse sinuses* commence at the internal occipital protuberance and run in the tentorium cerebelli on either side along its attached margin. On reaching the mastoid part of the temporal bone each passes downwards, forwards and medially as the *sigmoid sinus* to emerge through the jugular foramen as the *internal jugular vein*.

The *cavernous sinuses* (Fig. 214) lie one on either side of the body of the sphenoid against the fibrous wall of the pituitary fossa and rest inferiorly on the greater sphenoid wing. They communicate freely with each other via the *intercavernous sinuses*.

Traversing the cavernous sinus are the internal carotid artery and the cranial nerves III, IV, V (ophthalmic and maxillary divisions) and VI. Lying above the cavernous sinus are three important structures – the optic tract, the uncus of the temporal lobe of the cerebrum and the internal carotid artery, which first pierces the roof of the sinus then doubles back to lie on top of it.

The *ophthalmic veins* drain into the anterior aspect of the cavernous sinus, which also links up, through these veins, with the pterygoid venous plexus and the anterior facial

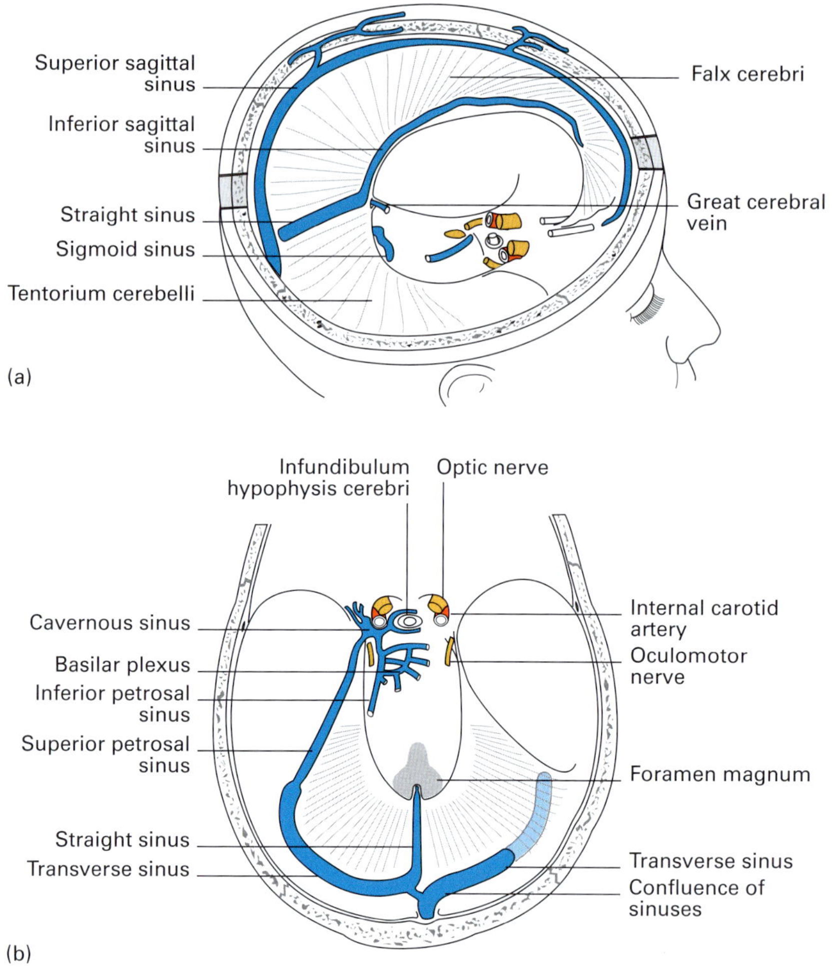

Fig. 213 The venous dural sinuses. (a) Lateral view. (b) Superior view.

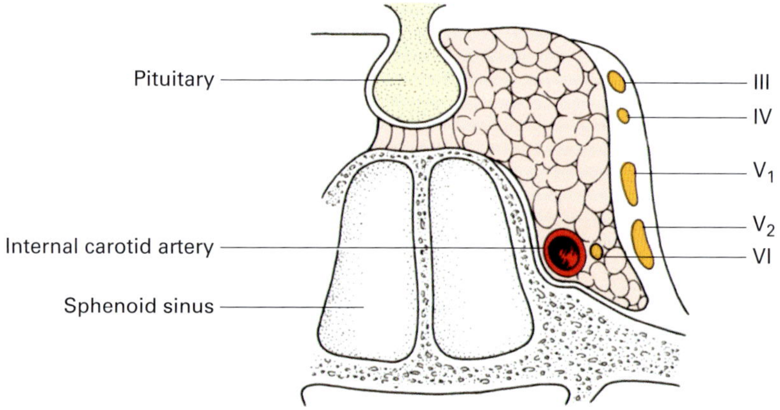

Fig. 214 The cavernous sinus – shown in coronal section.

vein. The cavernous sinus also receives venous drainage from the brain (the *superficial middle cerebral vein*) and from the dura (the *sphenoparietal sinus*).

Posteriorly, the *superior* and *inferior petrosal sinuses* drain the cavernous sinus, ipsilaterally, into the sigmoid sinus and into the commencement of the internal jugular vein, respectively.

CLINICAL FEATURES

1 The cavernous sinus is liable to sepsis and thrombosis as a result of spread of superficial infection from the lips and face via the anterior facial and ophthalmic veins, or from deep infections of the face via the pterygoid venous plexus around the pterygoid muscles, or from suppuration in the orbit or accessory nasal sinuses along the ophthalmic vein and its tributaries. A characteristic picture results – blockage of the venous drainage of the orbit causes oedema of the conjunctiva and eyelids and exophthalmos, which demonstrates transmitted pulsations from the internal carotid artery. Pressure on the contained cranial nerves results in ophthalmoplegia. Examination of the fundus shows papilloedema, venous engorgement and retinal haemorrhages, all resulting from the acutely obstructed orbital venous drainage.

2 Fractures of the skull or penetrating injuries of the skull base may cause rupture of the internal carotid artery within the cavernous sinus. This may result in a caroticocavernous arteriovenous fistula presenting with pulsating exophthalmos, a loud bruit easily heard over the eye and, again, ophthalmoplegia and marked orbital and conjunctival oedema due to the venous pressure within the sinus being raised to arterial level.

3 The sigmoid and transverse sinuses are often collectively termed *the lateral sinus* by clinicians. Close relationship to the mastoid air cells and middle ear renders these sinuses liable to infective thrombosis secondary to otitis media.

Spread of infection or thrombosis from the lateral sinus to the sagittal sinus may cause impaired CSF drainage into the latter and thereby the development of a hydrocephalus – this syndrome of raised CSF pressure associated with sinus thrombosis following ear infection is termed *otitic hydrocephalus*.

It is also possible for sagittal sinus thrombosis to result from infections of the skull, nose, face or scalp on account of its diploic and emissary vein connections. If there were no emissary veins, infections of the face and scalp would not arouse much clinical concern and would not carry the ominous clinical significance they do.

The internal jugular vein

The internal jugular vein runs from its origin at the jugular foramen (as the continuation of the sigmoid sinus) to its termination behind the sternal extremity of the clavicle, where it joins the ipsilateral subclavian vein to form the brachiocephalic vein.

It lies lateral first to the internal and then to the common carotid artery within the carotid sheath, and its relations are therefore practically identical to those of the carotid vessels within the carotid sheath (Fig. 209). The deep cervical chain of lymph nodes lies close against the vein and, if involved by malignant or inflammatory disease, may become densely adherent to the vein.

The tributaries of the internal jugular vein are:

1 the pharyngeal venous plexus;
2 the common facial vein;
3 the lingual vein;
4 the superior and middle thyroid veins.

Superficial veins

As might be expected there is considerable variation between individuals, in the manner in which the superficial veins of the head and neck are arranged. However, the usual broad plan is as follows (Fig. 215).

The *superficial temporal* and *maxillary veins* (corresponding to the terminal branches of the external carotid artery) join to form the *retromandibular vein*. This branches while traversing the parotid gland into a posterior division and an anterior division. The posterior division, together with the *posterior auricular vein*, forms the external jugular vein, while the anterior division joins the *facial vein* to form the *common facial vein* which in turn, opens into the internal jugular vein.

The *external jugular vein* crosses the sternocleidomastoid in the superficial fascia, pierces the deep fascial roof of the posterior triangle about 2.5 cm (1 in) above the clavicle to enter the subclavian vein. You can observe this vein in your own neck in the mirror when you perform a Valsalva manoeuvre. At times the vein is a double vessel.

The *anterior jugular vein* runs down one on either side of the midline of the neck, crossing the thyroid isthmus. Just above the sternum it communicates with its fellow then passes outwards, deep to the sternocleidomastoid, to enter the external jugular vein before the latter joins the subclavian vein.

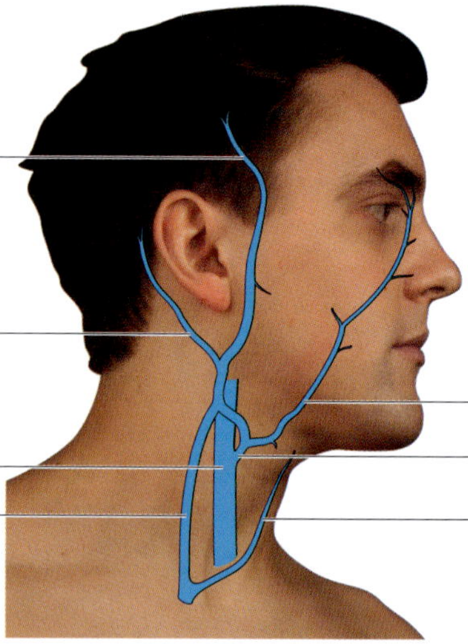

Fig. 215 The usual arrangement of the veins in the neck.

The subclavian vein

This is the continuation of the axillary vein and extends from its commencement at the outer border of the first rib to the medial border of scalenus anterior, where it joins the internal jugular vein to form the brachiocephalic vein. During its short course it crosses, and lightly grooves, the superior surface of the first rib. It arches upwards and then passes medially, downwards and slightly forwards to its termination behind the sternoclavicular joint. On the left side it receives the termination of the thoracic duct. Its only tributary is the external jugular vein. Anteriorly the vein is related to the clavicle and subclavius muscle (Fig. 216).

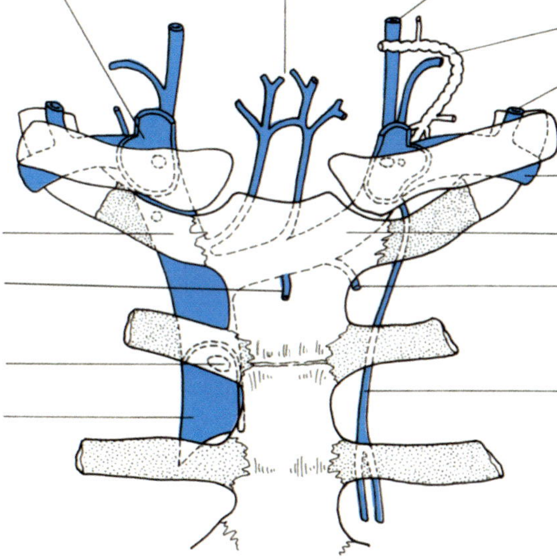

Fig. 216 The great veins of the neck and their tributaries.

CLINICAL FEATURES

Techniques of central venous catheterization are of great clinical importance as a means of measuring central venous pressure (which in turn reflects right atrial filling pressure). Central venous cannulation also allows rapid fluid and blood replacement and serves as a conduit for long-term intravenous parenteral nutrition. The internal jugular vein can be cannulated by direct puncture in the triangular gap between the sternal and clavicular heads of the sternocleidomastoid immediately above the clavicle. Feel this landmark on yourself. The needle is inserted near the apex of this triangle at an angle of 30–40° to the skin surface and is advanced caudally towards the inner border of the anterior end of the first rib behind the clavicle. A reflux of blood confirms venepuncture.

More commonly, these days, internal jugular venous cannulation is performed under ultrasound guidance, which aids accuracy, precision and safety.

Subclavian venepuncture can be carried out most effectively by the infraclavicular approach (Fig. 217). The needle is inserted obliquely below the junction of the medial and middle thirds of the clavicle. The needle is advanced medially and upwards behind the clavicle in the direction of the sternoclavicular joint to puncture the subclavian vein at its junction with the internal jugular. When a free flow of blood is obtained by syringe aspiration, a radio-opaque plastic catheter is threaded through the needle to pass into the brachiocephalic vein.

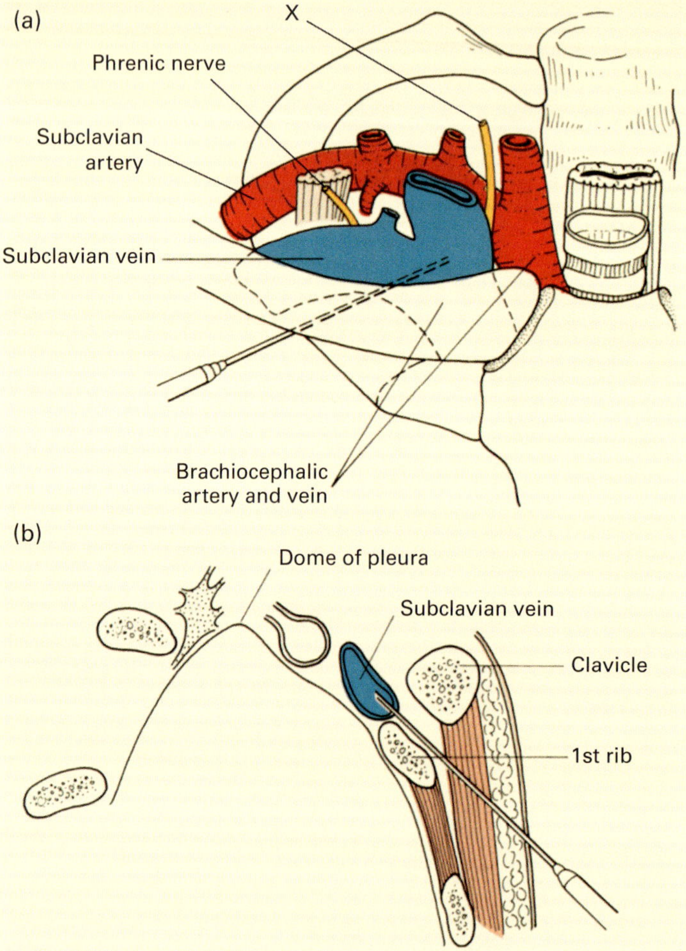

Fig. 217 The anatomy of the infraclavicular approach to the subclavian vein. (a) Anterior view. (b) In sagittal section.

The lymph nodes of the neck

The cervical lymph nodes are of great importance in the context of neoplastic and inflammatory disease involving viscera in the head and neck. Although the lymphatic drainage of individual viscera is dealt with under appropriate headings (tongue, larynx, etc.), it may be helpful to summarize, here, the general arrangement of the lymph nodes of the head and neck as a whole (Fig. 218). Cervical lymph nodes may be classified broadly into two groups: superficial and deep, depending on whether the lymph nodes lie superficial or deep to the investing layer of deep cervical fascia. Each of these two categories is further subdivided into groups on the basis of location and territory of drainage.

It is the deep cervical lymph nodes that are most commonly involved in visceral neoplasia. It is unusual for the superficial nodes to be involved in cervical visceral malignancies, except perhaps at a very late stage of the disease.

The conventional system of naming superficial and deep cervical lymph nodes according to topographical location is shown in Fig. 218. Thus the cervical lymph nodes can be grouped into horizontally and vertically disposed aggregates.

The *horizontal nodes* form a number of small clusters which encircle the junction of the head with the neck and which are named, according to their location, the *submental*, *submandibular*, *superficial parotid* (or *preauricular*), *mastoid* and *suboccipital* nodes. Some of these nodes drain the superficial tissues of the head and efferents then pass to the deep cervical nodes (although some lymph vessels pass directly to the deep cervical nodes).

The *vertical nodes* are exemplified by the jugular lymph nodes (alongside the carotid sheath), under cover of the sternocleidomastoid muscle. Also in the vertical group are the prelaryngeal, pretracheal, paratracheal, parapharyngeal and retropharyngeal lymph nodes. All these nodes are situated in the central visceral column of the neck and drain the thyroid, larynx, trachea and part of the pharynx. The efferent lymphatics from these centrally located nodes empty into the deep cervical jugular lymph nodes on one or other side, from where lymph flows via the jugular trunk either to the thoracic duct or to the right lymphatic duct.

Thus all structures in the head and neck drain, eventually, to the deep cervical nodes, either directly or indirectly.

While useful in descriptive anatomy, the traditional system of naming deep cervical lymph nodes, according to topographical location, has its limitations when it comes to the clinical management of patients with head and neck cancers. The classification system favoured by all head and neck surgeons in the present day, and one that reflects actual clinical presentation and pattern of spread in upper aerodigestive tract cancers, is the one that was originally devised in the 1990s at the Memorial Sloan Kettering hospital in New York, United States of America. It has since been refined and enhanced.

According to this system, deep cervical lymph nodes are classified into eight levels indicated by roman numerals, as follows:

level I – nodes in submandibular and submental triangles
level II – nodes alongside upper third of internal jugular vein
level III – nodes alongside middle third of internal jugular vein
level IV – nodes alongside lower third of internal jugular vein
level V – nodes in the posterior triangle of neck
level VI – paratracheal (tracheo-oesophageal groove) nodes

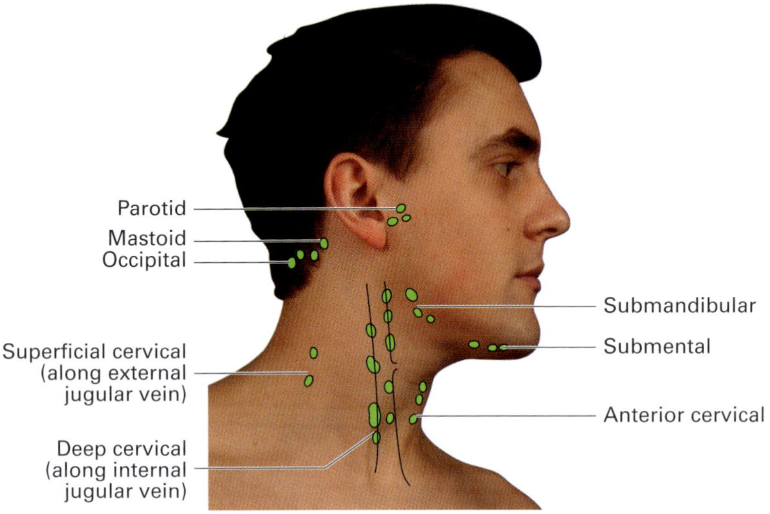

Fig. 218 Scheme of the lymph nodes of the head and neck.

level VII – pre-laryngeal, pre-tracheal and superior mediastinal nodes

level VIII – parapharyngeal and retropharyngeal nodes (on account of their deep location these are not palpable on clinical examination and are generally regarded as surgically inaccessible).

CLINICAL FEATURES

1 A constant lymph node lies at the junction of the internal jugular and common facial veins – the jugulodigastric or tonsillar node. This becomes enlarged in tonsillitis and is therefore a commonly encountered cervical lymphadenopathy.

2 *Radical neck dissection or block dissection of the neck* for malignant disease is an oncosurgical procedure which involves the removal of the lymph nodes of the anterior and posterior triangles of the neck and their associated lymph channels, as a *single block of tissue*. Also included in the same block are those structures which must be excised in order to make this lymphatic ablation possible. This elaborate procedure is sometimes combined with en bloc removal of the primary tumour.

One of a variety of incisions employed for the procedure is the Y-shaped incision, its centre being at the level of the upper border of the thyroid cartilage, its lower limb running downwards to the midpoint of the clavicle, its anterior limb extending to the symphysis menti and its posterior limb to the mastoid process. The block of tissue removed extends from the mandible above to the clavicle below and from the midline anteriorly to the anterior border of the trapezius behind. It consists of all the structures between the platysma and pretracheal fascia enclosed by these boundaries, preserving only the carotid arteries, the vagus trunk, the cervical sympathetic chain and the lingual and hypoglossal nerves. The sternocleidomastoid, omohyoid and digastric muscles are removed in the dissection. Excision also includes the external and internal jugular veins, around each of which lymph nodes are intimately related, and the submandibular gland and the lower pole of the parotid gland, since these both contain potentially involved lymph nodes.

The accessory nerve, passing across the posterior triangle, is usually sacrificed in the classical version of the procedure.

The cervical sympathetic trunk

The sympathetic chain continues upwards from the thorax by crossing the neck of the first rib, then ascends on the prevertebral fascia, behind the posterior wall of the carotid sheath to the base of the skull (Fig. 219). It bears three ganglia:

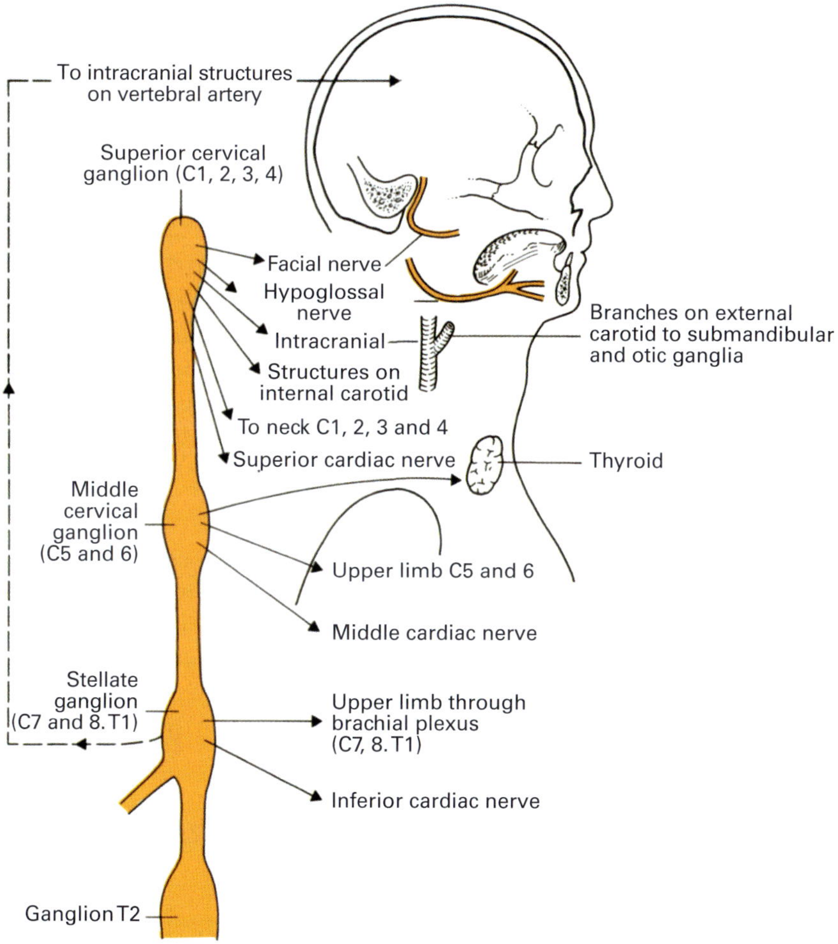

Fig. 219 The cervical sympathetic chain.

1 the *superior cervical ganglion* (the largest) lies opposite the C2 and C3 vertebrae and sends grey rami communicantes to the C1–C4 spinal nerves;
2 the *middle ganglion* lies level with the C6 vertebra and sends grey rami to the C5 and C6 nerves;
3 the *inferior ganglion* lies level with C7 and is tucked behind the vertebral artery. Frequently, it fuses with the first thoracic ganglion to form the *stellate ganglion* at the neck of the first rib. Grey rami pass from it to the C7 and C8 nerves.

Note that these ganglia receive no white rami from the cervical nerves; their preganglionic fibres originate from the upper thoracic white rami and then ascend in the sympathetic chain.

As well as *somatic branches* transmitted with the cervical nerves, the cervical chain gives off *cardiac branches* from each of its ganglia and also *vascular plexuses* along the carotid, subclavian and vertebral vessels. The sympathetic fibres to the dilator pupillae muscle travel in this plexus along the internal carotid artery. Grey rami pass from the superior ganglion to cranial nerves VII, IX, X and XII.

CLINICAL FEATURES

1 'Cervical sympathectomy' is a misnomer; it is an upper thoracic sympathectomy carried out through a cervical incision. The sympathetic chain is divided below the 3rd thoracic ganglion and the grey and white rami to the 2nd and 3rd ganglia are also cut. In this way the sudomotor and vasoconstrictor pathways to the head and upper limb (from segments T2, T3 and T4) are divided, preserving the T1 connection and the stellate ganglion, which are the sympathetic connections to the eyelid and pupil. The upper thoracic chain can also be removed via a transthoracic transpleural approach through the second intercostal space, or by fibreoptic endoscopy. The lung is allowed to collapse and the chain identified as it lies on the heads of the upper ribs. Resection of the T2–T4 segment results in a warm, dry hand.
2 *Horner's syndrome* results from interruption of the sympathetic fibres to the eyelids and pupil. The pupil is constricted (miosis, due to unopposed parasympathetic innervation via the oculomotor nerve), there is partial ptosis (due to paralysis of the smooth muscle component of levator palpebrae superioris) and the face on the affected side is dry and flushed (sudomotor and vasoconstrictor denervation). Enophthalmos is said to occur, but this is not confirmed by exophthalmometry. The syndrome may follow spinal cord lesions at the T1 segment (tumour or syringomyelia), closed, penetrating or operative injuries to the stellate ganglion or the cervical sympathetic chain, or pressure on the chain or stellate ganglion produced by enlarged cervical lymph nodes, an upper mediastinal tumour, a carotid aneurysm or a malignant mass in the neck.

The branchial system and its derivatives

Six visceral arches (pharyngeal or branchial arches) form on the lateral aspects of the fetal head separated from each other, on the outside, by ectodermal branchial clefts and, on the inside, by five endodermal pharyngeal pouches (Fig. 193). In the human embryo the 5th and 6th arches do not appear externally and are represented only by a mesodermal core.

Each arch has its own nerve supply, cartilage, muscle and artery, although considerable absorption and migration of these derivatives occur in development. The 5th arch disappears entirely.

The embryological significance of many of the branchial derivatives has already been discussed under appropriate headings (the development of the face, tongue, thyroid, parathyroid and aortic arch) but Table 4 serves conveniently to bring these various facts together.

Branchial cyst and fistula

The second branchial arch grows downwards to cover the remaining arches, leaving temporarily a space lined with squamous epithelium. This usually disappears but may persist and distend with cholesterol-containing fluid to form a *branchial cyst*. Another theory is that these cysts arise from squamous clefts in cervical lymph nodes.

If fusion fails to occur distally, a sinus persists at the anterior border of the origin of the sternocleidomastoid; this *branchial fistula* can be traced upwards between the internal and external carotids and may even open into the tonsillar fossa, demonstrating its association with the second branchial arch.

Surface anatomy and surface markings of the head

Many of the important landmarks of the skull are readily felt (see Figs 221, 222). Revise on your own skull the position of: the *external occipital protuberance* (the apex of this is termed the *inion*), the *nasion*, which is the depression between the two *supra-orbital margins*, and the *glabella*, which is the ridge above the nasion. Feel the sharp edge of the lateral margin of the orbit that is formed by the frontal process of the zygomatic bone; behind the zygomatic bone is the *zygomatic arch* with the *superficial temporal artery* crossing its posterior extremity and forming a convenient pulse which the anaesthetist can reach. Rather less easily felt is the *jugal point*, the junction between the zygomatic bone and the zygomatic process of the frontal bone; it is the mass of bone encountered by the finger running forwards along the upper border of the zygomatic arch. It is a useful aid in the surface marking of the middle meningeal artery. The anterior edge of the *mastoid* is easily palpable but its posterior aspect and its tip are rather obscured by the insertion of the sternocleidomastoid.

The whole of the superficial surface of the *mandible* is palpable apart from its coronoid process. The *condyloid process* can be felt by a finger placed immediately in front of, or within, the external auditory meatus while the mouth is opened and closed.

When the teeth are clenched, *masseter* and the *temporalis* can be felt contracting, respectively, over the ramus of the mandible and above the zygomatic arch. The *parotid duct* can be rolled over the tensed masseter and its orifice seen within the mouth at the level of the 2nd upper molar tooth.

Table 4 Derivatives of the branchial system (note the 5th arch disappears).

Arch	Nerve	Visceral	External cleft	Internal pouch	Floor	Cartilage	Muscle	Artery
I	V	Lower face	External auditory meatus	Eustachian tube, middle ear and mastoid antrum	Anterior 2/3 tongue	Meckel's, incus and malleus; sphenomandibular ligament	Muscles of mastication, anterior belly digastric, tensor palati, tensor tympani	Disappears
II	VII	Grows down to cover remaining clefts to form skin of neck		Palatine tonsil	Contributes to anterior tongue; thyroid forms as outgrowth between I and II	Stapes, styloid, stylohyoid ligament, upper body and lesser horn of hyoid	Muscles of facial expression, posterior belly digastric, stylohyoid, stapedius	Disappears
III	IX			Thymus, inferior parathyroid	Posterior 1/3 tongue	Greater horn and lower part of body of hyoid	Stylopharyngeus	Common and internal carotids
IV	X (superior laryngeal)			Superior parathyroid		Thyroid cartilage	Muscles of pharynx, larynx and palate	Right, subclavian; left, aortic arch
VI	X (inferior laryngeal)				Outgrowth of lung buds	Cricoid cartilage		Pulmonary artery and ductus arteriosus

The pulsation of the *facial artery* can be felt as it crosses the lower margin of the body of the mandible immediately in front of the masseter and again opposite the angle of the mouth. In the latter situation, if the cheek is gripped lightly with the finger placed within the mouth and the thumb placed on the skin surface, the pulse will be felt a little more than 1.25 cm (0.5 in) from the angle of the mouth.

A line drawn vertically between the first and second premolar teeth passes through the mental foramen, the infra-orbital foramen and the supra-orbital notch. Through these three orifices, lying in plumb-line, pass branches from each of the divisions of the trigeminal nerve; respectively, the mental branch of the inferior alveolar nerve (V_3), the infra-orbital nerve (V_2) and the supra-orbital nerve (V_1).

The *middle meningeal artery* can be represented by a line drawn upwards and somewhat forwards from a point along the zygomatic arch, two fingers' breadth behind the jugal point. The posterior branch of this artery passes backwards a thumb's breadth above, and roughly parallel to, the zygomatic arch.

The *central sulcus* of the cerebrum corresponds to a line drawn downwards and forwards from a point 1.25 cm (0.5 in) behind the midpoint between the nasion and the inion.

The scalp

The scalp is the name given to the soft tissues that cover the cranial vault. The eyebrows define the anterior limit of the scalp, while the posterior limit of the scalp is level with the superior nuchal line on the occipital bone. On either side the scalp may be said to extend down to the level of the zygomatic arch. The forehead, from eyebrows to the anterior hairline, is common to the face and scalp. The scalp is a many-layered structure and the five layers that constitute the scalp are easily and conveniently recalled, in the correct order, by the five letters that make up the word SCALP! Thus from the surface inwards the five layers are (Fig. 220):

S – skin;
C – connective tissue;
A – aponeurosis;
L – loose connective tissue;
P – periosteum.

Each of these layers has features of practical importance.

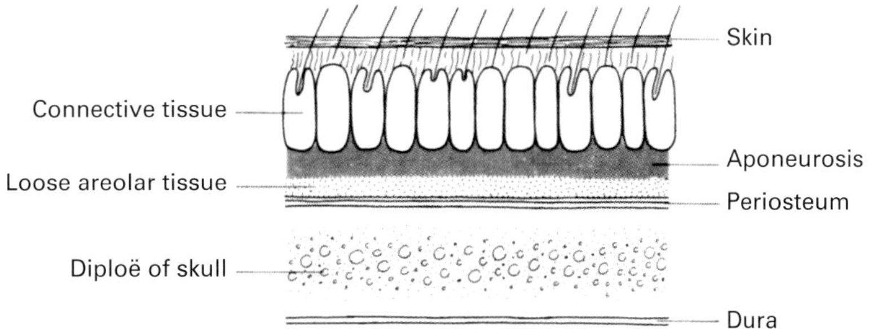

Fig. 220 The layers of the scalp.

The *skin* of the scalp is the thickest in the body. It is richly supplied with sebaceous glands and is the commonest site in the body for sebaceous cysts. It also has a large number of hair follicles.

The *subcutaneous connective tissue* consists of lobules of fat bound in tough fibrous septa, very much like the connective tissue of the palm and the sole. This dense encapsulation of fat makes it unsurprising that lipomata are extremely rare at these three sites and also that excess fat does not collect in any of these places even in the grossly obese.

The blood vessels of the scalp lie in this dense connective tissue layer. Firm adherence of the dense connective tissue to the walls of the arteries and veins prevents the vessels from retracting and constricting when severed – the usual response when skin vessels are severed elsewhere in the body. This is the reason for the profuse bleeding associated with scalp lacerations. When the scalp is lacerated, haemorrhage is arrested by pressing with the fingers firmly down onto the skull on either side of the wound (thus compressing the vessels), by placing a series of artery forceps on the divided aponeurotic layer and, finally, by suturing the laceration securely in two layers (aponeurotic and cutaneous). However scalp vessels anastomose richly with neighbouring vessels, and for this reason and also because the scalp has a rich blood supply, wounds of the scalp generally heal very well.

The veins of the scalp connect with the intracranial venous sinuses via numerous *emissary veins* that pierce the skull and that also link these two venous systems with the *diploic veins* between the tables of the skull vault. A superficial infection of the scalp may spread via this system, producing an osteitis of the skull, meningitis and venous sinus thrombosis.

The so-called *aponeurotic layer* is in fact aponeurotic only above the summit of the cranial vault. Both at the back and in front the aponeurosis is continuous with muscle. The muscles at the back are the right and left occipitalis muscles. These muscles arise side by side from a faint, curved ridge, the so-called *supreme nuchal line*, just above and parallel to the superior nuchal line of the occipital bone. Anteriorly the aponeurosis becomes continuous with the right and left frontalis muscles. The frontalis muscles have no attachment to bone. At their anterior ends the frontalis muscles insert into the dermis of the skin of the eyebrow region. It is the frontalis muscles that produce the transverse furrows on the forehead – the so-called 'worry lines'. On either side the lateral edge of the occipitofrontalis aponeurosis gains a fascial insertion into the corresponding zygomatic arch.

The layer of *loose connective tissue* beneath the aponeurosis accounts for the mobility of the scalp on the underlying bone.

Blood or pus collecting in this loose tissue tracks freely under the scalp but cannot pass into either the occipital or subtemporal regions because of the attachments of occipitofrontalis. Fluid can, however, track forwards into the eyelids and periorbital tissues, and this may account for the periorbital haematoma that may occasionally develop following a head injury or cranial operation.

The aponeurotic layer is under tension because of its muscular component and retracts on the underlying loose layer when divided; a gaping scalp wound must, therefore, have extended at least through the aponeurosis.

The *periosteum* adheres to the suture lines of the skull; collections of pus or blood beneath this layer, therefore, outline the affected bone. This is particularly well seen in birth injuries involving the skull (*cephalohaematoma*).

The skull (Figs 221, 222, 223)

The anatomy of the skull in relation to specific regions is dealt with under the appropriate headings (ear, nose, accessory sinuses, etc.). Collected together in this section are some general facts of clinical relevance followed by a general description of the floor of the cranial cavity.

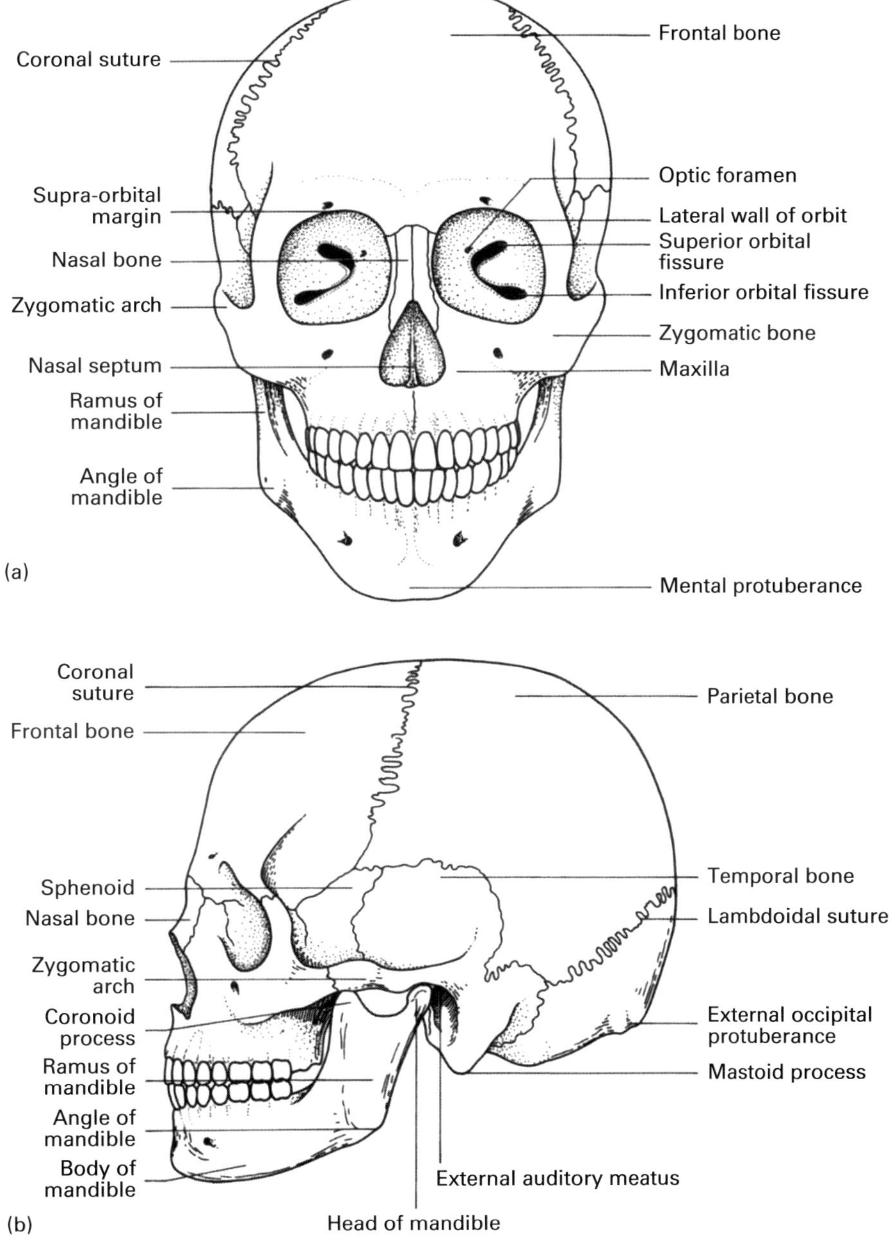

Fig. 221 The skull. (a) Anterior aspect. (b) Lateral aspect.

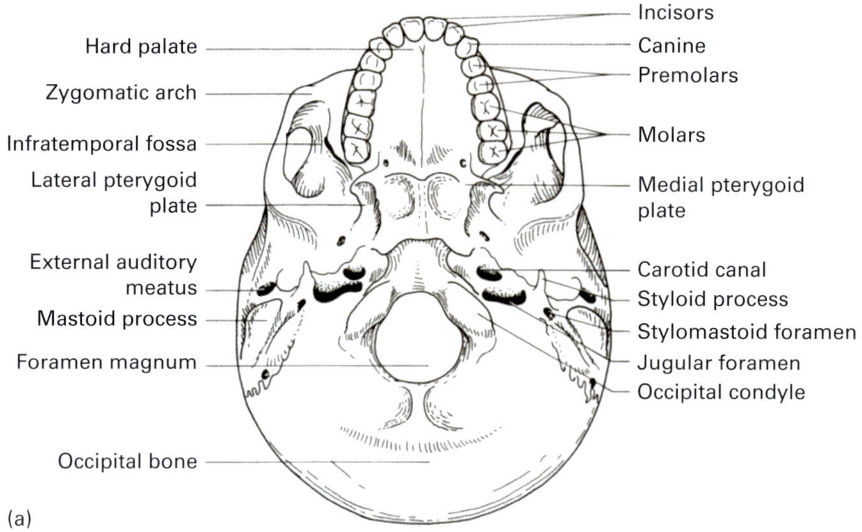

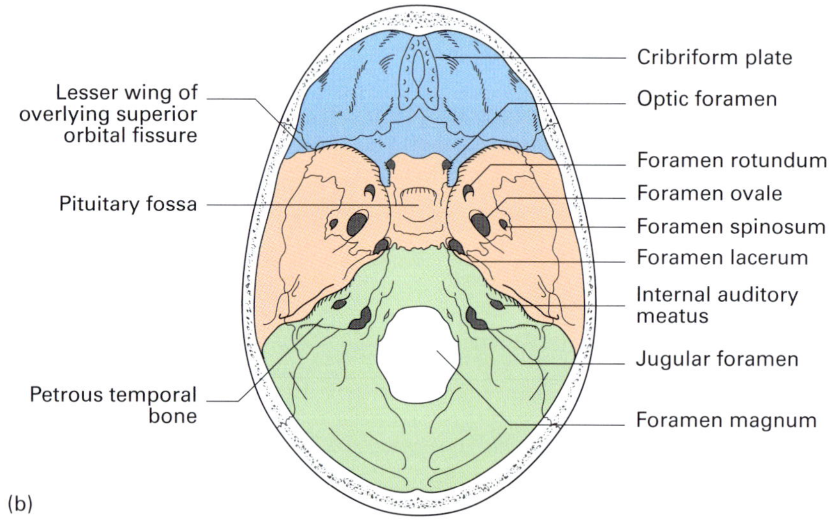

Fig. 222 The skull. (a) Inferior aspect. (b) Floor of the cranial cavity: the anterior, middle and posterior cranial fossae are colour coded.

The term ***skull*** in the strict anatomical sense of the word is made up of the *cranium* and the *mandible,* although in common usage the terms skull and cranium are used synonymously and interchangeably. The mandible articulates with the inferior surface of the cranial base at a pair of synovial joints, the right and left temporomandibular joints. The upper and posterior part of the cranium features the large cranial cavity which houses the brain and, to which, the cranium gives great support and protection. The roof of the cranial cavity is called the cranial vault (or calva or skull cap). The floor of the cranial cavity can be studied in detail only after removing the cranial vault. The floor of the cranial cavity is merely the upper surface of the skull base. The large

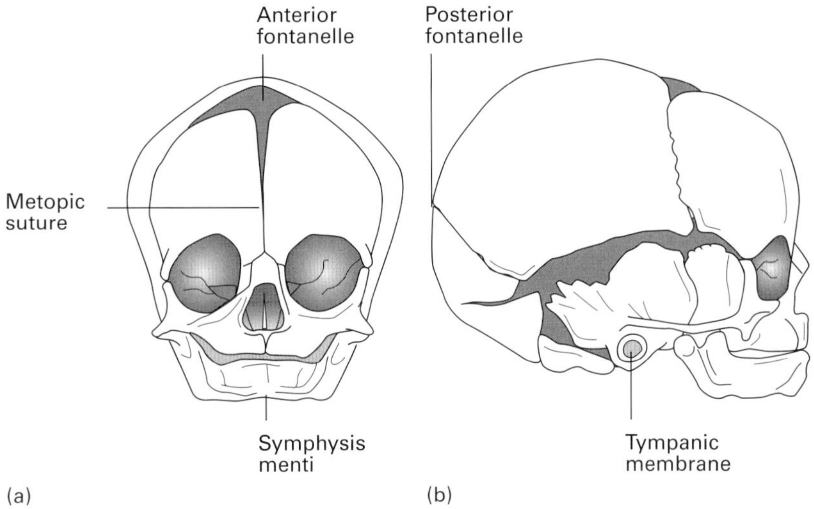

Fig. 223 The fetal skull. (a) Anterior aspect. (b) Lateral aspect.

opening in the floor of the cranial cavity is the *foramen magnum*. Viewed from below it is seen that, on either side of the foramen magnum, on the inferior surface of the skull base, there is a prominent ovoid condyle. These two condyles, termed the right and left occipital condyles, articulate with a pair of reciprocally concave facets on the upper surface of the atlas (the first cervical vertebra) to form the right and left atlanto-occipital joints. These are typical synovial joints.

The anterior aspect of the skull (Fig 221a) is the *facial skeleton*. The facial skeleton may be regarded as being made up of three horizontally orientated parallel zones: a lower zone, a middle zone and an upper zone, each connected to the zone immediately above.

The lower zone is represented by the mandible. The upper zone corresponds to the forehead and is made up of the squamous parts of the right and left frontal bones.

The middle zone may be said to extend from the superior orbital margins above, to the level of the maxillary teeth below. Of the three zones, the middle zone is the most complex in terms of design and architecture. It includes the nasal cavities, the orbital cavities, the maxillary and ethmoidal paranasal sinuses and the roof of the mouth. Thus it may be said that the oral cavity is located between the middle and lower zones.

The middle zone is made up largely of the right and left maxillae; the largest bones of the middle zone. By their palatal processes the two maxillae meet in the midline intermaxillary suture. Together the two palatal processes form most of the hard palate.

The medial surface of the body of the maxilla forms much of the lateral wall of the ipsilateral half of the nasal cavity. The upper surface of the body of the maxilla makes up much of the floor of the orbit.

On each side, immediately behind the maxilla and directly below the floor of the middle cranial fossa, are two important regions. Both of these regions communicate with the ipsilateral orbit. The lateral of the two regions is the larger of the two and is called the *infratemporal fossa*. It is closed laterally by the ramus of the mandible. The medial of the two regions is the *pterygopalatine fossa*. Separating the two regions is a downward projection of bone called the pterygoid process of the sphenoid.

Broadly speaking, the infratemporal fossa is concerned with the nerve supply and blood supply of the mandibular dentition, the floor of the mouth and tongue, while the pterygopalatine fossa is concerned with the blood supply and nerve supply of the maxillary dentition, roof of the mouth, nasal cavity and maxillary sinuses.

On each side of the midline, the anterior aspect of the facial skeleton displays a vertical arrangement of three significant foramina (Fig. 221a). The uppermost of the three is located just above the superior orbital margin and is called the supra-orbital foramen. The middle foramen is just below the inferior orbital margin and is called the infra-orbital foramen. The lowest of the three foramina is in the body of the mandible and is called the mental foramen. Each foramen transmits a sensory nerve and blood vessels, which share the name of the foramen they traverse – thus supra-orbital, infra-orbital and mental nerve and vessels.

The bony vault of the skull is relatively elastic in consistency (particularly in infancy and adolescence); thus a blow may injure the underlying brain without fracturing bone. Where the cranium is protected by thick muscle (the lower part of the occipital bone and the squamous temporal), the skull is correspondingly thin; if held up to the light it can, in some skulls, appear translucent at these sites.

Some of the palpable landmarks of the skull are enumerated in the section on the surface anatomy of the head (page 331). Radiologically, the *sutures* between the vault bones are important because they, as well as the vascular markings of the meningeal and diploic vessels, may be confused with fracture lines; however, unlike the usually straight lines of a fracture, suture lines are tortuous. The *coronal* suture divides the frontal from the parietal bones, the *sagittal* suture separates the parietal bones in the midline, the *lambdoid* suture marks off the occipital from the parietal and temporal bones and the *squamosal suture* separates the squamous temporal bone from the parietal bone and greater wing of sphenoid.

In about 8% of cases the *metopic suture* persists in the midline between the two frontal bones; in the rest, this suture fuses at about the 5th year.

Occasionally, small separate areas of ossification develop between the parietal and occipital bones termed *Wormian bones*, which, again, may cause radiological confusion.

The *lambda* is the point of junction of the lambdoid and sagittal sutures (the *posterior fontanelle* of infancy).

The *bregma* is the junction of the sagittal and coronal sutures (the infant's *anterior fontanelle*).

The *diploë*, between the inner and outer tables of the skull vault, is one of the sites of persistent red marrow in the adult skeleton. This distinction it shares with the pelvis, vertebrae, ribs, sternum, upper end of the humerus and upper end of the femur – a doubtful honour since these sites are almost confined secondary deposits of carcinoma in bone and multiple myelomata.

Floor of the cranial cavity (Fig. 222b)

The floor of the cranial cavity is the upper surface of the base of skull. In a dry skeleton it is revealed by removing the cranial vault. The cranial vault is made up of the following bones: right and left frontal bones, right and left parietal bones, the squamous part of the right and left temporal bones and the squamous part of the occipital bone.

The floor of the cranial cavity presents a terraced arrangement of three regions (areas): anterior cranial fossa, middle cranial fossa and posterior cranial fossa. The anterior fossa is the shallowest and the smallest, whereas the posterior fossa is the deepest and largest of the three areas.

The central part of the floor of the anterior cranial fossa is a thin, somewhat depressed and perforated plate of bone, the cribriform plate of ethmoid. This forms the highest part of the roof of the nasal cavity and is traversed on either side of the midline by the corresponding olfactory nerve filaments and corresponding anterior ethmoidal artery. On either side of the cribriform plate, the floor of the anterior cranial fossa is raised and undulant and constitutes the roof of the orbit of that side.

The anterior cranial fossa houses, in addition to the right and left olfactory pathways, the frontal lobes of the cerebral hemispheres and the anterior cerebral arteries as the latter course beneath the frontal lobes.

The middle cranial fossa floor shows a platform-like elevation in the centre. This is the body of the sphenoid bone; its upper surface being slightly concave and constituting the pituitary fossa. Situated above and projecting into the pituitary fossa is the pituitary gland suspended from the hypothalamus by the pituitary stalk. On either side of the central elevation, the floor is depressed and accommodates the corresponding temporal lobe of the cerebral hemisphere. Posterolateral to the pituitary fossa on either side lies the corresponding trigeminal ganglion, whereas lateral to the pituitary fossa on either side is the cavernous sinus (mentioned earlier).

Anteriorly, on either side of the midline, the middle cranial fossa communicates with the ipsilateral orbit by means of two openings: the larger and wider one being the superior orbital fissure and the smaller opening being the optic foramen (see Fig. 256). The latter transmits the optic nerve (ensheathed in the three meningeal layers) and ophthalmic artery, while the superior orbital fissure transmits the oculomotor (III), trochlear (IV) and abducent (VI) nerves, the ophthalmic nerve and the ophthalmic veins. On each side, the floor of the middle cranial fossa shows three significant foramina. From front to back these are the foramen rotundum, foramen ovale and foramen spinosum, which transmit, respectively, the maxillary nerve, mandibular nerve and the middle meningeal artery.

The posterior cranial fossa is the deepest and largest of the three fossae. It houses the entire cerebellum. Anterior to the cerebellum lies the brainstem comprising, from above downwards, the midbrain, pons and medulla oblongata. The medulla oblongata leaves the posterior cranial fossa through a large opening in the floor, the foramen magnum, to become the spinal cord. The 'slope' of bone which forms the anterior wall of the posterior cranial fossa, and lies in front of the brainstem, is called the *clivus*. The cerebellum is roofed by a large, thick and double-layered sheet of dura mater termed the *tentorium cerebelli*. Above the tentorium cerebelli (and therefore outside the posterior cranial fossa) lie the occipital lobes of the cerebral hemispheres.

Three significant openings, on each side, lead away from the posterior cranial fossa. These are the internal acoustic (auditory) meatus, the jugular foramen and the hypoglossal canal. The first of these transmits the VIIth (facial) and VIIIth (vestibulocochlear) cranial nerves. The jugular foramen transmits the IXth (glossopharyngeal), Xth (vagus) and XIth (accessory) cranial nerves, and also the sigmoid and inferior petrosal venous sinuses. The hypoglossal canal transmits the XIIth (hypoglossal) cranial nerve.

Development

The skull vault develops in membrane, the skull base in cartilage.

At birth (Fig. 223), the diamond-shaped anterior fontanelle and triangular posterior fontanelle are fairly wide. The posterior fontanelle closes at about 3 months; the anterior fontanelle closes at about 18 months. Until then, blood can be obtained by puncturing the sagittal sinus immediately below the anterior fontanelle in the midline, and CSF aspirated by passing a needle obliquely into the lateral ventricle.

The face at birth is considerably smaller proportionate to the skull, than in the adult; this is due to the teeth being non-erupted and rudimentary and the nasal accessory sinuses being undeveloped; the sinuses are evident at about 8 years but fully developed only in the late teens.

The mastoid and its air cells develop at the end of the 2nd year; until then the facial nerve is relatively superficial in its location and may be damaged by quite trivial injuries.

With advancing age, the relative vertical measurement of the face again diminishes as a result of loss of teeth and subsequent absorption of the alveolar margins.

Development of the mandible and the teeth are considered on pages 345 and 346, respectively.

CLINICAL FEATURES

Fractures of the skull

Imagine the skull as a rather elastic sphere completely filled by semifluid material; a violent blow to such a structure will produce a splitting effect commencing at the site of the blow and tending to travel along the lines of least resistance. The base of the skull is more fragile than the vault and is thus commonly involved in such fractures. The petrous part of the temporal bone, however, forms a firm and less commonly involved buttress of the skull base, the fracture line passing through less resistant areas, particularly the middle cranial fossa, the pituitary fossa and the various basal foramina.

A localized severe injury, in the adult, may produce a depressed comminuted fracture; the infant's skull is much more elastic and a similar injury here will result in a 'pond' depressed fracture, rather like the dimple produced by squeezing on a ping-pong ball.

Localizing signs in cranial fractures

Fractures of the anterior cranial fossa may involve the frontal, ethmoidal and sphenoidal sinuses and be accompanied by bleeding into the nose or mouth. In such cases CSF leakage from the nose implies an associated tear of the meninges; the subarachnoid space is thus put in communication with the exterior via the nasal cavity with consequent risk of meningitis.

Fractures involving the roof of the orbit are frequently associated with blood tracking forwards beneath the conjunctiva (subconjunctival haemorrhage); this must be differentiated from a small flame-shaped haemorrhage of the conjunctiva caused by direct injury to it.

A 'black eye' is not necessarily indicative of an anterior fossa fracture; it may be produced also by direct contusion of the soft tissues or by blood tracking down deep to the aponeurotic layer of the scalp (see 'The scalp', page 333).

Anterior basal fractures may involve the cribriform plate (with anosmia – loss of smell – due to rupture of fibres of the olfactory bulb) or the optic foramen (with primary optic atrophy and blindness).

Fractures of the middle cranial fossa may produce bleeding into the mouth (sphenoid involvement), bleeding or CSF leakage from the ear and facial and auditory nerve injury. Aural bleeding may, of course, be produced by direct injury to the ear – for example, rupture of the drum – without an associated skull fracture. Because of its long course, the abducent (VI) nerve may be damaged with paralysis of the lateral rectus muscle and resultant diplopia on lateral gaze.

Posterior fossa fractures are occasionally accompanied by cranial nerve involvement. These fractures are suggested clinically by bruising over the mastoid region extending downwards over the sternocleidomastoid.

The paranasal sinuses (accessory nasal sinuses)

(The nose and nasal cavities are described in the section on special senses in Part 6, p 406.)

The paranasal sinuses are air-containing cavities lying within bone adjacent to the nasal cavity. They are lined with respiratory, ciliated epithelium and communicate with the nasal cavity through narrow, and therefore easily occluded, openings (termed ostia) (Fig. 224). The paranasal sinuses are paired structures, each member of a pair opening into the lateral wall of its half of the nasal cavity. The paranasal sinuses are named for the bone in which each is located; thus maxillary, frontal, sphenoidal and ethmoidal sinuses. The maxillary sinus (maxillary antrum) and sphenoidal sinus are present in a rudimentary state at birth; the other two become evident at about the 8th year. All become fully formed only in adolescence.

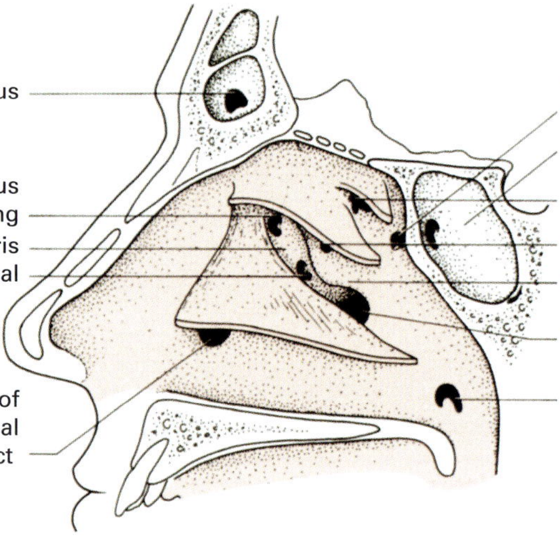

Fig. 224 The lateral wall of the right nasal cavity; the conchae have been partially removed to show structures that drain into the nose.

The frontal sinuses

The frontal sinuses are contained in the frontal bone. They vary greatly in size and one or both are occasionally absent. In section, each is roughly triangular, its anterior wall forming the prominence of the forehead, its posterosuperior wall lying adjacent to the frontal lobe of the brain, and its floor abutting the ethmoid cells, the roof of the nasal fossa and the orbit.

The frontal sinuses are separated from each other by a median bony septum, and each in turn is further broken up by a number of incomplete septa. Each sinus drains into the anterior part of the middle nasal meatus via the infundibulum into the hiatus semilunaris.

CLINICAL FEATURES

1 The proximity of the frontal sinus to the frontal lobe of the brain explains how infection of this sinus may result in the development of a frontal lobe abscess.
2 A fracture, involving the sinus, severe enough to tear the dura and pia-arachnoid, will place the subarachnoid space in communication with the nasal cavity and CSF may then be detected trickling through the nostril, usually on the affected side (CSF rhinorrhoea), although, as these sinuses may communicate, a contralateral leak sometimes occurs.
3 The neurosurgeon must take into account the considerable variations in size and extent of the frontal sinus when proposing to turn down a frontal skull flap, obviously, taking care to avoid opening the sinus because of the risk of infection. The surgeon must therefore consult the radiographs and other images (CTs and MRIs) of the patient's skull preoperatively, which will clearly show the configuration of the sinuses.

The maxillary sinus (antrum of Highmore) (Fig. 225)

This is a pyramidal-shaped sinus occupying the body of the maxilla. Its medial wall forms part of the lateral wall of the nasal cavity and bears on it the superior and middle conchae (property of the maxilla) and the inferior concha (a separate bone). Above the inferior concha is the opening, or *ostium*, of the maxillary sinus into the middle meatus in the hiatus semilunaris (Fig. 224). This opening, unfortunately, is not appropriately located for efficient and adequate drainage.

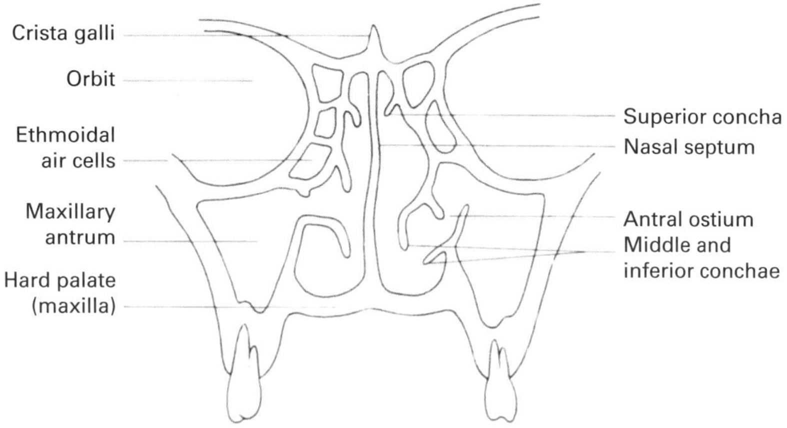

(a)

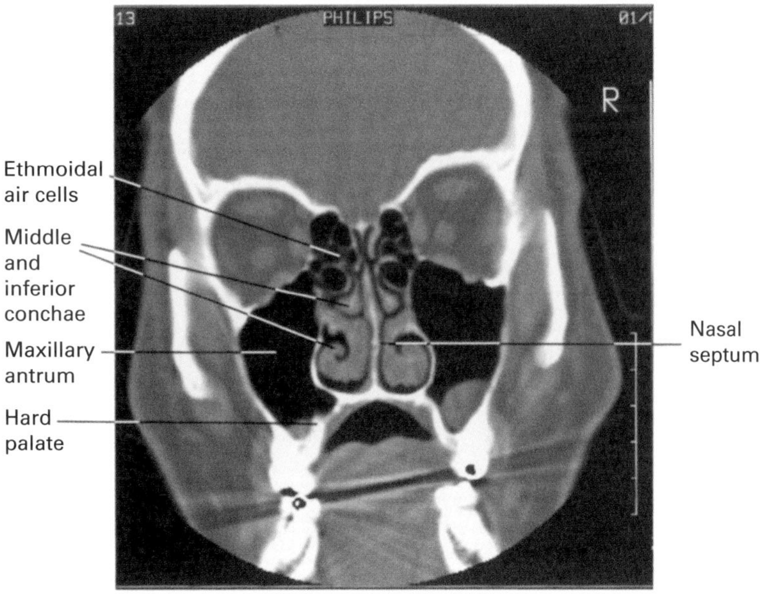

(b)

Fig. 225 (a) The maxillary antrum in coronal section. (Note the inefficient drainage of this antrum and its close inferior relationship to the teeth.) (b) The corresponding computed tomography (CT) scan.

The infra-orbital nerve lies in a groove that bulges down into the roof of the sinus, while its floor bears the impressions of the upper premolar and molar roots. These roots are separated only by a thin layer of bone which may, in fact, be deficient so that uncovered dental roots project into the sinus. Note that the floor of the sinus, therefore, corresponds to the level of the alveolus and not to the floor of the nasal cavity – it actually extends about 1.25 cm (0.5 in) lower than the latter.

CLINICAL FEATURES

1 The maxillary sinus, or antrum, may become infected (*maxillary sinusitis*) either from the nasal cavity or from caries of the upper molar teeth. Chronic maxillary sinusitis, inadequately responsive to antibiotic treatment, may require antral lavage. This is usually accomplished, these days, under vision through a fibreoptic endoscope.

   Drainage and lavage of the maxillary sinus may also be undertaken by fenestrating the antrum in the gingivolabial fold (Caldwell–Luc operation).

2 The numerous symptoms and signs which may be produced by a carcinoma of the maxillary sinus, are easily remembered anatomically.

   a Medial invasion encroaches on the nasal cavity, producing obstruction of the nares and epistaxis. Blockage of the nasolacrimal duct in this wall may cause epiphora (leakage of tears down the face).

   b Invasion of the orbit displaces the globe and causes diplopia. If the infra-orbital nerve becomes involved, there will be facial pain and then anaesthesia of the skin over the maxilla.

   c Invasion of the sinus floor may produce a visible bulge or even ulceration in the palatal roof.

   d Lateral spread may produce a swelling of the face or a palpable mass in the gingivolabial fold.

   e Posterior spread may involve the palatine nerves and produce severe pain referred to the teeth of the upper jaw.

The ethmoid sinuses

The ethmoid sinuses are made up of a group of 8–10 air cells within the lateral mass of the ethmoid and lie between the side-walls of the upper nasal cavity and the orbits (Fig. 225). Superiorly, they lie on each side of the cribriform plate and are related above to the frontal lobes of the brain. The ethmoidal air cells are divided into three clusters termed the anterior, middle and posterior ethmoidal air sinuses. The posterior sinus drains into the superior meatus of the nasal cavity, while the anterior and middle sinuses drain into the middle meatus (Fig. 224).

CLINICAL FEATURES

As with the frontal sinus, infection (ethmoiditis) may result in a frontal cerebral abscess and an ethmoidal fracture may cause a CSF leakage into the nasal cavity.

The sphenoidal sinuses

These lie one on either side of the midline, within the body of the sphenoid (Fig. 224). They vary a good deal in size and may extend laterally into the greater wing of the sphenoid or backwards into the basal part of the occipital bone.

Each sinus drains into the nasal cavity above the superior concha (at the sphenoethmoidal recess).

CLINICAL FEATURES

In patients with a pituitary tumour the pituitary gland may be approached endoscopically via a transnasal, trans-sphenoidal route and the tumour excised.

The mandible (Fig. 226)

The mandible (the bone of the lower jaw) is the largest and strongest bone of the facial skeleton. It comprises a horizontal horseshoe-shaped *body*. From the posterior extremity of the body on each side, projecting upwards is a plate of bone, the *ramus* which, at

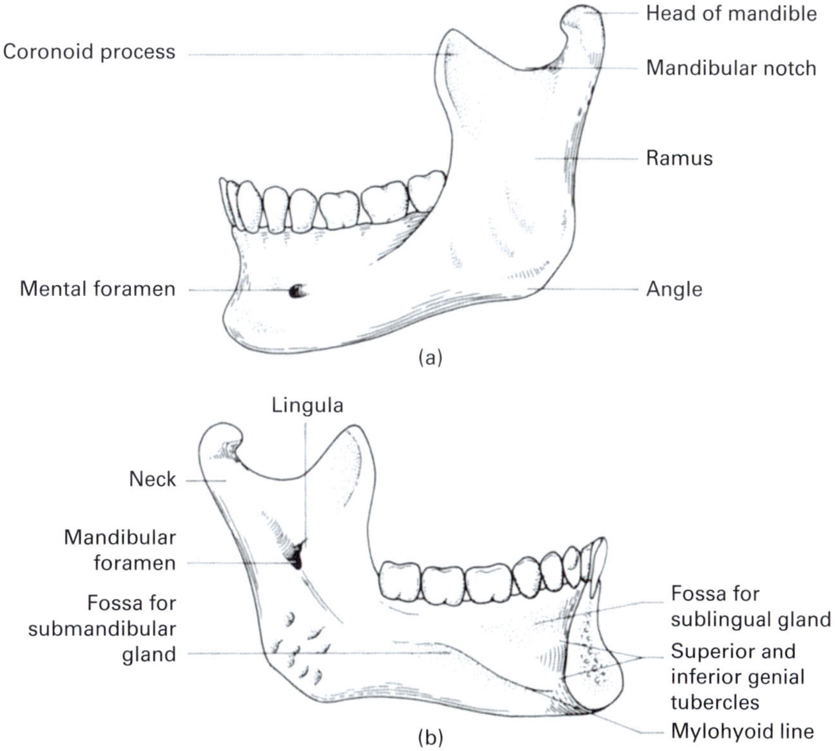

Fig. 226 The mandible. (a) Lateral aspect. (b) Medial aspect.

its upper end, bears an anterior *coronoid* and a posterior *condylar* process; the latter being made up of the *head* and *neck*. Between the coronoid and condylar processes is the *mandibular notch*. Developmentally, the body of the mandible represents the fusion of two similar halves in the anterior midline at the *symphysis menti* (fusion occurring at the 2nd year).

On the medial aspect of the ramus is the *mandibular foramen* for the inferior alveolar branch of the mandibular division of the trigeminal nerve, which traverses the body within the *mandibular canal*, then emerges as the mental nerve through the *mental foramen* on the lateral surface of the body below and between the two premolars. The nerve supply to the incisors and canine runs forwards within the mandible beyond this point in the *incisive canal*.

The upper border of the body bears the *alveolar border* with sixteen dental sockets or *alveoli*. The angle between the posterior and inferior borders of the ramus is called the *angle of the mandible*. In the adult it is almost always somewhat everted; the degree of eversion usually being greater in the male.

Development

The mandible develops as membrane bone in the fibrous sheath of Meckel's cartilage (the cartilage of the first branchial arch, which also gives rise to the malleus and incus). The cartilage itself is completely absorbed. Bony union of the two halves of the mandible occurs in the 2nd year.

The temporomandibular joint (TMJ)

This synovial joint is an articulation between the condylar process of the mandible and the articular fossa and articular eminence of the temporal bone. The articular surfaces are covered with fibrous (*not* hyaline) cartilage, and there is also a fibrocartilaginous *articular disc* dividing the joint cavity into upper and lower compartments. Thus, the TMJ, like the sternoclavicular and acromioclavicular joints, is an atypical synovial joint.

The fibrous capsule surrounding the joint is reinforced by a lateral *temporomandibular ligament* and by the *sphenomandibular ligament* which passes from the spine of the sphenoid to the *lingular process* immediately in front of the mandibular foramen; this ligament represents part of the primitive 1st arch, or Meckel's cartilage.

The lower jaw can be depressed, elevated, protruded, retracted and moved from side to side.

The muscles effecting these movements are:

- *elevation* – temporalis, masseter and medial pterygoid;
- *depression* – lateral pterygoid, together with digastric, mylohyoid and geniohyoid (assisted by gravity – your jaw drops open when you fall asleep at a lecture);
- *retraction* – posterior fibres of temporalis;
- *protraction* – lateral and medial pterygoids acting together;
- *side to side* – lateral and medial pterygoids acting together, and alternating in action with the contralateral pterygoids.

CLINICAL FEATURES

Dislocation of the jaw, when uncomplicated, occurs only in a forwards direction. When the mouth is widely open, the condylar process of the mandible slides forwards onto the articular eminence; thence, a blow, or even a yawn, may cause forward dislocation into the infratemporal fossa on one or both sides. Upward dislocation can occur only in association with extensive comminution of the skull base, and backward dislocation can occur with communition of the bony external auditory canal and tympanic cavity that lie immediately behind the joint.

Reduction is effected by pressing down on the molar teeth with the thumbs placed in the mouth, at the same time pulling up the chin; the former stretches the masseter and temporalis muscles which are in spasm, the latter levers the mandibular head back into place.

The teeth

There are twenty deciduous or 'milk' teeth replaced by thirty-two permanent teeth made up, in each half jaw, thus:

- *deciduous*: two incisors, one canine and two molars;
- *permanent*: two incisors, one canine, two premolars and three molars.

The times of eruption of the teeth are clinically useful milestones in a child's development as well as being of forensic interest.

As a rough guide, these times can be thought of in multiples of 6, thus:

• the 1st lower incisor deciduous tooth appears at	6 months
• all the deciduous teeth have appeared by	24 months
• the permanent 1st molar • the permanent 1st incisor } appears at	6 years
• the second permanent molar appears at	12 years (approx.)
• the third permanent molar appears at	18–24 years

The lower teeth appear somewhat before their corresponding upper neighbours.

Each tooth is fixed in its socket by the *periodontal membrane*, which is, in fact, periosteum. This layer is radiotranslucent and is the dark line seen around the root of each tooth on radiography.

Development

The enamel crown of the tooth develops from a downgrowth of the alveolar epithelium and represents the toughest tissue in the human body. The rest of the tooth (pulp, dentine and cement) differentiates from the underlying mesodermal connective tissue.

CLINICAL FEATURES

Osteomyelitis of the jaw following dental extractions is confined to the lower jaw and occurs only with the permanent dentition. The explanation for this is an anatomical one.

The lower jaw is supplied *only* by the inferior alveolar (dental) artery, which runs with the nerve in the mandibular canal; damage to this artery at extraction, or its thrombosis in subsequent infection, therefore, produces bone necrosis. The upper jaw, on the other hand, receives segmental vertical branches from the superior dental vessels and ischaemia does not follow injury to an individual artery. The deciduous teeth of the lower jaw are placed well clear of the mandibular canal which is, in any case, protected by the unerupted permanent teeth; damage to the artery cannot therefore occur during their removal.

Inferior alveolar nerve (inferior dental nerve) block

This is a useful procedure for the dental surgeon because it produces complete anaesthesia of all the lower teeth on the ipsilateral side of the mandible. The needle is advanced past the last molar tooth on to the inner aspect of the ramus of the mandible, and local anaesthetic solution is injected in the region of the mandibular foramen. Anaesthesia is produced in the lower teeth, the skin and mucosa of the lower lip (via the mental branch of the inferior alveolar nerve) and, because of spread of the anaesthetic solution to the lingual nerve in the vicinity, there is loss of sensation over the anterior two-thirds of the tongue ipsilaterally, owing to involvement of the lingual nerve, which lies immediately anteromedial to the inferior alveolar nerve (see Fig. 254).

The vertebral column

The vertebral column, synonymous with spinal column or spine, and known colloquially as the backbone, forms the central axis of the body's skeleton. Along with the sternum and the twelve pairs of ribs, it forms the skeleton of the trunk. The vertebral column is a very strong, yet flexible midline strut. At its upper end, the vertebral column articulates with the skull base and thereby supports the skull. The inferior part of the vertebral column articulates on each side, with the corresponding hip bone. The two hip bones are united in front at the pubic symphysis to form the pelvic girdle. Each hip bone, in turn, articulates with the head of the corresponding femur to form the hip joint.

The vertebral column contains the delicate spinal cord within the vertebral canal (spinal canal) and thereby confers much protection to the spinal cord from external trauma.

Powerful muscles attached to the posterior part of the vertebral column provide support for the column and play an indispensable role in maintaining the posture of the individual.

For descriptive purposes the vertebral column is divided into five regions. In sequence, from above downwards these are the cervical, thoracic, lumbar, sacral and coccygeal regions. The thoracic vertebral column articulates, on either side, with the posterior ends of all of the twelve ribs, and thus forms the posterior wall of the thoracic skeleton (thoracic cage).

The adult vertebral column makes up about two-fifths of the total height of the body and is formed of a vertical chain of individual bony elements termed vertebrae. From above downwards, this chain comprises seven cervical vertebrae, twelve thoracic vertebrae, five lumbar vertebrae, the sacrum and the coccyx. The cervical, thoracic and lumbar vertebrae are termed *moveable vertebrae*, on account of the fact that the individual vertebrae can move relative to their neighbouring vertebrae. The sacrum and coccyx, by contrast, are formed by the fusion of vertebrae (five individual vertebrae fuse to form the sacrum and four vertebrae fuse to form the coccyx). The sacrum and coccyx are therefore spoken of as immoveable, implying the immobility of the individual vertebrae in these two regions.

In the fetus the spine is curved into a gentle C shape (concave ventrally and reciprocally convex dorsally). This ventral concavity is termed the primary curvature of the spine and is retained throughout life in the thoracic, sacral and coccygeal regions of the column. However, after birth, secondary curvatures with an anterior convexity (lordosis) appear gradually in the cervical and lumbar regions, resulting eventually, in the permanent sinuous curves of the fully developed spinal column that is evident when the spinal column is viewed in profile. The cervical lordosis is the consequence of sustained extension of the head and neck produced by the postvertebral muscles when the child first holds up its head. The lumbar lordosis appears much later and is associated with the muscular support of the trunk provided by the powerful postvertebral muscles when the infant learns to sit, stand and walk.

Morphology of a typical vertebra

With the exception of the first two cervical vertebrae (atlas and axis respectively), all moveable vertebrae whether from the cervical, thoracic or lumbar region, share a more-or-less common morphological design (Fig. 227). Thus, each typical moveable vertebra features a cylindroid vertebral body, anteriorly. Attached to the back of the body is a bony arch, termed the vertebral arch (neural arch). Between the two is the vertebral foramen. In the articulated vertebral column all the vertebral foramina 'stacked' one on top of another constitute, collectively, the vertebral canal (spinal canal). Occupying the upper two-thirds of the length of the vertebral canal is the spinal cord, which in the adult ends at the level of the first lumbar vertebra.

Projecting laterally from the vertebral arch on either side is the corresponding transverse process (Fig. 231). Projecting backwards from the posterior midline of the vertebral arch is the spinous process (spine). On either side of the midline, the part of the vertebral arch that lies between the roots of the transverse and spinous processes is called the lamina, on account of its thick and plate-like shape (Figs 227b and 231). The right and left laminae meet in the posterior midline at the root of the spinous process.

The most anterior part of the vertebral arch on each side where the arch adjoins the back of the vertebral body is termed the pedicle. The height of each pedicle is approximately half the height of the vertebral body. Thus, there is a substantial gap between successive pedicles. This is called the *intervertebral foramen*. Each intervertebral foramen transmits a spinal nerve with accompanying radicular arteries and veins.

Projecting upwards from the vertebral arch on either side of the midline, at approximately the junction of the lamina, pedicle and the root of the transverse process

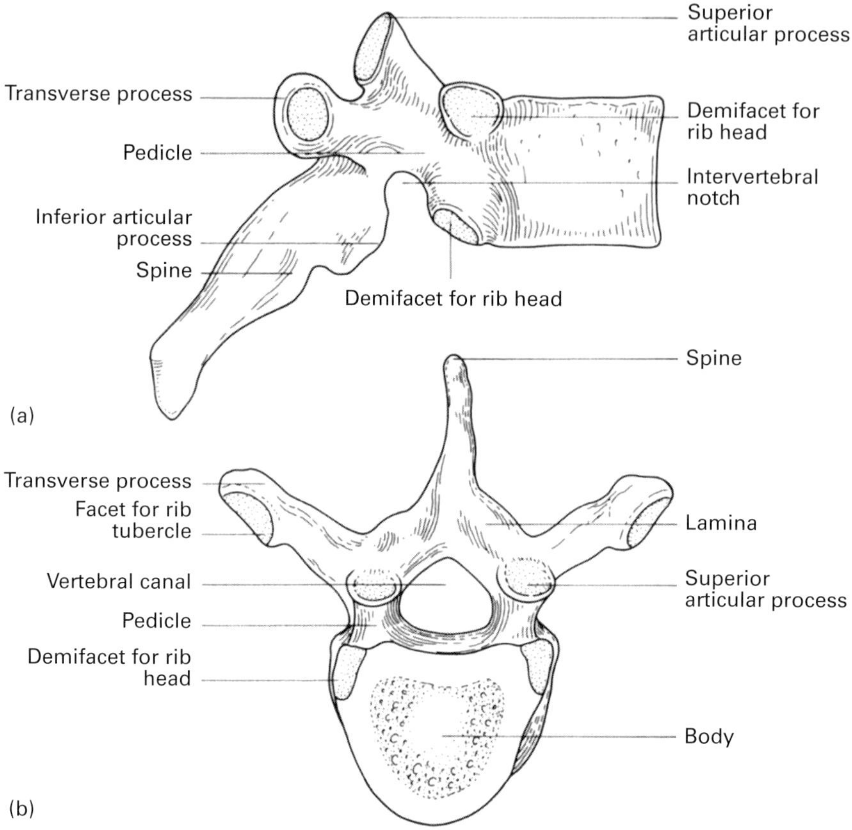

Fig. 227 A 'typical' thoracic vertebra. (a) Lateral aspect. (b) Superior aspect.

is the superior articular process, while projecting inferiorly from the vertebral arch in line with the superior articular process is the inferior articular process. Each articular process features a smooth articular facet that, in life, is covered by a layer of articular hyaline cartilage. Each superior articular process articulates with the inferior articular process of the superjacent vertebra, and each inferior articular process articulates with the superior articular process of the subjacent vertebra. These articulations are typical synovial joints and are known as the *intervertebral facet joints*.

Spinal motion segment

While the vertebra is the morphological unit of the vertebral column, the *spinal motion segment* is the name given to the *functional* or biomechanical unit of the vertebral column. The spinal motion segment may be defined as any *two successive, moveable vertebrae* including the structures and articulations that unite them. Thus, for example, C7 and T1 vertebrae together constitute a spinal motion segment as do T9 and T10, or L4 and L5. Contained within the boundaries of each spinal motion segment is a complementary pair of intervertebral foramina.

Three factors serve to confer physical stability, structural integrity and flexibility to a spinal motion segment, and thereby, to the entire length of the vertebral column. The three factors are as follows:

The intervertebral disc (reinforced by the anterior and posterior longitudinal ligaments);

The intervertebral facet joints;

Vertebral arch ligaments (ligaments between adjacent vertebral arches).

The intervertebral disc is the principal bond between adjacent vertebral bodies (Fig. 232a). There are 23 intervertebral discs in all; the first disc being situated between the bodies of C2 and C3, and the last disc being situated at the lumbosacral junction. The upper and lower surfaces of each vertebral body are covered by thin plates of hyaline cartilage. The intervertebral disc is interposed between these hyaline cartilage covered surfaces and is thus an example of a secondary cartilaginous joint.

Collectively, the discs make up about a quarter of the height of the vertebral column. The discs are thinnest in the upper thoracic region of the vertebral column and thickest in the lumbar region. In the lower lumbar region the discs tend to be prominently wedge-shaped, i.e. thick anteriorly and tapered posteriorly.

Each intervertebral disc is made up of two elements: an outer lamellated (multi-layered) fibrous ring called the *annulus fibrosus* and a gelatinous and inner zone termed the *nucleus pulposus*. The annulus possesses high tensile strength and extensibility, and by virtue of the manner in which the fibres are arranged in each layer, the annulus is able to withstand all manner of torsional and shearing forces to which it is subjected. The nucleus pulposus by contrast, functions as a hydrated gel and possesses compressibility. Thus, together, the two components of the intervertebral disc make the disc a most effective shock absorber.

The strong union between adjacent vertebral bodies, effected by the intervertebral disc, is reinforced by the anterior and posterior longitudinal ligaments (known also as the anterior and posterior spinal ligaments). Running down the entire length of the vertebral column, these ligaments fuse with the anterior and posterior aspects of the circumference of the intervertebral disc (Fig. 249b).

The intervertebral facet joints (properly and formally called zygapophyseal joints) collectively form a vertical row of articulations on either side of the midline (Fig. 249a).

Each facet joint is a typical synovial joint between the inferior articular process of one vertebra and the superior articular process of the subjacent vertebra. The shape and contour of the articular facet differs between one vertebral region and another and is the principal determinant of the type of movement that takes place between adjacent vertebrae in a given vertebral region.

It is the presence of such a large number of closely spaced synovial joints arranged in a linear order on either side of the midline that gives the vertebral column such an impressive degree of flexibility and so much versatility of movement. In common with other typical synovial joints, the facet joints are susceptible to both common forms of arthritis; osteoarthritis and rheumatoid arthritis.

Vertebral arch ligaments (ligaments between adjacent vertebral arches) (Figs 232a & 249b)

In addition to the facet joints that connect adjacent vertebrae, there are strong and biomechanically important ligaments that run between adjacent vertebral arches, providing considerable stability to the vertebral column. Three ligaments are particularly significant, namely, the *supraspinous ligament, interspinous ligament* and *ligamentum flavum*. The supraspinous and interspinous ligaments are midline structures, while the ligamenta flava are symmetrically arranged on either side of the midline. The supraspinous ligaments run between the tips of adjacent spinous processes. They are dense and strong bands of fibrous tissue that become taut during flexion of the vertebral column and lax during extension. In the cervical region the supraspinous ligament is represented by the ligamentum nuchae. The interspinous ligaments are sheets of fibrous tissue that run vertically in the midline between the facing margins of adjacent spinous processes and blend with the deep surface of the overlying supraspinous ligament. The interspinous ligaments are especially dense and strong in the lumbar region.

The *ligamenta flava* (ligamentum flavum in the singular) span the gap between adjacent laminae. Each ligament is a relatively short structure. Its superior attachment is to the anterior surface of the lower border of the lamina above, while its inferior attachment is to the posterior surface of the upper border of the subjacent lamina. This arrangement resembling the arrangement of tiles on a roof is termed imbrication.

The ligamenta flava are elastin-rich structures and become elongated on flexion of the vertebral column, the length of the ligaments being restored on extension.

The ligamenta flava constitute an important anti-gravity support mechanism to the vertebral column.

Now to consider the individual vertebrae.

The cervical vertebrae (*n* =7)

These are readily identified by the *foramen transversarium* present in the transverse processes of each and every one of the seven cervical vertebrae. These foramina transmit the vertebral artery (except that of C7), the vertebral veins and sympathetic fibres. The spinous processes are small and bifid (except C1 which has no spinous process at all, and C7, whose spinous process is not bifid) and the articular facets show a slight slope (Fig. 228).

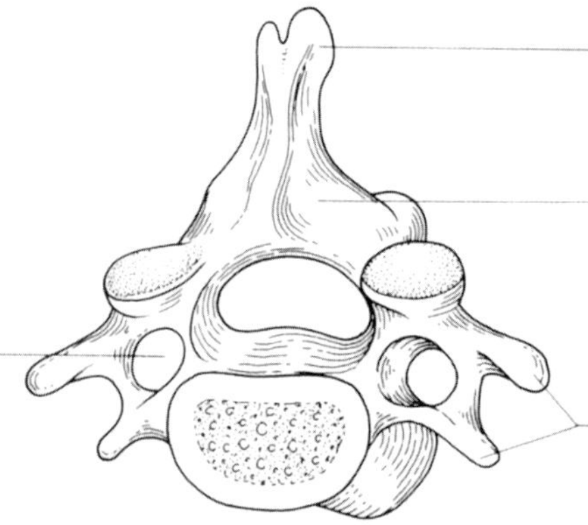

Fig. 228 A 'typical' cervical vertebra.

The *atlas* (C1) (Fig. 229) is a ring of bone and has no body. It possesses a pair of lateral masses joined to each other by a short anterior arch of bone and a long and slender posterior arch. The upper and lower surfaces of the lateral mass of the atlas bear respectively, a superior articular facet and inferior articular facet; the former for articulation with the occipital condyle and the latter for articulation with a facet on the upper surface of the axis.

The upper aspect of the posterior arch of the atlas, immediately posteromedial to the lateral mass, is grooved by the vertebral artery as the latter passes medially and upwards to enter the posterior cranial fossa through the foramen magnum.

The *axis* (C2) (Fig. 230) bears the *dens* (*odontoid process*) on the superior aspect of its body. The dens is thought to represent the detached body of C1 incorporated in the axis.

Nodding and lateral flexion movements occur at the atlanto-occipital joint, whereas rotation of the skull occurs at the atlanto-axial joint around the dens, which acts as a pivot.

C7 is the *vertebra prominens*, so-called because of its relatively long and easily felt non-bifid spine; it is the first clearly palpable spine on running one's fingers downwards along the posterior midline of the neck, although the spine of T1 immediately below it is, often, equally, if not more, prominent.

The vertebral artery enters its vertebral course nearly always at the foramen transversarium of C6; it is not surprising, therefore, that the foramen transversarium of C7, which transmits only the vein, is small.

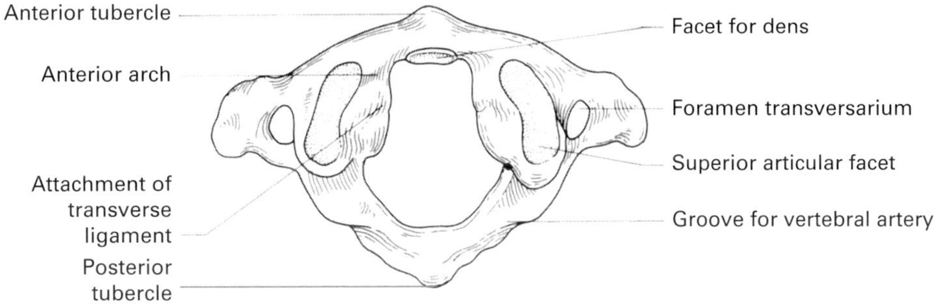

Fig. 229 The atlas in superior view.

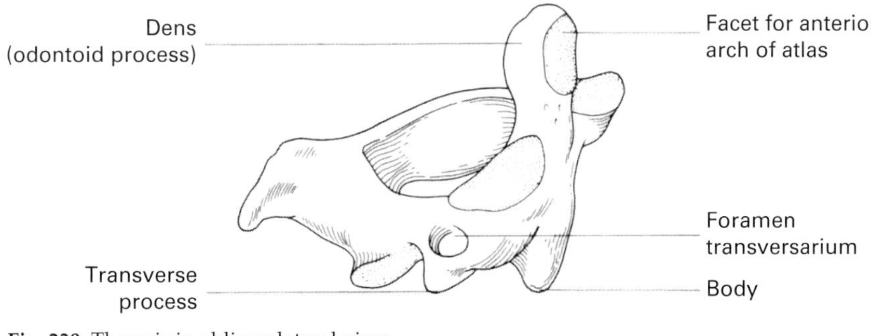

Fig. 230 The axis in oblique lateral view.

The thoracic vertebrae ($n = 12$)

These vertebrae (Fig. 227) are characterized by demifacets on the sides of their bodies for articulation with the heads of the ribs and by facets on their transverse processes (apart from those of the lower two or three vertebrae) for the rib tubercles. The spines are long and downward sloping and the articular facets are also relatively vertical. The lowest two or three thoracic vertebrae have a single facet on each side of the body for articulation with the head of the numerically corresponding rib and no facet on the transverse process.

The bodies of T5 and T8 are worth noting; they come into relationship with the descending aorta and are a little flattened by it on their left flank. If the descending aorta becomes aneurysmally dilated, these four vertebral bodies become eroded by its pressure, although their avascular intervertebral discs remain intact. You can make this diagnosis when shown a specimen of four partly worn-away vertebrae with normal intervening discs.

The lumbar vertebrae ($n = 5$)

These are of great size with strong, thick rectangular, horizontal spinous processes and with articular facets that lie in the sagittal plane (Fig. 231).

L5 is distinguished by its massive, conical transverse process, the root of which connects with the entire lateral aspect of the pedicle and practically abuts the vertebral body; the transverse processes of the other lumbar vertebrae attach to the junction of the pedicle with the lamina.

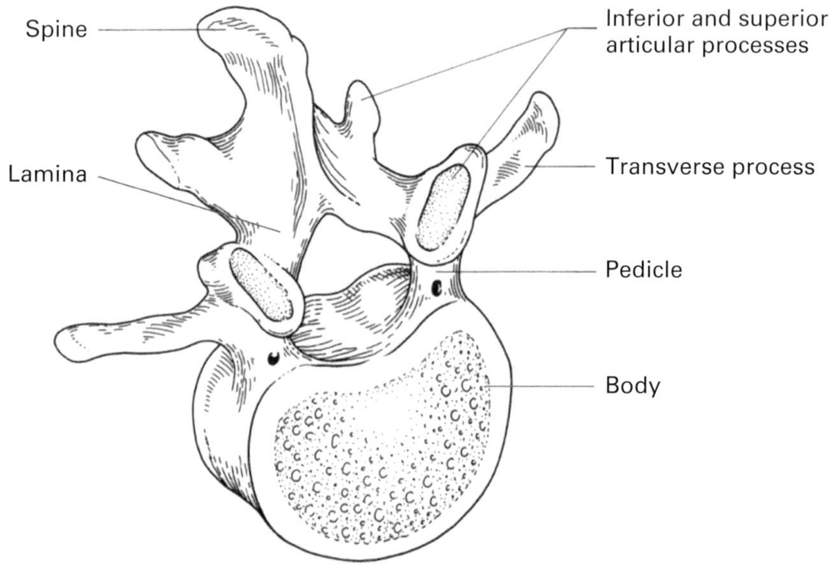

Fig. 231 A lumbar vertebra (superior aspect).

The sacrum (comprising 5 fused vertebrae)

The sacrum is a triangular bone whose upper surface articulates with the body of L5 and whose lower end articulates with the coccyx. Laterally, the sacrum articulates with the corresponding hip bone at the sacro-iliac joint.

The coccyx (comprising 3, 4 or 5 fused vertebrae)

These are considered with the bony pelvis (see page 129).

Development

Each vertebra ossifies from three primary centres, one for each side of the arch and one for the body. The body occasionally develops from two centres and failure of one of these to form results in formation of a hemivertebra with a consequent congenital scoliosis. Failure of the two arch centres to fuse posteriorly results in the condition of spina bifida, which occurs particularly in the lumbar region. Usually this is not associated with any neurological abnormality (spina bifida occulta), although in such cases there is often an overlying dimple, lipoma or tuft of hair to alert the observant clinician to the possibility of an underlying bony abnormality. More rarely, there is a gross defect of one or several arches with protrusion of the meninges, with or without elements of the cauda equina or spinal cord; this anomaly may be associated with hydrocephalus.

L5 may occasionally fuse wholly or in part with the sacrum (sacralization of the 5th lumbar vertebra) or, more rarely, the 1st segment of the sacrum may differentiate as a separate vertebra (lumbarization of S1).

Extensor muscles of the vertebral column

Running along the posterior aspect of the entire length of the vertebral column, from sacrum to skull, is a layered arrangement of powerful muscles. Some of these muscles are considerably bulky, exemplified by erector spinae.

Known collectively as the postvertebral muscles, these muscles are principally extensors of the vertebral column and extensors of the skull on the vertebral column. They are innervated, segmentally, by the posterior rami of spinal nerves. These muscles provide tremendous support to the vertebral column and are important postural muscles.

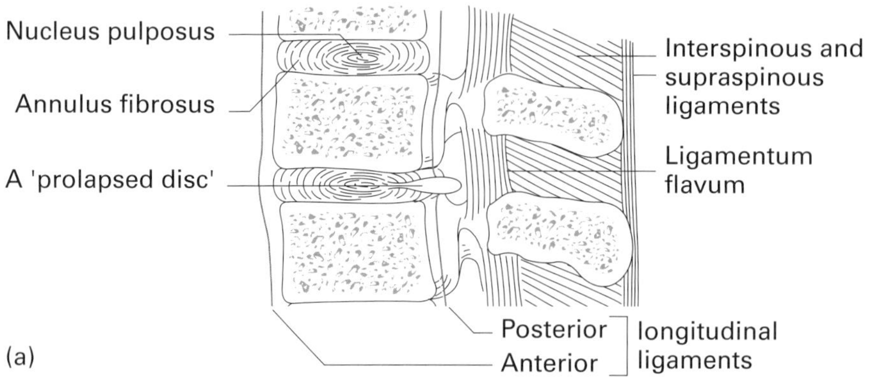

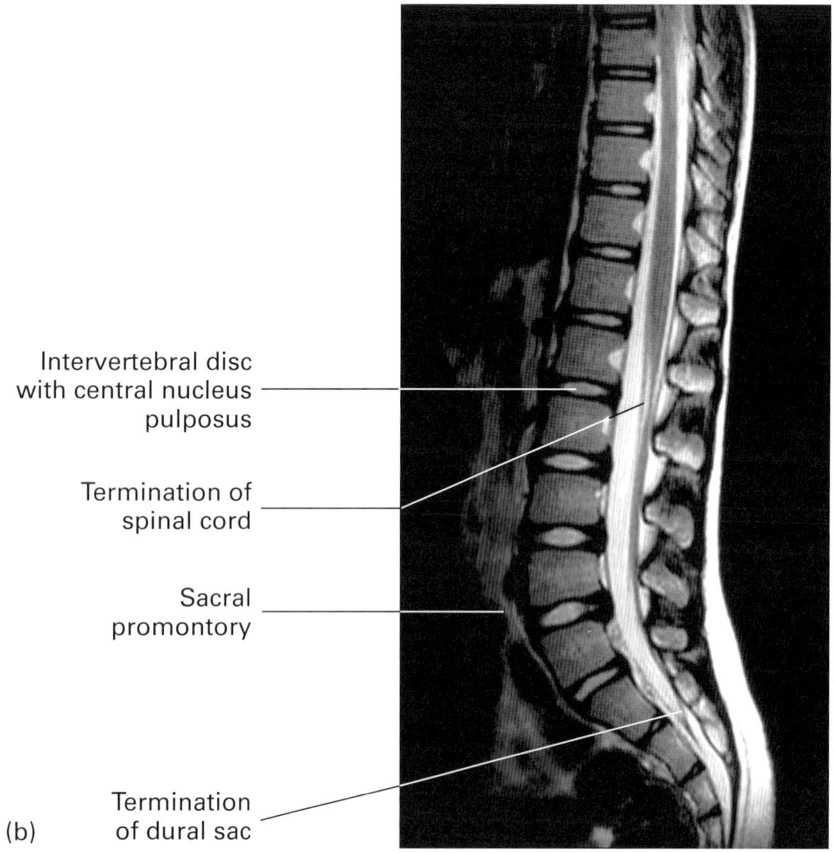

Fig. 232 (a) Longitudinal section through the lumbar vertebrae showing a normal and a prolapsed intervertebral disc. (b) Magnetic resonance imaging (MRI) through a normal lumbar spine and sacrum. Note the excellent anatomical details.

CLINICAL FEATURES

1 Fractures of the spine most commonly involve T12, L1 and L2. The cause is usually a flexion–compression type of injury (for example, a fall from a height landing on the feet or buttocks, or a heavy weight falling on the shoulders), with resultant wedging of the involved vertebrae. If, in addition to compression, there is forceful forward movement, one vertebra may displace forwards on its neighbour below, with either dislocation or fracture of the articular facets between the two (fracture dislocation) and with rupture of the interspinous ligaments.

The cervical vertebrae (particularly C7) may be fractured or, more commonly, dislocated by a fall on the head with acute flexion of the neck, as might happen on diving into shallow water. Dislocation may even result from the sudden forward jerk that may occur when a motor car or aeroplane crashes. Note that the relatively horizontal intervertebral facets of the cervical vertebrae allow dislocation to take place without their being fractured, whereas the relatively vertical thoracic and lumbar intervertebral facets nearly always fracture in forward dislocation of the dorsolumbar region.

2 The comparatively thin posterior part of the annulus fibrosus may rupture, either because of trauma or because of degenerative changes, allowing the nucleus pulposus to protrude posteriorly into the vertebral canal – the so-called 'prolapsed intervertebral disc' (Fig. 232), and also known as 'slipped disc' and 'disc herniation'. This may sometimes occur in the lower cervical intervertebral discs (C5/6 and C6/7), very rarely in the thoracic and upper lumbar region, and most commonly in the L4/5 or L5/S1 disc. The diagnosis of this and other spinal conditions has been greatly facilitated by the introduction of magnetic resonance imaging (MRI), which gives excellent anatomical details of this region (Fig. 232b).

A prolapsed L4/5 disc, protruding posterolaterally, to one or other side of the tough posterior longitudinal ligament, will produce pressure effects on the root of the corresponding 5th lumbar nerve. There may be consequent weakness of ankle dorsiflexion and numbness over the lower and lateral part of the leg and dorsum of the foot (L5). L5 involvement may also cause noticeable weakness of extension of the great toe (extensor hallucis longus).

A similar prolapse of the L5/S1 disc will press on the 1st sacral nerve. In the latter case, pain is referred to the back of the leg and foot along the distribution of the sciatic nerve. Hip flexion with the leg extended ('straight leg raising') is painful and limited because of the traction that this movement puts upon the already irritated and stretched nerve root. The ankle jerk may be diminished or absent and there may be weakness of plantarflexion.

Occasionally, the disc prolapses directly backwards, and, if this is extensive, may compress the whole cauda equina, producing paraplegia. Degenerative changes in the intervertebral disc are invariable in old age and result in atrophy, loss of hydration and loss of height of the disc and, thereby, a significant reduction in the height of the individual and exaggeration of the dorsal curvature of the spine.

3 Lumbar puncture – see page 386.

Part 6
The Nervous System

Introduction

For descriptive purposes, the nervous system can be divided, topographically, into two parts: the central nervous system (CNS) and the peripheral nervous system.

The *CNS* comprises the brain and spinal cord, which are located, respectively, in the cranial cavity and the vertebral (spinal) canal, and are continuous with each other at the foramen magnum (where the medulla oblongata of the brain stem adjoins the spinal cord).

The *peripheral nervous system* comprises the twelve pairs of cranial nerves, thirty-one pairs of spinal nerves, the ganglia associated with the cranial and spinal nerves and the right and left ganglionated sympathetic chains.

This division into central and peripheral systems is somewhat arbitrary, as the two 'systems' are physically connected and normally function in an integrated and co-ordinated manner.

The brain

On a functional basis, the brain may be pictured as being made up of four major divisions:

1 brainstem (comprising, from below upwards, the medulla oblongata, pons and midbrain);
2 cerebellum;
3 diencephalon (comprising, mainly, the thalamus and hypothalamus);
4 cerebral hemispheres.

By another convention, based on embryological development, the brain may be divided into the forebrain (comprising the cerebral hemispheres and diencephalon), midbrain and hindbrain (made up of the pons, medulla oblongata and cerebellum).

The brainstem

Extending from just above the tentorial hiatus to just below the foramen magnum, the brainstem is a stalk-like structure that is continuous superiorly with the diencephalon, and inferiorly with the spinal cord. As has been stated previously, the brainstem and the cerebellum are situated in the posterior cranial fossa.

The brainstem serves three major functions by:

1 housing the nuclei of all but two of the twelve pairs of cranial nerves (the exceptions being the cranial nerve pairs I and II which may both be regarded as peripheral extensions of the forebrain);
2 acting as a 'thoroughfare' for the various ascending and descending nerve tracts running to and from the cerebral cortex, and for other tracts that project to the cerebellum;
3 containing the reticular formation (a fine and diffuse network of nerve cells and nerve fibres) and the reticular activating system. The reticular formation spans the

entire length of the brainstem and harbours the 'vital centres' – important reflex centres that regulate respiratory and cardiovascular function. The reticular formation and reticular activating system regulate the individual's level of awareness and wakefulness. Damage to the reticular formation in the upper part of the brainstem may cause the patient to be in a state of prolonged coma.

The medulla oblongata

The medulla oblongata is 2.5 cm (1 in) in length and about 1.8 cm (0.75 in) in diameter. It is continuous below, through the foramen magnum, with the spinal cord and above with the pons; posteriorly, it is connected to the cerebellum by way of the right and left inferior cerebellar peduncles.

External features (Fig. 233)

The anterior surface of the medulla is grooved by a median fissure, on either side of which are longitudinal prominences termed pyramids which contain the pyramidal tracts. These *pyramids*, in turn, are separated from the *olivary eminences* by the anterolateral sulcus along which the rootlets of the XIIth cranial nerve emerge. Emerging from the posterolateral aspect of the olivary eminences are the rootlets of cranial nerves IX, X and XI. The posterior median sulcus of the cord is continued halfway up the medulla, where it widens out to form the inferior limits of the diamond-shaped outline of the 4th ventricle. On either side of the sulcus the posterior columns of the spinal cord expand to form two distinct tubercles, corresponding to the gracile and cuneate nuclei.

The *blood supply* of the medulla is derived from the vertebral arteries directly and from their posterior inferior cerebellar branches.

CLINICAL FEATURES

The medulla contains the respiratory, cardiac and vasomotor centres – the 'vital centres'. The respiratory centre is particularly vulnerable to compression, injury or poliomyelitis with consequent respiratory failure.

The pons

External features (Fig. 233)

The pons lies between the medulla and the midbrain and is connected to the right and left cerebellar hemispheres by the right and left middle cerebellar peduncles, respectively. It is 2.5 cm (1 in) in length and 3.8 cm (1.5 in) in width. Its ventral surface presents a shallow, vertical median groove and numerous transverse ridges, which are continuous laterally on either side with the corresponding middle cerebellar peduncle. The dorsal surface of the pons forms part of the floor of the 4th ventricle. Ventrally, its junction with the medulla is marked close to the midline by the emergence of the VIth cranial nerves and, in the angle between the pons and the cerebellum, by the VIIth and

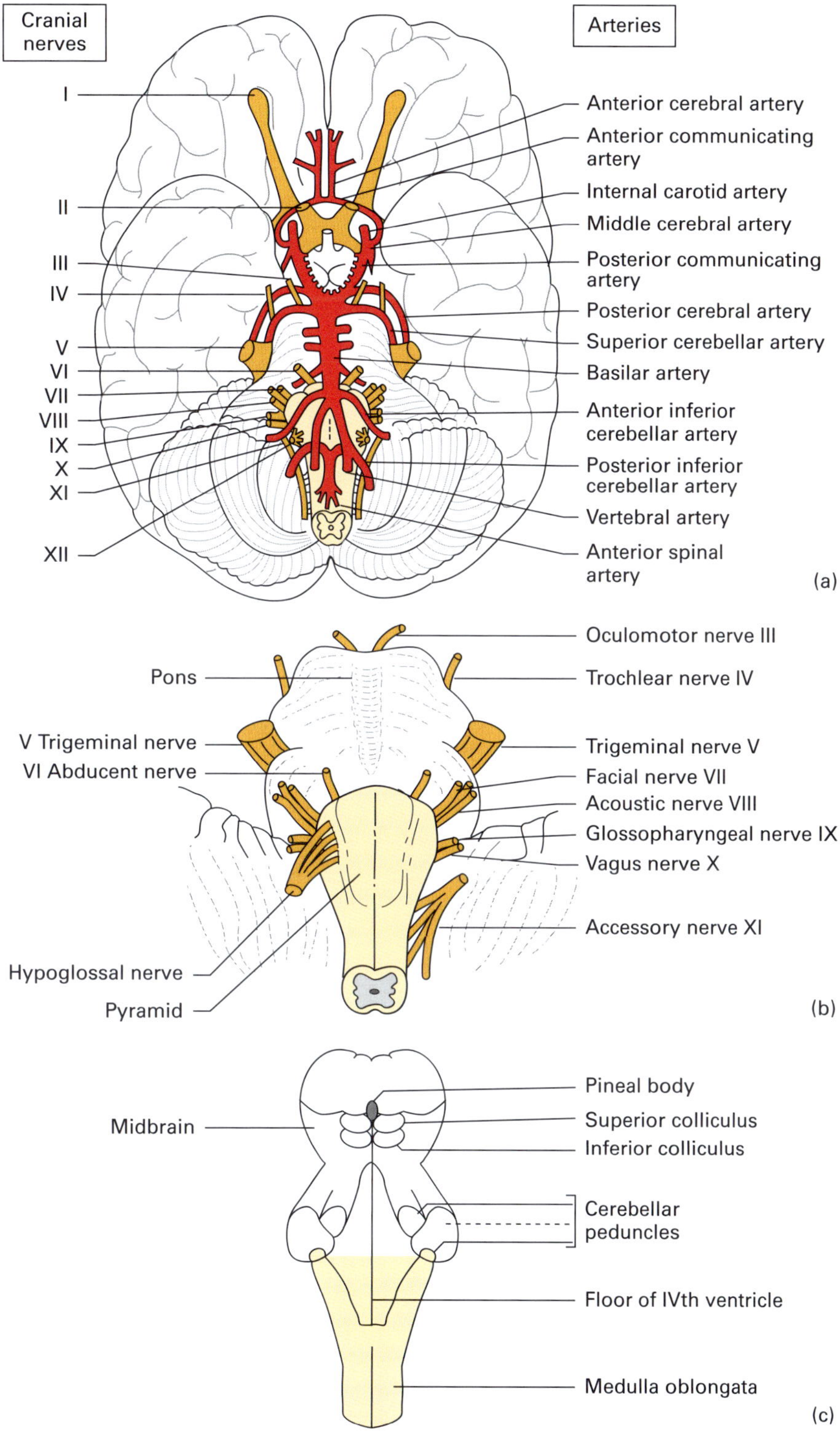

Fig. 233 (a) The base of the brain showing the cranial nerve roots and their relationships to the circle of Willis. (b) Anterior aspect of the brainstem. (c) Posterior aspect of the brainstem.

VIIIth cranial nerves. Both the motor and sensory roots of the Vth cranial nerve leave the anterolateral part of the pons near its upper border.

The *blood supply* of the pons is derived from multiple small pontine branches of the basilar artery (Fig. 233), which in turn is formed by the confluence of the two vertebral arteries.

The midbrain

The midbrain is the shortest part of the brainstem; it is just under 2.5 cm (1 in) long and connects the pons and cerebellum to the diencephalon. It lies within the tentorial hiatus (the gap in the tentorium cerebelli) and is largely hidden by the surrounding structures.

External features (Fig. 233)

The only parts of the midbrain visible from the ventral aspect of the brain are the two *cerebral peduncles*, which emerge from the substance of the cerebral hemisphere and pass downwards and medially, connecting the internal capsule to the pons. The right and left oculomotor nerves (cranial nerve III) emerge between the two cerebral peduncles in the *interpeduncular fossa*. Viewed from the lateral aspect, the midbrain is seen to consist of three distinct portions: the basis pedunculi ventrally, the midbrain *tegmentum* centrally and the *tectum* dorsally. The trochlear nerve (IV), the optic tract and the posterior cerebral artery wind around this aspect of the midbrain. The dorsal aspect of the midbrain (Fig. 233c) presents the four *colliculi* (or *corpora quadrigemini*) and the superior *medullary velum* between the two superior cerebellar peduncles. The *pineal body* is a midline structure. It rests between the two superior colliculi and is attached by a stalk to the posterior part of the thalamus. The pineal secretes melatonin and has an important role in setting the circadian rhythm. When calcified, the pineal gland is easily identified on skull radiographs. It may then give the important radiological sign of lateral displacement by a space-occupying lesion of the cerebral hemisphere.

The cerebellum

External features (Fig. 233; see Fig. 235)

The cerebellum is the largest part of the hindbrain and occupies most of the posterior cranial fossa. It is made up of the right and left *cerebellar hemispheres* and a median *vermis*. Inferiorly, the vermis is clearly separated from the two hemispheres and lies at the bottom of a deep cleft, the *vallecula*; superiorly, it is marked off from the hemispheres only as a low median elevation. A small ventral portion of each cerebellar hemisphere lies on the middle cerebellar peduncle of its side and is almost completely separated from the rest of the cerebellum. It is termed the *flocculus*. The surface of the cerebellum is divided into numerous narrow *folia* and, by a few deep fissures, into a number of lobules. The effect of this fissuring is to give the cerebellum in section the appearance of a many-branched tree (the *arbor vitae*) (see Fig. 242).

Internal structure

The structure of the cerebellum is remarkably uniform. It consists of a *cortex* of grey matter (in which all the afferent fibres terminate) covering a mass of white matter, in which deep nuclei of grey matter are buried.

The cerebellum is connected to the brainstem by way of three pairs of *cerebellar peduncles*. The *inferior peduncles* connect it to the dorsolateral aspect of the medulla; the *middle cerebellar peduncles* to the pons; and the *superior peduncles* to the caudal midbrain. Ventrally, the cerebellum is related to the 4th ventricle and to the medulla and pons; laterally, to the sigmoid venous sinus and the mastoid antrum and air cells; and posterosuperiorly, it is separated from the cerebral hemispheres by the *tentorium cerebelli*.

The *blood supply* of the cerebellum is derived from three pairs of arteries (Fig. 211); the *posterior inferior cerebellar* branches of the vertebral arteries supply the posterior aspect of the vermis and hemispheres, and the *anterior inferior* and *superior cerebellar branches of the basilar artery* supply the anterolateral part of the undersurface and the superior aspect of the cerebellum, respectively.

Functions of the cerebellum

The principal function of the cerebellum is to regulate and maintain balance and to co-ordinate timing and precision of body movements. The cerebellum has multiple connections with the cerebral cortex, reticular formation in the brainstem, thalamus and vestibular nuclei. Through these intricate connections, the cerebellum constantly monitors proprioceptive sensory input from joints, muscles and tendons and accordingly refines and co-ordinates the contractions of skeletal muscles.

However, unlike the cerebral cortex of the primary motor area, the cerebellum is neither incapable of initiating movement nor involved in the conscious perception of somatic or visceral sensations.

CLINICAL FEATURES

1 As the cerebellum is principally concerned with balance and the regulation of posture, muscle tone and muscular co-ordination, it is not surprising that cerebellar lesions result in disturbance of one or more of these motor functions, manifesting as any one or more of the following: unsteady gait, ataxia, hypotonia, tremor, nystagmus, dysarthria and dysdiadokokinesia (the inability to perform alternating movements rapidly, e.g. supination/pronation).

Lesions of the cerebellum give rise to symptoms and signs on the *same side of the body*.

Destruction of the dentate nucleus (a large collection of cells within the cerebellar white matter) or the superior cerebellar peduncle results in a disability almost as severe as ablation of the entire cerebellar hemisphere.

2 Thrombosis of the posterior inferior cerebellar artery (PICA) gives rise to a characteristic syndrome (PICA syndrome) marked by ataxia and hypotonia of the ipsilateral limbs owing to involvement of the inferior cerebellar peduncle and cerebellar cortex, signs of cranial nerve involvement (V to X) and contralateral loss of pain and thermal sensibility (spinothalamic tract involvement).

The diencephalon

The diencephalon comprises principally the hypothalamus and thalamus, which are continuous with each other. A vertically disposed, median, cleft-like space is present between the right and left halves of the diencephalon and is called the 3rd ventricle (Fig. 234). In addition to the thalamus and hypothalamus, the diencephalon includes two small but functionally important regions: the epithalamus and ventral thalamus. The epithalamus is the dorsal portion of the diencephalon and contains the pineal body. The ventral thalamus (also known as the subthalamus) contains the subthalamic nucleus, which is one of the basal nuclei (basal ganglia). It is believed to be the main regulator and modulator of the other basal nuclei, and thus is a significant influence on motor activity.

The hypothalamus (Figs 233a, 234)

The hypothalamus forms the floor of the 3rd ventricle, and also the lower part of its lateral wall. Viewed from below, the hypothalamus is seen to include, from before backwards, the *optic chiasma*, the *tuber cinereum*, the *infundibular stalk* (leading down to

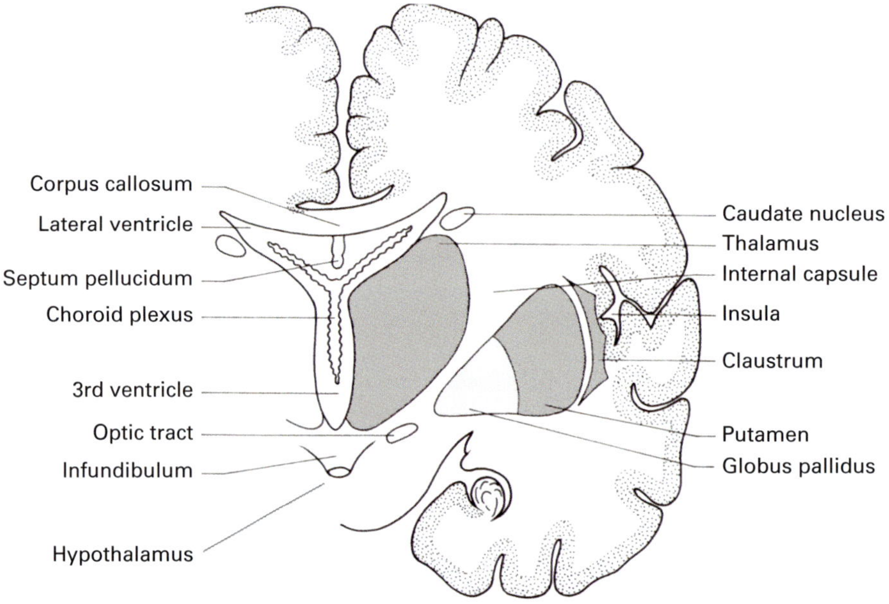

Fig. 234 The thalamus and 3rd ventricle in coronal section.

the posterior lobe of the pituitary), the *mamillary bodies* and the posterior *perforated substance*. In each of these there is a number of cell masses or nuclei and a fibre pathway – the medial forebrain bundle – which runs throughout the length of the hypothalamus and serves to link it with the midbrain postero-inferiorly and the basal forebrain areas anterosuperiorly.

Sherrington described the hypothalamus as the head ganglion of the autonomic system. It is largely concerned with autonomic activity and can be divided into a posteromedial sympathetic area and an anterolateral area concerned with parasympathetic activity.

The hypothalamus plays an important role in endocrine control by the formation of releasing factors or release-inhibiting factors. These substances, following their secretion into the hypophyseal portal vessels, influence the production by the cells of the anterior pituitary of adrenocorticotrophin, follicle-stimulating hormone, luteinizing hormone, prolactin, somatotrophin, thyrotrophin and melanocyte-stimulating hormone.

The hormones oxytocin and vasopressin (antidiuretic hormone) are produced by two distinct aggregations of neurones (the paraventricular and supra-optic nuclei, respectively) in the hypothalamus and released at their axon terminals in the posterior pituitary. Oxytocin and antidiuretic hormone are thus neurosecretions.

In addition to its major influence on the autonomic nervous system and on pituitary function, the hypothalamus also plays a significant role in temperature regulation, water and electrolyte balance, regulation of appetite and sleep–wake patterns.

CLINICAL FEATURES

1 Given its manifold functions, lesions of the hypothalamus may present to the clinician as a variety of autonomic and non-autonomic disturbances, e.g. somnolence, disturbances of temperature regulation and obesity, as well as a variety of endocrine abnormalities, e.g. hypogonadism and hypothyroidism.
2 Damage to the supra-optic nucleus or the infundibular stalk leads to diabetes insipidus, through loss of production of antidiuretic hormone.

The thalamus (Fig. 234; see Fig. 236)

The thalamus is an oval mass of grey matter that forms the upper part of the lateral wall of the 3rd ventricle; it extends from the interventricular foramen rostrally, to the midbrain caudally. Laterally, it is related to the internal capsule (and through it to the basal ganglia) and dorsally to the floor of the lateral ventricle. Medially, it is frequently connected with its fellow of the opposite side through the *massa intermedia* (interthalamic connexus). Posteriorly, it presents five distinct eminences: the *pulvinar* in the midline, flanked on each side by the corresponding *medial* and *lateral geniculate bodies*.

The medial and lateral geniculate bodies are the thalamic relay nuclei of hearing and vision, respectively.

The thalamus is the principal sensory relay nucleus that projects impulses from the main sensory pathways onto the cerebral cortex. It does this via a number of thalamic radiations in the internal capsule.

The blood supply of the thalamus is derived principally from the posterior cerebral artery through its thalamostriate branches, which pierce the posterior perforated substance to supply also the posterior part of the internal capsule. Thalamic damage, by occlusion of this blood supply, results in contralateral sensory loss of the face and body.

The pituitary gland (hypophysis cerebri)

This is an example of a 'two-in-one' organ, of which nature appears so keen; compare the two glandular components of the suprarenal cortex and medulla and the exocrine and endocrine parts of the pancreas, testis and ovary. The pituitary comprises a larger anterior and smaller posterior lobe, the latter connected by the hollow infundibulum (pituitary stalk) to the tuber cinereum in the floor of the 3rd ventricle. The two lobes of the pituitary are connected by a narrow zone termed the pars intermedia.

The pituitary lies in the cavity of the pituitary fossa covered over by the diaphragma sellae, which is a fold of dura mater. This fold has a central aperture through which passes the infundibulum. Below the pituitary is the body of the sphenoid; laterally on either side lies the corresponding cavernous sinus and its contents separated by dura mater (Fig. 214), with intercavernous sinuses running in front, behind and below the pituitary. The optic chiasma lies above, immediately in front of the infundibulum.

Structure

The anterior lobe is extremely cellular and consists of chromophobe, eosinophilic and basophilic cells. The pars intermedia contains large colloid vesicles reminiscent of the thyroid. The posterior lobe is made up of nerve fibres whose cell bodies lie in the hypothalamus.

Development

The posterior lobe is a diverticulum of the diencephalon. The anterior lobe and the pars intermedia develop from Rathke's pouch in the roof of the embryonic buccal cavity. Occasionally, a tumour grows from remnants of the epithelium of this pouch (craniopharyngioma). These tumours are often cystic and calcified.

Owing to their strikingly different histological appearances and different embryological origins, the anterior and posterior lobes of the pituitary are also referred to as the adenohypophysis and neurohypophysis, respectively.

CLINICAL FEATURES

Tumours of the pituitary, as well as forming intracranial space-occupying lesions, may have two special features: their endocrine disturbances and their relationship to the optic chiasma.

Chromophobe adenoma is a commonly occurring tumour that arises in the anterior pituitary. As it enlarges, it expands the pituitary fossa (sella turcica) and this may be demonstrated radiologically. Compression of the optic chiasma produces the very rapid typical bitemporal hemianopia (see 'The optic nerve (II) and the visual pathway', page 393, and Fig. 250). The tumour itself is non-secretory and gradually destroys the normally functioning gland. The patient develops hypopituitarism with loss of sex characteristics, hypothyroidism and hypoadrenalism. In childhood there is an arrest of growth. As the tumour extends there may be involvement of the hypothalamus with diabetes insipidus and obesity.

The *eosinophil adenoma* secretes the pituitary growth hormones. If it occurs before puberty, which is unusual, it produces gigantism; after puberty, it results in acromegaly.

The *basophil adenoma* is small, produces no pressure effects and may be associated with Cushing's syndrome, although this more often results from hyperplasia or tumour of the suprarenal cortex.

The close relationship of the pituitary to the sphenoid sinus makes it possible to insert fibreoptic instruments into the pituitary gland by a transnasal, trans-sphenoidal approach. This is now the preferred approach to surgery of pituitary tumours, rather than through a frontal bone flap.

The cerebral hemispheres

The cerebral hemispheres, which, in man, have developed out of all proportion to the rest of the brain, comprise the cerebral cortex, the basal ganglia and their afferent and efferent connections. The lateral ventricles, containing cerebrospinal fluid (CSF), occupy the centre of each cerebral hemisphere.

The cerebral cortex

The cortex of the cerebral hemispheres is divided on topographical and functional grounds into four lobes – frontal, parietal, temporal and occipital (Fig. 235).

Frontal lobe

This includes all the cortex anterior to the central sulcus of Rolando. Its important cortical areas are as follows:

1 *The motor cortex*. The primary motor area occupies a large part of the precentral gyrus. It receives afferents from the premotor cortex, thalamus and cerebellum and is concerned with voluntary movements. Stimulation of this area results in discrete muscle movements. Details of localization of function in the motor cortex are considered on page 372.

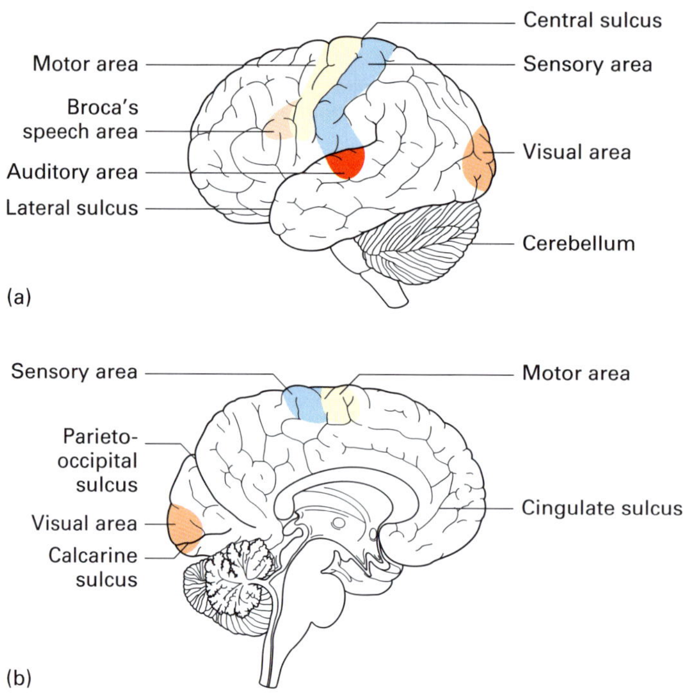

Fig. 235 Localization of function in the cerebral cortex. (a) Lateral aspect. (b) Medial aspect.

2 *The premotor cortex*. This lies anterior to the precentral gyrus and the adjoining lower part of the frontal gyri. It, too, is concerned with voluntary movement, but its stimulation results in movements of groups of muscles with a common function, and thus lacks the precise definition of muscle movement that is a feature of stimulation of the precentral gyrus.

3 *Eye motor field*. This lies in the middle frontal area anterior to the premotor cortex. Lesions of this area result in impaired eye movement with deviation of gaze to the side of the lesion.

4 *Broca's speech area*. Lesions of the area around the posterior part of the inferior frontal gyrus of the dominant hemisphere (the left hemisphere in 98% of individuals) were shown by Broca to affect the motor element in speech.

5 *Frontal association cortex (clinically called the prefrontal cortex)*. This comprises a considerable part of the frontal lobe and is one of the remarkable, evolutionary advances seen in the human brain. Its afferents are derived from the thalamus, limbic area and also from other cortical areas; it probably sends efferents to the thalamus and hypothalamus. From a functional point of view the lateral aspect of the frontal lobe appears to be related to 'intellectual activity' (i.e. cognitive functions – analysis, judgement and planning), the medial and orbital surfaces to affective (or emotional) behaviour and the control of autonomic activity.

Parietal lobe

The parietal lobe is bounded anteriorly by the central sulcus and behind by a line drawn from the parieto-occipital sulcus to the posterior end of the lateral (Sylvian) sulcus. The important cortical areas of the parietal lobe are as follows.

1 The *primary somatosensory cortex*. The postcentral gyrus receives afferent fibres from the thalamus and is concerned with all forms of somatic sensation. Details of localization along the sensory cortex are considered on pages 370 and 371.
2 The *parietal association cortex*, comprising the remainder of the parietal lobe, is concerned largely with the recognition of somatic sensory stimulation and its integration with other forms of sensory information. It also receives afferents from the thalamus and, when damaged, gives rise to more complex defects than simple loss of sensation. An example of this is the inability to recognize somatic stimuli, which is called *astereognosis*; put a pen or a coin in the patient's hand – he is aware of the object but is unable to recognize what it is. The lower part of the parietal lobe in the subject's dominant hemisphere interacts with the somatosensory visual and auditory associations and has a key role in language.

The temporal lobe

This is arbitrarily separated from the occipital lobe by a line drawn vertically downwards from the upper end of the lateral sulcus.

The important cortical areas of the temporal lobe are the following.

1 The *auditory cortex*. This lies in the superior temporal gyrus on the lateral and superior surfaces of the hemisphere. Its afferent fibres are from the medial geniculate body, and it is concerned with the perception of auditory stimuli.
2 The *temporal association cortex*. The area surrounding the auditory cortex is responsible for the recognition of auditory stimuli and for their integration with other sensory modalities. Lesions of this area result in auditory agnosia, i.e. the inability to recognize or to understand the significance of meaningful sounds. The cortical region just above and behind this area on the dominant hemisphere (Wernicke's area) is of considerable importance in the sensory aspects of language comprehension. This visual area of the occipital lobe connects with the temporal lobe and is concerned with visual recognition. The antero-inferior aspect of the frontal lobe connects with the medial aspect of the temporal lobe and is concerned with behaviour.

The parahippocampal gyrus The cortex of the most medial part of the undersurface of the temporal lobe is known as the parahippocampal gyrus, much of which is referred to as the *entorhinal cortex*. It receives widespread association cortical afferents and is a significant source of inputs to the hippocampus. Anteriorly, it is related to the olfactory cortex of the uncus. Medially, it is in direct continuity with the layer of in-rolled cortex which is the *hippocampus* and which is one of the most important sources of afferents to this structure. The hippocampus occupies the whole length of the floor of the inferior horn of the lateral ventricle and extends to the amygdala. It sends its efferents into the overlying layer of white matter known as the *alveus*. The fibres of the alveus collect on the medial margin of the hippocampus to form a compact bundle, the *fimbria*, which, as it arches under the corpus callosum, becomes known as the *fornix*. The fornix passes forwards and then downwards in front of the interventricular foramen and finally backwards into the hypothalamus to terminate in the *mamillary body*. It also gives fibres to the thalamus and the hypothalamus.

Projection of the hippocampus to the hypothalamus is part of the *limbic system*. This is an important substrate for emotions, behaviour and memory. The circuit is completed by projections of the hypothalamus to the thalamus, from the thalamus to the cingulate gyrus and from thence back to the hippocampus. Bilateral hippocampal damage results in inability to form new long-term memories.

The amygdaloid nuclear complex The amygdaloid nuclear complex is also a prominent temporal lobe structure, situated immediately rostral to the hippocampus. It is conveniently divided into three groups of nuclei: corticomedial, central and basolateral, which receive largely olfactory, gustatory and association cortical afferents, respectively. These divisions also have more or less separable projections to the hypothalamus and septum, brainstem autonomic centres and ventral striatum. The amygdala is involved in the control of emotional behaviour and conditioned reflexes. Its neuroanatomical connections are clearly appropriate for such a role, since it is in a position to affect emotional responses in endocrine, autonomic and motor domains. Destruction of the amygdala is particularly associated with reduced aggressive behaviour, whereas the very high density of benzodiazepine receptors here has suggested amygdaloid involvement in anxiety and stress and their treatments.

Occipital lobe

The occipital lobe lies behind the parietal and temporal lobes. On its medial aspect it presents the Y-shaped *calcarine* and *postcalcarine sulci* (Fig. 235). The following cortical areas are noteworthy.

1 The *visual cortex* surrounds the calcarine and postcalcarine sulci and receives its afferent fibres from the lateral geniculate body of the thalamus of the same side; it is concerned with vision of the opposite (contralateral) half field of sight (Fig. 236).
2 The *occipital association cortex* lies anterior to the visual cortex. This area is particularly concerned with the recognition and integration of visual stimuli.

The insula (Figs 234, 236)

If the lips of the lateral sulcus are separated, it is seen that there is a considerable area of cortex buried in the floor of this sulcus. This area is known as the *insula of Reil*. It is divided into a number of small gyri and is crossed by the middle cerebral artery. Apart from its upper part, which abuts on the sensory cortex and probably represents the taste area of the cerebral cortex, the function of the insula is unknown. Its stimulation excites visceral effects such as belching, increased salivation, gastric movements and vomiting.

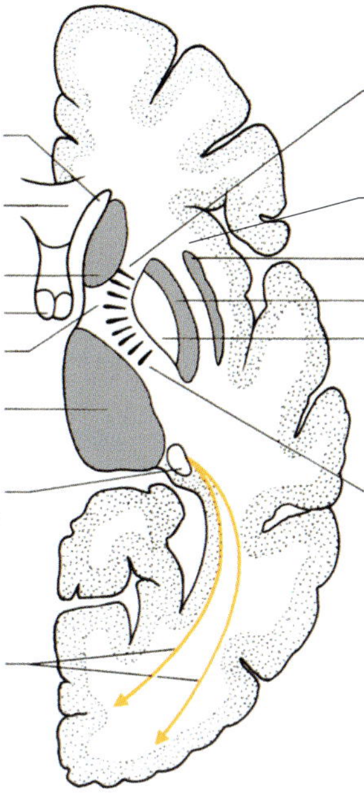

Fig. 236 The basal nuclei (basal ganglia) and internal capsule shown in horizontal section through the cerebrum.

The connections of the cerebral cortex

As has been indicated, most areas of the cerebral cortex receive their main afferent input from the thalamus, but, in addition to this, there are well-established *commissural connections* with the corresponding area of the opposite hemisphere by way of the *corpus callosum*. *Intracortical association fibres* also link neighbouring cortical areas on the same side and, in some cases, connect distant cortical areas; thus, the frontal, occipital and temporal lobes within the same hemisphere are directly connected by long association pathways.

CLINICAL FEATURES

It is convenient to summarize here the clinical effects of lesions affecting the principal cortical areas.

1 *Frontal cortex* – impairment of higher mental functions and emotions.

2 *Precentral (motor) cortex* – weakness of the opposite side of the body; lesions low down the cortex affecting the face and arm, high lesions affecting the leg. Midline lesions (meningioma, sagittal sinus thrombosis or a gunshot wound) may produce paraplegia by involving both leg areas.

3 *Sensory cortex* – contralateral hemianaesthesia (distributed in the same pattern as the motor cortex) affecting especially the higher sensory modalities such as stereognosis and two-point position sense.

(For area localizations along the motor and sensory cortex, see page 372.)

4 *Occipital cortex* – contralateral homonymous hemianopia.

5 Lesions adjacent to the *lateral sulcus* in the frontal, parietal or temporal lobes of the dominant hemisphere result in aphasia.

The basal nuclei (basal ganglia) (Figs 234, 236)

These compact masses of grey matter are situated deep in the substance of the cerebral hemisphere and comprise the *corpus striatum* (composed of the caudate nucleus, the putamen and the globus pallidus) and the *claustrum*. Together with the cerebellum, they are involved in co-ordination and control of movement.

The corpus striatum

The *caudate nucleus* is a large homogeneous mass of grey matter consisting of a *head*, anterior to the interventricular foramen and forming the lateral wall of the anterior horn of the lateral ventricle; a *body*, forming the lateral wall of the body of the ventricle; and an elongated *tail*, which forms the roof of the inferior (temporal) horn of the ventricle. It is largely separated from the putamen by the *internal capsule*, but the two structures are connected anteriorly. The *putamen* is a roughly ovoid mass closely applied to the lateral aspect of the *globus pallidus*; together, they are called the *lentiform nucleus*. The corpus striatum receives afferent connections from the cerebral cortex and sends efferents to the globus pallidus. From there, fibres project to the thalamus and, thence, back to the premotor cortex. Dopaminergic fibres project from the substantia nigra to the corpus striatum and efferent fibres also pass to the thalamus, hypothalamus, red nucleus, substantia nigra and the inferior olivary nucleus.

The long ascending and descending pathways

The somatic afferent pathways (Fig. 237)

1 Proprioceptive and tactile impulses pass uninterruptedly through the posterior root ganglia, through the ipsilateral *posterior columns* of the spinal cord to the *gracile* and *cuneate nuclei* in the lower part of the medulla. In the posterior columns there is a fairly precise organization of the afferent fibres; those from sacral and lumbar segments are situated medially in the tracts whereas fibres from thoracic and cervical levels are successively added to their lateral aspect. This arrangement according to body segments is maintained in the gracile and cuneate nuclei and in the efferents from these nuclei to the contralateral thalamus. The fibres arising from the gracile and cuneate nuclei immediately cross over to the opposite side in the *sensory decussation* of the medulla and continue up to the thalamus as a compact contralateral bundle – the *medial lemniscus*.
2 Dorsal root fibres subserving pain and temperature, together with some tactile afferents, end ipsilaterally in the *substantia gelatinosa* of the posterior horn. They then synapse and cross to the contralateral anterior lateral columns of the cord and are relayed to the contralateral thalamus. The fibre crossing occurs in the anterior white commissure of the spinal cord. In the brainstem these fibres come to lie immediately lateral to the medial lemniscus and are sometimes known as the *spinal lemniscus* (Fig. 237). They terminate in the thalamus.

These somatic afferents are relayed from the thalamus, through the posterior limb of the internal capsule (Fig. 236) to the somatic sensory cortex of the *postcentral gyrus*. In the internal capsule the fibres are arranged in the sequence 'face, arm, trunk and leg'

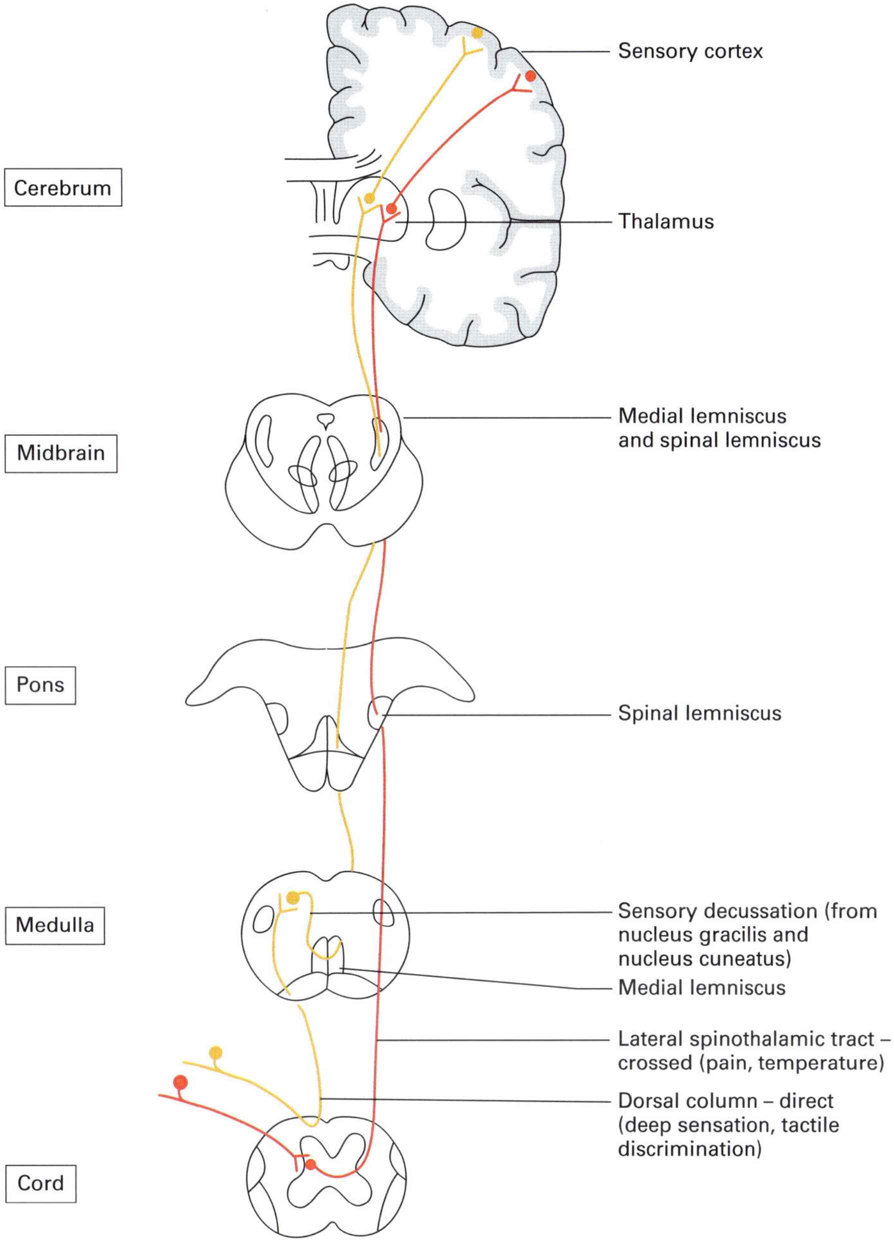

Fig. 237 The long ascending pathways of the dorsal columns (yellow lines) and spinothalamic tracts (red lines).

from before backwards, and this segregation persists in the sensory cortex, where the leg is represented on the dorsal and medial part of the cortex, the trunk and arm in its middle portion and the face most inferiorly. Since the size of the area of cortical representation reflects the density of the peripheral innervation and hence complexity of the function being performed rather than the area of the receptive field, there is a good deal of distortion of the body image in the cortex, the cortical representation of the face and hand being much greater than that of the limbs and trunk.

CLINICAL FEATURES

1 Lesions of the sensory pathway most commonly occur in the internal capsule following some form of cerebrovascular accident. If complete, these result in a total hemianaesthesia of the opposite side of the body. In partial lesions the area of sensory loss will be determined by the site of the injury/ischaemia in the internal capsule and, from a knowledge of the sensory (and motor) loss, it is usually possible to determine with some degree of accuracy the site of a lesion in the capsule.

2 Since there is modality segregation below the decussation of the medial lemniscus, lesions of the sensory pathways at cord level result in dissociation of sensation, with an area of analgesia contralaterally together with impairment of tactile sensibility ipsilaterally (for further details, see pages 381–383).

The auditory, visual and olfactory pathways are dealt with later under the appropriate cranial nerves.

The motor pathways (Fig. 238)

It is customary to divide the motor pathways of the brain and spinal cord into pyramidal and extrapyramidal systems. Although the latter is an imprecise term, it nevertheless provides a useful collective term for the many motor structures not confined to the pyramidal tracts in the medulla.

The pyramidal tract The pyramidal system is the main 'voluntary' motor pathway and derives its name from the fact that projections to the motor neurones in the spinal cord are grouped together in the medullary pyramids. The fibres in this pathway arise from a wide area of the cerebral cortex. About two-thirds derive from the motor and premotor cortex of the frontal lobes; however, about one-third arise from the primary somatosensory cortex. In both the motor and premotor cortex there is an organization comparable to that seen in the sensory area. Again, the body is inverted so that the 'leg area' is situated in the dorsomedial part of the precentral gyrus encroaching on the medial surface of the hemisphere, supplied by the anterior cerebral artery. The 'face area' is near the lateral sulcus, while the 'arm area' occupies a central position, both supplied by the middle cerebral artery. Again, the body image is greatly distorted; the areas representing the hand, lips, eyes and foot are exaggerated out of proportion to the rest of the body and in accordance with the complexity of the tasks they perform.

From the cortex, the motor fibres pass through the posterior limb of the internal capsule (Fig. 236) where they are again organized in the sequence of 'face, arm, leg', anteroposteriorly. From the internal capsule the fibres form a compact bundle that occupies the central third of the cerebral peduncle. From there they pass through the ventral pons, where they are broken up into a number of small bundles between the cells of the pontine nuclei and the transversely disposed pontocerebellar fibres. Near the lower

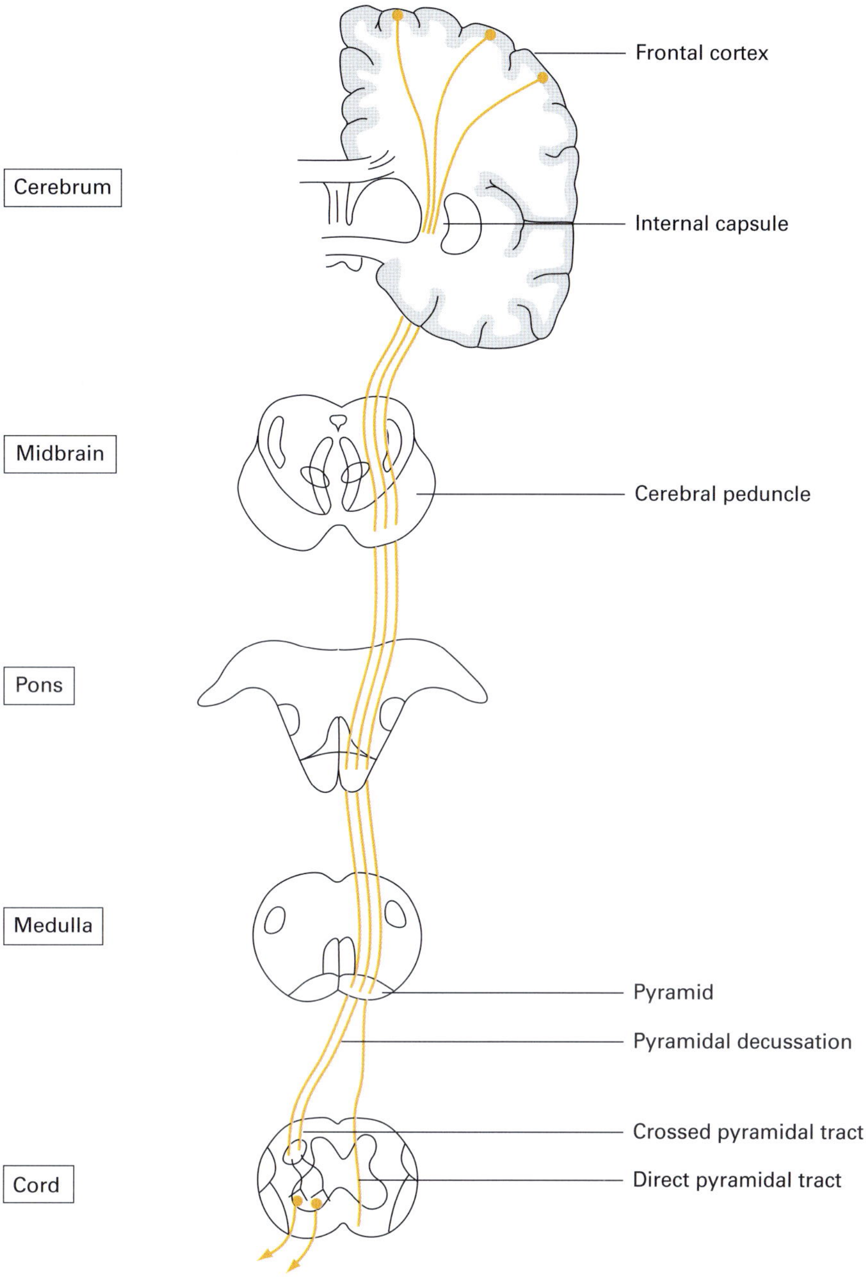

Fig. 238 The long descending pathway of the pyramidal tract.

end of the pons they again collect to form a single bundle, which comes to lie on the ventral surface of the medulla and forms the elevation known as the 'pyramid'. As it passes through the brainstem, the pyramidal system gives off, at regular intervals, contributions to the somatic and branchial arch efferent nuclei of the cranial nerves. Most of these *corticobulbar fibres* cross over in the brainstem, but many of the cranial nerve nuclei are bilaterally innervated.

Near the lower end of the medulla the great majority of the pyramidal tract fibres cross over to the opposite side and come to occupy a central position in the lateral white column of the spinal cord. This is the so-called 'crossed pyramidal tract' shown in Fig. 244. A small proportion of the fibres of the medullary pyramid, however, remain uncrossed until they reach the segmental level at which they finally terminate. This is the *direct* or *uncrossed pyramidal tract*, which runs downwards close to the anteromedian fissure of the cord, with fibres passing from it at each segment to the opposite side.

In view of the frequent involvement of the pyramidal tract in cerebrovascular accidents, its blood supply is listed here in some detail:

- *motor cortex* – leg area: anterior cerebral artery; face and arm areas: middle cerebral artery;
- *internal capsule* – branches of the middle cerebral artery;
- *cerebral peduncle* – posterior cerebral artery;
- *pons* – pontine branches of basilar artery;
- *medulla* – anterior spinal branches of vertebral artery;
- *spinal cord* – segmental branches of anterior and posterior spinal arteries.

CLINICAL FEATURES

1 It is important to remember that, in the motor cortex, movements are represented rather than individual muscles; lesions of this pathway result in paralysis of voluntary movement on the opposite side of the body, although the muscles themselves are not paralysed and may cause involuntary movements. This is the essential difference between an 'upper motor neurone' lesion (i.e. a lesion of the central motor pathway) and a 'lower motor neurone' lesion (i.e. a lesion affecting the cranial nerve nuclei, or the anterior horn cells or their axons). In both types of lesion muscular paralysis results, in the latter, reflex activity is abolished and flaccidity and muscular atrophy follow, whereas, in pyramidal lesions, there is spasticity, increased tendon reflexes and an extensor plantar response.

2 Experimental lesions strictly confined to the pyramidal tract are not followed by increased muscular tone in the affected part (spasticity), but clinically this is a feature of upper motor neurone lesions; it is attributable to concomitant involvement of the extrapyramidal system, hence demonstrating the oversimplification of the pyramidal and extrapyramidal concept.

3 The pyramidal tract is most frequently involved in cerebrovascular accidents where it passes through the internal capsule. Indeed, the artery supplying this area – the largest of the perforating branches of the middle cerebral artery – has been termed the *artery of cerebral haemorrhage*.

4 A list of the more important related signs is given here for involvement of the pyramidal tract at each level.

a *Cortex* – isolated lesions may occur here, resulting in loss of voluntary movement in, say, only one contralateral limb, but often the sensory cortex is also involved. Aphasia in dominant hemisphere lesions (usually left), involving Broca's and Wernicke's areas and the cortex between them, is not uncommon.

b *Internal capsule* – usually all parts of the tract are involved, giving a complete contralateral hemiplegia with associated sensory loss. The lesion may extend back to involve the visual radiation, giving a contralateral homonymous field defect (hemianopia).

c *Cerebral peduncle and midbrain* – the fibres from the IIIrd nerve are often concomitantly involved so that there are the associated signs of a IIIrd nerve palsy.

d *Pons* – here the VIth nerve is often involved, alone or together with the VIIth cranial nerve. There may then be a hemiplegia affecting the arm and leg of the opposite side, an ipsilateral facial palsy of the lower motor neurone type and failure to abduct the ipsilateral eyeball.

e *Medulla* – because of the proximity of the pyramids to one another, medullary lesions often affect both sides of the body. Paralysis of the tongue on the side of the lesion is due to involvement of the XIIth nerve or its nucleus. The respiratory, vasomotor and swallowing centres may also be affected.

f *Spinal cord* – the paralysis following lesions of the spinal cord is ipsilateral and accurately depends on the level at which the pyramidal tract is involved. Lower motor neurone lesion signs can be detected at the level of the spinal trauma (direct injury) and upper motor neurone lesion signs below. The proximity of the pyramidal tracts to the ascending sensory pathways accounts for the concomitant sensory changes which are usually found.

The extrapyramidal motor system This should, by definition, include all those motor projections that do not pass physically through the medullary pyramids. It was once thought to control movement in parallel with and, to a large extent, independently of the pyramidal motor system and the pyramidal/extrapyramidal division was used clinically to distinguish between two motor syndromes: one characterized by spasticity and paralysis and the other characterized either by involuntary movements or by immobility without paralysis. It is now clear that many 'extrapyramidal' structures, particularly the basal nuclei (basal ganglia), actually control movement by altering activity in the premotor cortex and, thus, the pyramidal motor projections. This indicates the lack of any sharp distinction between the functional pathways underlying the two systems.

Components of the extrapyramidal system include the red nuclei, vestibular nuclei, superior colliculus and reticular formation in the brainstem, all of which project via discrete pathways to influence spinal cord motor neurones. Cerebellar projections (see page 361) are also included since they influence not only these brainstem motor pathways but also the motor cortex itself via the dentatothalamic projection.

Perhaps the most important structures to retain an extrapyramidal definition are the basal nuclei (basal ganglia) (see page 370). The neostriatum (caudate and putamen) receives widespread cortical afferents, including those from high-order sensory association and motor areas, and projects mainly to the globus pallidus. The latter nucleus is the major outflow for the basal ganglia and, via the ventral anterior thalamus, exerts its major influence on premotor and hence the motor cortices. This pattern of connections suggests that the basal ganglia are involved in complex aspects of motor control, including motor planning and the initiation of movement.

A variety of motor disorders are associated with basal nuclei (basal ganglia) pathology and, in some instances, neuroanatomically discrete deficits in specific neurotransmitters. For example, Parkinson's disease involves the degeneration of dopaminergic neurones in the substantia nigra in the midbrain. This pigmented nucleus provides the neostriatum with a dense dopaminergic innervation which may be completely lost in severe cases of Parkinsonism. Knowledge of this selective chemical neuropathology has resulted in the development of a treatment of the disease which involves the oral administration of the dopamine precursor L-DOPA.

The membranes of the brain and spinal cord (the meninges)

Three concentrically arranged membranes, known as meningeal layers or meninges, surround the brain and spinal cord. From outside in, these three layers are the dura mater, arachnoid mater and pia mater.

The *dura* is a dense membrane which, within the cranium, is often described as being made up of two layers. This description requires some qualification. The so-called outer layer of the dura is intimately adherent to the inner surface of the skull; the inner layer, which is the true dural layer, is for the most part fused with the outer layer except where the two layers are separated by the intracranial dural venous sinuses and where the inner layer projects inwards to form four, prominent, reduplicated sheets (Fig. 213):

- the falx cerebri;
- the falx cerebelli;
- the tentorium cerebelli;
- the diaphragma sellae.

These dural reduplications serve to compartmentalize the cranial cavity and act as partitions between different parts of the brain, thereby performing the hugely important function of minimizing the considerable torsional stresses to which the brain is normally subjected.

The *arachnoid* is a delicate membrane applied, throughout, to the inner surface of the dura, and separated from the dura by the potential *subdural space*.

The *pia* is closely moulded to the surface of the brain and spinal cord. It dips down into all the cerebral sulci. The interval between the pia mater and the overlying arachnoid is termed the *subarachnoid space*. This space contains CSF and is traversed by trabeculae of fine fibrous strands that run from the arachnoid to the pia.

The ventricular system and the cerebrospinal fluid circulation

The CSF is formed by the secretory activity of the epithelium covering the choroid plexuses (delicate vascular tufts that invaginate the pia) in the lateral, 3rd and 4th ventricles; it circulates through the ventricular system of the brain and drains into the subarachnoid space from the roof of the 4th ventricle before being reabsorbed into the dural venous system.

The general appearance of the ventricular system is indicated in Fig. 239. The two *lateral ventricles*, which are by far the largest components of the system, occupy a considerable part of the cerebral hemispheres. Each has an *anterior horn* (in front of the interventricular foramen), a *body*, above and medial to the body of the caudate nucleus, a *posterior horn* in the occipital lobe and an *inferior horn* reaching down into the temporal lobe. The choroid plexuses of the lateral ventricles, which are responsible for the production of most of the CSF, extend from the inferior horn, through the body, to the interventricular foramen where they become continuous with the plexus of the 3rd ventricle (Fig. 234).

The *3rd ventricle* is a narrow midline slit-like cavity between the two halves of the diencephalon. Thus the upper part of the 3rd ventricle lies between the two halves of the thalamus, while the lower part of the ventricle is between the two halves of the hypothalamus. The floor of the 3rd ventricle is formed, from front to back, by the optic chiasma, tuber cinereum, infundibulum and mamillary bodies. The hypothalamus thus contributes to both the lateral wall and floor of the 3rd ventricle. From the 3rd ventricle the CSF passes through the narrow *cerebral aqueduct* (*of Sylvius*) in the midbrain to reach the 4th ventricle.

The *4th ventricle* is diamond-shaped when viewed from above and tent-shaped as seen from the side. Its floor is formed caudally by the medulla and rostrally by the

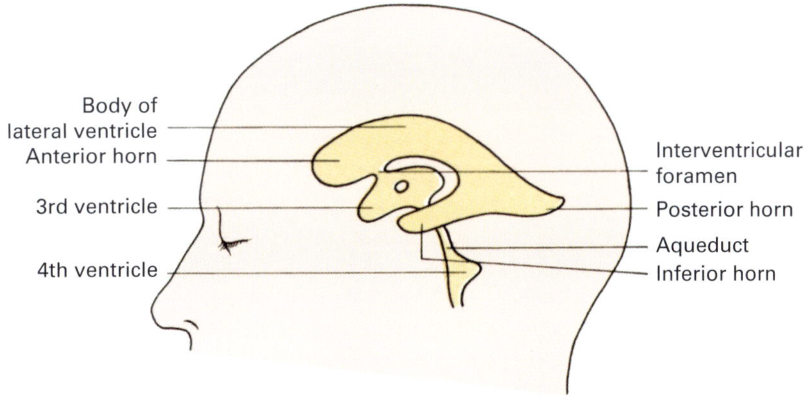

Fig. 239 The ventricular system.

pons. Its roof is formed by the cerebellum overlying the superior and inferior medullary vela. The CSF escapes from the 4th ventricle into the subarachnoid space by way of the *median aperture of Magendie* and the two *lateral apertures* of *Luschka* and then flows over the surface of the brain and spinal cord.

In certain areas the subarachnoid space is considerably enlarged to form distinct cisterns. The most important of these are the *cisterna magna* between the cerebellum and the dorsum of the medulla; the *cisterna pontis* over the ventral surface of the pons; the *interpeduncular cistern* between the two cerebral peduncles; the *cisterna ambiens* between the splenium of the corpus callosum and the superior surface of the cerebellum (containing the great cerebral vein and the pineal gland); and the *chiasmatic cistern* around the optic chiasma. Reabsorption of CSF is principally by way of the superior sagittal sinus and to a lesser extent by the other dural venous sinuses, the modified arachnoid of the arachnoid granulations piercing the dura and bringing the CSF into direct contact with the sinus endothelium. Along the superior sagittal sinus these granulations (or arachnoid villi) clump together to form the Pacchionian bodies, which produce the pitted erosions readily seen along the median line of the inner aspect of the skull cap.

About one-fifth of the CSF is absorbed along similar spinal villi or escapes along the nerve sheaths into the lymphatics. This absorption of CSF is passive, depending on its hydrostatic pressure being higher than that of the venous blood.

CLINICAL FEATURES

1 Computed tomography (CT scanning) has revolutionized the investigation of intracranial space-occupying lesions (post-traumatic haematoma, abscesses and neoplasms), both by delineating the lesion itself and by demonstrating displacement of the ventricular system. Figures 240 and 241 are representative transverse cuts through the skull to illustrate normal anatomical features; note that the details of the anatomy of the ventricles are clearly visualized.

2 Magnetic resonance imaging (MRI) is particularly valuable in producing high-quality images of the CNS (Fig. 242).

3 The CSF serves several purposes, including the provision of a protective water-jacket and a regulating mechanism of intracranial pressure with changing cerebral blood flow.

4 The total capacity of the CSF in the adult is about 150 ml, of which some 25 ml is contained within the spinal theca; it is normally under a pressure of about 100 mm of water (with a range of 80–180) in the lateral horizontal position. The dural theca acts as a simple hydrostatic system, so that, when the patient sits up, the CSF pressure in the lumbar theca rises to between 350 and 550 mm, whereas the ventricular fluid pressure falls to below atmospheric.

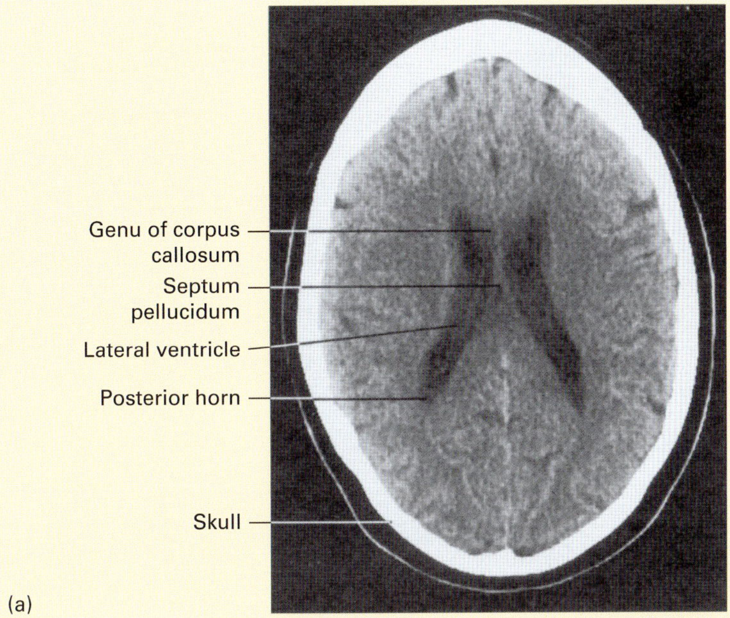

(a)

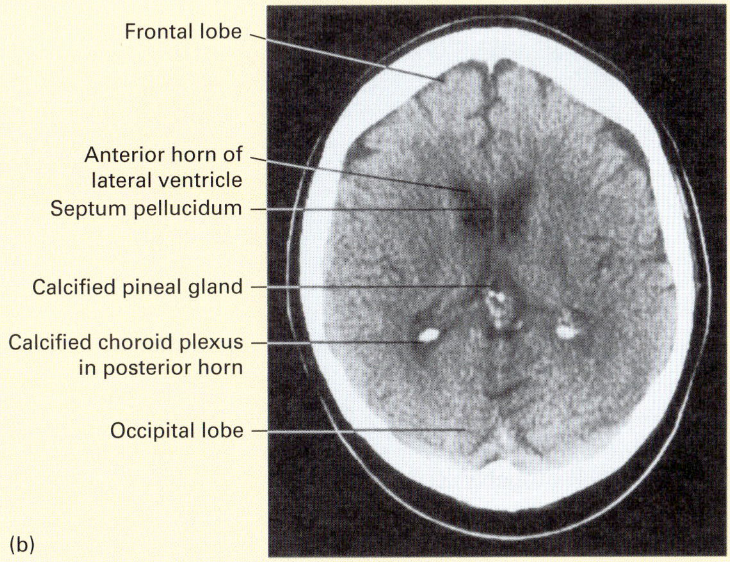

(b)

Fig. 240 (a) Computed tomography (CT) scan of the skull through the level of the bodies of the lateral ventricles. (b) CT scan cut through the level of the anterior horns of the lateral ventricles.

5 Certain parts of the CSF pathway are narrow and easily obstructed. These sites are the interventricular foramina, the 3rd ventricle, the aqueduct, the exit foramina of the 4th ventricle and the subarachnoid space around the midbrain in the tentorial notch.

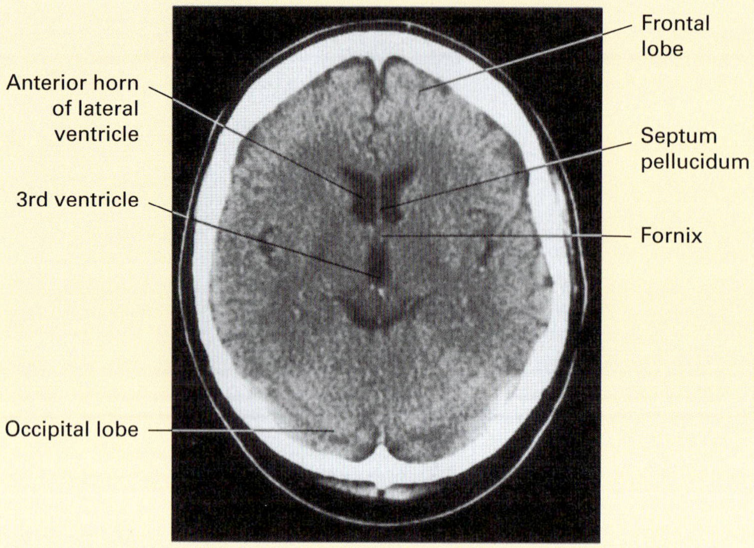

Fig. 241 Computed tomography (CT) scan cut through the level of the 3rd ventricle.

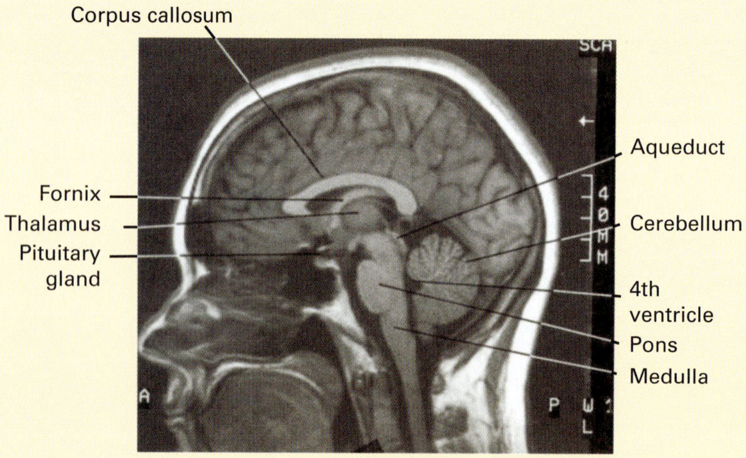

Fig. 242 Magnetic resonance imaging (MRI) sagittal section of the head. Note the fine details of brain structure which can be visualized by this technique.

Obstruction to the system causes increased intracranial pressure and ventricular dilatation (hydrocephalus).

6 The meningeal coverings, together with the subarachnoid space, are prolonged along the optic nerve. Raised CSF pressure is transmitted along this space and may compress the venous drainage of the eye, thus producing *papilloedema*. This swelling of the optic disc can be detected by ophthalmoscopic examination of the fundus.

7 Lumbar puncture – see page 386.

The spinal cord

The spinal cord is 45 cm (18 in) long. It is continuous above with the medulla oblongata at the level of the foramen magnum and ends below at the level of the lower border of the 1st lumbar vertebra. Inferiorly, it tapers into the *conus medullaris*, from which a prolongation of pia mater, the *filum terminale*, descends to be attached to the back of the coccyx.

The cord bears a deep longitudinal *anterior fissure*, a narrower *posterior septum* and, on either side, a *posterolateral sulcus* along which the *posterior (sensory) nerve roots* are serially arranged (Fig. 243).

These posterior roots each bear a *ganglion*, which constitutes the first cell-station of the sensory nerves (see Fig. 268).

The *anterior (motor) nerve roots* emerge serially along the anterolateral aspect of the cord on either side. Both the anterior and posterior nerves arise by a series of rootlets from the cord.

At each intervertebral foramen the anterior and posterior nerve roots unite to form a *spinal nerve* that immediately divides into its *anterior* and *posterior (primary) rami*, each transmitting both motor and sensory fibres.

The length of the roots increases progressively from above downwards owing to the disparity between the length of the cord and the vertebral column; the lumbar and sacral roots below the termination of the cord at vertebral level L2 continue as a leash of nerve roots termed the *cauda equina* (from its fanciful resemblance to a horse's tail). Thirty-one complementary and symmetrically arranged, pairs of spinal nerves emerge from the spinal cord as follows: 8 cervical, 12 thoracic, 5 lumbar, 5 sacral and one coccygeal.

A ***spinal cord segment*** is defined as a horizontal segment of spinal cord giving attachment to a complementary pair of spinal nerves. Based on this definition the spinal cord possesses thirty-one segments.

Structure (Fig. 243)

In transverse section of the cord is seen the *central canal* around which is the 'H'-shaped *grey matter*, surrounded in turn by the *white matter,* which contains the long ascending and descending tracts.

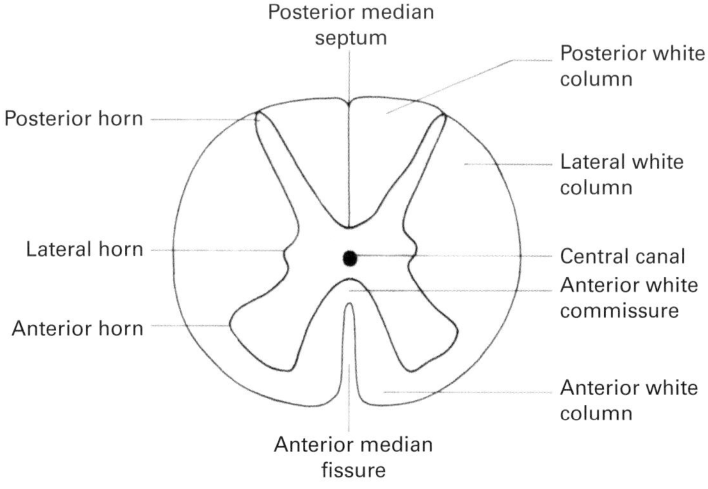

Fig. 243 The spinal cord – transverse section through a thoracic segment.

Within the *posterior horns* of the grey matter, capped by the *substantia gelatinosa*, terminate many of the sensory fibres entering from the posterior nerve roots. In the large *anterior horns* lie the motor cells that give rise to the fibres of the anterior roots.

In the thoracic and upper lumbar cord are found the *lateral horns* on each side, containing the cells of origin of the sympathetic system.

The more important long tracts in the white matter will now be dealt with.

Descending tracts (Fig. 244)

1 *The pyramidal (lateral cerebrospinal* or *crossed motor) tract*. The motor pathway commences at the pyramidal cells of the motor cortex, decussates in the medulla and then descends in the pyramidal tract on the contralateral side of the cord. At each spinal segment, fibres enter the anterior horn and connect with the motor cells there – the tract therefore becomes progressively smaller as it descends.
2 *The direct pyramidal (anterior cerebrospinal* or *uncrossed motor) tract* is a small tract descending without medullary decussation. At each segment, however, fibres pass from it to the ventral horn (anterior) motor cells of the opposite side.

Ascending tracts (Fig. 244)

1 The *posterior* and *anterior spinocerebellar tracts* ascend on the same side of the cord and enter the cerebellum through the inferior and superior cerebellar peduncles, respectively.
2 The *lateral* and *anterior spinothalamic tracts*. Pain and temperature fibres enter the posterior roots, ascend a few segments, relay in the substantia gelatinosa and then cross

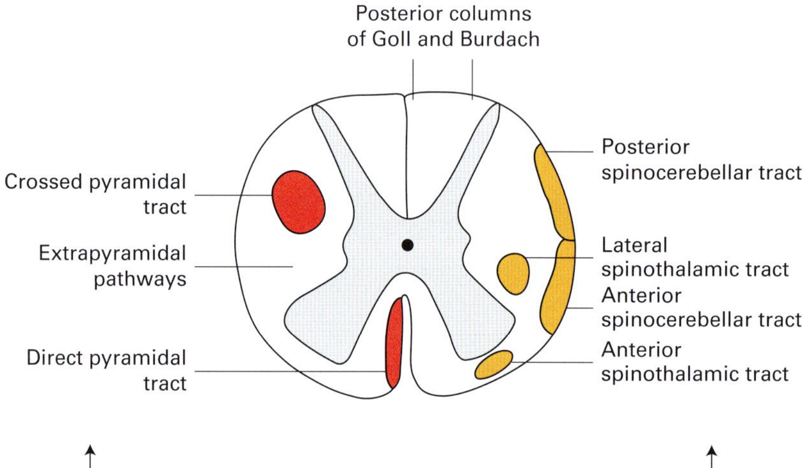

Fig. 244 The location of the important spinal tracts. (The descending tracts are shown on the left, the ascending tracts on the right.)

to the opposite side to ascend in these tracts to the thalamus, where they are relayed to the sensory cortex.

3 The *posterior columns* comprise a medial and lateral tract, termed, respectively, the *fasciculus gracilis* (*of Goll*) and *fasciculus cuneatus* (*of Burdach*). They convey 1st-order sensory fibres subserving fine touch, vibration sense and proprioception (position sense), mostly uncrossed, to the gracile and cuneate nuclei in the medulla where, after synapse, the 2nd-order fibres decussate, pass to the thalamus and, after further synapse, 3rd-order fibres are relayed to the sensory cortex. Some fibres pass from the medulla to the cerebellum along the inferior cerebellar peduncle.

Blood supply

The *anterior* and *posterior spinal arteries* descend in the subarachnoid space from the intracranial part of the vertebral artery. They are reinforced serially by spinal branches from the ascending cervical, the cervical part of the vertebral, the posterior intercostal arteries and the lumbar arteries.

CLINICAL FEATURES

1 Complete transection of the cord is followed by total loss of sensation in the regions supplied by the cord segments below the level of injury together with flaccid muscle paralysis. As the cord distal to the section recovers from a period of spinal shock, the paralysis becomes spastic, with exaggerated reflexes. Voluntary sphincter control is lost but reflex emptying of bladder and rectum subsequently return, provided that the cord centres situated in the sacral zone of the cord are not destroyed.

2 Destruction of the centre of the cord, as occurs in syringomyelia and in some intramedullary tumours, first involves the decussating spinothalamic fibres so that initially there is bilateral loss of pain and temperature sense below the level of the lesion; proprioception and fine touch are preserved until late in the uncrossed posterior columns.

3 Hemisection of the cord is followed by the *Brown-Séquard syndrome*; there is paralysis on the affected side below the lesion (pyramidal tract) and also loss of proprioception and fine discrimination (dorsal columns). Pain and temperature senses are lost on the *opposite* side below the lesion because the affected spinothalamic tract carries fibres which have decussated below the level of cord hemisection.

4 *Tabes dorsalis*, once common but a rare condition today, is a syphilitic degenerative lesion of the posterior columns and posterior nerve roots and is characterized by loss of proprioception; the patient becomes ataxic, particularly if he closes his eyes, because he has lost his position sense for which he can partially compensate by visual knowledge of his spatial relationship (Romberg's sign).

5 Intractable pain can be treated in selected cases by cutting the appropriate posterior nerve roots (posterior rhizotomy) or by division of the spinothalamic tract on the side opposite the pain (cordotomy). A knife passed 3 mm (0.125 in) into the cord anterior to

the denticulate ligament and then swept anteriorly from this point will sever the spinothalamic tract but preserve the pyramidal tract lying immediately posterior to it.

6 Cauda equina syndrome is the term for a condition in which there is extrinsic compression of the nerve roots which make up the cauda equina. The cause is often a prolapsed intervertebral disc (at L4–L5 level or L5–S1 level). The condition may also be caused by tumours or trauma. Less common causes include arteriovenous malformations in the spinal canal, abscesses and haematomas. The clinical presentation of the condition includes urinary and/or recto-anal dysfunction, saddle anaesthesia, lower limb motor weakness and low back pain.

Age differences

Up to the 3rd month of fetal life the spinal cord occupies the full extent of the vertebral canal. The vertebrae then outpace the cord in the rapidity and extent of their growth so that, at birth, the cord reaches the level of only the 3rd lumbar vertebra (Fig. 245).

Further differential growth up to the time of adolescence brings the cord to its definitive position at the approximate level of the disc between the 1st and 2nd lumbar vertebrae (Fig. 246).

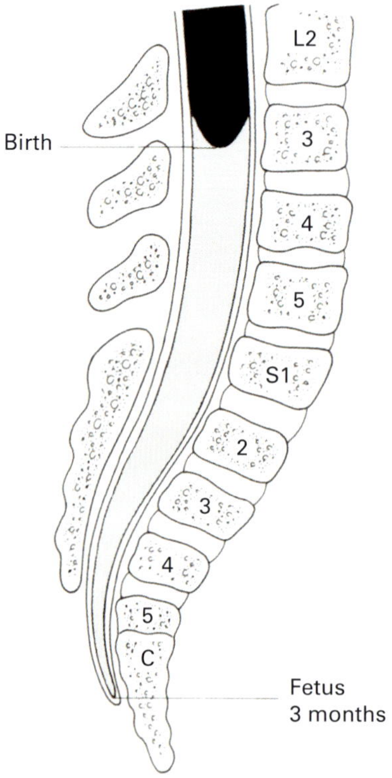

Fig. 245 The relationship between the spinal cord and the vertebrae in the 3-month fetus and in the newborn child.

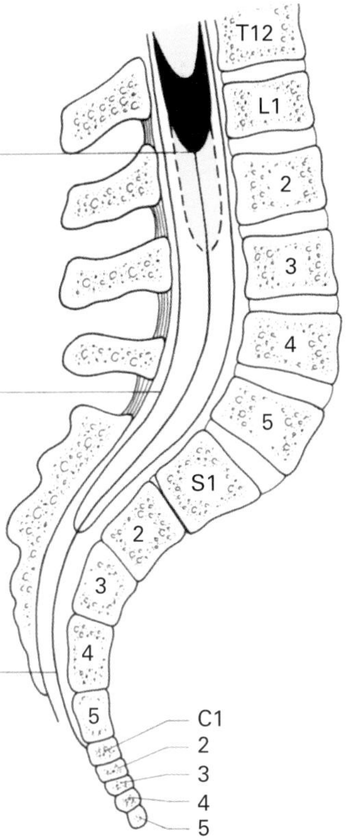

Fig. 246 The range of variation in the termination of the spinal cord in the adult.

The membranes of the cord (the meninges) (Fig. 247)

The spinal cord, like the brain, is closely ensheathed by the *pia mater*. This is thickened on either side between successive nerve roots to form a series of tooth-like lateral extensions, collectively termed the *denticulate ligament*, which passes laterally to adhere to the dura. Inferiorly, the pia continues as the *filum terminale*, which pierces the distal extremity of the dural sac and becomes attached to the coccyx.

The *arachnoid mater* lines the *dura mater*, leaving an extensive *subarachnoid space*, containing CSF, between it and the pia. Both pia and arachnoid are continued along the spinal nerve roots.

The dura itself forms a tough sheath surrounding the cord. It ends distally at the level of the 2nd sacral vertebra. It also continues along each nerve root and blends with the sheaths of the peripheral nerves.

The *extradural* (or *epidural*) *space* is the compartment between the dural sheath and the spinal canal. It extends downwards from the level of the foramen magnum to the level of the sacral hiatus. It is filled with semiliquid fat and contains lymphatics (although there are no lymphatics within the nervous system deep to the dura), together with arteries and large, thin-walled veins.

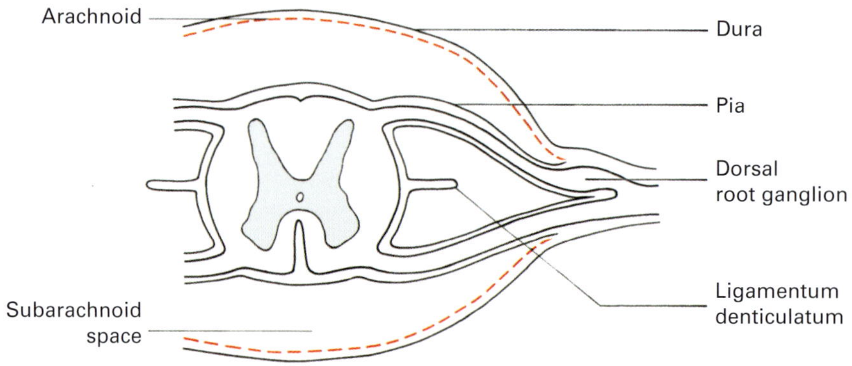

Fig. 247 The membranes of the spinal cord.

Whereas the arteries of this space are not especially prominent, the extradural veins form a rich network of intercommunicating vessels termed the internal vertebral venous plexus. This plexus receives the *basivertebral veins*, which emerge from the posterior aspect of each vertebral body. In addition, the internal vertebral venous plexus links up with both the pelvic veins below and the cerebral veins above – thereby allowing a pathway for the spread of both bacteria and tumour cells. This accounts, for example, for the ready spread of prostatic cancer to the sacrum and vertebrae (Batson's 'valveless vertebral venous plexus'), the spread of aggressive carcinomas of the breast to the thoracic vertebrae and the spread of follicular cancers of the thyroid to the cervical vertebrae.

CLINICAL FEATURES

Lumbar puncture to withdraw CSF from the spinal subarachnoid space must be performed well clear of the termination of the cord. A line joining the summits of the iliac crests corresponds to the level of the 4th lumbar vertebra (Fig. 40); therefore the intervertebral spaces immediately above or below this landmark can be used with safety. The spine must be fully flexed (with the patient either seated or lying in the left or right lateral position) so that the vertebral interspinous spaces are opened to their maximal extent (Fig. 248). The needle is passed inwards and somewhat cranially exactly in the midline and at right angles to the spine; the supraspinous and interspinous ligaments are traversed and then the dura is penetrated, the latter with a distinct 'give'. Occasionally, root pain is experienced if a root of the cauda equina is impinged upon, but usually these float clear of the needle.

At spinal puncture CSF can be obtained for examination; antibiotics, radio-opaque contrast medium or anaesthetics may be injected into the subarachnoid space, and the CSF pressure can be estimated (normal, when lying on the side, 80–180 mm CSF). A block in the subarachnoid space above the point of puncture, produced, for example, by a spinal tumour, can be revealed by *Queckenstedt's test* as follows.

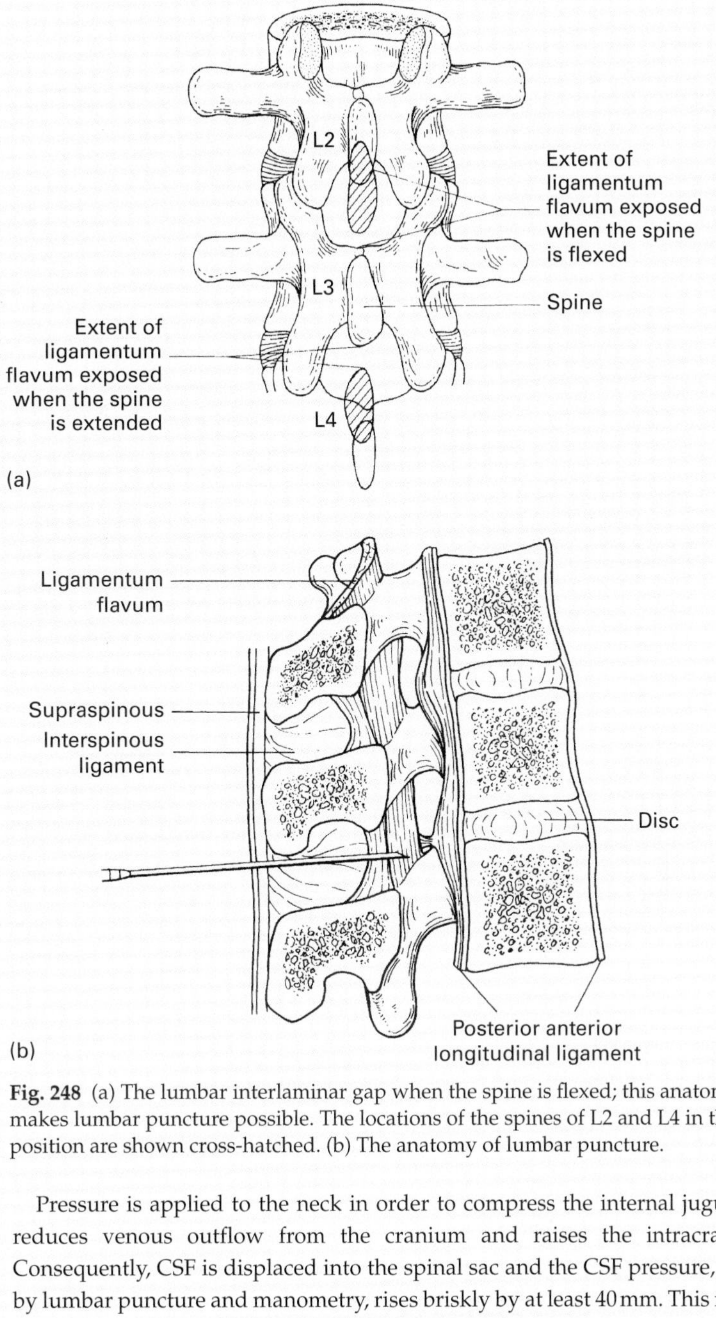

Fig. 248 (a) The lumbar interlaminar gap when the spine is flexed; this anatomical fact makes lumbar puncture possible. The locations of the spines of L2 and L4 in the extended position are shown cross-hatched. (b) The anatomy of lumbar puncture.

Pressure is applied to the neck in order to compress the internal jugular veins; this reduces venous outflow from the cranium and raises the intracranial pressure. Consequently, CSF is displaced into the spinal sac and the CSF pressure, as determined by lumbar puncture and manometry, rises briskly by at least 40 mm. This rise in pressure is not seen if a block is present in the subarachnoid space.

Extradural block. The extradural space can be entered by a needle passed either between the spinal laminae or via the sacral hiatus (caudal or sacral anaesthesia, see page 137).

The cranial nerves

Just as the thirty-one pairs of spinal nerves are regarded as the peripheral nerves of the spinal cord, so may the twelve pairs of cranial nerves be considered the peripheral nerves of the brain. The name of each cranial nerve suggests either the main function of the nerve or some characteristic anatomical feature of the nerve. It is also conventional to refer to the twelve cranial nerves by Roman numerals. Thus, cranial nerve I (olfactory nerve) is the uppermost one to emerge from the brain, and cranial nerve XII (hypoglossal nerve) the lowermost. Cranial nerves I and II are generally regarded as extensions of the forebrain, while the remaining cranial nerves (III–XII) originate in, and emerge from, the brainstem.

Clinically it is helpful to categorize the cranial nerves into one or other of the following three groups (as this classification determines the approach to the clinical testing of the cranial nerve): (1) exclusively sensory (cranial nerves I, II, VIII); (2) exclusively motor (cranial nerves III, IV, VI, XI, XII); and (3) mixed motor and sensory (V, VII, IX, X).

The olfactory nerve (I)

The fibres of the olfactory nerve, unlike other afferent fibres, are unique in being the central processes of the olfactory cells and not the peripheral processes of a central group of ganglion cells.

The central processes of the olfactory receptors pass upwards from the olfactory mucosa in the upper part of the superior nasal concha and septum, through the cribriform plate of the ethmoid bone to end by synapsing with the dendrites of mitral cells in the olfactory bulb. The mitral cells in turn send their axons back in the olfactory tract to terminate in the cortex of the uncus (on the inferior aspect of the anterior pole of the temporal lobe), the adjacent inferomedial temporal cortex and the region of the anterior perforated space. The further course of the olfactory pathway is uncertain in man, but it is now clear that the hippocampus–fornix system is not directly concerned with olfaction.

CLINICAL FEATURES

1. The sense of smell is not highly developed in man and is easily disturbed by conditions affecting the nasal mucosa generally (e.g. the common cold). However, unilateral anosmia may be an important sign in the diagnosis of frontal lobe tumours. Tumours in the region of the uncus may give rise to the so-called 'uncinate' type of fit, characterized by olfactory hallucinations associated with impairment of consciousness and involuntary chewing movements.
2. Bilateral anosmia due to interruption of the olfactory nerve may occur after head injuries, particularly in association with anterior cranial fossa fractures, when leakage of CSF through the cribriform plate may present as rhinorrhoea.

The optic nerve (II) and the visual pathway

(For a description of the eye itself, see the section on special senses, page 411.)

The optic nerve is the nerve of vision. It is not a true cranial nerve but should be thought of as a brain tract that has become drawn out from the cerebrum. Embryologically, it is developed, together with the retina, as a lateral diverticulum of the forebrain. Devoid of neurilemmal sheaths, its fibres, like other brain tissues, are incapable of regeneration after division.

From a *functional* point of view the retina can be regarded as consisting of three cellular layers: a layer of receptor cells – the *rods* and *cones*; an intermediate layer of *bipolar cells*; and a layer of *ganglion cells*, whose axons form the optic nerve (Fig. 249). From all parts of the retina these axons converge on the *optic disc*, whence they pierce the sclera to form the optic nerve.

The optic nerve passes backwards and medially to the optic foramen (situated between the body and lesser wing of the sphenoid bone) (Fig. 222b), through which it reaches the optic groove on the dorsum of the body of the sphenoid. Here, all the fibres from the medial half of the retina (i.e. those concerned with the temporal visual field) cross over in the *optic chiasma* to the optic tract of the opposite side, while the fibres from the lateral half of the retina (nasal visual field) pass back in the optic tract of the same side. The great majority of the fibres in the optic tract end in the *lateral geniculate body* of the thalamus. From the lateral geniculate body the fibres of the optic radiation sweep laterally to the temporal lobe before passing backwards to the occipital visual cortex (the striate area surrounding the calcarine fissure) where they terminate in such a way that the upper and lower halves of the retina are represented on the upper and lower lips of the fissure, respectively (Figs 235, 250).

However, a small proportion of fibres in the optic tract, subserving pupillary, ocular and head and neck reflexes, bypass the geniculate body to reach the superior colliculus and pretectal nucleus of the midbrain. From the pretectal nucleus, fibres connect with

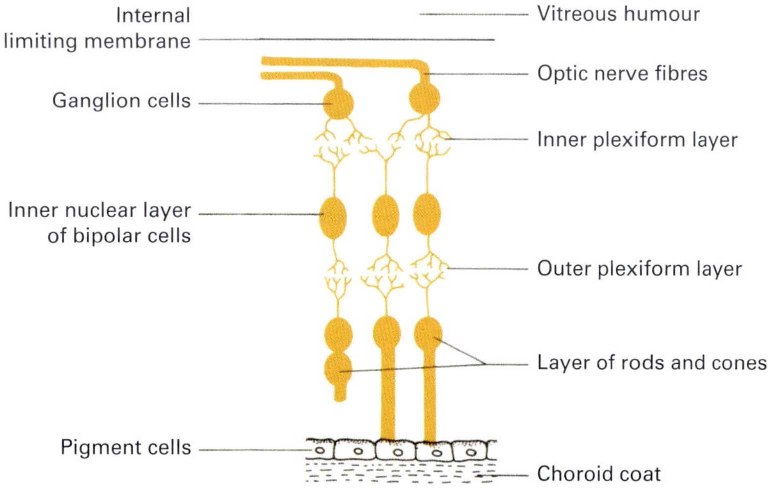

Fig. 249 The layers of the retina.

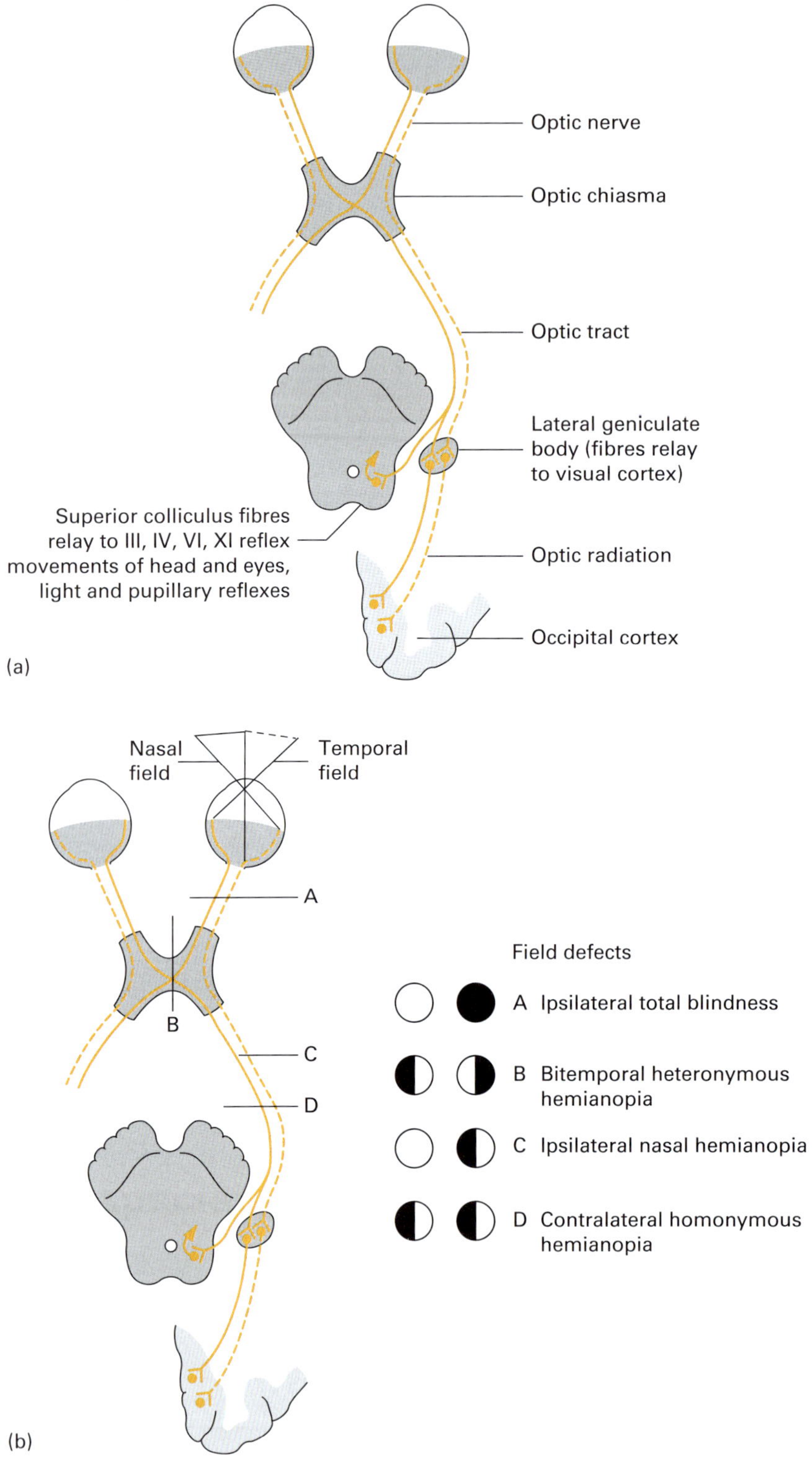

Fig. 250 (a) The optic pathway. (b) Scheme of field defects. A–D denote sites of interruption of the visual pathway.

the Edinger–Westphal nucleus of both sides. This pathway explains the direct and consensual pupillary response (i.e. a light shone into one eye causes contraction of both pupils).

CLINICAL FEATURES

1 Lesions of the retina or optic nerve result in *ipsilateral blindness* in the affected segment, but lesions of the optic tract and central parts of the visual pathway result in contralateral *homonymous defects*. Similarly, lesions of the optic chiasma (e.g. from an expanding pituitary tumour) will give rise to a *bitemporal hemianopia*, i.e. there will be a loss of vision in both temporal eye-fields.

2 The lesion responsible for the *Argyll Robertson pupil* is thought to be in the vicinity of the pretectal area. The pupil is constricted, does not respond to light but responds to accommodation; there is no satisfactory explanation why the pupillary reaction to light should be abolished while the convergence–accommodation reflex is preserved. It is classically seen in syphilis affecting the CNS.

The oculomotor nerve (III)

In addition to supplying most of the extrinsic eye muscles, the oculomotor nerve conveys the preganglionic parasympathetic fibres for the sphincter of the pupil via the ciliary ganglion. Its nucleus of origin lies in the midbrain and consists essentially of two components: the *somatic efferent nucleus*, which supplies the extrinsic ocular muscles, and the *Edinger–Westphal nucleus*, from which the preganglionic parasympathetic fibres are derived. The former is referred to as the main oculomotor nucleus, and the latter is termed the accessory oculomotor nucleus.

From these nuclei, fibres pass vertically through the midbrain tegmentum to emerge just medial to the cerebral peduncle. Passing forwards between the superior cerebellar and posterior cerebral arteries, the nerve pierces the dura mater to run in the lateral wall of the cavernous sinus (Fig. 251) as far as the superior orbital fissure. Before entering the fissure it divides into a superior branch and an inferior branch; both branches enter the orbit through the tendinous ring from which the recti arise (see Fig. 255). The superior branch passes lateral to the optic nerve to supply the superior rectus muscle and levator palpebrae superioris; the inferior branch supplies three muscles, the medial rectus, the inferior rectus and the inferior oblique, the nerve to the last conveying the parasympathetic fibres to the ciliary ganglion.

The ciliary ganglion

This small but important ganglion lies near the apex of the orbit just lateral to the optic nerve. It receives, in addition to the preganglionic parasympathetic fibres from the Edinger–Westphal nucleus, a sympathetic (postganglionic) root ultimately from the plexus on the internal carotid artery and a sensory root from the nasociliary nerve (a branch of the ophthalmic division of the trigeminal nerve). Of these fibres,

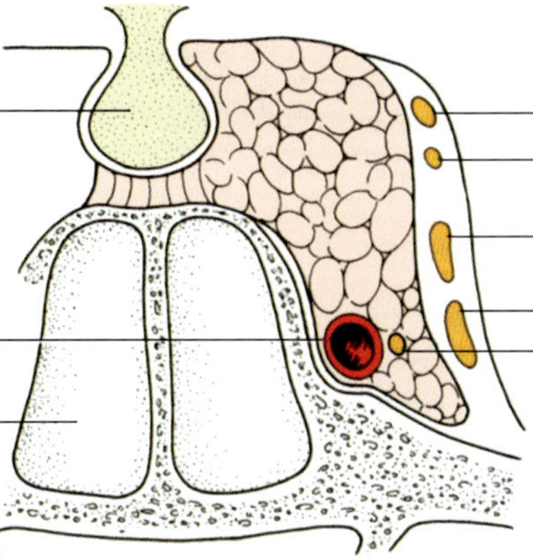

Fig. 251 The cavernous sinus – showing the relations of the IIIrd, IVth, Vth and VIth cranial nerves.

only the *parasympathetic* synapse in the ganglion, the others pass directly through it. The postganglionic efferent fibres from the ganglion pass to the ciliary muscle and the muscles of the iris by way of about ten *short ciliary nerves*. Stimulation results in pupillary constriction and in accommodation of the lens. The sympathetic and sensory fibres are, respectively, vasoconstrictor and pupillodilator, and sensory to the globe of the eye.

(Note that the majority of sympathetic dilator pupillae nerve fibres are transmitted to the eye in the long ciliary branches of the nasociliary nerve.)

CLINICAL FEATURES

Complete division of the IIIrd nerve results in a characteristic group of signs:

- *ptosis* – due to paralysis of the levator palpebrae superioris;
- a *divergent squint* – due to the unopposed action of the superior oblique and lateral rectus muscles, rotating the eyeball laterally;
- *dilatation of the pupil* – the dilator action of the sympathetic fibres being unopposed;
- *loss of the accommodation–convergence* and *light reflexes* – due to constrictor pupillae paralysis;
- diplopia (*double vision*).

The trochlear nerve (IV)

The trochlear nerve is the most slender of the cranial nerves and supplies only one eye muscle, the *superior oblique*.

Emerging on the dorsum of the pons (being the only cranial nerve to arise from the dorsal aspect of the brainstem), the nerve winds around the cerebral peduncle and then passes forwards between the superior cerebellar and posterior cerebral arteries to pierce the dura. It then runs forwards in the lateral wall of the cavernous sinus (Fig. 251) between the oculomotor and ophthalmic nerves to enter the orbit through the superior orbital fissure, lateral to the tendinous ring from which the recti take origin. It then passes medially over the optic nerve to enter the superior oblique muscle.

CLINICAL FEATURES

A lesion of the trochlear nerve results in paralysis of the superior oblique muscle, resulting in diplopia that occurs when the patient attempts to look downwards and laterally. This can be remembered as 'the tramp's nerve' – it makes the eye go 'down and out'!

The trigeminal nerve (V) (Figs 252, 253)

As the name suggests, this nerve consists of three divisions. Together they supply sensory fibres to the greater part of the skin of the head and face, the mucous membranes of the mouth, nose and paranasal air sinuses and, by way of a small motor root, the muscles of mastication. In addition it is associated with four autonomic (parasympathetic) ganglia, the ciliary, pterygopalatine, otic and submandibular.

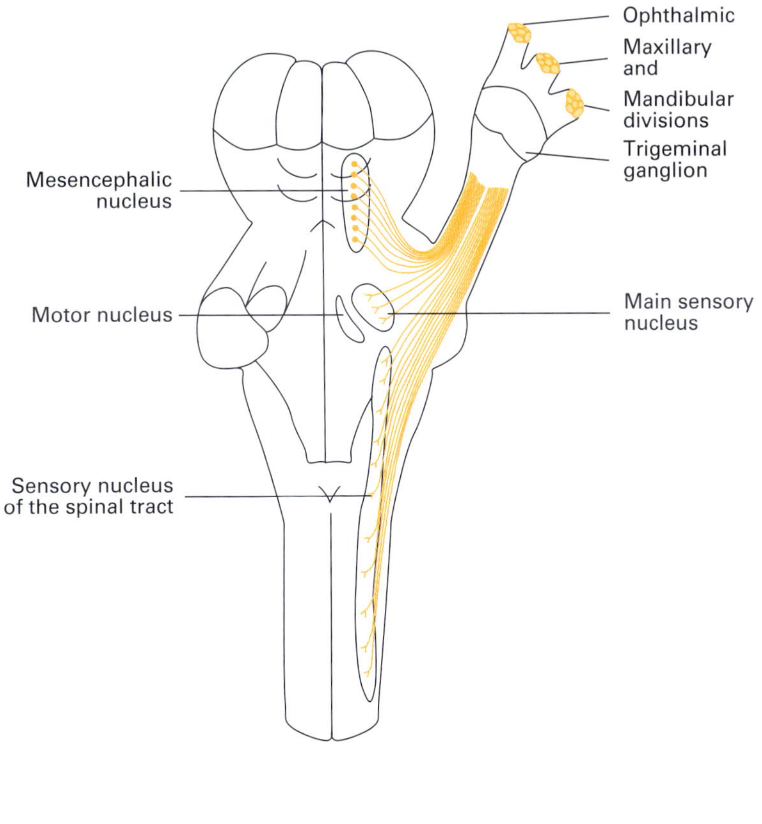

Fig. 252 Plan of the trigeminal nerve and its nuclei in dorsal view.

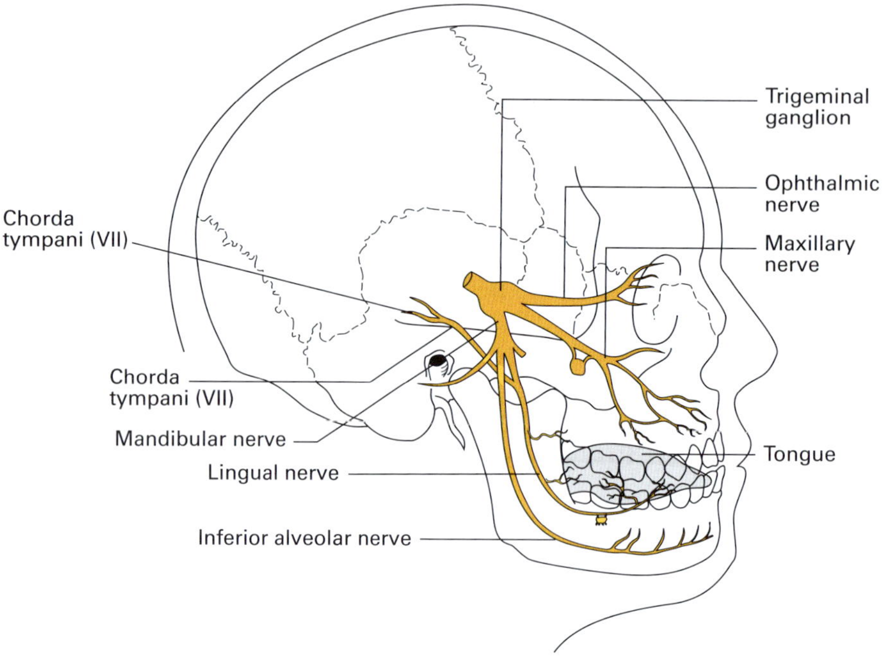

Fig. 253 Distribution of the trigeminal nerve.

The trigeminal ganglion

This ganglion, which is also termed the *semilunar ganglion*, is equivalent to the dorsal root sensory ganglion of a spinal nerve. It is crescent-shaped and is situated within an invaginated pocket of dura in the middle cranial fossa. It lies near the apex of the petrous temporal bone, which is somewhat hollowed for it. The motor root of the trigeminal nerve and the greater superficial petrosal nerve both pass deep to the ganglion. Above the ganglion, lies the hippocampal gyrus of the temporal lobe of the cerebrum; medially lies the internal carotid artery and the posterior part of the cavernous sinus. The trigeminal ganglion represents the first cell-station for all sensory fibres of the trigeminal nerve except those subserving proprioception.

V_1: the ophthalmic division (Fig. 253)

This is the smallest division of the trigeminal nerve; it is wholly sensory and is responsible for the innervation of the skin of the forehead, the upper eyelid, cornea and part of the nose. Passing forwards from the trigeminal ganglion, it immediately enters the lateral wall of the cavernous sinus where it lies beneath the trochlear nerve (Fig. 251). Just before entering the orbit it divides into three branches; frontal, lacrimal and nasociliary.

The *frontal nerve* runs forwards just beneath the roof of the orbit for a short distance before dividing into its two terminal branches, the *supratrochlear* and *supraorbital nerves*, which supply the upper eyelid and the scalp as far back as the lambdoid suture.

The *lacrimal nerve* supplies the lacrimal gland (with postganglionic parasympathetic fibres from the pterygopalatine ganglion which reach it by way of the maxillary nerve) and the lateral part of the conjunctiva and upper lid.

The *nasociliary nerve* gives branches to the ciliary ganglion, the eyeball, cornea and conjunctiva, the medial half of the upper eyelid, the dura of the anterior cranial fossa and to the mucosa and skin of the nose.

V_2: the maxillary nerve (Fig. 253)

The maxillary nerve is also purely sensory. Passing forwards from the central part of the trigeminal ganglion, close to the cavernous sinus, it leaves the skull by way of the *foramen rotundum* and emerges into the upper part of the pterygopalatine fossa. Here, it gives off a number of branches before continuing through the inferior orbital fissure and the infra-orbital canal as the *infra-orbital* nerve, which supplies the skin of the cheek and lower eyelid. The maxillary nerve has the following named branches:

1 the *zygomatic nerve*, whose zygomaticotemporal and zygomaticofacial branches supply the skin of the temple and cheek, respectively;
2 *superior alveolar (dental) branches* to the teeth of the upper jaw; and
3 the *branches from the pterygopalatine ganglion*, which run a descending course and are distributed as follows: the *greater* and *lesser palatine nerves*, which pass through the corresponding palatine foramina to supply the mucous membrane of the hard and soft palates, the uvula and the tonsils, and the mucous membrane of the nose and a *pharyngeal branch* supplying the mucosa of the nasopharynx. The *nasopalatine nerve* (long sphenopalatine) supplies the nasal septum then emerges through the incisive canal of the hard palate to supply the gum behind the incisor teeth. The *posterior superior lateral nasal nerves* (short sphenopalatine) supply the posterosuperior lateral wall of the nose.

The pterygopalatine ganglion

Associated with the maxillary division of V as it lies in the pterygopalatine fossa is the relatively large pterygopalatine ganglion. This receives its parasympathetic or secretomotor root from the greater superficial petrosal branch of VII, its *sensory* component from two pterygopalatine branches of the maxillary nerve and its *sympathetic* root from the internal carotid plexus. Its parasympathetic efferents pass to the lacrimal gland through a communicating branch to the lacrimal nerve. Parasympathetic efferents from the pterygopalatine ganglion are also distributed to the mucous and serous glands of the nose, palate and paranasal sinuses. Sensory and sympathetic (vasoconstrictor) fibres are distributed to nose, nasopharynx, palate and orbit.

V_3: the mandibular nerve (Fig. 253)

This is the largest of the three divisions of the trigeminal nerve and the only one to convey motor fibres. In addition to supplying the skin of the temporal region, part of the auricle and the lower face, the mucous membrane of the anterior two-thirds of the tongue and the floor of the mouth, it also provides motor innervation to the muscles of mastication and secretomotor fibres to the salivary glands.

Passing forwards from the trigeminal ganglion, it almost immediately enters the foramen ovale through which it reaches the infratemporal fossa. Here, it divides into a small anterior and a larger posterior trunk, but before doing so it gives off the *nervus spinosus* to supply the dura mater and the *nerve to the medial pterygoid muscle* from which the *otic ganglion* is suspended and through which motor fibres are transmitted to tensor palati and tensor tympani.

The anterior trunk gives off:

1 a sensory branch, the *buccal nerve*, which supplies part of the skin of the cheek and the mucous membrane on its inner aspect; and
2 motor branches to the masseter, temporalis and lateral pterygoid muscles.

The posterior trunk, which is principally sensory, divides into three branches:

1 the *auriculotemporal nerve*, which conveys sensory fibres to the skin of the temple and auricle and secretomotor fibres from the otic ganglion to the parotid gland;
2 the *lingual nerve*, which passes downwards under cover of the ramus of the mandible to the side of the tongue (Fig. 196), where it supplies the mucous membrane of the floor of the mouth, the anterior two-thirds of the tongue (including the taste buds by way of fibres which join it from the chorda tympani) and the sublingual and submandibular salivary glands;
3 the *inferior alveolar* (*dental*) *nerve*, which passes down into the mandibular canal and supplies branches to the teeth of the lower jaw. A side branch, *the mental nerve,* emerges from the mental foramen to supply the outer gingiva of the lower jaw, skin of the chin and lower lip. The inferior alveolar nerve is the only branch of the posterior trunk that carries motor fibres. These motor fibres are conveyed in the nerve to mylohyoid, a branch of the inferior alveolar nerve given off before the latter enters the mandibular foramen. The *nerve to the mylohyoid* supplies the muscle of that name and the anterior belly of the digastric.

The otic ganglion

The otic ganglion lies immediately below the foramen ovale medial to the trunk of the mandibular nerve. Its *parasympathetic* fibres reach the ganglion by the lesser (superficial) petrosal branch of the glossopharyngeal nerve; these fibres relay in the ganglion and the postganglionic (post-synaptic) fibres pass via the auriculotemporal nerve to the parotid gland and are the secretomotor nerve supply of the latter. The *sympathetic* fibres that course through the otic ganglion are derived from the plexus which surrounds the middle meningeal artery. These sympathetic fibres are, of course, derived from the superior cervical ganglion and are vasoconstrictors to the parotid gland.

The submandibular ganglion

This is suspended from the lower aspect of the lingual nerve. Its *parasympathetic* supply is derived from the chorda tympani branch of the facial nerve (see Fig. 256) by which it is conveyed to the lingual nerve. It carries the secretomotor supply to the submandibular and sublingual salivary glands.

Sympathetic fibres are transmitted from the superior cervical ganglion via the plexus on the facial artery and supply vasoconstrictor fibres to these same two salivary glands. The *sensory* component is contributed by the lingual nerve itself, which provides sensory fibres to these salivary glands and also to the mucous membrane of the floor of the mouth.

The central connections of the trigeminal nerve

The central processes of the trigeminal ganglion cells enter the lateral aspect of the pons and divide into ascending and descending branches, which terminate in one or other component of the sensory nucleus of V (Fig. 252). This nucleus consists of three parts, each of which appears to subserve different sensory modalities: a chief sensory nucleus in the pontine tegmentum concerned with touch; a descending, or spinal, nucleus subserving pain and temperature; and a mesencephalic nucleus receiving proprioceptive afferents. The *motor root of the trigeminal nerve* lies just medial to the sensory nucleus in the upper part of the pons; its efferents pass out with the sensory fibres and are distributed by way of the mandibular division of the nerve.

CLINICAL FEATURES

1 Section of the whole trigeminal nerve results in ipsilateral anaesthesia of the face and anterior part of the scalp, the auricle and the mucous membranes of the nose, mouth and anterior two-thirds of the tongue, together with paralysis and wasting of the ipsilateral muscles of mastication. Lesions of individual divisions of the trigeminal nerve give rise to corresponding sensory deficits in the area of distribution of the affected nerve. Injury to the mandibular division will result in sensory and motor deficits.

2 Trigeminal neuralgia may affect any one or more of the three divisions, giving rise to the characteristic acute, lancinating and episodic pain over the appropriate area (Fig. 254).

3 Pain is frequently referred from one segment to another. Thus, a patient with a carcinoma of the tongue (lingual nerve) frequently complains of severe earache (auriculotemporal nerve). The classical description of such a case is an old gentleman sitting in the outpatients department spitting blood and with a piece of cotton wool in his ear.

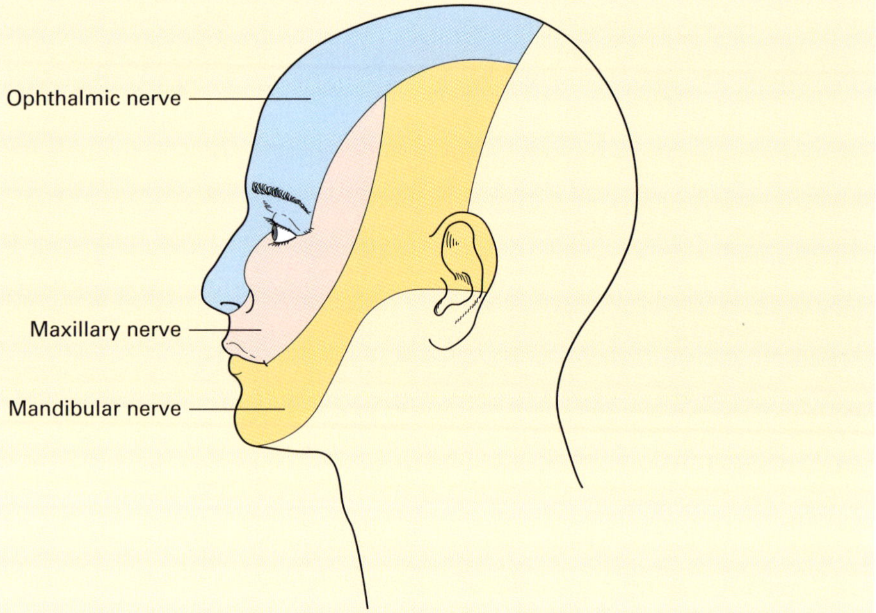

Fig. 254 Areas of the face and scalp supplied by the three divisions of the trigeminal nerve.

The abducent nerve (VI)

Like the trochlear nerve, the abducent nerve supplies only one extrinsic ocular muscle, the *lateral rectus*. Its nucleus lies in the pons and from there its fibres emerge on the base of the brain at the junction of the pons and medulla. The nerve then passes forwards to enter the cavernous sinus (Fig. 251). Here, it lies lateral to the internal carotid artery and medial to the IIIrd, IVth and Vth nerves. Passing through the tendinous ring just below the IIIrd nerve, it enters the orbit to pierce the medial surface of the lateral rectus (Fig. 255).

CLINICAL FEATURES

On account of its long intracranial course, the VIth nerve is frequently involved in injuries to the base of the skull. When damaged, it gives rise to diplopia and a convergent squint. The patient is unable to deviate the affected eye laterally.

The facial nerve (VII)

In addition to supplying the muscles of facial expression, the facial nerve conveys secretomotor fibres to the sublingual and submandibular salivary glands and the lacrimal gland as well as to the nasal mucosa; it also carries taste fibres from the anterior two-thirds of the tongue.

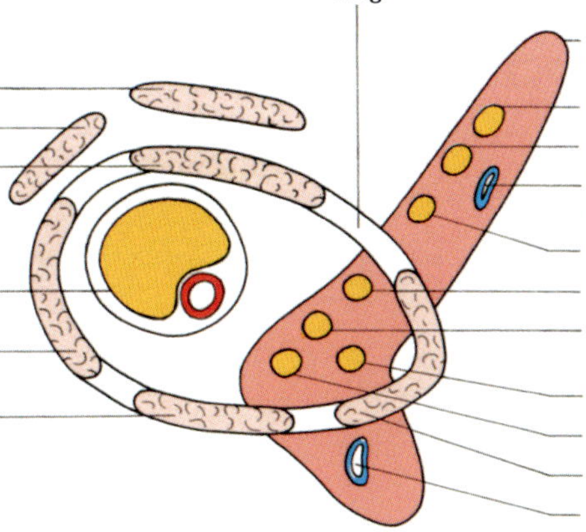

Fig. 255 The superior orbital fissure and tendinous ring of origin of the extrinsic orbital muscles, showing the relations of the cranial nerves as they enter the orbit (schematic; left orbit viewed from the front).

The fibres innervating the facial muscles have their nucleus of origin in the ventral part of the caudal pons; the parasympathetic secretomotor fibres for the salivary glands are derived from the superior salivary nucleus. The sensory fibres associated with the nerve have their cells of origin in the facial (geniculate) ganglion. The sensory fibres of the facial nerve and the parasympathetic secretomotor fibres group together to form the *nervus intermedius*. This nerve emerges from the pontomedullary junction lateral to, and quite separate from the motor root of the facial nerve.

Originating in the motor nucleus, the motor root of the facial nerve runs a tortuous course within the pons before emerging from the lateral aspect of the pons together with the nervus intermedius and cranial nerve VIII in the *cerebellopontine angle*.

The nervus intermedius and motor root of the facial nerve pass together into the internal auditory meatus, at the bottom of which they unite to form a single nerve. The facial nerve parts company with the VIIIth nerve and enters the facial canal. Here, it runs laterally over the vestibule before bending sharply backwards over the promontory of the middle ear. This bend, or *genu of the facial nerve*, as it is called, marks the site of the facial ganglion and the point at which the secretomotor fibres for the lacrimal gland leave to form the greater (superficial) petrosal nerve. The facial nerve then passes downwards, medial to the middle ear, to reach the stylomastoid foramen (Fig. 256).

Just before entering this foramen it gives off the branch, known as the *chorda tympani*, which runs forwards within the tympanic membrane, between the incus and malleus, exits via the fissure between the tympanic and petrous parts of the temporal bone to enter the infratemporal fossa where it joins the lingual nerve. Hence its taste fibres reach the anterior two-thirds of the tongue, and its secretomotor fibres are conveyed to the submandibular ganglion, thence to the submandibular and sublingual salivary glands.

On emerging from the stylomastoid foramen, the facial nerve supplies the stylohyoid and the posterior belly of digastric muscle. It then enters the parotid gland, where it eventually divides into five divisions for the supply of the muscles of facial expression (mimetic muscles): the temporal, zygomatic, buccal, mandibular and cervical branches (Figs 207, 257).

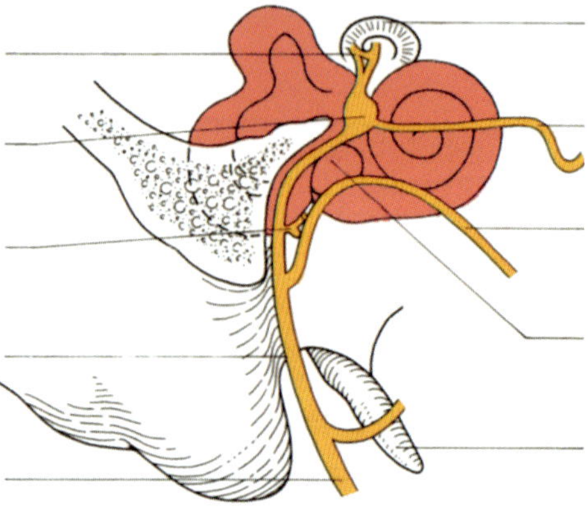

Fig. 256 Distribution of the facial nerve within the temporal bone.

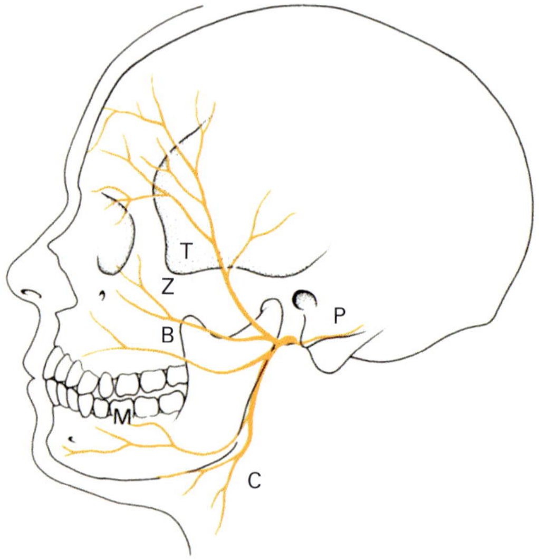

Fig. 257 Distribution of the facial nerve: B, buccal; C, cervical; M, mandibular; P, posterior auricular branch; T, temporal; Z, zygomatic.

CLINICAL FEATURES

1 It is important to distinguish between 'nuclear' and 'infranuclear' facial palsies on the one hand and 'supranuclear' palsies on the other. Both nuclear and infranuclear palsies result in a facial paralysis that is complete and affects *all* the muscles of the face, ipsilaterally. In supranuclear palsies there is no involvement of the muscles above the palpebral fissure since the portion of the facial nucleus supplying these muscles receives fibres from both cerebral hemispheres. Furthermore, in such cases the patient may involuntarily use the facial muscles but will be unable to do so on request.

2 Supranuclear facial palsies most frequently result from vascular involvement of the corticobulbar pathways, e.g. in cerebral haemorrhage. Nuclear palsies may occur in

poliomyelitis or other forms of bulbar paralysis, while infranuclear palsies may result from a variety of causes including compression in the cerebellopontine angle (as by an acoustic neuroma), fractures of the temporal bone and invasion by a malignant parotid tumour. However, by far the commonest cause of infranuclear facial paralysis is *Bell's palsy*, which is generally described as a condition of unknown aetiology. Nevertheless, there is, in many cases, a fairly strong association between Bell's palsy and viral infections (particularly herpes simplex infections and influenza).

When the intracranial part of the nerve is affected or when it is involved in fractures of the base of the skull there is usually loss of taste over the anterior two-thirds of the tongue and an associated loss of hearing (VIIIth nerve damage).

The auditory (vestibulocochlear) nerve (VIII)

The VIIIth nerve consists of two sets of fibres: cochlear and vestibular. The *cochlear fibres* (concerned with hearing) represent the central processes of the bipolar spiral ganglion cells of the cochlea which traverse the internal auditory meatus to reach the lateral aspect of the medulla, at the cerebellopontine angle (together with VII), where they terminate in the *dorsal* and *ventral cochlear nuclei* (Fig. 233b). The majority of the projection fibres from these nuclei cross to the opposite side and ascend to reach the *inferior colliculus* and the *medial geniculate body*; from the former, fibres reach the motor nuclei of the cranial nerves and form the pathway of auditory reflexes; from the latter, fibres sweep laterally in the *auditory radiation to the auditory cortex* in the superior temporal gyrus (Fig. 235).

The *vestibular fibres* (concerned with equilibrium) enter the medulla just medial to the cochlear division and terminate in the *vestibular nuclei*. Many of the fibres from these nuclei pass to the cerebellum in the inferior cerebellar peduncle together with fibres bypassing the vestibular nuclei and passing directly to the cerebellum.

Other vestibular connections are to the nuclei of III, IV, VI and XI and to the upper cervical cord (via the vestibulospinal tract). These connections bring the eye and neck muscles under reflex vestibular control.

CLINICAL FEATURES

1 Lesions of the cochlear division result in deafness which may, or may not, be accompanied by tinnitus. The differential diagnosis between middle ear deafness and cochlear (inner ear) or auditory nerve lesions can be made clinically by the use of a tuning fork. Air conduction (the fork being held beside the ear) is normally louder than bone conduction (the fork being held against the mastoid process). If the middle ear is damaged, the reverse will hold true.
2 Apart from injury to the cochlear nerve itself, unilateral lesions of the auditory pathway do not greatly affect auditory acuity because of the bilaterality of the auditory projections.

3 Temporal lobe tumours may give rise to auditory hallucinations if they encroach upon the auditory (superior temporal) gyrus.

4 Lesions of the vestibular division of the labyrinth or of the vestibulocerebellar pathway result in vertigo, a subjective feeling of rotation, together with nausea, ataxia and nystagmus.

The glossopharyngeal nerve (IX) (Fig. 209)

The glossopharyngeal nerve contains sensory fibres for the pharynx and the posterior one-third of the tongue (including the taste buds), motor fibres for the stylopharyngeus muscle and secretomotor fibres for the parotid gland. It also supplies the carotid sinus (baroreceptor) and carotid body (chemoreceptor). It is attached to the upper part of the medulla by four or five rootlets along the groove between the olive and the inferior cerebellar peduncle (Fig. 233b) and leaves the skull by way of the jugular foramen in which it gives off its tympanic branch.

Below the jugular foramen the nerve courses downwards and forwards between the internal carotid artery and the internal jugular vein to reach the styloid process. From here it passes along the stylopharyngeus muscle to enter the pharynx between the superior and middle constrictors. Here, it breaks up into its terminal branches, which supply the posterior one-third of the tongue and the mucous membrane of the pharynx (including the tonsil).

The *tympanic branch*, which is continued as the *lesser superficial petrosal nerve*, conveys the preganglionic parasympathetic fibres to the otic ganglion (parotid secretomotor fibres).

The only other branch of significance is the *carotid nerve*, which arises just below the skull and runs down on the internal carotid artery to supply both the carotid body and carotid sinus. This small twig serves as the afferent limb of the baroreceptor and chemoreceptor reflexes from the carotid sinus and body, respectively. Although small, this branch is, in a physiological sense, perhaps the most important component of the glossopharyngeal nerve.

CLINICAL FEATURES

Complete section of the glossopharyngeal nerve results in sensory loss in the pharynx, loss of taste and common sensation over the posterior one-third of the tongue, some pharyngeal weakness and loss of salivation from the parotid gland. However, such lesions are frequently difficult to detect and rarely occur as isolated phenomena since there is so often associated involvement of the vagus or its nuclei.

The vagus nerve (X)

The vagus has the most extensive distribution of all the cranial nerves, innervating the heart and the major part of the respiratory and alimentary tracts (*vagus* = wanderer)

Central connections

The *dorsal nucleus* of the vagus in the medulla is a mixed visceral afferent and efferent nucleus. It receives sensory fibres from the heart, the lower respiratory tract and the alimentary tract as far as the distal transverse colon; in addition, it gives rise to preganglionic parasympathetic motor fibres to the heart and to the smooth muscles of the bronchi and gut.

From the *nucleus ambiguus* efferent fibres pass to the striped muscles of the pharynx and larynx.

Distribution

The nerve is connected to the side of the medulla by about ten filaments that lie in series with the glossopharyngeal nerve along the groove between the olive and the inferior cerebellar peduncle (Fig. 233b). These filaments unite to form a single bundle that passes beneath the cerebellum to the jugular foramen. Two sensory ganglia are associated with this part of the nerve: a superior, within the jugular foramen, and an inferior, immediately beneath the skull.

The vagus then passes vertically downwards to the root of the neck, lying in the posterior part of the carotid sheath between the internal jugular vein and the internal and then common carotid arteries (Fig. 212). There are a number of important branches in the neck: *pharyngeal* to the pharyngeal and palatal musculature by way of the pharyngeal plexus; *superior laryngeal*, supplying the interior of the larynx above the vocal folds and the cricothyroid and inferior constrictor muscles; and the superior and inferior *cardiac branches* which are inhibitory to the heart.

Below the level of the subclavian arteries the course and relations of the nerve on the two sides differ.

On the *right side* the *recurrent laryngeal branch* is given off as the vagus crosses the subclavian artery; beyond this, the vagus descends through the superior mediastinum in close association with the great veins. Behind the root of the lung it takes part in the formation of the *pulmonary plexus* and then passes on to the oesophagus to form, with its fellow, the *oesophageal plexus*.

The *left vagus* enters the thorax in close association with the great arteries, lying at first lateral to the common carotid and then crossing the arch of the aorta (Fig. 38). The *left recurrent laryngeal branch*, which is given off as the vagus crosses the aortic arch, passes below the ligamentum arteriosum, behind the arch, and then ascends in the groove between the trachea and the oesophagus (Fig. 34a). The vagus then passes behind the root of the lung, enters into the formation of the pulmonary plexus and passes on to the oesophagus to form a plexus from which emerge two trunks, named anterior and posterior vagal trunks, each comprising fibres from both the left and right vagus.

The two vagal trunks then enter the abdomen through the oesophageal opening in the diaphragm, the anterior vagus passing on to the anterior surface and the posterior passing to the posterior aspect of the stomach (Fig. 53). Beyond this it is difficult to trace the course of the nerves, but branches are given to the *coeliac*, *hepatic* and *renal plexuses* and, by way of these plexuses, are distributed to the fore- and midgut and to the kidneys.

CLINICAL FEATURES

1 Isolated lesions of the vagus nerve are uncommon, but it may be involved in injuries or disease of related structures.
2 A simple test for the integrity of the vagus relies on its innervation of the muscles of the palate. In unilateral paralysis, the uvula deviates to the normal side when the patient says 'Ah'.
3 Vagotomy – see pages 78–79.
4 Injuries to the recurrent laryngeal nerve – see page 307.

The accessory nerve (XI) (Figs 209, 233b)

The accessory nerve is conventionally described as having a cranial and a spinal root. According to standard descriptions, the cranial root is formed by a series of rootlets that emerge from the medulla between the olive and the inferior cerebellar peduncle. These rootlets are considered to join the spinal root, travel with it briefly, then separate within the jugular foramen and are distributed with the vagus nerve to supply the musculature of the palate, pharynx and larynx.

A detailed dissection study undertaken a few years ago demonstrated that all the medullary rootlets that do not join to form the glossopharyngeal nerve (IX) join the vagus nerve at the jugular foramen. All the rootlets that form the accessory nerve arise caudal to the olive and no connections can be demonstrated between the accessory nerve and the vagus in the jugular foramen. Thus, according to this study the accessory nerve has no cranial component and consists only of the structure hitherto referred to as the spinal root of the accessory nerve.

This spinal root is formed by the union of fibres from an elongated nucleus in the anterior horn of the upper five cervical segments, which leave the cord midway between the anterior and posterior roots, join, then pass upwards through the foramen magnum. The accessory nerve and the converging rootlets of the vagus nerve then enter the jugular foramen in a shared sheath of dura. The glossopharyngeal nerve enters the jugular foramen anterior to the vagus through a separate dural sheath.

The accessory nerve passes backwards over the internal jugular vein to the sternocleidomastoid muscle, which it pierces (and supplies), and then crosses the posterior triangle of the neck to enter and supply the deep surface of the trapezius.

Surface marking of the spinal accessory nerve

The extracranial course of the spinal accessory nerve can be marked out by a line which runs from the tragus of the ear to a point at the junction of the middle and lower thirds of the anterior border of the trapezius. This line will be seen to cross the palpable transverse process of the atlas (which lies immediately inferior to the mastoid process) and also the junction of the upper and middle thirds of the posterior border of the sternocleidomastoid muscle. There is, however, a good deal of variation in the precise position of the nerve as it crosses the posterior triangle of the neck.

CLINICAL FEATURES

Division of the accessory nerve results in paresis of the sternocleidomastoid and trapezius muscles. This follows, for example, most block dissections of the lymph nodes of the neck, the nerve being sacrificed in clearing the posterior triangle. The accessory nerve may also be damaged inadvertently during a supraclavicular lymph node biopsy or other relatively minor operative procedures in this region. Great care must be exercised to avoid this complication.

Division of the accessory nerve results in paralysis of sternocleidomastoid and trapezius. Sternocleidomastoid is tested clinically by asking the patient to turn his/her chin to the opposite side against the resistance of the examining clinician's hand, while trapezius is tested by asking the patient to elevate his/her shoulder against the resistance applied by the clinician's hand. (A paralysed trapezius results in flattening and drooping of the ipsilateral shoulder.)

Injury to the accessory nerve in the posterior triangle will result in paralysis of trapezius with the sternocleidomastoid being spared.

The hypoglossal nerve (XII)

The hypoglossal nerve is entirely motor and supplies all the intrinsic and extrinsic muscles of the ipsilateral half of the tongue (with the exception of the palatoglossus). From its nucleus, which lies in the floor of the 4th ventricle, a series of about a dozen rootlets leave the side of the medulla in the groove between the pyramid and the olive (Fig. 233b). These rootlets unite to leave the skull by way of the hypoglossal canal (also known as the anterior condylar canal) in the floor of the posterior cranial fossa just above the lateral margin of the foramen magnum. Lying at first deep to the internal carotid artery and the jugular vein, the nerve passes downwards between these two vessels to just above the level of the angle of the mandible. Here, it passes forwards over the internal and external carotid arteries and gives off its descending and thyrohyoid branches. It then crosses the hyoglossus and genioglossus muscles to enter the tongue (Fig. 258). Its descending branch (*descendens hypoglossi*) actually derives from a twig of the 1st cervical nerve and therefore transmits C1 fibres. It passes more or less vertically downwards upon the internal carotid artery to join the descending cervical nerve (C2 and C3) to form a loop known as the *ansa cervicalis* (or *ansa hypoglossi*) just

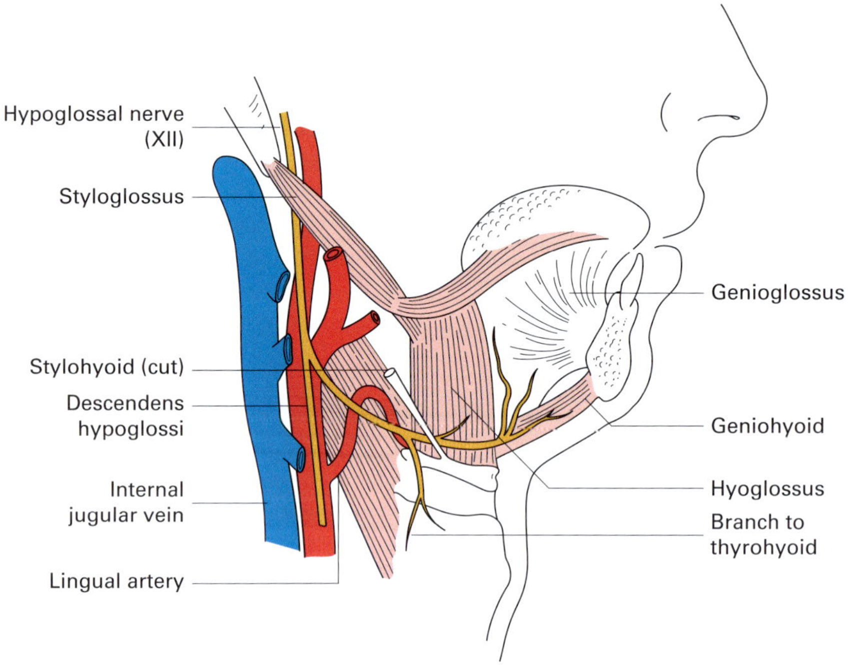

Fig. 258 The distal course of the hypoglossal nerve.

above the omohyoid muscle. From this loop branches are given to three infrahyoid muscles – sternothyroid, sternohyoid and omohyoid.

CLINICAL FEATURES

1 Division of the hypoglossal nerve, or lesions involving its nucleus, results in an ipsilateral paralysis and wasting of the muscles of the tongue. This is detected clinically by deviation of the protruded tongue to the affected side.
2 Supranuclear paralysis (due to an upper motor neurone lesion involving the corticobulbar pathways) leads to paresis but not atrophy of the muscles of the contralateral side.

The special senses

The nose (see also 'The paranasal sinuses (accessory nasal sinuses)', page 340)

The *external nose* consists of a bony and cartilaginous framework closely overlaid by skin and fibrofatty tissues. The bones are the two nasal bones and the frontal processes of the maxilla. The *ala* (*the lateral margin*) is composed solely of fatty tissue at its lower free edge.

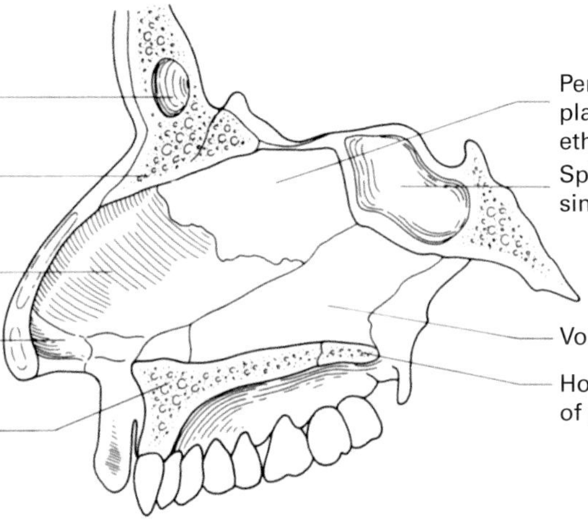

Fig. 259 The septum of the nose.

The *nasal cavity* is divided into right and left halves by a median *nasal septum* formed by the *perpendicular plate* of the *ethmoid bone*, the *septal cartilage* and the *vomer* (Fig. 259). Each cavity extends from the nostril (or anterior nares) in front to the posterior nasal aperture behind, communicating through the latter with the nasopharynx. The *lateral wall* is very irregular, owing to the projection of the three *conchae* (superior, middle and inferior) and the underlying meatuses (Figs 224, 225).

The superior meatus receives the opening of the posterior ethmoidal air cells. Opening into the middle meatus are (from before backwards) the frontal and maxillary sinuses and the anterior and middle ethmoidal air cells. Only the nasolacrimal duct opens, in splendid isolation, into the inferior meatus. The roof of the cavity is horizontal in its central portion, where it is formed by the cribriform plate of the ethmoid, but slopes downwards both anteriorly (the frontal and nasal bones) and posteriorly (the sphenoid). The *floor* corresponds to the roof of the mouth; it comprises the palatine process of the maxilla and the horizontal process of the palatine bone.

Mucous membrane

The *olfactory portion*, which is confined to the superior concha and the adjacent upper part of the septum, is thin and dull yellow in colour; it contains the olfactory receptors and supporting cells. The remaining *respiratory portion* is thick, vascular and moist with secretions of mucous glands; its epithelium is ciliated.

The upper part of the nasal cavity receives its arterial supply from the ethmoidal branches of the ophthalmic artery, a branch of the internal carotid. The sphenopalatine branch of the maxillary artery, a terminal of the external carotid, supplies the lower part of the cavity. Just within the vestibule of the nose, on the antero-inferior part of the septum, it links with a septal branch of the facial artery and it is from this zone, *Little's area*, that 90% of nosebleeds occur. The veins drain downwards into the facial vein and upwards to the ethmoidal tributaries of the ophthalmic veins.

CLINICAL FEATURES

1 The skin of the external nose and its surrounds contains many sebaceous glands and hair follicles that may become blocked and infected. The significance of this fact is that the facial veins, which may become secondarily infected, communicate directly with the ophthalmic veins and hence with the cavernous sinus. For this reason, this zone is often known as the 'danger area of the face'.
2 The extensive relations of the nasal cavity are important in the spread of infection. Observe that it is in direct continuity with (1) the anterior cranial fossa (via the cribriform plate of the ethmoid bone); (2) the nasopharynx and, through the pharyngotympanic tube, the middle ear; (3) the paranasal air sinuses; and (4) the lacrimal apparatus and conjunctiva.
3 The septum is frequently deviated to one or other side, interfering both with inspiration and with drainage of the nose and accessory sinuses.

The ear

The external ear (Fig. 260)

This comprises the auricle and external auditory meatus. The *auricle*, for the most part, consists of a cartilaginous framework to which the skin is closely applied. The intrinsic and extrinsic muscles described for the ear are of no significance in man.

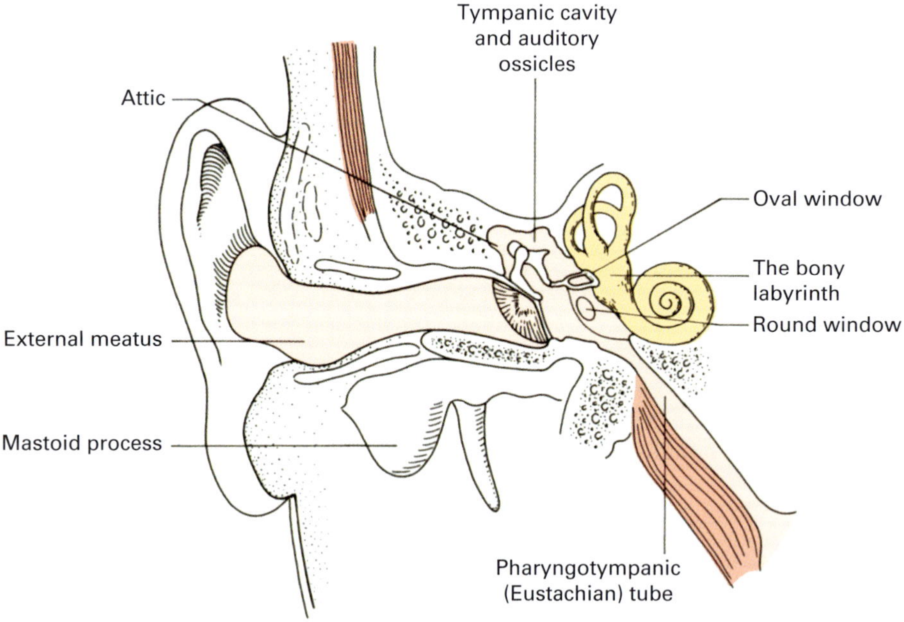

Fig. 260 General view of the ear.

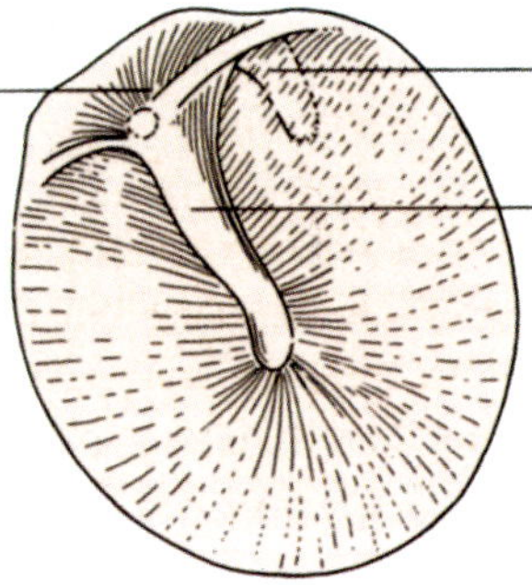

Fig. 261 The tympanic membrane as seen through an otoscope.

The *external auditory meatus* extends inwards to the tympanic membrane. It is about 3.7 cm (1.5 in) long and has a peculiar 'S'-shaped course, being directed first medially upwards and forwards, then medially and backwards and, finally, medially forwards and downwards. The outer third of the canal is cartilaginous and somewhat wider than the medial osseous portion. The whole canal is lined by skin, which is closely adherent to the osseous portion but is separated from the cartilaginous part by the ceruminous glands in the subcutaneous tissue.

The *tympanic membrane*, or *ear drum* (Figs 260, 261), separates the middle ear from the external auditory meatus. It is made up of an outer cutaneous layer, continuous with the skin of the external auditory meatus, a middle fibrous layer and an inner mucous layer continuous with the mucoperiosteum of the rest of the tympanic cavity. It is oval in outline, a little less than 1.25 cm (0.5 in) in its greatest (vertical) diameter, and faces laterally, downwards and forwards; it is slightly concave outwards. Since it is translucent (except at its margin where it is attached to the medial aspect of the external auditory meatus), it is possible on examination to see the underlying malleus and part of the incus. The greater part of the membrane is taut and is known as the *pars tensa*, but above the lateral process of the malleus there is a small triangular area where the membrane is thin and lax – the *pars flaccida*. This area is bounded by two distinct malleolar folds that reach down to the lateral process of the malleus. The point of greatest concavity of the membrane is known as the *umbo*; this marks the attachment of the handle of the malleus to the membrane.

The middle ear

The *middle ear*, or *tympanic cavity*, is the narrow slit-like cavity in the petrous part of the temporal bone containing the three auditory ossicles: malleus (the hammer), incus (the anvil) and stapes (the stirrup) (Fig. 260).

The walls of the cavity and its important relations are as follows.

The *lateral wall* is formed mainly by the tympanic membrane, which separates the tympanic cavity from the external auditory meatus, and above this by the squamous part of the temporal bone; the part of the cavity above the tympanic membrane is known as the *epitympanic recess* or *attic*; this part of the cavity contains the incus and the head of the malleus.

The *medial wall*, which separates the cavity from the internal ear, presents the *fenestra cochleae* (round window), closed by the secondary tympanic membrane; the *fenestra vestibuli* (oval window), occupied by the base (foot-piece) of the stapes; the *promontory*, formed by the first turn of the cochlea; and the *prominence* caused by the underlying canal for the facial nerve (Fig. 256).

The *floor* is a thin plate of bone separating the cavity from the bulb of the jugular vein.

The *roof* is formed by the thin sheet of bone known as the *tegmen tympani*, which separates it from the middle cranial fossa and the temporal lobe of the brain.

Anteriorly, the cavity communicates with the pharynx by way of the pharyngotympanic or Eustachian tube.

Posteriorly, it communicates with the mastoid or tympanic antrum and the mastoid air cells.

The *mastoid antrum* is a small cavity in the posterior part of the petrous temporal bone connected to the epitympanic recess of the middle ear by way of the narrow *aditus*. Its importance is twofold: it is in communication with the mastoid air cells (hence the portal through which infection may spread to these spaces from the middle ear) and it is intimately related posteriorly to the sigmoid sinus and the cerebellum, both of which may be involved from a middle ear infection.

The *mastoid air cells* arise postnatally as diverticula from the tympanic antrum, becoming obvious first at 2 years. They may invade not only the mastoid process but also the squamous part of the temporal bone. They are lined by a mucoperiosteum continuous anteriorly with that of the tympanic cavity.

The *pharyngotympanic* (*Eustachian*) *tube* reaches downwards, forwards and medially from the anterior part of the tympanic cavity to the lateral walls of the nasopharynx. In all it is about 3.7 cm (1.5 in) long, the first 1.25 cm (0.5 in) being bony while the rest is cartilaginous. It is lined by a ciliated columnar epithelium. The mucous membrane is thin in its bony part but the cartilaginous segment contains numerous mucous glands and, near its pharyngeal orifice, a considerable collection of lymphoid tissue termed the *tubal tonsil*. This may become swollen in infection, producing blockage of the tube. The tube is widest at its pharyngeal end and narrowest at the junction of the bony and cartilaginous portions.

Conduction of sound through the middle ear is by way of the malleus, incus and stapes. The *malleus* is the largest of the three and is described as having a handle, attached to the tympanic membrane, a rounded head, which articulates with the incus, and a lateral process, which can be seen through the tympanic membrane and from which the malleolar folds radiate. The *incus* comprises a body, which articulates with the malleus, and two processes, a short process attached to the posterior wall of the middle ear and a long process for articulation with the stapes. The shadow of the long process can often be seen through an auroscope running downwards behind the handle of the malleus. The *stapes* has a head for articulation with the incus, a neck and a base, which is firmly fixed in the fenestra vestibuli (the oval window).

Two small muscles are associated with these ossicles: the *stapedius*, which is attached to the neck of the stapes and is supplied by the facial nerve, and the *tensor tympani*, which is inserted into the handle of the malleus and is supplied by the mandibular division of V. Both serve to damp high-frequency vibrations.

The internal ear (Fig. 262)

The internal ear consists essentially of a complicated bony labyrinth made up of a central *vestibule*, which communicates posteriorly with three semicircular ducts and anteriorly with the spiral cochlea. This cavity contains a fluid known as *perilymph* and encloses the *membranous labyrinth*, comprising the *utricle* and *saccule*, which communicate, respectively, with the semicircular canals and the cochlear canal. The duct system is filled with *endolymph*.

In each component of the membranous labyrinth there are specialized sensory receptor areas known as the *maculae* of the utricle and saccule, the *ampullary crests* of the semicircular canals and the *spiral organ of Corti* in the cochlea.

The disposition of the semicircular canals in three planes at right angles to each other renders this part of the labyrinth particularly well suited to signal changes in position of the head. The organ of Corti is adapted to record the sound vibrations transmitted by the stapes at the oval window.

The eye and associated structures (for optic nerve and visual pathway, see page 389).

The eyeball (Fig. 263)

The eyeball, which is just under 2.5 cm (1 in) in all diameters, is formed by segments of two spheres of different size: a prominent anterior segment, which is transparent and forms about one-sixth of the eyeball, and a larger posterior segment, which is opaque and constitutes five-sixths of a sphere. The optic nerve enters the eye about 3 mm (0.125 in) to the nasal (medial) side of the posterior pole.

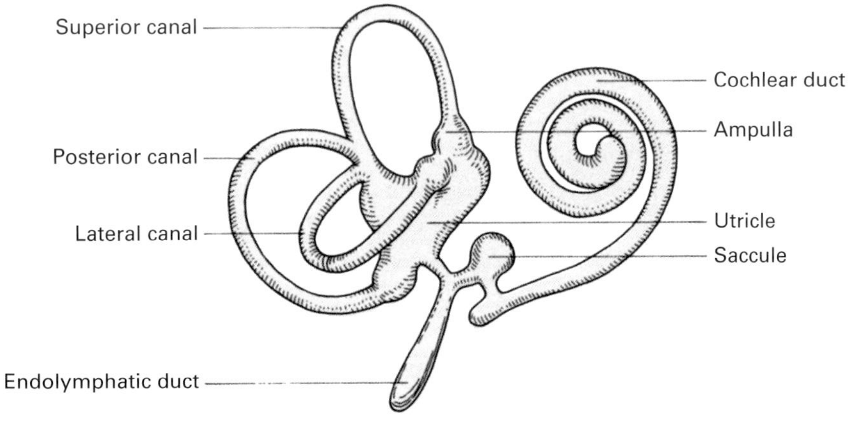

Fig. 262 Detail of the membranous labyrinth.

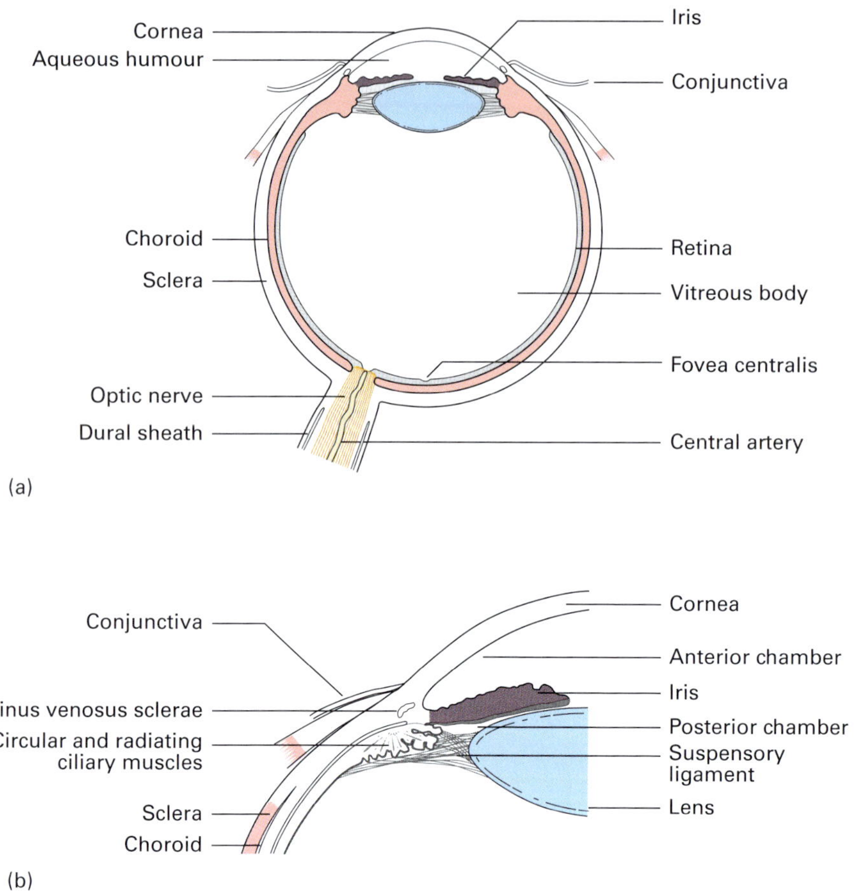

Fig. 263 (a) The eyeball in section. (b) Detail of the ciliary region.

The eyeball is made up of three coats: a fibrous outer coat, a vascular middle coat and an inner neural coat – the retina.

The fibrous coat

The fibrous coat comprises a transparent anterior part, the cornea, and an opaque posterior portion, the sclera. Peripherally, the *cornea* is continuous with the sclera at the *sclerocorneal junction*. The *sclera* is a tough, fibrous membrane which is responsible for the maintenance of the shape of the eyeball and which receives the insertion of the extra-ocular muscles. Posteriorly, it is pierced by the optic nerve, with whose dural sheath it is continuous.

The vascular coat

This is made up of the choroid, the ciliary body and the iris.

The *choroid* is a thin but highly vascular membrane lining the inner surface of the sclera. Posteriorly it is pierced by the optic nerve and anteriorly it is connected to the iris by the ciliary body.

The *ciliary body* includes the *ciliary ring*, a fibrous ring continuous with the choroid, the *ciliary processes*, a group of 60–80 folds arranged radially between the ciliary ring and the iris and connected posteriorly to the suspensory ligament of the lens, and the *ciliary muscles*, an outer radial and inner circular layer of smooth muscle responsible for the changes in convexity of the lens in accommodation and supplied by parasympathetic fibres transmitted in the oculomotor nerve (III).

The *iris* is the contractile disc surrounding the pupil. It consists of four layers:

1 an anterior mesothelial lining;
2 a connective tissue stroma containing pigment cells;
3 a group of radially arranged smooth muscle fibres – the dilator of the pupil (supplied by the sympathetic system) and a circular group, the pupillary sphincter (supplied by the parasympathetic fibres in the oculomotor nerve);
4 a posterior layer of pigmented cells which is continuous with the ciliary part of the retina.

The neural coat

The *retina* is formed by an outer pigmented and an inner nervous layer and is interposed between the choroid and the hyaloid membrane of the vitreous. Anteriorly, it presents an irregular edge, the *ora serrata*, while posteriorly the nerve fibres on its surface collect to form the optic nerve. Its appearance as seen through an ophthalmoscope is shown in Fig. 264. Near its posterior pole there is a pale yellowish area, the *macula lutea*, the site of central vision, and just medial to this is the pale *optic disc* formed by the passage of nerve fibres through the retina, corresponding to the 'blind spot'. The *central artery of the retina* emerges from the disc and then divides into upper and lower branches; each of these in turn divides into a nasal and temporal branch. Histologically, the retina consists of a number of layers but from a functional point of view only three need be considered: an inner receptor cell layer – the layer of rods and cones; an

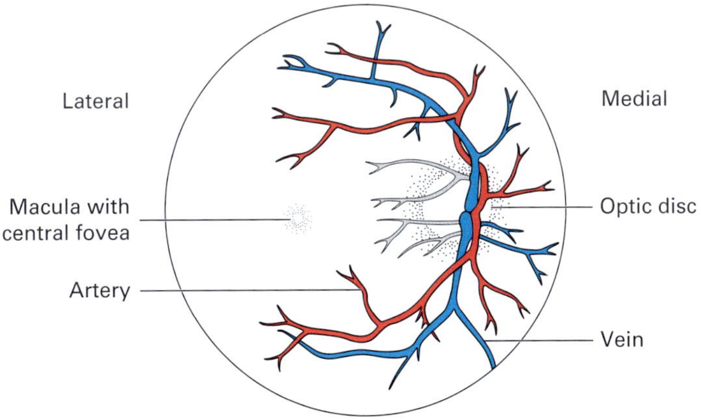

Fig. 264 The right fundus oculi as seen through an ophthalmoscope.

intermediate layer of bipolar neurones; and the layer of ganglion cells, whose axons form the superficial layer of optic nerve fibres (Fig. 249).

Contents of the eyeball

Within the eyeball are found the lens, the aqueous humour and the vitreous body. The *lens* is biconvex and is placed between the vitreous and the aqueous humour, just behind the iris. The *aqueous humour* is a filtrate of plasma secreted by the vessels of the iris and ciliary body into the *posterior chamber* of the eye (i.e. the space between the lens and the iris). From here it passes through the pupillary aperture into the *anterior chamber* (between the cornea and the iris) and is reabsorbed into the ciliary veins by way of the *sinus venosus sclerae* (or *canal of Schlemm*). The *vitreous body*, which occupies the posterior four-fifths of the eyeball, is a thin transparent gel contained within a delicate membrane – the *hyaloid membrane* – and pierced by the lymph-filled *hyaloid canal*. The anterior part of the hyaloid membrane is thickened, receives attachments from the ciliary processes and gives rise to the *suspensory ligament of the lens*. This ligament is attached to the capsule of the lens in front of its equator and serves to retain it in position. It is relaxed by contraction of the radial fibres of the ciliary muscle and so allows the lens to assume a more convex form in accommodation (close reading).

The orbital muscles (Fig. 255; see Fig. 266)

These are the levator palpebrae superioris and the extra-ocular muscles; the medial, lateral, superior and inferior recti and the superior and inferior obliques. The four *recti* arise from a tendinous ring around the optic foramen and the medial part of the superior orbital fissure and are inserted into the sclera anterior to the equator of the eyeball. The lateral rectus is supplied by the VIth nerve, the others by the IIIrd. The *superior oblique* arises just above the tendinous ring and is inserted by means of a long tendon that loops around a fibrous pulley on the medial part of the roof of the orbit into the sclera just lateral to the insertion of the superior rectus. It is supplied by the IVth nerve. The *inferior oblique* passes like a sling from its origin on the medial side of the orbit around the undersurface of the eye to insert into the sclera between the superior and lateral recti; it is supplied by III.

Both the oblique muscles insert behind the equator of the eyeball.

The eyeball can be elevated, depressed, adducted, abducted and rotated. The medial and lateral recti move the eyeball about just one axis, the vertical axis.

The other four extra-ocular muscles move the eyeball simultaneously on all three axes:

- superior rectus – elevation, adduction and medial rotation;
- inferior rectus – depression, adduction and lateral rotation;
- superior oblique – depression, abduction and medial rotation;
- inferior oblique – elevation, abduction and lateral rotation.

Pure elevation and depression of the eyeball are produced by one rectus acting with its opposite oblique – rectus superior with inferior oblique producing pure elevation and rectus inferior with the superior oblique producing pure depression.

A useful mnemonic is that the superior oblique is 'the tramp's muscle' – it moves the eye 'down and out'!

The actions of these muscles are shown in Fig. 265.

The *fascial sheath of the eye* (*Tenon's capsule*) is the membrane enclosing the eyeball from the optic nerve behind to the sclerocorneal junction in front. It is pierced by the vessels and nerves of the eye and by the tendons of the extra-ocular muscles. It is thickened inferiorly, where it forms the suspensory ligament.

The eyelids and conjunctiva (Fig. 266)

Of the two eyelids, the upper is the larger and more mobile, but, apart from the presence of the levator palpebrae superioris in this lid, the structure of the eyelids is essentially the same. Each consists of the following layers, from without inwards:

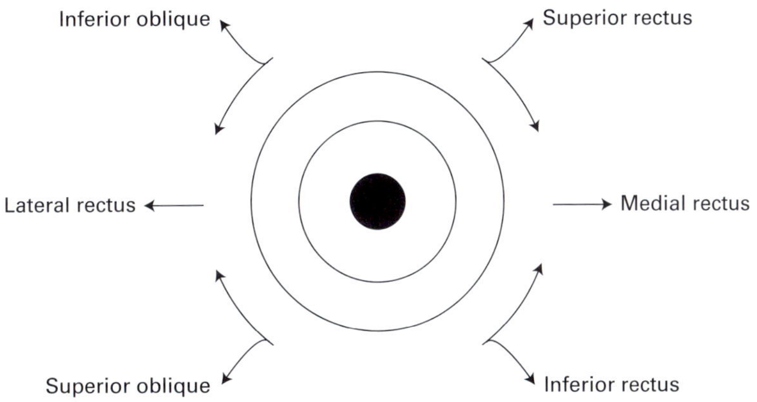

Fig. 265 The direction of action of the muscles acting on the eyeball from the primary position (i.e. looking directly forwards).

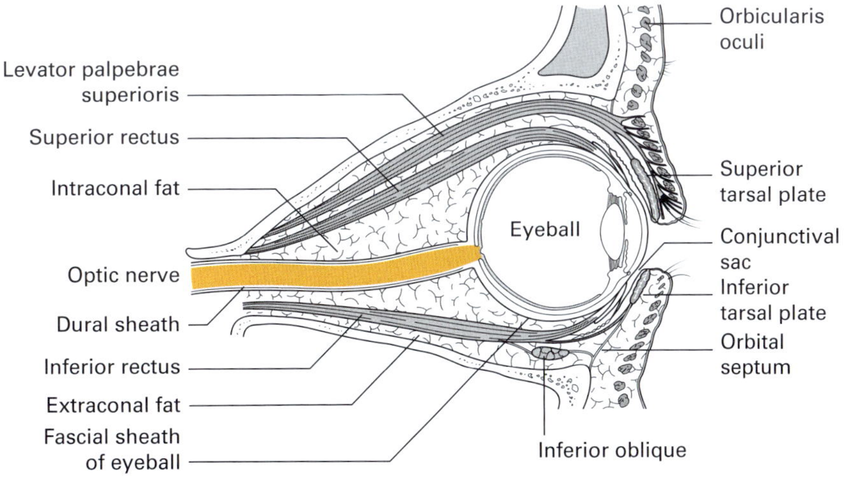

Fig. 266 Compartments of the orbit.

skin, loose connective tissue, fibres of the orbicularis oculi muscle, the tarsal plates, of very dense fibrous tissue, tarsal glands and conjunctiva. The eyelashes arise along the mucocutaneous junction and immediately behind the lashes there are the openings of the *tarsal* (*Meibomian*) *glands*. These are large sebaceous glands whose secretion helps to seal the palpebral fissure when the eyelids are closed and forms a thin layer over the exposed surface of the open eye; if blocked, they distend into Meibomian cysts.

The *conjunctiva* is the delicate mucous membrane lining the inner surface of the lids from which it is reflected over the anterior part of the sclera to the cornea. Over the lids it is thick and highly vascular, but over the sclera it is much thinner and over the cornea it is reduced to a single layer of epithelium. The line of reflection from the lid to the sclera is known as the conjunctival fornix; the superior fornix receives the openings of the lacrimal glands.

Movements of the eyelids are brought about by the contraction of the orbicularis oculi and levator palpebrae superioris muscles. The width of the palpebral fissure at any one time depends on the tone of these muscles and the degree of protrusion of the eyeball.

The lacrimal apparatus (Fig. 267)

The *lacrimal gland* is situated in the upper, lateral part of the orbit in what is known as the lacrimal fossa. The main part of the gland is about the size and shape of an almond, but it is connected to a small terminal process that extends into the posterolateral part

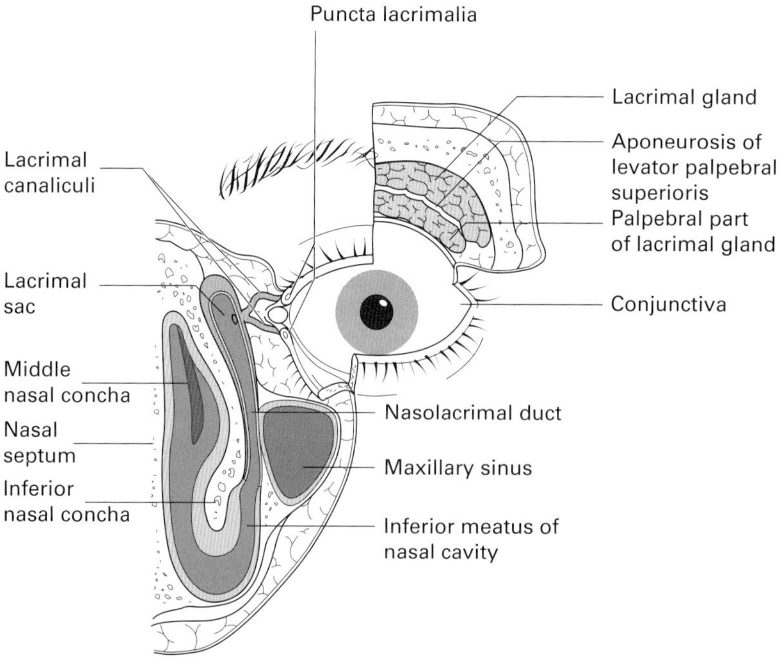

Fig. 267 The lacrimal gland and its drainage system.

of the upper lid. The gland is drained by a series of 8–12 small ducts that open into the lateral part of the superior conjunctival fornix whence its secretion is spread over the surface of the eye by the action of the lids.

The tears are drained by way of the *lacrimal canaliculi*, whose openings, the *lacrimal puncta*, can be seen on the small elevation near the medial margin of each eyelid known as the *lacrimal papilla*. The two canaliculi, superior and inferior, open into the *lacrimal sac*, which is situated in a small depression on the medial surface of the orbit. This in turn drains through the nasolacrimal duct into the anterior part of the inferior meatus of the nose. The nasolacrimal duct, which not uncommonly becomes obstructed, is about 2 cm (0.75 in) in length and lies in its own bony canal that leads from the fossa for the lacrimal sac along the lateral wall of the nasal cavity.

The autonomic nervous system

The nervous system may be pictured as being divided into two broad functional groups: the *cerebrospinal system*, made up of the brain, spinal cord and the peripheral cranial and spinal nerves, and the *autonomic system* (also termed the *vegetative, visceral* or *involuntary system*), comprising the autonomic ganglia and nerves. Broadly speaking, the cerebrospinal system is concerned with the responses of the body to the external environment. In contrast, the autonomic system is concerned with the control of the internal environment, exercised through the innervation of the non-skeletal muscle of the heart, blood vessels, bronchial tree, gut and the pupils and the secretomotor supply of many glands, including those of the alimentary tract and its outgrowths, the sweat glands and, as a rather special example, the suprarenal medulla.

The two systems should not be regarded as being independent of each other, for they are linked anatomically and functionally. Anatomically, autonomic nerve fibres are transmitted in all of the peripheral and some of the cranial nerves; moreover, the higher connections of the autonomic system are situated within the spinal cord and brain. Functionally, the two systems are closely linked within the brain and spinal cord.

The characteristic feature of the autonomic system is that its efferent nerves emerge as medullated fibres from the brain and spinal cord, are interrupted in their course by a synapse in a peripheral ganglion and are then relayed for distribution as fine non-medullated fibres. In this respect they differ from the somatic efferent nerves, which pass without interruption to their terminations (Fig. 268).

The autonomic system is subdivided into the sympathetic and parasympathetic systems on anatomical, functional and, to a considerable extent, pharmacological grounds.

Anatomically, the sympathetic nervous system has its motor cell-stations in the lateral grey column of the thoracic and upper two lumbar segments of the spinal cord. The parasympathetic system is less neatly defined anatomically since it is divided into a cranial outflow, which passes along the cranial nerves III, VII, IX and X, and a sacral outflow, with cell-stations in the 2nd, 3rd and sometimes 4th sacral segments of the cord.

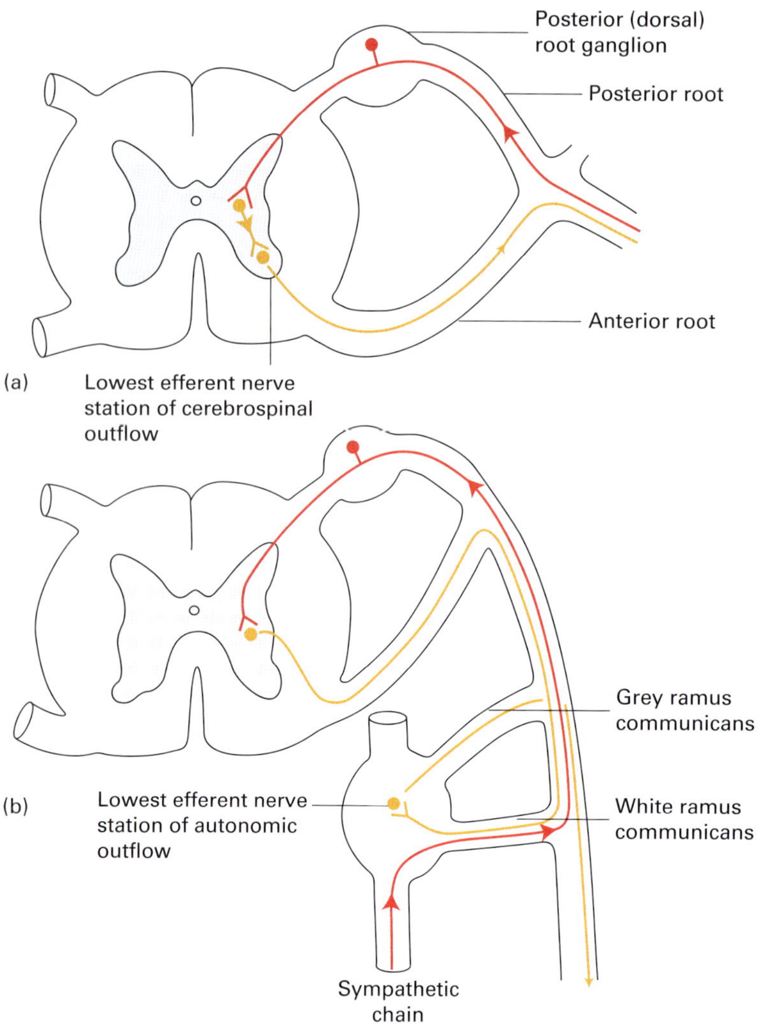

Fig. 268 The essential difference between the cerebrospinal and autonomic outflows: (a) the cerebrospinal system has its lowest efferent nerve cell-stations within the central nervous system; (b) the autonomic system has its lowest efferent cell-stations in a peripheral ganglion (here illustrated by a typical sympathetic nerve ganglion). Red, afferent pathway; yellow, efferent pathway.

Functionally, the sympathetic system is concerned principally with stress reactions of the body. When this system is stimulated, the pupils dilate, peripheral blood vessels constrict, the force, rate and oxygen consumption of the heart increase, the bronchial tree dilates, visceral activity is diminished by inhibition of peristalsis and increase of sphincter tone, glycogenolysis takes place in the liver, the suprarenal medulla is stimulated to secrete and there is cutaneous sweating and pilo-erection. The sympathetic pelvic nerves inhibit bladder contraction and are motor to the internal vesical sphincter.

Coronary blood flow is increased, partly by a direct sympathetic effect and partly produced by indirect factors, which include more vigorous cardiac contraction, reduced systole, relatively increased diastole and an increased concentration of vasodilator metabolites.

Table 5 Summary of effects of sympathetic and parasympathetic stimulation

	Sympathetic stimulation	Parasympathetic stimulation
Eye	Pupil dilates	Pupil constricts; accommodation of lens
Lacrimal gland	Vasoconstrictor	Secretomotor
Heart	Increase in force, rate, conduction and excitability	Decrease in force, rate, conduction and excitability
Lung	Bronchi dilate	Bronchi constrict; secretomotor to mucous glands
Skin	Vasoconstrictor Pilo-erection Secretomotor to sweat glands	
Salivary glands	Vasoconstrictor	Secretomotor
Musculature of alimentary canal	Peristalsis inhibited	Peristalsis activated; sphincters relax
Acid secretion of stomach	–	Secretomotor
Pancreas	–	Secretomotor
Liver	Glycogenolysis	–
Suprarenal	Secretomotor	–
Bladder	Detrusor inhibited Sphincter stimulated	Detrusor stimulated Sphincter inhibited
Uterus	Uterine contraction Vasoconstriction	Vasodilatation

The parasympathetic system tends to be antagonistic to the sympathetic system (Table 5). Its stimulation results in constriction of the pupils, diminution in the rate, conduction and excitability of the heart, an increase in gut peristalsis with sphincter relaxation and enhanced alimentary glandular secretion. In addition, the pelvic parasympathetic nerves inhibit the vesical internal sphincter and are motor to the detrusor muscle of the bladder.

The sympathetic system tends to have a 'mass action' effect; stimulation of any part of it results in a widespread response. In contrast, parasympathetic activity is usually discrete and localized. This difference can be explained, at least in part, by differences in anatomical peripheral connections of the two systems, as will be described in the section on 'The parasympathetic system'.

It is useful to think of the two systems as acting synergistically. For example, reflex slowing of the heart is effected partly from increased vagal and partly from decreased sympathetic stimulation. In addition, some organs receive their autonomic innervation from one system only; for example, the suprarenal medulla and the cutaneous arterioles receive only sympathetic fibres, whereas neurogenic gastric secretion is entirely under parasympathetic control via the vagus nerve.

Pharmacologically, the sympathetic postganglionic terminals release adrenaline (epinephrine) and noradrenaline (norepinephrine), with the single exception of the terminals to the sweat glands which, in common with all the parasympathetic postganglionic terminations, release acetylcholine.

The sympathetic system

The efferent fibres of the sympathetic system arise in the lateral grey column of the spinal cord (Figs 268, 269) from segments T1–L2. From each of these segments small medullated axons emerge into the corresponding anterior primary ramus and pass via a white ramus communicans into the sympathetic trunk.

The spinal segments responsible for the sympathetic innervation of the various parts of the body are approximately as follows:

- head and neck, T1–T2;
- upper limb, T2–T5;
- thoracic viscera, T1–T5;
- abdominal viscera, T4–L2;
- pelvic viscera, T10–L2;
- lower limb, T11–L2.

Stimulation of a single white ramus communicans would thus obviously have widespread effects – the anatomical basis of the 'mass action' response of sympathetic stimulation.

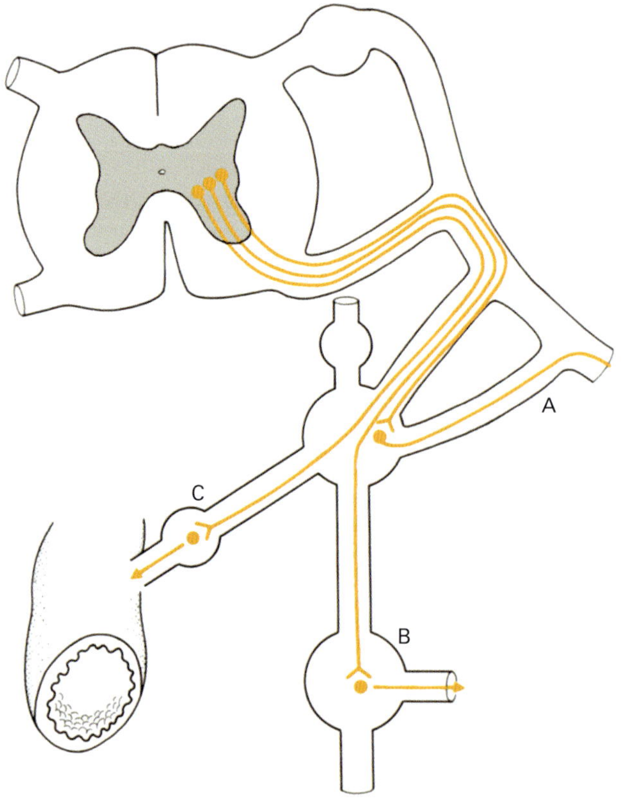

Fig. 269 The three fates of sympathetic white rami. These may (A) relay in their corresponding ganglion and pass to their corresponding spinal nerve for distribution, (B) ascend or descend in the sympathetic chain and relay in higher or lower ganglia or (C) pass without synapse to a peripheral ganglion for relay.

The sympathetic trunk

The sympathetic trunk on each side is a ganglionated nerve chain that extends from the base of the skull to the coccyx in close relationship to the vertebral column, maintaining a distance of about 2.5 cm (1 in) from the midline throughout its course. Commencing in the superior cervical ganglion beneath the skull base, the chain descends closely behind the posterior wall of the carotid sheath, enters the thorax anterior to the neck of the first rib, descends over the heads of the upper ribs and then on the sides of the bodies of the last three or four thoracic vertebrae. The chain then passes into the abdomen behind the medial arcuate ligament of the diaphragm and descends in a groove between psoas major and the sides of the lumbar vertebral bodies, overlapped by the abdominal aorta on the left and the inferior vena cava (IVC) on the right. The chain then passes behind the common iliac vessels to enter the pelvis anterior to the ala of the sacrum and then descends medial to the anterior sacral foramina. The sympathetic trunks end below by meeting each other at the *ganglion impar* on the anterior face of the coccyx.

The details of the cervical, thoracic and lumbar portions of the trunk are given on pages 329, 52 and 160, respectively.

The sympathetic trunk bears a series of ganglia along its course that contain motor cells with which preganglionic medullated fibres enter into synapse and from which non-medullated postganglionic axons originate. Developmentally, there was originally one ganglion for each peripheral nerve, but by a process of fusion these have been reduced in man to three cervical, twelve or fewer thoracic, two to four lumbar and four sacral ganglia. Only the ganglia of T1–L2 receive white rami directly; the higher and lower ganglia must receive their preganglionic supply from medullated nerves that travel through their corresponding ganglia without relay and that then ascend or descend in the sympathetic chain. Still other preganglionic fibres pass intact through the ganglia to peripheral visceral ganglia for relay.

There are thus three fates which may befall white rami (Fig. 269):

1 to enter the sympathetic trunk and synapse within a corresponding sympathetic ganglion at the level of entry (this applies only to the T1–L2 segments);
2 to ascend or descend in the sympathetic chain with relay in higher or lower ganglia;
3 to traverse the ganglia intact and relay in peripheral ganglia.

Pharmacologically, the sympathetic postganglionic terminals release adrenaline (epinephrine) and noradrenaline (norepinephrine), with a single exception of the sweat glands, which, in common with all the parasympathetic postganglionic terminations, release acetylcholine.

Distribution

The branches of the sympathetic ganglionic chain have somatic and visceral distribution.

Somatic distribution

Each spinal nerve receives one or more grey rami from a sympathetic ganglion that distributes postganglionic non-medullated sympathetic fibres to the segmental skin area supplied by the spinal nerve. These fibres are vasoconstrictor to the skin arterioles, sudomotor to sweat glands and pilomotor to the cutaneous hairs.

Visceral distribution

Postganglionic fibres to the head and neck and to the thoracic viscera arise from the ganglion cells of the sympathetic chain. Those to the head ascend along the internal carotid and vertebral arteries, whereas those to the thoracic organs are distributed by the cardiac, pulmonary and oesophageal plexuses.

The abdominal and pelvic viscera, however, are supplied by postganglionic fibres that have their cell-stations in more peripherally placed prevertebral ganglia – the coeliac, hypogastric and pelvic plexuses – which receive their preganglionic fibres from the splanchnic nerves (Fig. 270). These nerves are detailed on page 52, and shown in Fig. 38a,b.

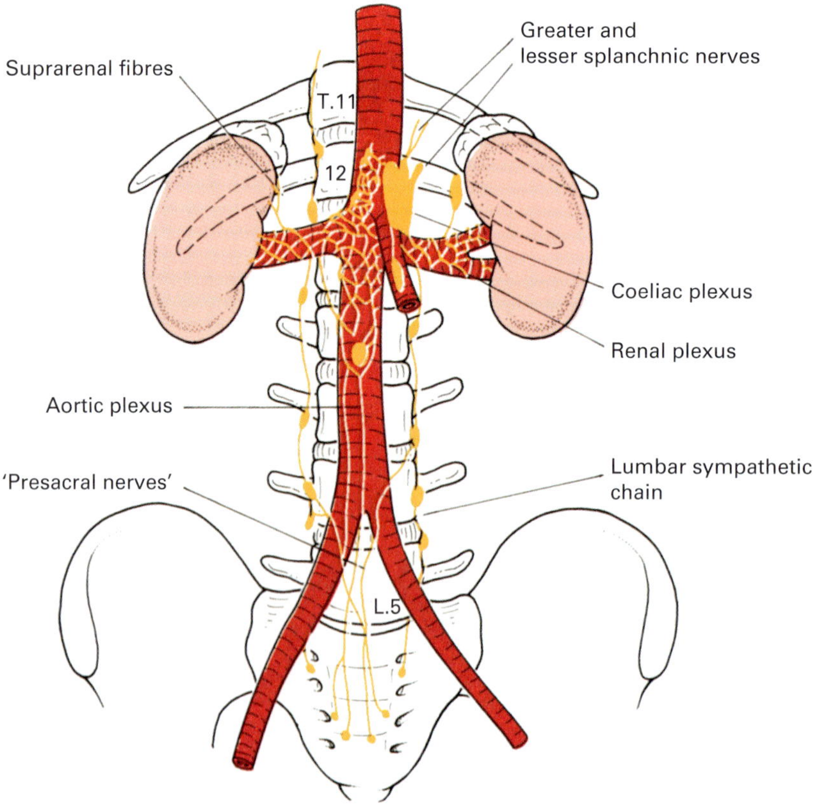

Fig. 270 The abdominal sympathetic plexuses.

The suprarenal medulla has a unique nerve supply comprising a rich plexus of preganglionic fibres that pass without relay from the coeliac ganglion to the gland. These fibres end in direct contact with the chromaffin medullary cells and liberate acetylcholine (as in all autonomic ganglia), which stimulates the secretion of adrenaline (epinephrine) and noradrenaline (norepinephrine) by the suprarenal medulla.

The chromaffin cells of the suprarenal medulla may thus be regarded as sympathetic cells that have not developed postganglionic fibres; indeed, embryologically both the medulla and the sympathetic nerves have a common origin from the neural crest.

Afferent sympathetic fibres

As well as the efferent sympathetic system, there are also important *afferent sympathetic fibres*. These arise from the thoracic, abdominal and pelvic viscera and are concerned with the afferent arc of the autonomic reflexes and also – of great importance from the clinical point of view – with the conduction of visceral pain sensation to the higher centres. The afferent sympathetic fibres pass from receptors in the walls of the viscera and ascend in the autonomic sympathetic plexuses. The afferent course from any viscus is therefore along the same pathway as the efferent autonomic fibres which supply that organ. They have their cell-stations in the dorsal root ganglia of the spinal nerves (Fig. 268).

(Note that, although afferent fibres are conveyed in both sympathetic and parasympathetic nerves, they are independent – they do not relay in the autonomic ganglia and terminate, just like somatic sensory fibres, in the dorsal ganglia of the spinal and cranial nerves. They merely use the autonomic nerves as a convenient anatomical conveyor system from the periphery to the brain.)

The afferent sympathetic fibres ascend centrally to the hypothalamus and thence to parts of the cerebral cortex and the limbic system along as yet undefined pathways.

Normally we are unaware of the afferent impulses from our viscera. Indeed, the thoracic, abdominal and pelvic organs are insensitive to cutting or burning. Thus, haemorrhoids can be injected, polyps in the stomach or colon biopsied and oesophageal varices or bleeding peptic ulcers injected without the patient being aware of this. Visceral pain may be provoked by distension, traction, excessive involuntary muscle contraction, inflammation or ischaemia; hence, the pain of coronary artery occlusion, intestinal obstruction, biliary or ureteric colic and the uterine contractions in childbirth.

In contrast to somatic pain, which is usually sharp and well localized, visceral pain is poorly localized and dull, and difficult to describe. Of considerable diagnostic importance, however, is referral of pain to the cutaneous areas that correspond to the segments of visceral nerves involved.

Referred pain can be from:

- heart (T1–T5) – to the front of the left chest, epigastrium, or medial side of the left arm;
- stomach, adnexae, foregut and midgut (T5–T12) – to the epigastrium and upper and mid-abdomen (the gall bladder typically gives referred pain to the lower pole of the scapula, T7);
- kidney and ureter (T10–T12, L1) – lumbar region, flank, groin and, in the male, the testis;

- gonads (T10–T11) – to the iliac fossa and loin;
- pelvic viscera (S2–S4) – sacral area, the buttocks and posterior aspects of the thighs.

CLINICAL FEATURES

- *Coeliac plexus block* – may be used to treat the intractable pain of chronic pancreatitis or upper gastrointestinal malignancy.
- *Presacral nerve block* – may similarly be used in the management of pain from pelvic malignant disease.
- *Cervical sympathectomy* – see page 330.

The parasympathetic system

As already stated, this system has a cranial and a sacral component. Its medullated preganglionic fibres synapse with ganglion cells that lie close to, or actually in the walls of, the viscera supplied. Postganglionic fibres therefore have only a short and direct course to their effector cells, and there is thus the anatomical pathway of a local discrete response to parasympathetic stimulation (Fig. 271).

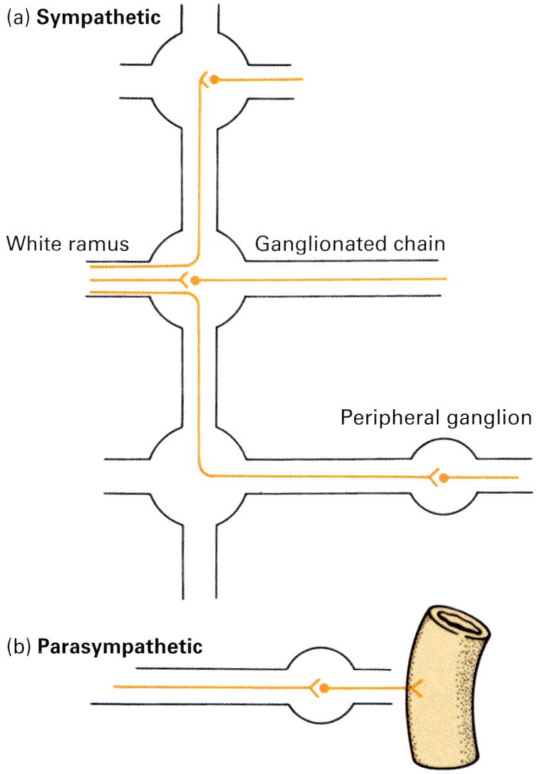

Fig. 271 The anatomical basis of widespread sympathetic and local parasympathetic response. (a) The widespread distribution of postganglionic fibres from a single sympathetic white ramus. (b) The localized distribution of postganglionic parasympathetic fibres.

Cranial outflow

The cranial component of the parasympathetic system is conveyed in cranial nerves III, VII, IX and X, of which X (the vagus) is the most important and the most widely distributed. The functions of this group of nerves can be summarized as follows:

1 pupils – constrictor to pupil, motor to ciliary muscle (accommodation);
2 salivary glands – secretomotor;
3 lacrimal glands – secretomotor;
4 heart – inhibitor of cardiac conduction, contraction, excitability and impulse formation (with consequent slowing of the heart and diminution of its contraction force);
5 lungs – bronchoconstrictor, secretomotor to mucous glands;
6 alimentary canal – motor to gut muscles as far as the region of the ascending colon; inhibitor to the pyloric sphincter; secretomotor to the glands and adnexae of the stomach and intestine.

The parasympathetic distribution of III, VII and IX is carried out via four ganglia from which postganglionic fibres relay. These ganglia also transmit (without synapse and therefore without functional connection) sympathetic and sensory fibres which have similar peripheral distribution. These ganglia are the ciliary (see page 391), pterygopalatine (see page 395), submandibular (see page 397) and otic (see page 396).

The Xth (vagal) distribution conveys by far the most important and largest contributions of the parasympathetic system. It is responsible for all the functions of the parasympathetic cranial outflow enumerated previously, apart from the innervation of the eye and the secretomotor supply to the salivary and lacrimal glands. The efferent fibres are derived from the dorsal nucleus of X and are distributed widely in the cardiac, pulmonary and alimentary plexuses. Postganglionic fibres are relayed from tiny ganglia that lie in the walls of the viscera concerned; in the gut, these constitute the submucosal *plexus of Meissner* and the myenteric *plexus of Auerbach*.

The sacral outflow

The anterior primary rami of S2, S3 and occasionally S4 give off nerve fibres termed the *pelvic splanchnic nerves* or *nervi erigentes*, which join the sympathetic pelvic plexus for distribution to the pelvic organs. Tiny ganglia in the walls of the viscera then relay postganglionic fibres.

The sacral parasympathetic system has been termed by Cannon 'the mechanism for emptying'. It supplies visceromotor fibres to the muscles of the rectum and inhibitor fibres to the internal anal sphincter, motor fibres to the bladder wall and inhibitor fibres to the internal vesical sphincter. In addition, vasodilator fibres supply the erectile cavernous sinuses of the penis and the clitoris.

Afferent parasympathetic fibres

Parasympathetic afferent fibres are conveyed in the glossopharyngeal nerve (IX), transmitting baroreceptor fibres from the carotid sinus and chemoreceptor fibres from the carotid body, afferent fibres of the vagus nerve (X) from the heart, lungs and alimentary tract, and along the pelvic splanchnic nerves (S2, S3 and S4) from the pelvic viscera.

Like the afferent fibres conveyed in the sympathetic system (see page 423), these do not relay in the autonomic ganglia and have their cell-stations, just like somatic sensory fibres, in the dorsal ganglia of the spinal and cranial nerves. They simply use the autonomic nerves as a convenient anatomical pathway from the viscera to the brain.

Autonomic control of micturition, defecation and sexual function

The detrusor muscle in the urinary bladder is innervated by the parasympathetic fibres. These originate in the 2nd, 3rd and possibly 4th sacral segments of the spinal cord and reach the bladder via the pelvic splanchnic nerves and inferior hypogastric plexuses. Thus, detrusor contractility is exclusively under parasympathetic control. The smooth muscle in the bladder neck and the superficial trigonal muscle are, however, innervated by sympathetic fibres. Normal bladder emptying is the result of pelvic parasympathetic stimulation and reciprocal sympathetic inhibition. Damage to the pelvic parasympathetic fibres will therefore result in an atonic bladder with neither voluntary nor reflex control.

The autonomic control of sexual function in the male is as follows: penile erection is mediated by pelvic parasympathetic fibres (an alternative name for the pelvic parasympathetics is *nervi erigentes*, the nerves of erection; of course, the parasympathetics mediate a great deal more than just penile erection!). The penile branches of the pelvic parasympathetics, upon stimulation, produce vasodilatation of the arteries in the penile erectile tissue, i.e. corpora cavernosa and corpus spongiosum. Ejaculation is, by contrast, essentially mediated by sympathetic nerves. These nerves, when stimulated, result in contraction of the bladder neck muscle (thereby preventing retrograde ejaculation) and simultaneous contraction of seminal vesicles, prostatic muscle and the muscle in the walls of the vas deferens and epididymis.

The initiation of defecation is brought on by stimulation of receptors in the rectal wall. This provokes a parasympathetic reflex response resulting in peristalsis. The urge to defecate can, up to a point, be overridden by higher (cortical) centres. The anal sphincter complex has two components:

1 an internal anal sphincter, which is a smooth muscle sphincter and is under sympathetic control (L1–L2 segments); the internal anal sphincter normally accounts for 40–50% of the resting anal tone;
2 an external anal sphincter, which is the larger of the two sphincters. It is a striated muscle sphincter and thus under voluntary control. It is innervated by a somatic nerve – the inferior rectal branch of the pudendal nerve.

Glossary of eponyms

In spite of their being 'unscientific', eponymous terms are still commonly used – more so among clinicians, it is true, than among professional anatomists. This glossary gives brief biographical details of the names mentioned in the text. Entries appear alphabetically according to the person whose name is used adjectivally in the term: *valves of Ball* under Ball, *column of Burdach* under Burdach, and so on.

transpyloric plane of Addison A transverse (horizontal) plane halfway between the sternal notch and the upper edge of the pubic symphysis. It corresponds to the level of the lower border of the 1st lumbar vertebra.
Christopher Addison (1869–1951), Professor of Anatomy, University of Sheffield. He subsequently took up a full-time career in politics, becoming a member of parliament in 1910. Shortly after the end of the First World War, he became Britain's first ever Minister of Health.

Alcock's canal Fascial tunnel on the lateral wall of the ischiorectal fossa that conveys the pudendal vessels and nerve.
Benjamin Alcock (1801–?), Professor of Anatomy, first in Dublin and then Cork. He emigrated to America and disappeared from the scene.

Argyll Robertson pupil The pupil does not respond to light but reacts to accommodation. It is classically seen in neurosyphilis.
Douglas Argyll Robertson (1837–1909), ophthalmic surgeon at the Royal Infirmary, Edinburgh.

Auerbach's plexus Nerve plexus between the circular and longitudinal muscle coats of the intestine.
Leopold Auerbach (1828–1897), Professor of Pathology, Breslau.

valves of Ball Valve-like folds that connect the distal extremities of the columns of Morgagni (q.v.) in the upper half of the anal canal.
Sir Charles Ball (1851–1916), Regius Professor of Surgery, Dublin, and an early pioneer of rectal surgery.

Bartholin's gland The greater vestibular gland. Mucus-secreting gland in the posterior labium majus.
Caspar Bartholin (1655–1738), Professor of Anatomy, Copenhagen.

Batson's venous plexus The 'valveless vertebral veins' communicate with the prostatic plexus of veins and explain the readiness with which carcinoma of the prostate spreads to the pelvis and lumbar vertebrae.
Oscar Batson (1894–1979), Professor of Anatomy, University of Pennsylvania.

Bell's palsy Viral infection of the facial (VII) nerve.
Sir Charles Bell (1774–1842), surgeon at the Middlesex Hospital, London.

Bennett's fracture Fracture dislocation of the base of the metacarpal of the thumb.
Edward Hallaran Bennett (1837–1907), Professor of Surgery at Trinity College, Dublin. He described this fracture in 1882.

Bigelow's Y-shaped ligament The tough iliofemoral ligament of the hip joint.
Henry James Bigelow (1818–1890), surgeon at Harvard Medical School, Boston, MA.

Blalock's operation The right subclavian artery is anastomosed end-to-side into the right pulmonary artery in order to overcome the pulmonary stenosis of the tetralogy of Fallot (q.v.).
Alfred Blalock (1899–1964), Professor of Surgery, Johns Hopkins Hospital, Baltimore, MD.

Bochdalek's foramen The pleuroperitoneal canal of the developing diaphragm.
Vincent Bochdalek (1801–1883), anatomist in Prague.

Broca's area The anterior portion of the inferior frontal gyrus; on the dominant side it is the motor area for speech.
Pierre Broca (1824–1880), Professor of Clinical Surgery, Paris.

Brown-Séquard syndrome Produced by hemisection of the spinal cord.
Charles Edouard Brown-Séquard (1817–1894), born in Mauritius, practised as a neurologist in Paris, at Harvard and at the National Hospital, Queen's Square, London.

Brunner's glands The characteristic submucosal acinar glands of the duodenum.
Johann Brunner (1653–1727), Swiss anatomist who became Professor of Anatomy at Heidelberg and later at Strasbourg. It is said that his father-in-law, J. J. Wepfer, actually discovered these glands!

Bryant's triangle Used in measurement of the hip.
Thomas Bryant (1828–1914), surgeon at Guy's Hospital, London; President of the Royal College of Surgeons of England.

column of Burdach The lateral tract (fasciculus cuneatus) of the posterior column of the spinal cord.
Charles Burdach (1776–1847), Professor of Anatomy and Medicine, Konigsberg.

Caldwell–Luc operation For drainage of the maxillary sinus.
George Walter Caldwell (1866–1946), ENT surgeon in New York.
Henri Luc (1855–1925), ENT surgeon in Paris.

Calot's triangle Triangle formed by the liver, common hepatic duct and cystic duct.
Jean Francois Calot (1861–1941), surgeon at the Rothschild Hospital, Paris, where he specialized in the surgical treatment of tuberculosis in children.

Camper's fascia The superficial fatty layer of the superficial fascia of the lower abdominal wall.
Peter Camper (1722–1789), Professor of Medicine, Amsterdam, and then Professor of Medicine, Surgery, Anatomy and Botany, Groningen.
Cannon's description of the sacral parasympathetic system as the 'mechanism for emptying'.
William Bradford Cannon (1871–1945), George Higginson Professor of Physiology, Harvard University, Boston, MA.

Cloquet's gland Lymph node situated in the femoral canal.
Jules Cloquet (1790–1883), Professor of Anatomy and Surgery, Paris.

Colles' fascia The perineal fascia.

Colles' fracture Fracture of the lower end of the radius with dorsal displacement.
Abraham Colles (1773–1843), Professor of Anatomy and Surgery, Royal College of Surgeons in Ireland, Dublin.

ligament of Cooper The iliopectineal fascia.

ligaments of Cooper Fibrous septa in the breast.
Sir Astley Paston Cooper (1768–1841), surgeon at Guy's Hospital, London; President of the Royal College of Surgeons.

organ of Corti The sound receptor organ in the cochlea.
Alfonso Corti (1822–1888), Italian histologist who worked mainly on the retina and the ear.

Cowper's glands Two glands situated in the deep perineal pouch which drain into the bulbous urethra.
William Cowper (1666–1698), surgeon in London.

Cushing's syndrome Endocrine abnormality associated with hyperplasia or tumour of the adrenal cortex or of a basophil adenoma of the anterior pituitary.
Harvey Cushing (1869–1939), pioneer neurosurgeon at the Peter Bent Brigham Hospital, Boston, MA.

fascia of Denonvilliers Fascia which separates the prostate from the rectum.
Charles Pierre Denonvilliers (1808–1872), Professor of Anatomy, Paris.

Dormia basket A small collapsible basket, which can be passed down the side-channel of an endoscope and used to entrap, and then remove, a stone lodged in the biliary duct system or urinary tract.
Enrico Dormia (1928–2009), Professor of Urology, University of Milan, Italy. Acknowledged to be the first practitioner of minimally invasive surgery in Italy.

arcuate line of Douglas The lower margin of the posterior rectus sheath.

pouch of Douglas The recto-uterine peritoneal pouch.
James Douglas (1675–1742), anatomist and obstetrician in London.

marginal artery of Drummond The continuous arterial arcade that lies alongside the inner (mesenteric) border of the entire colon and is formed by a series of anastomoses between the successive colic branches of the superior and inferior mesenteric arteries.
Hamilton Drummond (1882 – 1925), Surgeon, Royal Victoria Infirmary, Newcastle upon Tyne.

Dupuytren's contracture Contraction and fibrosis of the palmar (and occasional plantar) fascia.
Baron Guillaume Dupuytren (1777–1835), surgeon at the Hôtel Dieu, Paris.

Edinger–Westphal nucleus Supplies the parasympathetic fibres of the oculomotor nerve.
Ludwig Edinger (1855–1918), German anatomist and neurologist.
Karl Westphal (1833–1890), neurologist in Berlin. Described the nucleus in the adult 2 years after this had been demonstrated in the fetus by Edinger.

Erb–Duchenne paralysis Results from injury to the C5 and C6 roots of the brachial plexus.
Wilhelm Erb (1840–1921), Professor of Neurology, Heidelberg.
G. B. A. Duchenne (1806–1875), neurologist in Paris; also described Duchenne's muscular dystrophy.

Eustachian tube The pharyngotympanic tube.
Bartolomeo Eustachi (1524–1574), Professor of Anatomy, Rome.

Fallopian tube The uterine tube.
Gabrielle Fallopio (1523–1562), Professor of Anatomy, Padua, and a pupil of Vesalius.

Fallot's tetralogy Congenital heart disease comprising pulmonary stenosis, right ventricular hypertrophy, ventricular septal defect and overriding of the aorta.
Etienne Fallot (1850–1911), Professor of Medicine, Marseilles.

Galen's vein The great cerebral vein.
Claudius Galen (130–200), physician to the emperor Marcus Aurelius. Taught anatomy in Rome and prolific author of text books.

duct of Gartner Mesonephric duct remnant in the female.
Hermann Gartner (1785–1827), Danish surgeon.

Gimbernat's ligament The lacunar portion of the inguinal ligament.
Manuel Gimbernat (1734–1816), Professor of Anatomy, Barcelona.

column of Goll The medial tract of the posterior column of the spinal cord (fasciculus gracilis).
Friedrich Goll (1829–1903), both a neurologist and anatomist; Professor of Anatomy, Zurich.

Graafian follicle Maturing ovarian follicle.
Regnier de Graaf (1641–1673), physician and anatomist in Delft.

Hartmann's pouch Dilatation of the gall bladder proximal to its neck.
Henri Hartmann (1860–1952), Professor of Surgery, Faculty of Medicine, Paris.

Henry's method A method of locating the posterior interosseous branch of the radial nerve in the forearm.
Arnold Henry (1886–1962), Professor of Surgery, Cairo University, and subsequently, Professor of Anatomy, the Royal College of Surgeons in Ireland, Dublin.

antrum of Highmore The maxillary sinus.
Nathaniel Highmore (1613–1685), physician in Sherborne, Dorset. His claim to fame is tenuous since the maxillary sinus was well known to previous anatomists and was illustrated by Leonardo da Vinci.

Hilton's law Nerves crossing a joint supply the muscles acting on the joint and the joint itself.
John Hilton (1805–1878), surgeon at Guy's Hospital, London.

Hippocratic method For reduction of dislocation of the shoulder.
Hippocrates (*c*. 460–375 BC) lived on the Greek island of Cos. He is generally acknowledged as the *Father of Medicine*.

bundle of His Atrioventricular conduction fibres in the heart.
Wilhelm His, Jr (1863–1934), Swiss-born anatomist and cardiologist. Professor of Medicine, University of Berlin.

Horner's syndrome Ptosis and constriction of the pupil resulting from interruption of the sympathetic innervation to the eyelids and pupil.
Johann Horner (1831–1886), Professor of Ophthalmology, Zurich.

Houston's valves The three lateral folds of the rectum.
John Houston (1802–1845), lecturer in surgery, Dublin.

Hunter's canal The subsartorial canal.
John Hunter (1728–1793), surgeon at St George's Hospital, London. He described ligation of the femoral artery in the subsartorial canal for popliteal aneurysm.

Killian's dehiscence The potential gap between the two parts of the interior constrictor muscle through which a pharyngeal pouch protrudes.
Gustav Killian (1860–1921), ENT surgeon in Berlin.

Klumpke's paralysis Injury to the lowest root of the brachial plexus.
Augusta Dejerine-Klumpke (1859–1927), neurologist in Paris. Married another famous neurologist, Joseph Dejerine.

Kocher's incision The subcostal approach to the gall bladder.

Kocher's manoeuvre Mobilization of the duodenum by incising its lateral peritoneal attachment.

Kocher's method For reduction of dislocation of the shoulder.
Theodore Kocher (1841–1917), Professor of Surgery in Berne. Winner of the Nobel Prize for Medicine or Physiology in 1909. The first surgeon ever to receive this accolade.

islets of Langerhans Clumps of insulin-secreting cells in the pancreas.
Paul Langerhans (1847–1888), Professor of Pathology, Freiburg. He described the islet cells in his doctorate studies in 1869, at the age of 22.

nerve of Latarjet The fibres of the vagus nerve that supply the gastric antrum.
André Latarjet (1876–1947), Professor of Anatomy, Lyons.

dorsal tubercle of Lister A palpable prominence on the dorsal surface of the distal radius. Immediately to its ulnar side lies the tendon of extensor pollicis longus.
Joseph (Lord) Lister (1827–1912), Professor of Surgery, successively at the Universities of Glasgow and Edinburgh, and at King's College Hospital, London.

Little's area Area of arterial anastomosis on the antero-inferior part of the nasal septum.
James Lawrence Little (1836–1885), Professor of Surgery, University of Vermont, New England.

angle of Louis The angulated articulation between the manubrium sterni and mesosternum.
Pierre Charles Louis (1787–1872), Physician to the Hôpital de la Pitié, Paris. He was, in his day, a leading authority on pulmonary tuberculosis.

Ludwig's angina Infection of the submandibular region.
Wilhelm Ludwig (1790–1865), Professor of Surgery, Tubingen.

foramina of Luschka The lateral openings of the fourth ventricle.
Hubert Luschka (1820–1875), Professor of Anatomy, Tubingen.

Mackenrodt's ligaments The transverse cervical (or cardinal) ligaments of the female pelvis.
Alwin Mackenrodt (1859–1925), Professor of Gynaecology, Berlin.

foramen of Magendie The midline opening of the fourth ventricle.
François Magendie (1783–1855), physician at the Hotel Dieu, Paris.

vein of Mayo A constant vein that crosses the junction of the pylorus with the duodenum.
Charles Mayo (1865–1939), with his father and his brother, William, founded the Mayo Clinic, Rochester, MN. The vein of Mayo was described earlier by Latarjet (q.v.).

McBurney's point Two-thirds of the way laterally along the line from the umbilicus to the anterior superior iliac spine; the usual site of maximum tenderness in acute appendicitis and the centre of the skin incision for appendicectomy.
Charles McBurney (1845–1913), Professor of Surgery, New York. A pioneer of early surgery in acute appendicitis.

Meckel's cartilage The cartilage of the first branchial arch.

Meckel's diverticulum The remains of the embryonic vitellointestinal duct and present in approximately 2% of subjects.
Johann Meckel (1781–1833), Professor of Anatomy, Halle. His grandfather, who was Professor of Anatomy in Berlin, described the pterygopalatine ganglion and the dural space which contains the ganglion of the trigeminal nerve. Johann's father was also Professor of Anatomy in Halle.

Meibomian glands The tarsal glands of the eyelid. If blocked, they distend into Meibomian cysts.
Heinrich Meibom (1638–1700), Professor of Medicine, Helmstadt.

Meissner's plexus The nerve plexus in the submucosal layer of the intestine.
George Meissner (1829–1905), anatomist and physiologist, Professor successively in Basle, Freiburg and Gottingen. He also described Meissner's corpuscles, the cutaneous sensory end-organs.

glands of Montgomery The modified sebaceous glands of the areola of the nipple.
William Montgomery (1797–1859), practised obstetrics in Dublin.

columns of Morgagni Vertical columns of mucosa in the anal canal.

foramen of Morgagni Gap between the xiphoid and costal origins of the diaphragm.

hydatid of Morgagni The appendix epididymis, the remnant of the mesonephros.
Giovanni Morgagni (1682–1771), Professor of Anatomy, Padua – a post he held for 59 years!

Morison's pouch The right subhepatic space.
James Rutherford Morison (1853–1939), Professor of Surgery, University of Durham. He had served as a surgical dresser to Joseph Lister.

Müllerian duct The paramesonephric duct.
Johannes Müller (1801–1858), Professor of Anatomy, Berlin.

Naegele's pelvis Absence or underdevelopment of one-half of the sacrum resulting in a contracted, ovate pelvis.
Franz Karl Naegele (1778–1851), obstetrician, Düsseldorf.

Nelaton's line A line joining the anterior superior iliac spine to the ischial tuberosity. The greater trochanter normally lies distal to this line.
Auguste Nelaton (1807–1873), Professor of Surgery, Paris, and surgeon to Napoleon III.

sphincter of Oddi The sphincter around the termination of the common bile duct.
Ruggero Oddi (1845–1906), surgeon in Rome. The sphincter had already been described by Glisson in the seventeenth century!

Pacchionian bodies Clumps of arachnoid villi along the superior sagittal sinus.
Antoine Pacchioni (1665–1726), Professor of Anatomy, Rome.

Pancoast's syndrome Invasion of the brachial plexus by an apical tumour of the lung.
H. K. Pancoast (1875–1939), Professor of Radiology, University of Pennsylvania, the first such appointment in the USA.

Parkinson's disease Tremor and rigidity due to lesions of the substantia nigra.
James Parkinson (1755–1824), medical practitioner, Shoreditch, London. His small book *An Essay on the Shaking Palsy* in 1817 was based mainly on close observation of one case.

Passavant's ridge Produced by contraction of the superior pharyngeal constrictor in deglutition. Philipp Passavant (1815–1893), surgeon in Frankfurt.

Perthes' disease Avascular necrosis of the femoral head in children.
Georg Perthes (1869–1927), Professor of Surgery, Tubingen.

Pfannenstiel incision Transverse lower abdominal incision employed usually for pelvic surgery.

Hermann Johannes Pfannenstiel (1862–1909), gynaecologist in Breslau (then part of Prussia).

Pott's disease Spinal tuberculosis.

Pott's fracture Fracture–dislocation of the ankle.
Percival Pott (1714–1789), surgeon at St Bartholomew's hospital, London.

Poupart's ligament The inguinal ligament.
Francois Poupart (1661–1708), surgeon at the Hotel Dieu, Paris.

Pringle's manoeuvre Compression of the hepatic artery at the foramen of Winslow (q.v.) in the control of haemorrhage.
James Hogarth Pringle (1863–1941), surgeon at the Royal Infirmary, Glasgow.

Purkinje's fibres Specialized large, striated cardiac muscle lying beneath the ventricular endocardium.
Johannes Purkinje (1787–1869), Professor of Physiology in Breslau and later at Prague.

Queckenstedt's test Compression of the internal jugular vein during lumbar puncture produces a rise in cerebrospinal fluid pressure.
H. H. G. Queckenstedt (1876–1918), neurologist in Rostock. He described his test in 1916 while serving in the German army during the First World War. He was killed in a road accident 2 days before the armistice.

Rathke's pouch Origin of the anterior pituitary in the root of the embryonic buccal cavity.
Martin Heinrich Rathke (1793–1860), Professor of Zoology and Anatomy, Königsberg, Prussia.

island of Reil The insula of the cerebral cortex.
Johann Reil (1759–1813), Professor of Medicine, Halle and, later, Berlin.

cave of Retzius The retropubic space.
Andreas Retzius (1797–1860), Professor of Anatomy, Karolinska Institute, Stockholm.

sulcus of Rolando The central cerebral fissure.
Luigi Rolando (1773–1831), Professor of Anatomy, Turin.

Romberg's sign Ataxia when the eyes are closed because of loss of position sense. Characteristic of posterior column lesions.
Moritz Romberg (1795–1873), Director of the University Hospital in Berlin and author of the first systematic book on neurology.

duct of Santorini The accessory pancreatic duct.
Giovanni Santorini (1681–1737), Professor of Anatomy, Venice.

Sappey's plexus The plexus of lymphatics below the nipple.
Marie Sappey (1810–1896), Professor of Anatomy, Paris.

Scarpa's fascia The fibrous layer of superficial fascia of the lower abdomen.
Antonio Scarpa (1747–1832), Professor of Anatomy and Surgery, Pavia. His name is also attached to the femoral triangle.

canal of Schlemm The sinus venosus sclerae, draining the aqueous humour from the anterior chamber of the eye.
F. S. Schlemm (1795–1858), Professor of Anatomy, Berlin.

Seldinger technique A method of percutaneous puncture and catheterization of arteries and other hollow tubes (under radiological control), using a guidewire over which is passed a Seldinger catheter.
Sven-Ivar Seldinger (1921–1998), radiologist, Mora (near Uppsala).

Semon's law In partial damage of the recurrent laryngeal nerve, the abductors of the vocal cords are affected more than the adductors.
Felix Semon (1849–1921), graduated in Berlin but emigrated to England and became a laryngologist at St Thomas' Hospital, London.

Sherrington's description of the hypothalamus As the 'head ganglion of the autonomic nervous system'.
Charles Scott Sherrington (1857–1952), Waynfleet Professor of Physiology, University of Oxford.

Stensen's duct The duct of the parotid gland.
Niels Stensen (1638–1686), Professor of Anatomy, University of Copenhagen.

aqueduct of Sylvius Between the third and fourth ventricles.

sulcus of Sylvius The lateral cerebral fissure. Francois de la Boë Sylvius (1614–1672), Professor of Medicine, Leyden.

Tenon's capsule The fascial sheath of the eye.
Jacques Tenon (1724–1816), surgeon at the Salpetrière, Paris.

suspensory ligament of Treitz Peritoneal fold from the right crus of the diaphragm to the duodenal termination.
Wenzel Treitz (1819–1872), Professor of Pathology, Prague.

Trendelenburg's test A clinical test for hip stability.
Friedrich Trendelenburg (1844–1924), Professor of Surgery, Leipzig. He attempted a pulmonary embolectomy (unsuccessfully) in 1908.

bloodless fold of Treves The ileocaecal fold.
Sir Frederick Treves (1853–1923), surgeon at the London Hospital. Drained the appendix abscess of King Edward VII in 1902.

Valsalva manoeuvre Forcible exhalation of inhaled air against a closed airway (nose and mouth).
Antonio Mario Valsalva (1666–1723), physician and anatomist, Bologna.

ampulla of Vater The ampulla of the common bile duct.
Abraham Vater (1684–1751), Professor of Anatomy, Wittenberg.

Volkmann's contracture Produced by ischaemic fibrosis of the forearm muscles.
Richard von Volkmann (1830–1889), Professor of Surgery, Halle, and one of the pioneers of Lister's antiseptic surgical technique.

Waldeyer's ring The ring of lymphoid tissue comprising the nasopharyngeal tonsil, the palatine tonsils and the lymphoid nodules on the dorsum of the tongue.
Heinrich Waldeyer (1836–1921), Professor of Anatomy, first in Strasbourg and then Berlin. He also described the plasma cell in 1875.

Wernicke's speech area Superior area of the temporal lobe of the cerebral cortex.
Karl Wernicke (1848–1904), psychiatrist, first in Breslau then Halle.

Wharton's duct The duct of the submandibular salivary gland.
Thomas Wharton (?1616–1673), physician at St Thomas' Hospital, London. His name is also given to the mucoid substance of the umbilical cord (Wharton's jelly).

circle of Willis The arterial anastomosis at the base of the brain.
Thomas Willis (1621–1675), practised medicine in Oxford and then London. Buried in Westminster Abbey.

foramen of Winslow The opening into the lesser sac (epiploic foramen).

ligament of Winslow Oblique popliteal ligament of the knee.
Jacob Winslow (1669–1760), born in Denmark and became Professor of Anatomy and Surgery, Paris.

Wirsung's duct The main pancreatic duct.
Johann Wirsung (1600–1643), Professor of Anatomy, Padua, where he was assassinated!

Wolffian body and ducts The mesonephros and its ducts.
Caspar Wolff (1733–1794), born in Berlin; Professor of Anatomy, St Petersburg. One of the pioneers of embryology.

Wormian bones Occasional accessory bones between the parietal and occipital bones.
Ole Worm (1588–1654), Professor of Anatomy, Copenhagen.

Index

Note: Index entries for major specific anatomical structures (such as individual bones, muscles) have been grouped under these main entries ('Bones', 'Muscles'), in addition to individual entries, e.g. 'Biceps' is included under 'Muscles' and also 'Biceps'. Page numbers in *italics* represent figures, those in bold represent tables.